CRITICAL PATHWAYS IN CARDIOVASCULAR MEDICINE

CRITICAL PATHWAYS IN CARDIOVASCULAR MEDICINE

SECOND EDITION

Edited By

Christopher P. Cannon, MD
and Patrick T. O'Gara, MD

Cardiovascular Division
Brigham and Women's Hospital
Harvard Medical School
Boston, MA

LIPPINCOTT WILLIAMS & WILKINS
A Wolters Kluwer Company

Philadelphia • Baltimore • New York • London
Buenos Aires • Hong Kong • Sydney • Tokyo

Acquisitions Editor: Fran DeStefano
Production Editor: David Murphy
Managing Editor: Joanne Bersin
Production Services: Maryland Composition Inc
Printer: Edwards Brothers

530 Walnut Street
Philadelphia, Pennsylvania 19106 USA

351 West Camden Street
Baltimore, Maryland 21201-2436 USA

Printed in the United States of America

Critical pathways in cardiovascular medicine / edited by Christopher
   P. Cannon and Patrick T. O'Gara.—2nd ed.
      p. ; cm.
   Includes bibliographical references.
   ISBN 0-7817-9439-0
   1. Cardiology. 2. Critical path analysis. 3. Outcome assessment
(Medical care) 4. Medical protocols.   I. Cannon, Christopher P.
II. O'Gara, Patrick T.
   [DNLM: 1. Cardiovascular Diseases—diagnosis. 2. Cardiovascu-
lar Diseases—therapy. 3. Critical Care—standards. 4. Critical Path-
ways.   WG 141 C934 2007]
RC669.C755 2007
616.1'2—dc22
                                            2006021948

10 9 8 7 6 5 4 3 2 1

Dedicated to our wives.

CPC & PO'G

CONTENTS

Preface ix
Contributors xi

1   Goals, Design, and Implementation of Critical Pathways in Cardiovascular Medicine 1
Christopher P. Cannon and Patrick T. O'Gara

PART I ■ PREHOSPITAL CRITICAL PATHWAYS

2   Prehospital Fibrinolysis 9
Freek W.A. Verheugt

3   Regional Transfer Programs for Primary Percutaneous Coronary Intervention 13
David M. Larson and Timothy D. Henry

4   Public Access Defibrillation 19
Joseph P. Ornato

PART II ■ CRITICAL PATHWAYS IN THE EMERGENCY DEPARTMENT

5   Non-ST Elevation ACS in the Emergency Department 27
Richard J. Ryan, Christopher P. Cannon, and W. Brian Gibler

6   Thrombolysis for ST-Elevation Myocardial Infarction in the Emergency Department 39
Joshua M. Kosowsky

7   Heart Failure in the Emergency Department 46
W. Frank Peacock

8   Atrial Fibrillation in the Emergency Department 53
Michael A. Ross and Antonio X. Bonfiglio

9   Stroke and Transient Ischemic Attack 63
Abdul Abdullah and Lee H. Schwamm

10   The Role of Exercise Testing in Chest Pain Units: Evolution, Application, Results 81
Ezra A. Amsterdam, J. Douglas Kirk, Deborah B. Diercks, William R. Lewis, and Samuel D. Turnipseed

PART III ■ CRITICAL PATHWAYS IN THE HOSPITAL

11   Critical Pathways Following Thrombosis 93
Christopher P. Cannon and Patrick T. O'Gara

12.   Primary PCI 100
Amr E. Abbas and Cindy L. Grines

13   Primary PCI at Community Hospitals without On-site Cardiac Surgery 108
Nancy Sinclair and Thomas P. Wharton, Jr.

14   Approach to the Patient with Complicated Myocardial Infarction 129
Richard C. Becker

15   Cardiac Catheterization and Percutaneous Coronary Intervention 155
Christopher P. Cannon and Patrick T. O'Gara

16   Pathways for Coronary Artery Bypass Surgery 160
Rashid M. Ahmad, Frances Wadlington, Tiffany Street, James P. Greelish, Jorge M. Balaguer, and John G. Byrne

17   Acute Aortic Syndromes 166
Piotr Sobieszczyk and Patrick T. O'Gara

18   Intensive Management of Hyperglycemia in Acute Coronary Syndrome 174
Vera T. Fajtova

19   Management of Atrial Fibrillation and Atrial Flutter 181
Eyal Herzog and Jonathan S. Steinberg

20   Heart Failure 190
Gregg C. Fonarow

21   Device Therapy in Heart Failure: Selection of Patients for ICD and CRT 210
Eli V. Gelfand and Peter J. Zimetbaum

22   Venous Thromboembolism 224
Samuel Z. Goldhaber

PART IV ■ CRITICAL PATHWAYS IN THE OUTPATIENT SETTING

23   Hyperlipidemia 241
Frederick F. Samaha and Daniel J. Rader

24   Diabetes and Metabolic Syndrome 249
Emily D. Szmuilowicz and Merri Pendergrass

25   Hypertension 260
Michael A. Weber

26   Smoking Cessation 273
Beth C. Bock

27   Secondary Prevention Overview 285
Sidney C. Smith, Jr.

28   Overview of the AHA "Get with the Guidelines" Programs 291
Yuling Hong and Kenneth A. LaBresh

29   Cardiac Rehabilitation 299
Daniel E. Forman

INDEX 307

Our goal in cardiovascular medicine, and indeed in all of medicine, is to provide the best possible care to our patients. Much progress has been made in the past ten years, especially in cardiovascular medicine, with countless clinical trials evaluating many new treatments for patients with cardiovascular disorders. Indeed, we practice in an era when new therapies and approaches to the management of patients with heart and vascular disease are introduced yearly. In this fashion, they serve as a readily available guide to the clinician.

But the process of improving the practice of medicine is more complicated than just doing a clinical trial of a new treatment. Although the basic researcher would see this as a culmination of years of research, for clinical care it is just the beginning. First, the Food and Drug Administration must review the clinical trial data pertaining to the new treatment for efficacy and safety, to ensure that there are sufficient data for the treatment's approval and use in patients. In parallel, guideline writing committees and experts review the clinical evidence and make recommendations on how and in which patients the new therapy should be added to existing treatments. Then, the pharmaceutical company generally will disseminate information to clinicians through various media, including continuing medical education forums. Medical societies will have symposia, and hospitals will have grand round lectures by investigators to inform cardiovascular clinicians on the new treatments.

Yet, even more work is required to ensure that new (or even standard) therapies are provided to patients according to recommended guidelines. In recent years, numerous registries have tabulated what treatments are given to patients in clinical practice. Uniformly, these have demonstrated that alarmingly high percentages of patients are not treated with even the basic medications, such as aspirin or lipid lowering drugs, for which strong recommendations have been formulated. Thus, we have all realized that more effort is needed to make sure that patients are treated with the right therapy, at the right time, by the right clinician.

A new field has emerged in medicine, and cardiovascular medicine has been in the forefront on this—Quality Improvement. This area comprises several different types of programs that aim to improve the quality of care provided to patients. One approach has been the development and utilization of critical pathways. These are standardized documents or computer order sets that incorporate proven therapies, and attempt to streamline care to make it more cost-effective. Although initially intended to reduce hospital length of stay, the use of critical pathways has grown exponentially. They offer a unique opportunity to raise the standard of care at institutions by including appropriate tests and treatments for patients with specific diagnoses.

In this book, we have solicited exemplary critical pathways from leading institutions around the country. These pathways are the "best practices" at these hospitals, developed by leaders in their areas of expertise. The authors have done a superb job of integrating the key clinical data into brief summaries, and of providing the critical pathways that they use at their hospitals. We have organized the book in a fashion to facilitate the reader's use of the information. We begin with an overview of what critical pathways are and how to develop them, then we present several pathways for management of patients in the pre-hospital setting as well as in the Emergency Department. The next section provides optimal treatment approaches for several major cardiovascular disorders, and the final section has several outpatient critical pathways, such as management of hypertension and lipid disorders. It is hoped that these pathways will allow clinicians to adopt routinely the embedded therapies as a means of improving the care of their cardiac patients.

Christopher P. Cannon, MD
Patrick T. O'Gara, MD

Amr E. Abbas, MD, FACC
Interventional Cardiology
William Beaumont Hospital
Royal Oak, Michigan

Abdul R. Abdullah, MD
Clinical Research Fellow and QI Fellow in Neurology
  (Acute Stroke Service)
Harvard Medical School
Massachusetts General Hospital
Boston, Massachusetts

Rashid M. Ahmad, MD
Assistant Professor of Cardiac Surgery
Vanderbilt Medical Center
Nashville, Tennessee

Ezra A. Amsterdam, MD
Professor of Internal Medicine
Associate Chief of Cardiology
University of California School of Medicine
Davis and Sacramento, California

Jorge Balaguer, MD
Assistant Professor of Cardiac Surgery
Vanderbilt University
Chief of Cardiac Surgery
Department of Veterans Affairs Medical Center
Nashville, Tennessee

Richard C. Becker, MD
Professor of Medicine
Director, Cardiovascular Thrombosis Center
Duke Clinical Research Institute
Durham, North Carolina

Beth C. Bock, PhD
Associate Professor of Psychiatry and Human Behavior
Brown Medical School
The Miriam Hospital
Providence, Rhode Island

Antonio X. Bonfiglio, MD, FACEP
Clinical Associate Professor of Emergency Medicine
Wayne State University
Detroit, Michigan

John G. Byrne, MD
William S. Stoney Professor of Surgery
Chairman of Cardiac Surgery
Vanderbilt University
Nashville, Tennessee

Deborah B. Dierks, MD
Associate Professor of Emergency Medicine
University of California
Davis, California

Vera T. Fajtova, MD
Assistant Professor
Harvard Medical School
Harvard Vanguard Medical Associates
Brigham and Women's Hospital
Beth Israel Deaconess Medical Center
Boston, Massachusetts

Gregg C. Fonarow, MD
Professor of Medicine
UCLA Division of Cardiology
The Eliot Corday Chair in Cardiovascular
  Medicine and Science
Director, Ahmanson-UCLA Cardiomyopathy Center
Director, UCLA Cardiology Fellowship Training
  ProgramLos Angeles, California

Daniel E. Forman, MS
Assistant Professor of Medicine
Harvard Medical School
Director of Cardiac Rehabilitation and Exercise Testing
  Laboratory
Brigham and Women's HospitalBoston, Massachusetts

Eli V. Gelfand, MD
Instructor in Medicine
Harvard Medical School
Section of Noninvasive Cardiology
Cardiovascular Division
Beth Israel Deaconess Medical Center
Boston, Massachusetts

W. Brian Gibler, MD, FACEP
Richard C. Levy Professor and Chair of Emergency
  Medicine
University of Cincinnati
Cincinnati, Ohio

Samuel Z. Goldhaber, MD
Professor of Medicine
Harvard Medical School
Director, Venous Thrombosis Research Group
Brigham and Women's Hospital
Boston, Massachusetts

James P. Greelish, MD
Assistant Professor of Cardiac Surgery
Vanderbilt University
Nashville, Tennessee

Cindy L. Grines, MD, FACC
Director, Cardiac Catheterization Laboratories
Director, Interventional Fellowship Program
William Beaumont Hospital,
Royal Oak, Michigan

Timothy D. Henry, MD, FACC
Associate Professor of Medicine
University of Minnesota School of Medicine
Interventional Cardiologist
Minneapolis Heart Institute
Minneapolis, Minnesota

Eyal Herzog, MD
Director, Cardiac Unit
St. Lukes-Roosevelt Hospital Center
Columbia University College of Physicians and Surgeons
New York, New York

Yuling Hong, MD, MSc, PhD, FAHA
Director of Biostatistics and Epidemiology
Senior Science and Medicine Advisor
American Heart Association National Center
Dallas, Texas

J. Douglas Kirk, MD
Associate Professor of Emergency Medicine
Director, Chest Pain Emergency Services
University of California
Davis, California

Joshua M. Kosowsky, MD
Instructor in Medicine
Harvard Medical School
Department of Emergency Medicine
Brigham and Women's Hospital
Boston, Massachusetts

Kenneth A. LaBresh, MD
Clinical Associate Professor of Medicine
Brown University School of Medicine
Senior Vice President and Chief Medial Officer
Masspro
Waltham, Massachusetts

David M. Larson, MD
Associate Clinical Professor
University of Minnesota Medical School
Minneapolis Heart Institute Research Foundation
Minneapolis, Minnesota

William R. Lewis, MD
Associate Professor of Internal Medicine
Director, Echocardiography and Exercise Testing
   Laboratories
University of California
Davis, California

Joseph P. Ornato, MD, FACP, FACC, FACEP
Professor and Chairman of Emergency Medicine
Virginia Commonwealth University Health System
Richmond, Virginia

W. Frank Peacock, MD, FACEP
Vice Chief of Research
Emergency Department
The Cleveland Clinic
Cleveland, Ohio

Merri Pendergrass, MD, PhD
Associate Professor of Medicine
Harvard Medical School
Director of Clinical Diabetes
Interim Chief, Diabetes Section
Brigham and Women's Hospital
Boston, Massachusetts

Daniel J. Rader, MD
University of Pennsylvania Medical Center
Philadelphia VA Medical Center
Philadelphia, PA

Michael A. Ross, MD, FACEP
Associate Professor of Emergency Medicine
Wayne State University School of Medicine
Medical Director, Chest Pain Center and Emergency
   Observation Unit
William Beaumont Hospital
Royal Oak, Michigan

Richard J. Ryan
Associate Professor of Emergency Medicine
Vice Chairman, Patient Care
Department of Emergency Medicine
University of Cincinnati
Cincinnati, Ohio

Frederick F. Samaha, MD
University of Pennsylvania Medical Center
Philadelphia VA Medical Center
Philadelphia, PA

Lee H. Schwamm, MD
Associate Professor of Neurology
Harvard Medical School
Director, Telestroke and Acute Stroke Services
Massachusetts General Hospital
Boston, Massachusetts

Nancy Sinclair, RN, MS
University of New Hampshire Graduate School
Durham, New Hampshire
Exeter Hospital
Exeter, New Hampshire

Sidney C. Smith, Jr, MD
Professor of Medicine
Director, Center for Cardiovascular Science and Medicine
University of North Carolina at Chapel Hill
Chapel Hill, North Carolina

Piot Sobieszczyk, MD
Instructor in Medicine
Harvard Medical School
Cardiovascular Division
Vascular Medicine Section and Cardiac Catheterization
   Laboratory
Brigham and Women's Hospital
Boston, Massachusetts

Jonathan S. Steinberg, MD
Professor of Medicine
Columbia University College of Physicians and Surgeons
Chief, Division of Cardiology
St. Lukes-Roosevelt Hospital Center
New York, New York

Tiffany Street, RN, MSN, ACNP
Methodist Hospital
Houston, Texas

Emily D. Szmuilowicz, MD
Postdoctoral Fellow in Endocrinology
Division of Endocrinology, Diabetes and Hypertension
Harvard Medical School
Brigham and Women's Hospital
Boston, Massachusetts

Samuel D. Turnipseed, MD
Professor of Emergency Medicine
Co-director of Chest Pain Emergency Services
University of California
Davis, California

Freek W.A. Verheugt, MD, FACC
Head of Department of Caridiology
University Hospital Nijmegen
Nijmegen, The Netherlands

Frances Wadlington, RN, BSN
Vanderbilt University Medical Center
Nashville, Tennessee

Michael A. Weber, MD
Professor of Medicine
SUNY Downstate College of Medicine
New York, New York

Thomas P. Wharton, Jr, MD
Director, Division of Cardiology and Cardiac
    Catheterization Laboratory
Exeter Hospital
Exeter, New Hampshire

Peter J. Zimetbaum, MD
Associate Professor of Medicine
Harvard Medical School
Director of Cardiac Care Unit
Beth Israel Deaconess Medical Center
Boston, Massachusetts

CHAPTER 1 ■ GOALS, DESIGN, AND IMPLEMENTATION OF CRITICAL PATHWAYS IN CARDIOVASCULAR MEDICINE

CHRISTOPHER P. CANNON AND PATRICK T. O'GARA

GOALS OF CRITICAL PATHWAYS
NEED AND RATIONALE FOR CRITICAL PATHWAYS
Reducing Hospital (and ICU) Length of Stay
Overutilization of Intensive Care
METHODS FOR THE DEVELOPMENT OF CRITICAL
   PATHWAYS
Methods of Implementation
Cardiac Checklist
EVIDENCE OF BENEFIT OF CRITICAL PATHWAYS
CONCLUSIONS AND FUTURE DIRECTIONS

With the numerous advances in all areas of medical science, the practice of medicine has become very complex and specialized. Each condition, fortunately, has many different tests that can help characterize the disease prognosis and sometimes even help in selecting treatment. Among the treatments, many exist, but registries of current practice repeatedly show underutilization of many lifesaving medications. Accordingly, a major focus of nearly every physician and health care group, including many governmental agencies, has been to try to improve appropriate use of medications and treatments. All this is especially true in cardiovascular medicine, where multiple lifesaving treatments exist for patients, but where underutilization is widespread, ironically in the highest-risk patients.

One approach to improving the practice of medicine has been the use of "critical pathways," which are standardized protocols for the management of specific disorders that aim to optimize and streamline patient care. Numerous other names have been developed for such programs, including "clinical pathways" (so as not to suggest to patients that they are in "critical" condition), or simply "protocols," such as acute ST-elevation myocardial infarction (STEMI) protocols used in emergency departments (EDs) to reduce time to treatment with thrombolysis (1,2). A broader name of "disease management" is currently used to denote that these pathways extend beyond the hospital phase of treatment to optimize medical management over the long term.

The complexity of the pathways has also been used to distinguish true "critical pathways" (e.g., coronary artery bypass surgery pathways) as tools that detail the processes of care and potential inefficiencies, from "clinical protocols," which are algorithms and treatment recommendations focused on improving compliance with "evidence-based" medicine. Different disease states lend themselves to more complex pathways, such as those that exist for coronary artery bypass surgery. In contrast, for medical conditions in which patients are treated as outpatients, such as hypertension or hypercholesterolemia, the critical pathways tend to be more algorithm-based documents. Notwithstanding these minor differences in terminology, a broader view of "critical pathways" is adopted in this book, where various types of pathways are presented by leading clinicians to summarize current state-of-the-art cardiovascular practice.

GOALS OF CRITICAL PATHWAYS

The use of critical pathways initially emerged from the interest of hospital administrators as a means to reduce length of hospital stay. However, clinicians have recognized many other goals for such pathways, the most important of which is the need to improve the quality of patient care (Table 1-1). Indeed, physicians involved in developing critical pathways should focus on the positive aspects of pathways and utilize them as a means to advance medical care. Other specific goals focus on (a) improving the use of medications and treatments, (b) improving patient triage to the appropriate level of care (1,3–5), (c) increasing participation in research protocols, and (d) limiting the use of unnecessary tests to reduce costs and allow savings to be allocated to other treatments that have been shown to be beneficial. With involvement of physicians, nurses, and other clinicians in the development of these pathways, those responsible for patient care can control how the patients are managed. Indeed, it is important to monitor their performance of pathways and to ensure that they are up to date with new advances in care.

TABLE 1-1

GOALS OF CRITICAL PATHWAYS

1. Improve patient care.
2. Increase use of recommended medical therapies (e.g., aspirin for all acute coronary syndromes, reperfusion therapy for STEMI).
3. Decrease use of unnecessary tests.
4. Decrease hospital length of stay.
5. Reduce costs.
6. Increase participation in clinical research protocols.

NEED AND RATIONALE FOR CRITICAL PATHWAYS

Despite wide dissemination of the clinical trial results, a large proportion of patients with acute coronary syndromes do not receive "evidence-based" medical therapies. Such a glaring deficiency has been seen most dramatically for aspirin (6–13), but it is also apparent with the use of thrombolytic therapy (10,14,15), beta-blockers (16), statins (8,17), and many other classes of drugs.

Another need addressed by critical pathways is the marked variation in the use of cardiac procedures following admission for acute MI and unstable angina. In acute MI, numerous studies have found wide differences in the use of invasive cardiac procedures but no differences in mortality (18–21), suggesting that some of these procedures may be unnecessary or inappropriate.

Other areas of potential overutilization of testing also exist (e.g., with laboratory tests and echocardiography) (22–24). Several studies have suggested that for patients with small non-Q wave MIs, assessment of LV function via echocardiography or ventriculography may not be necessary, a strategy that could have potential implications for more cost-effective care.

Reducing Hospital (and ICU) Length of Stay

Reduction in hospital length of stay has been the driving force behind the creation of critical pathways. As noted in the initial pathways for cardiac surgical patients, early discharge was the main outcome variable (25). In acute coronary syndromes, length of stay was quite long in the 1990s, where it was 9 days for patients with unstable angina and non-STEMI (UA/NSTEMI) (26) and in STEMI (27), even among patients who had an uncomplicated course (13). Over the subsequent decade, however, length of stay has steadily decreased (28), showing that this has been one way to improve efficiency of care.

Overutilization of Intensive Care

Overutilization of the intensive and coronary care unit (CCU) is another area in which critical pathways may reduce costs. In the 1980s and early 1990s, admission to the coronary care unit was standard for all unstable angina and MI (and frequently "rule out MI") patients (29,30). Even in 1996, 40% of patients with UA/NSTEMI in the multicenter GUARANTEE Registry conducted in the United States were admitted to the CCU (31). Because CCU admission is now generally recommended for higher-risk patients (i.e., those with STEMI and/or hemodynamic compromise or other complications), such data suggest opportunities may exist for reducing the number of patients admitted to intensive care units.

METHODS FOR THE DEVELOPMENT OF CRITICAL PATHWAYS

The process of developing a critical pathway derives first from identifying the problem (Table 1-2). Beginning with a specific diagnosis, the obstacles to the appropriate care of patients are delineated (e.g., low use of aspirin, as noted earlier) in parallel with the prevailing issues at the institutional level. For example, the use of blood tests might be higher than necessary when

TABLE 1-2

STEPS IN DEVELOPING AND IMPLEMENTING THE CRITICAL PATHWAY

1. Identify problems in patient care (e.g., underutilization of evidence-based therapies, excess resource use, long length of stay).
2. Identify committee to develop guidelines and critical pathway.
3. Distribute Draft Critical Pathway to all departments involved.
4. Revise pathway to reach a consensus.
5. Implement the pathway.
6. Collect and monitor data on critical pathway performance.
7. Periodically modify/update the pathway as needed to further improve performance, and keep current with new therapies and treatments.

left to an individual house officer or physician (e.g., multiple cholesterol measurements during a single hospital stay).

The next step is to establish a committee (comprised of clinicians recognized as local thought leaders) to create (or adapt) a critical pathway that would include recommended guidelines for the treatment of patients with specific diagnoses. The third step is to distribute the draft critical pathway(s) to all health care professionals and services who help manage for patients with those diagnoses, to ensure adequate input from all parties involved. For example, for a UA/NSTEMI pathway, one should include members of the cardiology, cardiac surgery, emergency medicine, nursing, noninvasive lab, cardiac rehabilitation, social services, case management, and dietary service teams. Comments from these parties are then included in the final pathway.

Implementation of the pathway can begin with a "pilot" and then be available for routine use. The fifth step in the process of establishing a critical pathway is to collect and monitor data regarding performance. This could include the number of patients for whom the pathway was used, use of recommended therapy, and the length of hospital stay. The final step is to interpret the initial data and modify the pathway as needed. These latter three steps collectively consist of the "continuous quality improvement" that must be ongoing during the implementation of any pathway. In addition, as new therapies become available, the data should be reviewed to determine which steps should be added or modified as part of optimal patient management. For example, clopidogrel has recently been shown to benefit patients with STEMI (32,33) and thus should be added to STEMI protocols.

Methods of Implementation

Several potential methods of implementation exist. First, one could have voluntary participation in a pathway. Although this appears to be an inefficient means of ensuring participation with a critical pathway, it is frequently all that can be accomplished with limited resources at individual hospitals. The pathway could be sent to physicians and nurses and presented at staff and house staff meetings. Another means of triggering pathway use is to use reminders via electronic mail messages triggered off the admission diagnosis or monthly reminders to physicians and nurses. Another approach is to have independent screening of all admissions, with copies of the pathway placed in the chart. Use of the pathway would be expected to be low with such a voluntary approach. On the other hand, if a pathway becomes implemented in an initial group of patients, that treatment strategy may become the standard of care at a particular hospital. Later, it may no longer be necessary to actually involve additional personnel to "implement" the pathway.

An alternate approach that some hospitals have used is to have a designated case manager evaluate each patient and ensure that all steps in the pathway are carried out. Such an approach would be expected to improve the use of the pathway. However, this approach obviously requires additional resources from the hospital or health care system. The approach used by individual hospitals for specific diagnoses needs to be individualized. The ultimate goal is to improve the care of patients and make such care more cost effective.

Cardiac Checklist

A very simplified version of a critical pathway is to use a "cardiac checklist." Although checklists exist for many purposes including admission tests and procedures, this format can be extended to medical treatments. It is a simple method to ensure that each patient receives all the recommended therapies. Table 1-3 shows an example "Cardiac Checklist" for a patient with UA/NSTEMI. This checklist could be used in two ways: physicians could keep a copy on a small index card in their pocket and scan down the list when writing admission orders, or the checklist could be used to develop standard orders for an MI patient, either printed or computerized, from which the physician can choose when admitting a patient. Such a system has worked well in ensuring extremely high compliance with evidence-based recommendations at Brigham and Women's Hospital. In the era of "scorecard medicine" (34), many outside observers, such as the Center for Medicare and Medicaid Services (CMS) or the Joint Commission for Accreditation of Hospital Organizations (JCAHO), tally up the use of recommended medications as quality-of-care measures. Thus, using tools to improve care will be closely monitored.

TABLE 1-3

"CARDIAC CHECKLIST" FOR UNSTABLE ANGINA AND NON-ST-ELEVATION MI

Medications

1. Aspirin ☐
2. Clopidogrel ☐
3. Heparin/LMWH ☐
4. IIb/IIIa inhibition ☐
5. Beta-blockers ☐
6. ACE inhibitors if low EF/CHF ☐

Interventions

7. Cath/Revascularization for recurrent ischemia or high-risk patients ☐

Secondary prevention

8. High-dose statin ☐
9. Smoking cessation ☐
10. Treat other risk factors (hypertension, diabetes) ☐

Updated with permission from Cannon CP. Optimizing the treatment of unstable angina. *J Thromb Thrombolysis* 1995;2:205–218.

EVIDENCE OF BENEFIT OF CRITICAL PATHWAYS

Many studies are now available showing the benefit of the use of critical pathways. The first example is the widely discussed pathways by the National Heart Attack Alert Program on "the 4 Ds": door, data, decision, and drug time (2). This pathway focuses on trying to administer thrombolytic therapy within 30 minutes of a patient arriving at the ED. The very simple pathway lists the four key steps in treating a patient in the ED. Data from the NRMI have shown a significant reduction in door-to-drug time, falling from over 60 minutes in the early 1990s to approximately 30 to 35 minutes on average (28). This is a simple pathway with really one parameter, but a successful one. Indeed, it is a good way to start implementing pathways: to begin with one focused problem area, and then to broaden to other areas and issues in care. A similar process has improved door-to-balloon times for patients treated with primary percutaneous coronary intervention (PCI) (35).

Several large, multicenter demonstrations of the benefits of critical pathway quality improvement efforts have come from the American College of Cardiology (ACC), the AHA, and the Veterans Affairs (VA) hospital system (36,37). The ACC sponsored the Guideline Applied in Practice (GAP) Program, lead by Kim Eagle in Michigan. In this program, 10 hospitals were identified to participate in the quality improvement effort. They each worked to implement pathways, including education of hospital staff through grand rounds programs, development and implementation of standardized order sets, and the use of pocket cards with treatment guidelines to be given to the physicians, shown in Figure 1-1, they found improvement in the use of guideline-recommended therapies and procedures; early use of aspirin and beta-blockers and measurement of low-density lipoprotein cholesterol were all improved after implementation of the GAP quality improvement effort (36). Most interestingly, the improvement was greatest in patients in whom they found evidence in the chart that the standardized pathway, the pocket tool, or one of the other tools rolled out at the individual hospitals had actually been used (36,38). This demonstrated that having tools available for clinicians to use as reminders really works and does improve the use of various therapies. This has provided evidence that it is critical for an individual institution to make sure that whatever tools are selected, they are adapted to fit into that hospital's standard clinical practice (36,38).

Most importantly, however, Eagle and colleagues demonstrated a significantly lower mortality at hospital discharge and through the following year among patients treated at hospitals after they implemented the GAP program as compared with the same hospital's results just the year prior to GAP (39) (Fig. 1-2). This closes the loop to show that pathways can improve the process of care, as well as improve outcomes.

The American Heart Association (AHA) has developed the Get with the Guidelines Program (40). This is a Web-based program that focuses on the time of discharge to help monitor in real time whether all the various guideline-recommended therapies have been used. It is a simple Web-based tool in which the targeted clinical information about the patient is entered. Reminders are built into the system that prompt compliance with the guidelines. For example, if a patient has high cholesterol, and no lipid-lowering agent is listed in the discharge medication, a prompt will suggest to the physician that the patient is a candidate for statin therapy. The tool is also linked to the ACC/AHA Guidelines, and thus the specific recommendations are available immediately. This program too has shown promising results with improvements in all aspects of the care of patients with coronary artery disease (40). New modules of

GAP Initiative: Adherence Improves With Tool Use

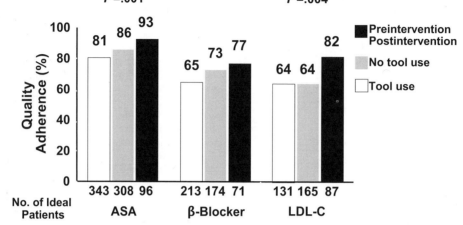

Early Quality Indicators and Standard Admission Orders

FIGURE 1-1. Implementation of the GAP initiative improved adherence to key treatments. When implementation tools such as standard admission orders were utilized (as indicated in the medical record), adherence to key treatments improved beyond the improvement seen without using tools. Implementation of guideline-based tools for acute MI may facilitate quality improvement among a wide variety of institutions, patients, and caregivers. (Adapted from Mehta RH, Montoye CK, Gallogly M, et al. Improving quality of care of acute myocardial infarction: The Guideline Applied in Practice (GAP) Initiative in Southeast Michigan. *JAMA* 2002;287:1269–1276, with permission.)

GAP Initiative: Changes in Mortality Before and After GAP Project

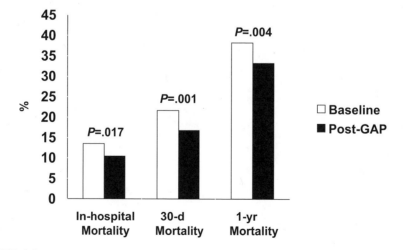

FIGURE 1-2. The American Heart Association's Guidelines Applied in Practice for the management of patients with acute myocardial infarction (GAP Initiative) followed 2,857 patients in 33 Michigan hospitals and compared patient care before and after implementation of the program. The GAP Initiative focused on changes in the use of evidence-based therapies, adoption of standardized admission and discharge tools, and effects on mortality. After the inception of the GAP Initiative, there were significantly lower rates of in-hospital mortality ($P = 0.017$), 30-day mortality ($P = 0.001$), and 1-year mortality ($P = 0.004$). (From Eagle KA, Montoye CK, Riba AL, et al. Guideline-based standardized care is associated with substantially lower mortality in medicare patients with acute myocardial infarction: the American College of Cardiology's Guidelines Applied in Practice (GAP) Projects in Michigan. *J Am Coll Cardiol* 2005;46(7):1242–1248, with permission.)

the program now aim to improve the care of patients with congestive heart failure and stroke.

A report from the VA system, which initiated a "re-engineering" of cardiology several years ago, focused on using standardized approaches and pathways and used information technology and computer order sets to build a system to help clinicians administer appropriate care (37). They did this broadly in congestive heart failure, pneumonia, and acute MI. A key part of this system was monitoring data and actually disclosing publicly the results at each of the individual hospitals. Thus each hospital was accountable for what their successes or failures were in terms of administering these therapies. They observed an improvement over the 4 years in the use of key therapies like aspirin and beta-blockers, admission, and discharge. All significantly improved and attained very high levels—greater than 90% to 95% for use of aspirin and beta-blockers—really the best that have been reported to date. It is encouraging that we can implement a pathway program, monitor data, and have a really meaningful improvement in outcome.

The most recent demonstration was from the CRUSADE registry. In this program, efforts were focused on improving implementation of the ACC/AHA Guidelines for UA/NSTEMI. In this registry, it was seen that the hospitals that had the best adherence to the guidelines had the lowest in-hospital mortality (41). Thus, as seen in the ACC's GAP program, better use of guideline-recommended therapies was associated with better outcomes.

CONCLUSIONS AND FUTURE DIRECTIONS

As the use of critical pathways continues to grow, the newest shift in the field (and since the first edition of this book) has been the evidence base of their benefit. Critical pathways have now clearly been shown in multiple studies to help improve patient care and, most importantly, improve outcomes. Standardized approaches with simple "checklists" to ensure the appropriate use of medications will be a significant improvement in the care of patients. However, use of pathways is itself an ongoing process, where monitoring of performance and periodic review and updating of the pathways is needed. In addition, as care shifts more broadly to electronic order entry and medical records, novel ways of implementing the pathways will need to be developed, but this area is one of great promise for greater benefits toward patient care.

References

1. Cannon CP, Antman EM, Walls R, et al. Time as an adjunctive agent to thrombolytic therapy. *J Thromb Thrombolysis* 1994;1:27–34.
2. National Heart Attack Alert Program Coordinating Committee–60 Minutes to Treatment Working Group. Emergency department: rapid identification and treatment of patients with acute myocardial infarction. *Ann Emerg Med* 1994;23:311–329.
3. Cannon CP. Optimizing the treatment of unstable angina. *J Thromb Thrombolysis* 1995;2:205–218.
4. Udelson JE, Beshansky JR, Ballin DS, et al. Myocardial perfusion imaging for evaluation and triage of patients with suspected acute cardiac ischemia: a randomized controlled trial. *JAMA* 2002;288(21):2693–2700.
5. Farkouh ME, Smars PA, Reeder GS, et al. A clinical trial of a chest-pain observation unit for patients with unstable angina. Chest Pain Evaluation in the Emergency Room (CHEER) Investigators. *N Engl J Med* 1998;339(26):1882–1888.
6. Rogers WJ, Bowlby LJ, Chandra NC, et al. Treatment of myocardial infarction in the United States (1990 to 1993). Observations from the National Registry of Myocardial Infarction. *Circulation* 1994;90:2103–214.
7. Ellerbeck EF, Jencks SF, Radford MJ, et al. Quality of care for medicare patients with acute myocardial infarction. A four-state pilot study from the Cooperative Cardiovascular Project. *JAMA* 1995;273:1509–1514.
8. Aronow WS. Underutilization of lipid-lowering drugs in older persons with prior myocardial infarction and a serum low-density lipoprotein cholesterol > 125 mg/dl. *Am J Cardiol* 1998;82(5):668–669, A6, A8.
9. Scirica BM, Moliterno DJ, Every NR, et al. Differences between men and women in the management of unstable angina pectoris (The GUARANTEE Registry). *Am J Cardiol* 1999;84(10):1145–1150.
10. Cannon CP, Bahit MC, Haugland JM, et al. Underutilization of evidence-based medications in acute ST elevation myocardial infarction: results of the Thrombolysis in Myocardial Infarction (TIMI) 9 Registry. *Crit Path Cardiol* 2002;1:44–52.
11. Spencer FA, Meyer TE, Gore JM, et al. Heterogeneity in the management and outcomes of patients with acute myocardial infarction complicated by heart failure: The National Registry of Myocardial Infarction. *Circulation* 2002;105(22):2605–2610.
12. Fox KA, Goodman SG, Klein W, et al. Management of acute coronary syndromes. Variations in practice and outcome; findings from the Global Registry of Acute Coronary Events (GRACE). *Eur Heart J* 2002;23(15):1177–1189.
13. Newby LK, Califf RM, Guerci A, et al. Early discharge in the thrombolytic era: an analysis of criteria for uncomplicated infarction from the Global Utilization of Streptokinase and t-PA for Occluded Coronary Arteries (GUSTO) trial. *J Am Coll Cardiol* 1996;27(3):625–632.
14. Barron HV, Bowlby LJ, Breen T, et al. Use of reperfusion therapy for acute myocardial infarction in the United States: data from the National Registry of Myocardial Infarction 2. *Circulation* 1998;97(12):1150–1156.
15. Eagle KA, Goodman SG, Avezum A, et al. Practice variation and missed opportunities for reperfusion in ST-segment-elevation myocardial infarction: findings from the Global Registry of Acute Coronary Events (GRACE). *Lancet* 2002;359:373–377.
16. Krumholz HM, Radford MJ, Wang Y, et al. Early beta-blocker therapy for acute myocardial infarction in elderly patients. *Ann Intern Med* 1999;131(9):648–654.
17. Fonarow GC, French WJ, Parsons LS, et al. Use of lipid-lowering medications at discharge in patients with acute myocardial infarction: data from the National Registry of Myocardial Infarction 3. *Circulation* 2001;103(1):38–44.
18. Every NR, Parson LS, Fihn SD, et al. Long-term outcome in acute myocardial infarction patients admitted to hospitals with and without on-site cardiac catheterization facilities. *Circulation* 1997;96:1770–1775.
19. Rouleau JL, Moye LA, Pfeffer MA, et al. A comparison of management patterns after acute myocardial infarction in Canada and the United States. *N Engl J Med* 1993;328:779–784.
20. Pilote L, Califf RM, Sapp S, et al. Regional variation across the United States in the management of acute myocardial infarction. *N Engl J Med* 1995;333:565–572.
21. Blomkalns AL, Chen AY, Hochman JS, et al. Gender disparities in the diagnosis and treatment of non-ST-segment elevation acute coronary syndromes: large-scale observations from the CRUSADE (Can Rapid Risk Stratification of Unstable Angina Patients Suppress Adverse Outcomes With Early Implementation of the American College of Cardiology/American Heart Association Guidelines) National Quality Improvement Initiative. *J Am Coll Cardiol* 2005;45(6):832–837.
22. Silver MT, Rose GA, Paul SD, et al. A clinical rule to predict preserved left ventricular ejection fraction in patients after myocardial infarction. *Ann Intern Med* 1994;121:750–756.
23. Tobin K, Stomel R, Harber D, et al. Validation of a clinical prediction rule for predicting left ventricular function post acute myocardial infarction in a community hospital setting. *J Am Coll Cardiol* 1996;27(Suppl. A):318A.
24. Krumholz HM, Howes CJ, Murillo JE, et al. Validation of a clinical prediction rule for left ventricular ejection fraction after myocardial infarction in patients ≥ 65 years old. *Am J Cardiol* 1997;80:11–15.
25. Nickerson NJ, Murphy SF, Kouchoukos NT, et al. Predictors of early discharge after cardiac surgery and its cost-effectiveness. *J Am Coll Cardiol* 1996;27:264A.
26. The TIMI IIIB Investigators. Effects of tissue plasminogen activator and a comparison of early invasive and conservative strategies in unstable angina and non-Q-wave myocardial infarction: results of the TIMI IIIB Trial. *Circulation* 1994;89:1545–1556.
27. Cannon CP, Antman EM, Gibson CM, et al. Critical pathway for acute ST segment elevation myocardial infarction: evaluation of the potential impact in the TIMI 9 registry. *J Am Coll Cardiol* 1998;31(Suppl. A):192A.
28. Rogers WJ, Canto JG, Lambrew CT, et al. Temporal trends in the treatment of over 1.5 million patients with myocardial infarction in the US from 1990 through 1999: the National Registry of Myocardial Infarction 1, 2 and 3. *J Am Coll Cardiol* 2000;36(7):2056–2063.
29. Goldman L, Cook EF, Brand DA, et al. A computer protocol to predict myocardial infarction in emergency department patients with chest pain. *N Engl J Med* 1988;318:797–803.
30. Pozen MW, D'Agostino RB, Mitchell JB, et al. The usefulness of a predictive instrument to reduce inappropriate admissions to the coronary care unit. *Ann Intern Med* 1980;92:238–242.
31. Cannon CP, Moliterno DJ, Every N, et al. Implementation of AHCPR guidelines for unstable angina in 1996: Unfortunate differences between men & women. Results from the multicenter GUARANTEE registry. *J Am Coll Cardiol* 1997;29(Suppl. A):217A.
32. Sabatine MS, Cannon CP, Gibson CM, et al. Addition of clopidogrel to

aspirin and fibrinolytic therapy for myocardial infarction with ST-segment elevation. *N Engl J Med* 2005;352(12):1179–1189.

33. Chen ZM, Jiang LX, Chen YP, et al. Addition of clopidogrel to aspirin in 45,852 patients with acute myocardial infarction: randomised placebo-controlled trial. *Lancet* 2005;366(9497):1607–1621.

34. Topol EJ, Califf RM. Scorecard cardiovascular medicine. Its impact and future directions. *Ann Intern Med* 1994;120:65–70.

35. Caputo RP, Ho KK, Stoler RC, et al. Effect of continuous quality improvement analysis on the delivery of primary percutaneous transluminal coronary angioplasty for acute myocardial infarction. *Am J Cardiol* 1997;79: 1159–1164.

36. Mehta RH, Montoye CK, Gallogly M, et al. Improving quality of care of acute myocardial infarction: The Guideline Applied in Practice (GAP) Initiative in Southeast Michigan. *JAMA* 2002;287:1269–1276.

37. Jha AK, Perlin JB, Kizer KW, et al. Effect of the transformation of the Veterans Affairs Health Care System on the quality of care. *N Engl J Med* 2003;348(22):2218–2227.

38. Mehta RH, Montoye CK, Faul J, et al. Enhancing quality of care for acute myocardial infarction: shifting the focus of improvement from key indicators to process of care and tool use. *J Am Coll Cardiol* 2004;43(12):2167–2173.

39. Eagle KA, Montoye CK, Riba AL, et al. Guideline-based standardized care is associated with substantially lower mortality in medicare patients with acute myocardial infarction: the American College of Cardiology's Guidelines Applied in Practice (GAP) Projects in Michigan. *J Am Coll Cardiol* 2005;46(7):1242–1248.

40. LaBresh KA, Ellrodt AG, Gliklich R, et al. Get with the guidelines for cardiovascular secondary prevention: pilot results. *Arch Intern Med* 2004;164(2): 203–209.

41. Peterson ED, Roe MT, Mulgund J, et al. Association between hospital process performance and outcomes among patients with acute coronary syndromes. *JAMA* 2006;295(16):1912–1920.

PART I ■ PREHOSPITAL CRITICAL PATHWAYS

CHAPTER 2 ■ PREHOSPITAL FIBRINOLYSIS

FREEK W. A. VERHEUGT

PREHOSPITAL REPERFUSION THERAPY
OPTIMAL PREHOSPITAL DIAGNOSIS
PREHOSPITAL DRUG ADMINISTRATION
ADJUNCTIVE THERAPY IN PREHOSPITAL FIBRINOLYSIS
ALTERNATIVE REPERFUSION STRATEGIES INITIATED IN
    THE AMBULANCE
CONCLUSION

INTRODUCTION

Reperfusion therapy for ST-elevation acute coronary syndromes aims at early and complete recanalization of the infarct-related artery to salvage myocardium and improve both early and late clinical outcomes. Prehospital diagnosis of ST-elevation acute coronary syndrome can be made by echocardiogram (ECG) with or without transtelephonic transmission, and subsequent fibrinolytic therapy can be instituted at home or in the ambulance. Prehospital fibrinolysis decreases time to treatment by about 1 hour compared to in-hospital therapy, resulting in a significant 15% relative risk reduction of early mortality. This may compare well with primary angioplasty for ST-elevation acute coronary syndrome, although more studies are necessary.

Reperfusion therapy has become the indisputable gold standard for the early management of acute ST-segment elevation coronary syndromes. The benefit of this strategy rises exponentially the earlier the therapy is initiated. The highest number of lives saved by reperfusion therapy is within the first hour after symptom onset: a window of opportunity aptly termed the golden hour (1). Clearly and logically, the mechanism of this benefit relates to maximizing myocardial salvage by early restoration of adequate coronary blood flow, resulting in preservation of left ventricular function, thereby enhancing both early and long-term survival.

According to the principle of the infarct wave front by Reimer and Jennings, a brief interruption of blood flow is associated with a small infarct size (2). The temporal dependence of the beneficial effect of coronary reperfusion has also been characterized by multiple metrics, including positron emission tomography (3). Irrespective of the methodology, however, the relationship between duration of symptoms and infarct size remains consistent.

The exponential form of the curve illustrating the benefit of reperfusion therapy on mortality and myocardial salvage has major implications for the timing of treatment. The impact of delay in time to treatment lessens as the duration of ischemia lengthens. Consequently, reducing delays will have a much more positive return in patients presenting early versus those presenting late (4). These considerations have provided strong incentive for the initiation of very early reperfusion therapy, including the use of prehospital fibrinolysis (5).

PREHOSPITAL REPERFUSION THERAPY

In 1985 Gotsman and coworkers implemented prehospital triage and treatment of patients with ST-segment elevation myocardial infarction in Jerusalem, Israel (6). They demonstrated the presence of minimal myocardial damage after the early administration of streptokinase. Nine years later, in a larger and randomized prehospital fibrinolysis study, prehospital treatment achieved significantly less Q wave infarctions, which may be correlated with a greater number of smaller infarctions (7). The same trial also demonstrated accelerated and more extensive ST-segment resolution with prehospital treatment suggesting enhanced myocardial perfusion (8). Subsequently, the large In-TIME-2 study demonstrated that with each additional hour of symptom onset to the start of fibrinolytic reperfusion therapy, the chance of achieving complete ST-segment resolution decreases by 6% (9). In an ASSENT-2 substudy, including 13,100 patients, the earlier lytic therapy was initiated, the higher the likelihood of ST-segment resolution on the ECG. Moreover, earlier therapy was inversely related to 1-year mortality (10).

Hence the ultimate objective of reperfusion therapy is early and effective treatment, which can only be established by prehospital treatment.

OPTIMAL PREHOSPITAL DIAGNOSIS

Clearly, medical history and appropriate electrocardiographic recording is necessary for the proper diagnosis of ST-elevation acute myocardial infarction. Transtelephonic or computer diagnosis can be used for this purpose and seems to be equivalent in accuracy (11). Also, the ambulance staff is important in the quality of prehospital triage. In The Netherlands a national ambulance protocol is used for the triage of patients with suspected acute myocardial infarction to initiate the optimal prehospital reperfusion strategy (Fig. 2-1). Usually ambulances are staffed with nurses with or without physicians. Importantly, nurses seem to work faster than physicians in the diagnosis of ST-elevation myocardial infarction and proper administration of a fibrinolytic agent (Fig. 2-2) (12). This is useful in reducing the treatment delay. In general, treatment delay can be shortened by about 55 minutes using prehospital thrombolysis versus in-hospital thrombolysis (13). This results in a 15% reduction of early mortality in comparison to in-hospital fibrinolysis (Fig. 2-3). This benefit applies to low-, middle-, and high risk patients to about the same extent as depicted in Figure 2-4.

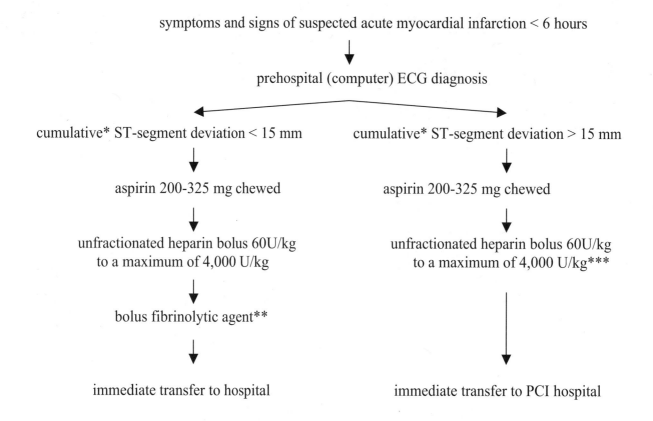

symptoms and signs of suspected acute myocardial infarction < 6 hours

prehospital (computer) ECG diagnosis

cumulative* ST-segment deviation < 15 mm	cumulative* ST-segment deviation > 15 mm
aspirin 200-325 mg chewed	aspirin 200-325 mg chewed
unfractionated heparin bolus 60U/kg to a maximum of 4,000 U/kg	unfractionated heparin bolus 60U/kg to a maximum of 4,000 U/kg***
bolus fibrinolytic agent**	
immediate transfer to hospital	immediate transfer to PCI hospital

*   sum of ST-segment elevation and reciprocal ST-segment depression

**   if contraindication(s) crossover to PCI

*** limited heparin dose in case of cross-over to firbinolytic therapy due to unexpected delay(s) during transfer and in-hospital

Abbreviations: PCI = primary coronary intervention

FIGURE 2-1. National ambulance protocol for the management of suspected acute myocardial infarction in the Netherlands.

PREHOSPITAL DRUG ADMINISTRATION

Both streptokinase and alteplase have been used in the prehospital setting but resulted in medication errors in more than 10% of cases, which was associated with more than doubling of the 24-hour and 30-day mortality rate (14). The most common medication error is miscalculation of dosing according to body weight. Especially patients with a low body weight may be overdosed, resulting in a high number of intracranial hemorrhages (14). The introduction of bolus lytic therapy has facilitated the use of prehospital thrombolysis, although the safety with regard to intracranial bleeding has been questioned (15). However, in later observations the safety looks excellent in patients under the age of 75 years (16). The first trial with a bolus lytic given in the prehospital setting was the ER TIMI-19 study in 315 patients in the Boston area, which showed a 30-minute reduction in treatment delay compared with in-hospital lytic therapy (17). Also in the ASSENT-3 PLUS trial a bolus lytic was given to 1,639 patients in a prehospital setting showing excellent safety, if combined with unfractionated heparin. However, in the elderly patients treated with enoxaparin, the intracranial hemorrhage rate was unacceptably high (18).

ADJUNCTIVE THERAPY IN PREHOSPITAL FIBRINOLYSIS

Immediately after the electrocardiographic diagnosis of acute ST-segment elevation acute coronary syndrome is made, aspi-

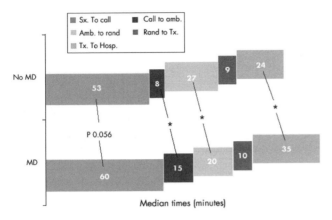

FIGURE 2-2. Time to fibrinolytic therapy in ambulances with (MD) and without (no MD) physicians on board. Abbreviations: Sx, symptoms; Amb, ambulance; Rand, randomization; Tx, thrombolysis; hosp, hospital). (Reproduced with permission from Welsh RC, Chang W, Goldstein P, et al. Time to treatment and the impact of a physician on prehospital management of acute ST-elevation myocardial infarction: insights from the ASSENT-3 PLUS trial. *Heart* 2005;91:1400–1406.)

rin should be given in a dose of 200 to 325 mg, preferably chewed. Before or immediately after the fibrinolytic has been given, a bolus of unfractionated heparin must be administered in a dose of 60 U/kg to a maximum of 4,000 U. Enoxaparin bolus as an alternative to unfractionated heparin should be avoided, especially in patients over 75 years of age (see earlier discussion). Recently, it was shown that an oral loading dose of 300 mg clopidogrel together with aspirin, heparin, and a bolus fibrinolytic is safe and is associated with earlier and more complete reperfusion of the infarct-related artery (19).

ALTERNATIVE REPERFUSION STRATEGIES INITIATED IN THE AMBULANCE

In the primary angioplasty era the CAPTIM trial in France was carried out in 845 patients showing that prehospital thrombolytic therapy is not inferior to primary percutaneous coronary intervention (PCI) provided the patients are triaged in the ambulance (20). In the patients treated within 2 hours mortality was nearly significantly lower in the prehospital thrombolysis group compared to those treated with primary PCI (Fig. 2-5) (21). Thus, the use of modern bolus lytic therapy in the

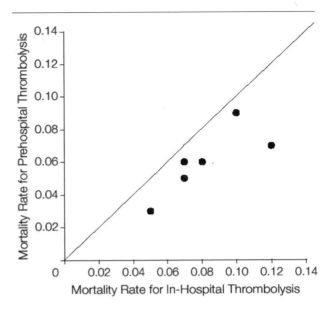

FIGURE 2-4. Relation of early mortality of prehopital versus in-hospital fibrinolysis in various risk categories in ST-elevation myocardial infarction. (Reproduced with permission from Morrison LJ, Verbeek PR, McDonald AC, et al. Mortality and prehospital thrombolysis for acute myocardial infarction. *JAMA* 2000;283:2686–2692.)

prehospital setting is a very attractive one, because of speed and ease of administration, which may challenge the benefit of primary PCI in ST-elevation acute myocardial infarction. However, the data from the CAPTIM trial should be confirmed in a larger trial comparing the best of two worlds: prehospital thrombolysis and primary PCI preferably triaged in the ambulance. Recently it was shown that prehospital diagnosis and subsequent immediate transfer to a PCI center results in shorter time delays than triage of these patients in non-PCI centers (22). Therefore, a new CAPTIM-like trial should be set up to compare prehospital thrombolysis versus primary PCI triaged in the ambulance with immediate transfer to a PCI center in

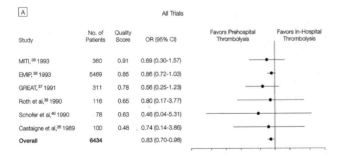

FIGURE 2-3. Meta-analysis of early mortality of prehopital versus in-hospital fibrinolysis in ST-elevation myocardial infarction. (Reproduced with permission from Morrison LJ, Verbeek PR, McDonald AC, et al. Mortality and prehospital thrombolysis for acute myocardial infarction. *JAMA* 2000;283:2686–2692.)

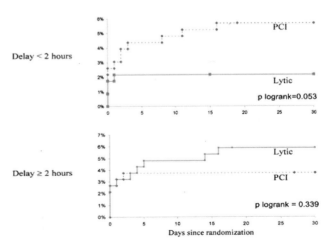

FIGURE 2-5. Early mortality of prehospital fibrinolysis versus primary angioplasty in relation to time from symptom onset to randomization. (Reproduced with permission from Steg PG, Bonnefoy E, Chabaud S, et al. Impact of time to treatment on mortality after prehospital fibrinolysis or primary angioplasty: data from the CAPTIM randomized clinical trial Circulation 2003;103:2851–2856.)

both arms. This is currently suggested in a study design in the United Kingdom.

Finally, agents other than fibrinolytics can be utilized in the prehospital setting to speed up coronary reperfusion. Platelet glycoprotein IIb/IIIa have been tested and showed better pre-angioplasty coronary patency in ST-elevation acute coronary syndrome than placebo. The earlier the drugs were given (in the ambulance or emergency department), the better the patency and clinical outcome (23).

CONCLUSION

The best results of reperfusion therapy of ST-elevation acute coronary syndromes can be obtained by prehospital initiation at home or in the ambulance. The introduction of ECG computer diagnosis and bolus formulation of fibrinolytic agents has further facilitated proper and timely prehospital treatment of ST-elevation acute coronary syndromes. In a singe trial, this strategy has shown to be not inferior to primary angioplasty with prehospital triage. However, more studies are needed to confirm these results.

References

1. Boersma E, Maas AC, Deckers JW, et al. Early thrombolytic therapy in acute myocardial infarction: reappraisal of the golden hour. *Lancet* 1996; 348:771–775.
2. Reimer KA, Lowe JE, Rasmussen MM, et al. The wavefront phenomenon of ischemic cell death. Myocardial infarct size versus duration of coronary occlusion in dogs. *Circulation* 1977;56:786–794.
3. Bergmann SR, Lerch RA, Fox KAA, et al. Temporal dependence of beneficial effects of coronary thrombolysis characterized by positron emission tomography. *Am J Med* 1982;73:573–580.
4. Gersh BJ, Stone GW, White HD, et al. Pharmacological facilitation of primary percutaneous coronary intervention for acute myocardial infarction: is the slope of the curve the shape of the future? *JAMA* 2005;293:979–986.
5. Huber K, De Caterina R, Kristensen SD, et al. Prehospital reperfusion therapy: a strategy to improve therapeutic outcome in patients with ST-elevation myocardial infarction. *Eur Heart J* 2005;26:2063–2074.
6. Koren G, Weiss AT, Hasin Y, et al. Prevention of myocardial damage in acute myocardial infarction by early treatment with intravenous streptokinase. *N Engl J Med* 1985;313:1384–1389.
7. Rawles J. Halving of mortality at 1 year by domiciliary thrombolysis in the Grampian Region Early Anistreplase Trial. *J Am Coll Cardiol* 1994;23:1–5.
8. Trent R, Adams J, Rawles J. Electrocardiographic evidence of reperfusion occurring before hospital admission. *Eur Heart J* 1994;15:895–897.
9. Antman EM, Cooper HA, Gibson CM, et al. Determinants of improvement of epicardial flow and myocardial perfusion for ST-elevation myocardial infarction. *Eur Heart J* 2002;23:928–933.
10. Fu Y, Goodman S, Wei-Ching C, et al. Time to treatment influences the impact of ST-segment resolution on one-year prognosis. *Circulation* 2001; 104:2653–2659.
11. Lamfers EJP, Hooghoudt TEH, Uppelschoten A, et al. Prehospital versus hospital fibrinolytic therapy using automated versus cardiologist ECG diagnosis of myocardial infarction: abortion of myocardial infarction and unjustified fibrinolytic therapy. *Am Heart J* 2004;147:509–515.
12. Welsh RC, Chang W, Goldstein P, et al. Time to treatment and the impact of a physician on prehospital management of acute ST-elevation myocardial infarction: insights from the ASSENT-3 PLUS trial. *Heart* 2005;91: 1400–1406.
13. Morrison LJ, Verbeek PR, McDonald AC, et al. Mortality and prehospital thrombolysis for acute myocardial infarction. *JAMA* 2000;283:2686–2692.
14. Cannon CP. Exploring the issues of appropriate dosing in the treatment of acute myocardial infarction: potential benefits of bolus fibrinolytic agents. *Am Heart J* 2000;140:154–160.
15. Metha SR, Eikelboom JW, Yusuf S. Risk of intracranial hemorrhage with bolus versus infusion thrombolytic therapy: a meta-analysis. *Lancet* 2000; 356:449–454.
16. ASSENT-3 Investigators. Efficacy and safety of tenecteplase with enoxaparin, abciximab or unfractionated heparin: the ASSENT-3 randomised trial in acute myocardial infarction. *Lancet* 2001;358:605–613.
17. Morrow DA, Antman EM, Sayah AJ, et al. Evaluation of the time saved by prehospital initiation of reteplase for ST-elevation myocardial infarction: results of the Early Retevase-Thrombolysis in Myocardial Infarction (ER-TIMI)-19 trial. *J Am Coll Cardiol* 2002;40:71–77.
18. Wallentin L, Goldstein P, Armstrong PW, et al. Efficacy and safety of tenecteplase in combination with the low-molecular weight heparin enoxaparin, or unfractionated heparin in the prehospital setting: the ASSENT-3 PLUS randomized trial in acute myocardial infarction. *Circulation* 2003;108: 135–142.
19. Montalescot G, Verheugt F, Sabatine MS, et al. Prehospital fibrinolysis with dual antiplatelet therapy in ST-elevation myocardial infarction. The prehospital CLARITY-TIMI-28 substudy. *Circulation* 2005;112:Suppl II:567 (abstract).
20. Bonnefoy E, Lapostolle F, Leizorovicz A, et al. Primary angioplasty versus prehospital fibrinolysis in acute myocardial infarction. *Lancet* 2002;360: 825–829.
21. Steg PG, Bonnefoy E, Chabaud S, et al. Impact of time to treatment on mortality after prehospital fibrinolysis or primary angioplasty: data from the CAPTIM randomized clinical trial *Circulation* 2003;103:2851–2856.
22. Terkelsen GJ, Lassen JF, Norgaard BL, et al. Reduction of treatment delay in patients with ST-elevation myocardial infarction: impact of prehospital diagnosis and direct referral to primary percutaneous coronary intervention. *Eur Heart J* 2005;26:770–777.
23. Montalescot G, Borentain M, Payot L, et al. Early vs late administration of glycoprotein IIb/IIIa inhibitors in primary percutaneous coronary intervention of acute ST-segment elevation myocardial infarction: a meta-analysis. *JAMA* 2004;292:362–366.

CHAPTER 3 ■ REGIONAL TRANSFER PROGRAMS FOR PRIMARY PERCUTANEOUS CORONARY INTERVENTION

DAVID M. LARSON AND TIMOTHY D. HENRY

TRANSFER FOR PRIMARY PCI TRIALS
IS TRANSFER FOR PRIMARY PCI FEASIBLE IN THE
 UNITED STATES?
ORGANIZING A SYSTEM FOR INTER-HOSPITAL
 TRANSFER
KEY COMPONENTS
Standardized Protocol
Empower the ED Physician
Individualize Transfer Agreements
Direct Admission to the Cardiac Catheterization Laboratory
Education/Training
Feedback and Quality Improvement
CHALLENGES TO IMPLEMENTING A REGIONAL
 TRANSFER PROGRAM
RESULTS OF A REGIONAL TRANSFER PROGRAM
CONCLUSIONS

Primary percutaneous coronary intervention (PCI) is the preferred reperfusion strategy in patients with ST-elevation myocardial infarction (STEMI) who present to hospitals with cardiac catheterization labs (1,2). Availability is the major limitation to widespread adoption of this strategy because 25% of hospitals in the United States have the ability to perform primary PCI (3). Delays resulting from the transfer of STEMI patients may offset the expected benefits of primary PCI in mortality and morbidity (4). One approach to expand the availability of primary PCI is the use of prehospital electrocardiogram (EKG) for early diagnosis of STEMI and to then bypass non-PCI hospitals (2). However, 50% of STEMI patients in the United States do not present by ambulance and would require ad hoc interhospital transfer to benefit from primary PCI (5). In rural communities, this strategy would result in long transfer times prior to the initial medical assessment, definitive diagnosis, and use of adjunctive medications. Therefore, an alternative approach is to transfer STEMI patients who present at rural and community hospitals without PCI capability to PCI centers. Recent data suggest an organized, integrated regional transfer system can expand the potential benefits of primary PCI to a large segment of the population (6).

TRANSFER FOR PRIMARY PCI TRIALS

Several European trials have demonstrated that transfer of STEMI patients from community hospitals for primary PCI is safe and effective. The first of these was the Primary Angioplasty After Transport of Patients from General Community Hospitals to Catheterization Units With/Without Thrombolysis Infusion (PRAGUE-1) study (7). In this trial, patients with STEMI from the Czech Republic were randomized to one of three groups. Patients in Group A received intravenous streptokinase (SK) and were admitted to the community hospital; Group B patients received SK and were transferred immediately for primary PCI; and Group C patients were transferred to the PCI center without fibrinolytics for primary PCI. The combined primary endpoint of death/reinfarction/stroke at 30 days was 23% in Group A, 15% in Group B, and 8% in Group C (P <0.02). There were no deaths during transfer, and the average door-to-balloon time from the community hospital in Group C was 95 minutes.

Subsequently a larger, multicenter, nationwide trial (PRAGUE-2) randomized 850 STEMI patients presenting to community hospitals without cardiac catheterization laboratory to SK versus immediate transfer for primary PCI (8). The primary endpoint was 30-day mortality, and the maximum transfer distance was 120 km. There was a trend toward reduction in mortality in the transfer group based on intent to treat (6.8% vs. 10.0%; $P = 0.12$). However, the mortality difference in the 360 patients who actually underwent primary PCI was 6.0% versus 10.4% in those who received fibrinolysis (P <0.05). Subgroup analysis demonstrated that those patients randomized <3 hours from symptom onset had no difference in mortality, and those patients randomized at >3 hours had a significant reduction in mortality favoring transfer for primary PCI (6.0% vs. 15.3%; P <0.02) (8).

A French multicenter study (CAPTIM) utilizing mobile emergency care units (SAMU) staffed by physicians randomized 840 STEMI patients to prehospital fibrinolysis with accelerated alteplase versus primary PCI (9). All patients were transferred immediately to PCI centers. The primary endpoint, the composite of death, nonfatal reinfarction, and nonfatal disabling stroke at 30 days was 6.2% in the primary PCI group versus 8.2% in the prehospital fibrinolysis group ($P = 0.29$). Mortality rates were not different in the two groups, but there was a trend toward increased stroke and nonfatal recurrent infarction in the fibrinolysis group. Rescue PCI was performed in 26% of the prehospital fibrinolysis patients. The median time from randomization to treatment was 27 minutes for fibrinolysis versus 82 minutes for primary PCI. At 1 year the composite endpoint was 16.4% for prehospital fibrinolysis versus 14% for primary PCI (P = NS); however, the overall costs were less for the primary PCI group both during the in-hospital period and at 1-year follow-up due to a high rate of subsequent revascularization in the fibrinolysis group (10).

The largest transfer for primary PCI trial, the Danish Multicenter Randomized Trial on Thrombolytic Therapy Versus Acute Coronary Angioplasty in Myocardial Infarction (DANAMI-2), randomized 1,572 STEMI patients presenting to both PCI centers and community hospitals to front-loaded alteplase versus primary PCI (11). The primary endpoint was the composite of death, reinfarction, or disabling stroke at 30 days. Of the 1,129 patients randomized at the non-PCI hospitals, the primary endpoint was 8.5% in the transfer for primary PCI group and 14.2% in the fibrinolysis group ($P = 0.002$). There was no significant difference in mortality (6.6% in the primary PCI group vs. 7.8% in the fibrinolysis group; $P = 0.35$) or stroke (1.1% vs. 2.0%; $P = 0.15$); however, there was a significant reduction in the rate of reinfarction (1.6% vs. 6.3%; $P < 0.001$). In the patients who were transferred for primary PCI (distance, 3–150 km), the median time from arrival at the community hospital to transfer was 50 minutes, transport time 32 minutes, and arrival at PCI center to balloon was 26 minutes. There were no deaths during transfer, but eight patients had ventricular fibrillation requiring cardioversion.

The Air Primary Angioplasty in Myocardial Infarction (Air-PAMI) Study was a predominantly U.S. trial that randomized high-risk STEMI patients to transfer for primary PCI versus on-site fibrinolysis (12). Difficulties in recruitment resulted in termination of the study after only 138 patients (32% of anticipated sample size) were randomized. The primary endpoint of major adverse cardiac events was 8.4% in the primary PCI group versus 13.6% in the fibrinolysis group. Because of the small sample size, this did not reach statistical significance ($P = 0.331$). Compared with the European trials, the Air-PAMI trials had greater delays in time to treatment (arrival at the community hospital to balloon inflation at PCI hospital was 155 min).

Each of the aforementioned trials was included in a recent meta-analysis of six trials (3,750 patients) comparing transfer for PCI versus fibrinolysis (13). The combined endpoint of death/reinfarction/stroke at 30 days was reduced by 42% (95% CI, 29% to 53%, $P < 0.001$) favoring transfer for primary PCI. There was also a trend toward reduction of all cause mortality by 19% (95% CI, −3% to 36%; $P = 0.08$) (Fig. 3-1A,B). If the CAPTIM trial (actually prehospital fibrinolysis with a high rate of rescue PCI) is excluded from this meta-analysis, the mortality benefit for transfer for primary PCI is also significant.

TABLE 3-1

30–30–30 GOAL

In-door-out-door at community hospital

Prehospital EKG and notification
Institution-specific STEMI protocol
STEMI team: emergency MD, RNs, lab, radiology
STEMI kit with laboratory supplies, transfer forms, adjunctive medications
One call to activate STEMI transfer protocol (see Fig. 3.3)
Dispatch transport team immediately

Transport time

Highest priority for transfer (same as trauma)
Rapid turnaround times (<10 minutes)
Air: hot loads
Ground: same crew, evaluation on gurney
Prearranged transfer agreements—no delays due to Emergency Medical Transport and Active Labor Act (EMTALA) restrictions
Community specific transfer plan

Door-to-balloon time at the PCI hospital

Cardiac catheterization laboratory team activated while the patient is en route
Direct admission to cardiac catheterization laboratory: bypass ED and ICU/CCU
Preregistration based on demographic information from community hospital
Clinical and laboratory data faxed directly to cardiac catheterization laboratory from community hospital

IS TRANSFER FOR PRIMARY PCI FEASIBLE IN THE UNITED STATES?

Transfer delays beyond 60 to 90 minutes may negate the benefit of primary PCI over fibrinolysis (14). As noted earlier,

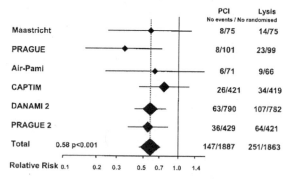

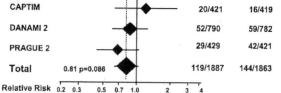

FIGURE 3-1. (A) Relative risk for the composite of death/reinfarction/stroke with thrombolysis and transfer for primary PCI in individual trials and the combined analysis (used by permission). (B) Relative risks for death with thrombolysis and transfer for primary PCI in individual trials and the combined analysis.

total door-to-balloon times in the Air-PAMI trial were longer than the European trials. Recent data from the National Registry of Myocardial Infarction (NRMI) indicate the median door-to-balloon time is 180 minutes in patients who are transferred for primary PCI in the United States (15). In fact, door-to-balloon times were <90 minutes in only 4.2% of patients and <120 minutes in 16.2%. These results have led many to believe that transfer for primary PCI is not a realistic alternative in the United States.

Using the trauma system as a model, several U.S. centers have demonstrated that STEMI patients can be transferred from community hospitals to tertiary cardiac centers in a timely and efficient manner. The Level 1 Heart Attack program at the Minneapolis Heart Institute in Minnesota recently reported a median total door-to-balloon time of 97 minutes in 11 hospitals up to 70 miles (Zone 1) from the PCI center using a standardized protocol and integrated transfer system for primary PCI. The median total door-to-balloon time was 117 minutes using a facilitated PCI protocol in 17 hospitals up to 210 miles (Zone 2) from the PCI center (16).

ORGANIZING A SYSTEM FOR INTERHOSPITAL TRANSFER

An organized, integrated system is needed to achieve the recommended door-to-balloon times for STEMI patients who are transferred for primary PCI. This system involves collaboration between cardiologists, emergency medicine, nursing, prehospital, and other ancillary medical personnel. Key components for organizing a regional system will be discussed in the next section.

When deciding which referral hospitals within a region are capable of transferring patients for primary PCI (door-to-balloon times of <90 minutes) consider the "30–30–30 goal" (Table 3-1):

> 30-minute in-door–out-door time at the referral hospital
> 30-minute interhospital transport time
> 30-minute door-to-balloon time at the PCI center

Hospitals that are not within the reach of these time goals should consider alternative strategies such as transfer for facilitated PCI with reduced-dose fibrinolytic or liberal use of rescue PCI after full-dose fibrinolysis.

KEY COMPONENTS

Standardized Protocol

A major step in development of a regional transfer program is the use of a standardized protocol for STEMI that is agreed on by all the cardiologists, emergency department (ED) physicians, and primary care physicians within the sys-

---

LEVEL 1 MI PROTOCOL

Criteria: ST Elevation Myocardial Infarction or new LBBB

Onset of symptoms less than 12 hours

- Activate team: Emergency MD and RNs, Lab, Radiology
- Dispatch transport team (Helicopter or Ground ALS)*
- Contact Minneapolis Heart Institute (One phone call to activate)
- Monitor, oxygen, IV and draw routine labs
- Aspirin 325 mg PO (4x81 mg chewable)
- Clopidogrel 600 mg PO (8x75 mg)
- Nitroglycerin 0.4 mg SL (repeat as needed or IV drip)
- Heparin loading dose 60u/kg (max 4000u), followed by continuous infusion 12u/kg/hr

  (max 1000u/hr)*
- Beta blocker: Metoprolol 5 mg IV q 5 minutes x 3 (unless contraindications)
- Morphine sulfate as needed for pain
- Chest x-ray: Portable
- Second IV (saline lock)
- Attach hands free defibrillation pads
- Consider anxiolytic for transport
- Transfer: In door-out door time goal less than 30 minutes

---

* Consider fibrinolytic if anticipated delay in transfer

FIGURE 3-2. Level 1 MI Protocol for a Zone 1 (within 70 miles) community hospital.

tem. Delays occur when the ED physician has to discuss the reperfusion strategy or which antithrombotic or antiplatelet regimen will be used with the on-call cardiologist. Each hospital should have a written, institution-specific critical pathway for STEMI that includes appropriate lab studies, initial diagnostic studies, and adjunctive medications, such as antiplatelet and antithrombin regimens, beta-blockers, nitrates, and pain control medications. Key details of the critical pathway should be available in checklists and standing orders in the ED. Tools such as laminated cards or posters with details of the standardized protocol are helpful (see sample protocol, Fig. 3-2).

Empower the ED Physician

The American College of Cardiology/American Heart Association (ACC/AHA) guidelines recommend that the ED physi-cian be responsible for making the initial diagnosis and treatment decision. The ED physician should be able to activate the transfer protocol with a single phone call leading to a group page (Fig. 3-3). This single phone call should mobilize the entire system, including the interventional cardiologist and cardiac catheterization laboratory staff, to be available within 30 minutes. Nondiagnostic EKGs or diagnostic dilemmas can be discussed with the cardiologist, but should be the exception not the rule.

Individualize Transfer Agreements

Each community hospital will have unique transfer issues based on distance and availability of air or ground ambu-lance. Therefore, individualized plans for transfer should be developed for each community hospital including prearranged transfer agreements with local ambulance or helicopter companies. Helicopter transport services need to be instructed to use a trauma transfer approach that includes 10-minute turnaround times and "hot loads" (keeping the rotors running).

Direct Admission to the Cardiac Catheterization Laboratory

Because the initial evaluation has been performed at the community hospital, the patient should be taken directly to the cardiac catheterization laboratory and not reevaluated in the ED or intensive care unit/coronary care unit (ICU/CCU). Patients can be preadmitted based on the initial demographic data from the community hospital. Key clinical and laboratory data collected at the community hospital along with the EKG should be faxed directly to the cardiac catheterization laboratory while the patient is being transferred (Fig. 3-4).

Education/Training

Education is an essential component of a successful transfer program. This includes education and training of the transport personnel, nursing and ancillary staff with the community and PCI hospital (ED, CCU, and cardiac catheterization laboratory), and primary care and ED physicians regarding EKG diagnosis and details of the critical pathway to facilitate

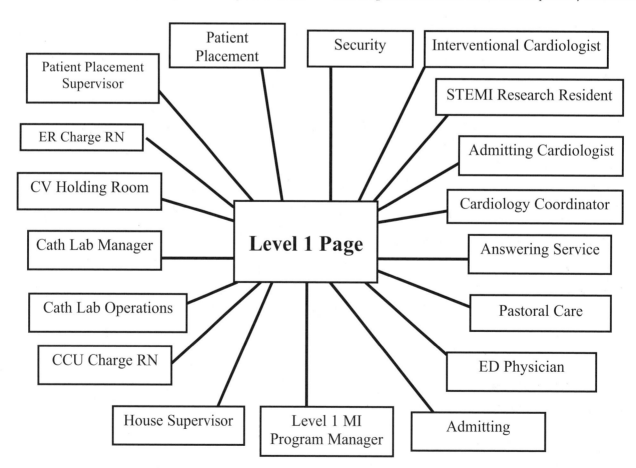

FIGURE 3-3. Team at Abbott Northwestern Hospital that is included in the group page to activate catheterization lab.

grand itasca
CLINIC & HOSPITAL

| Patient Name |
| Soc Sec # |
| DOB   Gender   M   F |
| Admit Date |

Level 1 Heart Attack Data Sheet
* = required information

Onset chest pain (Time)		*	ED arrival time		*	EKG time		*
Means of transport to ED*	Self/family		Ambulance					
Call to MCA (Time)		Receiving Cardiologist						
Call to transfer team		Mode	Ground ALS	Helicopter		Transfer team arrival		
Out-the-door time		Arrival time (to ANW)			Admit to:	CV Lab	ED	CCU

Presenting Clinical Data (ED Physician to complete)

ECG changes	Inferior (II, III, AVF)		Anterior (V1-V4)		Lateral (I, AVL, V5-V6)		Posterior	New LBBB
Pt Age		BP		HR		Rhythm		
History of CAD?	Yes	No	Previous PCI		Previous MI	Previous CABG		Date
Past Med Hx						Contraindication to lytics?		Yes No
Cardiac Risk Factors	HTN	Yes No	Diabetes	Yes No	Smoking	Current Recent Former Never		
Family Hx CAD	Yes No	Dyslipidemia	Yes No		Allergies			
Clinical signs of CHF?	Yes No	Rales	S3 gallop	Murmur	Killip Class	1 2 3 4		
Patient Weight		Patient Height		Allergy to IV Contrast	Yes	No		

Lab data (Fax copies of lab results) * = essential labs

Hgb *		Na		Glucose		PTT	
WBC		K *		Troponin I		INR	
Platelets *		Cr *		CK-MB		Serum HCG if child bearing age (12-50)	
Chest Xray							

Treatment (Nurse to complete)

Medications	Dose	Time	Administered by:
☐ Give the following SIX medications unless contraindicated:			
☐ Check allergies			
1. Aspirin (check with patient if already taken today)	324 mg (four, 81 mg chewable tabs)		
2. Clopidogrel (Plavix)	600 mg (eight, 75 mg tabs)		
3. ½ Dose TNKase IVP (Calculate full dose based on weight and give ½)			
4. Heparin (loading dose) 60 units/kg. (Max 4000 units)			
5. Heparin (Infusion) 12 units/kg. (Max of 1000 units/hr)			
6. Lopressor 5 mg every 5 minutes X 3 (Hold if systolic BP < 95 or pulse < 60)			
Administer as needed for pain:			
1. Nitroglycerin 0.4 mg SL, 1 tab every 15 minutes or..			
2. Nitroglycerin start @ 10 mcg and adjust PRN chest pain maintaining S.B.P greater than ____			
3. Morphine Sulfate			

ED Physician			Primary MD	
ED Phone	1218-326-7501	ED Fax	1-218-326-7780	General Phone	1-218-326-3401

Cath Lab Data (To be completed by ANW)

Arrive (Time)		Culprit Artery	LAD LCx RCA LM Graft Unknown
Procedure start		Culprit TIMI Flow	0 1 2 3
Balloon inflation (1st)		Post procedure TIMI Flow	0 1 2 3

When essential labs (noted with a *) are complete, please fax this sheet along with EKG to: <u>CV lab fax # 612-863-6292</u>

C:\WINNT\Profiles\A034226\Local Settings\Temporary Internet Files\OLK34\GR data.doc

FIGURE 3-4. Level 1 data sheet from a Zone 2 (within 70 to 210 miles) community hospital that is faxed to the catheterization lab.

rapid diagnosis and initial stabilization prior to transfer. This training should be facilitated by cardiovascular staff from the PCI hospital. Teamwork at the community and PCI hospitals is essential to achieve the goal of 30–30–30 times. Finally, local community education appears to decrease the time of symptom onset to arrival at the community hospital.

Feedback and Quality Improvement

After a patient is transferred, it is essential that the community hospital physician receive feedback from the PCI hospital. This includes the ED physician and nursing staff and primary care physicians. Communication fosters a sense of teamwork, and the immediate clinical and angiographic correlation will sharpen the diagnostic skills of the ED physician. We have adopted a system in which the interventionalcardiologist calls the ED physician following the procedure, the attending cardiologist calls the primary care physician, and the Level 1 MI nurse coordinator calls the community ED nursing staff. Cumulative data is provided quarterly to each community hospital. A STEMI database is helpful to follow trends in time to treatment, protocol compliance, and clinical outcomes. This data can be used for continuous quality improvement activities, as well as to meet JCAHO requirements. A sample database has been previously published (6).

CHALLENGES TO IMPLEMENTING A REGIONAL TRANSFER PROGRAM

The NRMI 3/4 median door-to-balloon time for patients transferred for primary PCI in the United States is unacceptably long at 180 minutes (15). Challenges to the development of a regional transfer program include the lack of an integrated system of health care, the lack of standardized treatment protocols, current reimbursement strategies, resource utilization issues in both the community and PCI hospitals, and the lack of an organized system for interfacility transfer (6). These challenges are real and will vary from hospital to hospital and from state to state, but the potential benefits of a successful transfer program should stimulate solutions to the problems.

RESULTS OF A REGIONAL TRANSFER PROGRAM

As noted earlier, the results of the Minneapolis Heart Institute's Level 1 myocardial infarction (MI) program demonstrate that an organized regional transfer program can be successful in decreasing the total door-to-balloon times. More important, these improvements in time to treatment were accompanied by improvements in outcomes with 30-day mortality of 4.3% in Zone 1 patients and 3.4% in Zone 2 patients. The overall length of stay was decreased to 3 days, and the number of "eligible but untreated" patients has been decreased substantially in the community hospitals. It is important to note that these results include all patients with ST elevation or new left bundle branch block with chest pain <24 hours after onset and therefore represent a very high risk patient population including 17% of patients >80 years old, 14% with cardiogenic shock, and 10% with cardiac arrest prior to the PCI. TIMI risk score ≥4 was present in 46% of the patients. The benefits of a regional transfer program clearly outweigh the challenges. There is increasing support for a national policy on treatment of STEMI patients similar to the U.S. trauma system, which will incorporate regional transfer protocols (17).

CONCLUSIONS

It has become increasing clear that primary PCI is the preferred reperfusion strategy if performed in a timely manner in high-volume centers. Transfer from community and rural hospitals to a PCI center can safely provide access to primary PCI to a wide segment of the U.S. population. Randomized trials using this strategy have demonstrated superiority to fibrinolytics if the transfer times are reasonable. Key components of the regional transfer program include standardized protocols, empowering the ED physician, a community-specific transfer plan, direct transfer to the cardiac catheterization laboratory, education, and quality improvement programs.

References

1. Keeley E, Boura J, Grines CL. Primary angioplasty versus intravenous thrombolytic therapy for acute myocardial infarction: a quantitative review of 23 randomized trials. *Lancet* 2003;361:13–20.
2. Antman EM, Anbe DT, Armstrong PW, et al. ACC/AHA guidelines for the management of patients with ST-elevation myocardial infarction—executive summary: a report of the American College of Cardiology/American Heart Association Task Force on Practice Guidelines (Writing Committee to Revise the 1999 Guidelines for the Management of Patients With Acute Myocardial Infarction). *Circulation* 2004;110:588–636.
3. Nallamothu BK, Bates ER, Wang Y, et al. Driving times and distances to hospitals with percutaneous coronary intervention in the United States: implications for prehospital triage of patients with ST-elevated myocardial infarction. *Circulation* 2006;113:1189–1195.
4. De Luca G, Suryapranata H, Ottervanger JP, et al. Time delay to treatment and mortality in primary angioplasty for acute myocardial infarction: every minute of delay counts. *Circulation* 2004;109:1223–1225.
5. Canto JG, Zalenski RJ, Ornato JP, et al. Use of emergency medical services in acute myocardial infarction and subsequent quality of care: observations from the National Registry of Myocardial Infarction 2. *Circulation* 2002; 106:3018–3023.
6. Henry TD, Unger BT, Sharkey SW, et al. Design of a standardized system for transfer of patients with ST-elevation myocardial infarction for percutaneous coronary intervention. *Am Heart J* 2005;150:373–384.
7. Widimsky P, Groch L, Zelizko M, et al. Multicentre randomized trial comparing transport to primary angioplasty vs immediate thrombolysis vs combined strategy for patients with acute myocardial infarction presenting to a community hospital without a catheterization laboratory. The PRAGUE study. *Eur Heart J* 2000;21:823–831.
8. Widimsky P, Budesinsky T, Vorac D, et al. Long distance transport for primary angioplasty vs immediate thrombolysis in acute myocardial infarction. Final results of the randomized national multicentre trial—PRAGUE-2. *Eur Heart J* 2003;24:94–104.
9. Bonnefoy E, Lapostolle F, Leizorovicz A, et al. Primary angioplasty versus prehospital fibrinolysis in acute myocardial infarction: a randomised study. *Lancet* 2002;360:825–829.
10. Machecourt J, Bonnefoy E, Vanzetto G, et al. Primary angioplasty is cost-minimizing compared with pre-hospital thrombolysis for patients within 60 min of a percutaneous coronary intervention center: the Comparison of Angioplasty and Pre-hospital Thrombolysis in Acute Myocardial Infarction (CAPTIM) cost-efficacy sub-study. *J Am Coll Cardiol* 2005;45:515–524.
11. Andersen HR, Nielsen TT, Rasmussen K, et al. A comparison of coronary angioplasty with fibrinolytic therapy in acute myocardial infarction. *N Engl J Med* 2003;349:733–742.
12. Grines CL, Westerhausen D, Weaver WD, et al. A randomized trial of transfer for primary angioplasty versus on-site thrombolysis in patients with high-risk myocardial infarction: the Air Primary Angioplasty in Myocardial Infarction study. *J Am Coll Cardiol* 2002;39:1713–1719.
13. Dalby M, Bouzamondo A, Lechat P, et al. Transfer for primary angioplasty versus immediate thrombolysis in acute myocardial infarction: a meta-analysis. *Circulation* 2003;108:1809–1814.
14. Nallamothu BK, Bates ER. Percutaneous coronary intervention versus fibrinolytic therapy in acute myocardial infarction: is timing (almost) everything? *Am J Cardiol* 2003;92:824–826.
15. Nallamothu BK, Bates ER, Herrin J, et al. Times to treatment in transfer patients undergoing primary percutaneous coronary intervention in the United States: National Registry of Myocardial Infarction (NRMI)-3/4 analysis. *Circulation* 2005;111:761–767.
16. Henry TD, Sharkey SW, Graham KJ, et al. Transfer for direct percutaneous coronary intervention for ST-elevation myocardial infarction: the Minneapolis Heart Institute Level 1 Myocardial Infarction Program. *Circulation* 2005;112:II-620.
17. Henry TD, Atkins JM, Cunningham MS, et al. ST elevation myocardial infarction: recommendations on triage of patients to cardiovascular centers of excellence. *J Am Coll Cardiol* 2006;47:1339–1345.

CHAPTER 4 ■ PUBLIC ACCESS DEFIBRILLATION

JOSEPH P. ORNATO

INTRODUCTION
THE IMPORTANCE OF TIME TO DEFIBRILLATION
EARLY DEFIBRILLATION BY PUBLIC SAFETY
   PERSONNEL
THE CONCEPT OF PUBLIC ACCESS DEFIBRILLATION
Early Defibrillation by Public Safety Personnel
Public Access Defibrillation by Laypersons
COST BENEFIT OF PUBLIC ACCESS DEFIBRILLATION
HOME DEFIBRILLATION
CONCLUSIONS

INTRODUCTION

Sudden out-of-hospital cardiac arrest (OOH-CA) results in the death of 400,000 to 460,000 Americans each year in the United States (1). Although the majority of these events occur in the home, up to 20% occur in public places (2). The majority of sudden, unexpected OOH-CA cases are caused by either ventricular fibrillation (VF) or ventricular tachycardia (VT) that degenerates rapidly to VF (3). Prompt defibrillation is a highly effective treatment if it can be delivered when the myocardium has not yet depleted its high-energy phosphate reserves. This early phase of cardiac arrest, which typically lasts only 3 to 4 minutes after cardiac arrest onset, is termed the "electrical phase" (4). Beyond this point, defibrillation may abolish the VF, but the heart is often unable to function adequately as a pump, resulting in either asystole or a pulseless electrical rhythm following defibrillation. This phase of resuscitation is termed the "circulatory phase" because a brief period of high-quality cardiopulmonary resuscitation (CPR) prior to attempting defibrillation may boost the heart's high-energy phosphates sufficiently to result in effective cardiac pumping activity post-defibrillation. Rescuers may be able to restore spontaneous circulation (ROSC) when there has been a very long delay (e.g., >8 minutes from onset of VF) until initiation of resuscitation, but the patient may suffer severe neurological impairment. This phase of resuscitation is termed the "metabolic phase," indicating that physical and/or pharmacological manipulation of cellular metabolism may be needed to mitigate long-term cellular impairment.

The purpose of this chapter is to review the current community approach to resuscitating OOH-CA patients using early defibrillation in the United States, with special focus on the use of automated external defibrillators (AEDs) by nonmedical personnel in public settings (i.e., "public access defibrillation" or "PAD").

THE IMPORTANCE OF TIME TO DEFIBRILLATION

The best outcomes from cardiac arrest because of VF in adults occur regularly in the electrophysiology laboratory, where prompt defibrillation (within 20 to 30 seconds) results in >99% survival (5). The next best reported outcomes are in cardiac rehabilitation programs, where defibrillation occurs typically in 1 to 2 minutes, and survival is approximately 85% to 90% (5). At Chicago's O'Hare and Midway airports, almost 70% of cardiac arrest patients whose initial rhythm is VF survive to hospital discharge (6). Survival from VF in Las Vegas casinos with victims treated by security officers equipped with AEDs varies from 75% when a shock is given in 3 minutes to 50% when a shock is given in 5 minutes (7). Outcomes in typical emergency medical service (EMS) systems that provide defibrillation in 8 to 8.5 minutes after patient collapse typically yield survival rates of about 16% (5). Thus, survival from cardiac arrest because of VF is highly dependent on the time interval from collapse to defibrillation. The chances for survival diminish by approximately 7% to 10% for every minute delay from the patient's collapse to defibrillation (5).

EARLY DEFIBRILLATION BY PUBLIC SAFETY PERSONNEL

The traditional community approach to optimizing survival from OOH-CA has been to train the public to recognize cardiac arrest, call 911, and perform CPR, while public safety personnel (fire or police first responders, emergency medical technicians (EMTs), and/or paramedics) rush to the scene to provide defibrillation and other advanced cardiac life support (ACLS) treatments. The American Heart Association (AHA) terms this sequence of events—early access, early CPR, early defibrillation, early ACLS—the "Chain of Survival" (5).

Early access to EMS is promoted by a 911 system currently available to more than 95% of the U.S. population. Enhanced 911 systems provide the caller's location to the dispatcher, which permits rapid dispatch of prehospital personnel to locations, even if the caller is not capable of verbalizing or the dispatcher cannot understand the location of the emergency. Such centers typically have intense quality-assurance programs to ensure that emergency medical dispatchers follow protocols and procedures correctly and consistently. This is particularly true for the prearrival instructions that are given to cardiac arrest bystanders to instruct them on how to perform CPR while awaiting arrival of emergency personnel (phone CPR).

Even though CPR performed by layperson bystanders improves the odds of neurologically intact survival from OOH-CA, only about 25% of bystanders in most U.S. cities are willing to perform CPR (a notable exception is Seattle, Washington, where 50% of layperson bystanders perform CPR) (8–12). Unwillingness of laypersons to perform mouth-to-mouth ventilation on strangers is a major part of the problem (13,14). Fortunately, increasing evidence suggests that chest compressions are much more important than artificial ventilation during the first 5 minutes after onset of OOH-CA in adults (12,15–18). Chest compressions alone cause changes in intrathoracic pressure that ventilate the victim adequately for the first 5 to 8 minutes after cardiac arrest. Chest compression-only CPR is being adopted for prearrival resuscitation instruction in many EMS systems.

To minimize time to treatment, most communities allow volunteer and/or paid firefighters and other first-aid providers to function as first responders, providing CPR and early defibrillation using AEDs until EMTs and paramedics arrive. Fire department personnel functioning as first responders are the backbone of the public safety primary response for most U.S. communities. Most of these personnel are trained either as first responders or basic EMTs.

Another approach has been to supplement the fire and EMS response with police officers who are trained and equipped to use AEDs. Such personnel can further enhance survival from out-of-hospital cardiac arrest compared to survival that can be achieved by conventional EMS services (7). White et al studied the outcome of all consecutive adult patients with nontraumatic cardiac arrest treated in Rochester, Minnesota, from November 1990 through July 1995. In that city, a centralized 911 center dispatched police and an ALS ambulance simultaneously for suspected cardiac arrest cases. The personnel who arrived first delivered the initial shock. Of 84 patients, 31 (37%) were shocked initially by police. Thirteen of the 31 demonstrated ROSC without need for ALS treatment. All 13 survived to discharge. The other 18 patients required ALS; 5 (27.7%) survived. Among the 53 patients first shocked by paramedics, 15 had ROSC after shocks only, and 14 survived. The other 38 needed ALS treatment; 9 survived. This study showed that a high discharge-to-home survival rate could be obtained when early defibrillation was provided by both police and paramedics. It is the rapidity of defibrillation that determines outcome, irrespective of who delivers the shock. When initial defibrillation attempts resulted in ROSC, the overwhelming majority of patients survived (96%). Even brief (e.g., 1 minute) decreases in the call-to-shock time interval increased the likelihood of ROSC from shocks only, with a consequent decrease in the need for further ALS intervention. Similar results have also been noted with the use of law enforcement early defibrillation in Miami-Dade County, Florida (19).

Most cities and larger suburban areas provide EMS ambulance services with providers from the fire department, a private ambulance company, and/or volunteers. The most common deployment pattern is a tiered system in which some of the ambulances are staffed and equipped at the basic EMT level (which includes first aid and early defibrillation with AEDs), and other units (either transporting or nontransporting) are staffed by paramedics or other intermediate-level EMTs (who can, in addition to basic care, start intravenous drips, intubate, and administer medications). In some systems, the advanced providers can also perform 12-lead ECGs, provide external pacing for symptomatic bradycardia, and perform other advanced techniques.

THE CONCEPT OF PUBLIC ACCESS DEFIBRILLATION

The concept of public access defibrillation emerged in 1990 from the AHA's Future of CPR Task Force led by Dr. Leonard

Cobb of Seattle, Washington. This group recognized that the majority of out-of-hospital cardiac arrests occur in the home. However, for those events occurring in a public place, they reasoned that the use of AEDs by laypersons could shave precious minutes off the time interval from collapse to defibrillation. Based on the Task Force's report, the AHA established an AED Task Force, led by Dr. Myron Weisfeldt.

The 1992 AHA Guidelines on Cardiopulmonary Resuscitation and Emergency Cardiac Care was the first to include the following statement regarding the PAD concept:

The placement of automated external defibrillators (AEDs) in the hands of large numbers of people trained in their use may be the key intervention to increase the survival chances of out-of-hospital cardiac arrest patients. . . . The widespread effectiveness and demonstrated safety of the AED have made it acceptable for nonprofessionals to effectively operate the device. Such persons must still be trained in CPR and use of defibrillators. In the near future, more creative use of AEDs by nonprofessionals may result in improved survival. . . . Participants in the national conference recommended that (a) AEDs be widely available for appropriately trained people, (b) all firefighting units that perform CPR and first aid be equipped with and trained to operate AEDs, (c) AEDs be placed in gathering places of more than 10,000 people, and (d) legislation be enacted to allow all EMS personnel to perform early defibrillation (20).

In 1994, the Task Force held its first PAD Conference in Washington, DC. At this landmark gathering, the conference participants affirmed the need for further research on the concept and encouraged the AHA to support additional discussion on the subject (21). The Task Force published an official AHA "Statement on Public Access Defibrillation" in 1995, declaring that

Early bystander cardiopulmonary resuscitation (CPR) and rapid defibrillation are the two major contributors to survival of adult victims of sudden cardiac arrest. The AHA supports efforts to provide prompt defibrillation to victims of cardiac arrest. Automatic external defibrillation is one of the most promising methods for achieving rapid defibrillation. In public access defibrillation, the technology of defibrillation and training in its use are accessible to the community. The AHA believes that this is the next step in strengthening the chain of survival. Public access defibrillation will involve considerable societal change and will succeed only through the strong efforts of the AHA and others with a commitment to improving emergency cardiac care.

Public access defibrillation will include (a) performance of defibrillation by laypersons at home and by firefighters, police, security personnel, and nonphysician care providers in the community, and (b) exploration of the use of bystander-initiated automatic external defibrillation in rural communities and congested urban areas where resuscitation strategies have had little success (22).

In 1996, the AHA worked with key members of the U.S. Congress to introduce legislation intended to remove legal barriers to implementation of early layperson defibrillation using AEDs. Termed the "Cardiac Arrest Survival Act," the bill underwent numerous modifications before it was finally passed into law in 2000.

The Second PAD Conference was held in 1997 in Crystal City, Virginia. This congress was truly international in scope and further defined the various "levels" of potential AED use in a community, the minimum training requirements, regulatory issues, likely cost versus benefit, and the need for a prospective, multicenter, randomized clinical trial. Four "levels" of PAD were identified at the 1997 AHA Conference:

Level 1: Traditional First-Responder Defibrillation
    This level includes defibrillation efforts by police, highway patrol personnel, and firefighter personnel. In many locations, firefighters are the first responders to cardiac emergencies, and yet they are often prohibited by regulations and state codes from providing early defibrillation.

Level 2: Nontraditional First-Responder Defibrillation
   This level includes defibrillation efforts by lifeguards, security personnel, and airline flight attendants.
Level 3: Citizen CPR Defibrillation
   This level refers to citizens and laypeople who have received AED training. These individuals are interested in providing emergency cardiac care, usually in the setting of a home in which a family member who is a high-risk patient resides.
Level 4: Minimally Trained Witness Defibrillation
   This level refers to individuals who happen to witness a cardiopulmonary emergency and have an AED available (for example, through a worksite defibrillation program). In general, this level occurs most commonly in the home or at a worksite where one group of people has been trained and other groups have not. The untrained witness wants to help out and assist, but she has not yet received formal AED training. Another example of this level is possible if AEDs become accessible in the so-called "fire-extinguisher mode," in which the AED location is displayed prominently and any witness to an emergency has access to these devices. At present, both Food and Drug Administration and state regulations permit physician prescription of AEDs to individual homes. This level will become more feasible with the introduction of newer technology that provides more voice prompts to the user, automatic 911 dialing, and possibly 911 dispatcher-assisted defibrillation (23).

Since this report was issued, numerous advances have been made in AED technology and training, and many of the previous regulatory barriers have been eliminated in the United States.

Early Defibrillation by Public Safety Personnel

One strategy for providing early defibrillation to a larger number of witnessed OOH-CA victims is to place AEDs in public places and to allow their use by nonmedical personnel. This concept, called public access defibrillation (PAD), has been shown to be safe and effective when used by trained public safety personnel who have a duty to respond to medical emergencies (e.g., airline flight attendants, airport personnel, and security officers in Las Vegas gaming casinos) (6,19,24–27).

Airline Flight Attendants

In 1988, 42 of 120 airline carriers who were members of the International Air Transport Association reported deaths during the preceding 8 years (28). A total of 577 in-flight deaths were recorded, for a reported average of 72 deaths per year. Deaths occurred at average rates of 0.31 per million passengers, 125 per billion passenger-kilometers, and 25.1 per million departures. The majority of those who died were men (66%, 382/577) and middle-aged (mean age, 53.8 years). Most of the individuals (77%, 399/515) reported no health problems prior to travel. Physicians aboard the aircraft offered medical assistance for 43% (247/577) of the deaths. More than half of the deaths (56%, 326/577) were related to cardiac problems. Sudden unexpected cardiac death was the cause of death in 63% (253/399) of the apparently healthy passengers and was the major cause of death during air travel.

Soon thereafter, Qantas Airlines began to install AEDs on their international aircraft and at major terminal buildings serving their fleet. Selected flight attendants were trained to use AEDs and to perform CPR. Supervision was provided by medical volunteers or remotely by airline physicians. During a 64-month period, AEDs were used on 109 occasions: 63 times for monitoring an acutely ill passenger and 46 times for cardiac arrest (29). Twenty-seven cardiac arrests occurred onboard aircraft, often unwitnessed (11/27), and they were usually associated with asystole or pulseless idioventricular

rhythm (21/27). In marked contrast, all 19 arrests that occurred in terminal buildings were witnessed, and VF was present initially in 17 (89%). Overall, defibrillation was successful initially in 21 of 23 cases (91%). Long-term survival from VF was achieved in 26% (2 of 6 in aircraft and 4 of 17 in terminals).

Other major airline carriers were somewhat slow to implement AED programs until there were a series of successful lawsuits against major U.S. carriers in the mid-1990s. AEDs are now found on virtually all larger commercial aircraft (26,29–31). American Airlines recently described their experience in which AEDs were attached to 200 patients (191 on the aircraft and 9 in the terminal), including 99 with documented loss of consciousness (26). Electrocardiographic data was available for 185 patients. A shock was advised in all 14 patients who had electrocardiographically documented VF, and no shock was advised in the remaining patients (sensitivity and specificity of the defibrillator in identifying ventricular fibrillation, 100%). The first shock successfully defibrillated the heart in 13 patients (defibrillation was withheld in one case at the family's request). The rate of survival to discharge from the hospital after shock with the AED was 40%. A total of 36 patients either died or were resuscitated after cardiac arrest. No complications arose from use of the AED as a monitor in conscious passengers.

Airport Personnel

In 1998, AEDs were installed throughout passenger terminals at O'Hare, Midway, and Meigs Field (now closed) airports, which together serve more than 100 million passengers per year. The use of defibrillators was promoted by public-service videos in waiting areas, pamphlets, and reports in the media. Over a 2-year period, 21 persons had nontraumatic cardiac arrest, 18 of whom had VF. In four patients with VF, defibrillators were neither nearby nor used within 5 minutes, and none of these patients survived. Three others remained in VF and eventually died, despite the rapid use of a defibrillator (<5 minutes). Eleven patients with VF were resuscitated successfully, including eight who regained consciousness before hospital admission. No shock was delivered in four cases of suspected cardiac arrest, and the device correctly indicated that the problem was not due to VF. The rescuers of 6 of the 11 successfully resuscitated patients had no training or experience in the use of automated defibrillators, although three had medical degrees. Ten of the 18 patients with VF were alive and neurologically intact at 1 year.

Security Officers in Las Vegas Gaming Casinos

In the mid-1990s, security officers were trained to use AEDs that were installed in 26 Las Vegas/Clark County gaming casinos. Between April 24, 1997, and October 31, 1999, the AEDs had been used on 105 individuals whose initial cardiac arrest rhythm was VF and whose collapse was witnessed. Survival to hospital discharge occurred in 56/105 cases (survival rate of 53%) (32). The collapse-to-first-shock time interval for the security officers using the AEDs was 4.4 + 2.9 minutes, whereas the collapse-to-arrival of traditional EMS responders was 9.8 + 4.3 minutes.

Public Access Defibrillation by Laypersons

Until recently, it was unknown whether trained volunteer laypersons without a duty to act could save more lives from OOH-CA by using an AED in addition to CPR. The PAD Trial was a large, prospective, randomized, controlled clinical trial designed to answer this question (33,34).

The PAD Trial compared the number of OOH-CA patients who survived to hospital discharge from community facilities with volunteer responders who were trained to (a) recognize the event, call 911, and perform CPR (CPR-only) versus (b) recognize the event, call 911, perform CPR, and provide early defibrillation with an on-site AED (CPR + AED) (33). The study was conducted in 21 U.S. and 3 Canadian cities. The sites chosen for inclusion had to provide a pool of potential volunteer responders and the ability to institute an emergency response plan capable of delivering an AED to the victim within 3 minutes. Potential sites that already had on-site personnel with a duty to respond to medical emergencies (e.g., law enforcement officers, firefighters, nurses, and physicians) and facilities with previous AED programs were excluded from participation.

Sites were randomized as a "community unit" if they had an expectation of at least one OOH-CA over the study period (the equivalent of ≥250 adults over age 50 for 16 hours a day, or a history of ≥1 witnessed OOH-CA in 2 years, on average). Eligible units were required to have clearly defined geographic boundaries and a typical EMS response time to defibrillation of 3 to 15 minutes. The primary patient study population consisted of individuals age >8 years with OOH-CA of cardiac etiology. Patients with OOH-CA due to trauma, drug overdose, or noncardiac causes of arrest were excluded from the primary comparison, but not from safety evaluation.

Volunteer layperson rescuers without a responsibility to provide medical assistance were trained to competency and retrained periodically following current AHA guidelines or equivalent. The study randomized 993 community units with an average data collection period of 22 ± 5.5 (SD) months. The majority of study units (84%) were in public locations, most of which were recreational facilities and shopping centers. Approximately twice as many OOH-CA victims, 31 versus 16, survived to hospital discharge in the CPR-AED versus CPR-only subgroups ($P = 0.03$) (34). Adverse events were rare and consisted mostly of transient psychological trauma to volunteers and stolen AEDs. No inappropriate shocks were given.

Although the PAD Trial demonstrated that trained volunteer use of AEDs is safe and effective when initiated in public locations with at least a moderate likelihood of having a witnessed OOH-CA (one per 7 years), the actual impact of widespread public AED implementation on survival from OOH-CA in similar locations is likely to be modest because the vast majority (79% to 84%) of OOH-CA cases occur in the home rather than a public place (2,35). For example, using the PAD Trial estimate that widespread implementation of public AED programs doubles survival, only 2,000 to 4,000 additional lives would be saved from the 400,000 to 460,000 OOH-CA cases in the United States each year. Although this is a significant step forward, additional measures are needed to affect the survival of individuals who arrest at home.

COST BENEFIT OF PUBLIC ACCESS DEFIBRILLATION

The true cost benefit of PAD is unclear, although preliminary analyses suggest that it may be reasonable. Nichol et al (36) used a decision model to compare the potential cost-effectiveness of standard EMS systems with that of EMS supplemented by PAD. They considered defibrillation by both lay responders and police, using an analysis with a U.S. health care perspective. Input data were derived from published data or fiscal databases. Monte Carlo simulation was performed to estimate the variability in the costs and effects of each program.

A standard EMS system yielded a median cost of $5,900 per cardiac arrest patient and a median of 0.25 quality-adjusted life years. PAD by lay responders generated a median incremental cost of $44,000 per additional quality-adjusted life year.

PAD by police was associated with a median incremental cost of $27,200 per additional quality-adjusted life year. The authors concluded that the PAD strategy may be economically viable, even though it is somewhat more expensive than standard EMS costs for treating OOH-CA victims. The effectiveness and cost-effectiveness of PAD should be assessed in a randomized, controlled trial. Although results have not yet been reported, investigators have recently described the method they will be using to estimate the cost benefit of this strategy based on the PAD Trial experience (37).

HOME DEFIBRILLATION

Clinical experience with the home use of AEDs by laypersons dates back to the late 1980s, when Dr. Mickey Eisenberg and his colleagues trained family members of 59 patients who had survived out-of-hospital cardiac arrest in King County, Washington, to use AEDs (38). Ninety-seven survivors of out-of-hospital VF were enrolled in the study; 59 patients received AEDs, and 38 patients were controls. During the study period, seven deaths occurred in the hospital without preceding out-of-hospital cardiac arrest or from noncardiac causes. There were 14 out-of-hospital cardiac arrests, 10 in the AED group and 4 in the control group. There was only one long-term survivor, who was actually in the control group. In the AED group, among the 10 cardiac arrests for which the device was available, it was applied to only 6 patients. Only 2 of these patients were in VF; 1 was resuscitated with residual neurological deficits and survived several months.

These study results suggested that there might be only a small potential for in-home layperson use of AEDs to save high-risk patients. However, the specific devices used in the project were early generation AED technology and not engineered for optimal layperson application based on today's standards. In contrast, Swenson et al (39) reported three successful resuscitations out of five cardiac arrests in 48 patients whose families had been trained to use an AED.

Dr. Gust Bardy is currently leading a National Institutes of Health-sponsored prospective, randomized, home AED trial (the "HAT trial") to determine whether a family member can save more victims of OOH-CA in the home when they have an AED in the house. Each study home contains survivors of anterior wall myocardial infarction who are not candidates for (or who have not consented to receive) an implantable defibrillator. Each home must have at least one other resident who is given a videotape containing instructions on CPR with (experimental group) or without (control group) AED instruction. Only experimental households are provided with a home AED. Results of this study are expected to provide guidance on whether home AED use can provide significant public health benefit.

CONCLUSIONS

OOH-CA claims the lives of almost a half million victims in the United States each year. In public locations, implementing an organized emergency response plan and training and equipping volunteers to provide early defibrillation using an AED can double the number of survivors to hospital discharge. The PAD Trial supports the concept that trained volunteers can use AEDs safely and effectively in a variety of public locations. The real challenge is whether similar results can be achieved by placing AEDs in the home setting, where the majority of OOH-CA incidents occur. The HAT trial is being conducted to determine the value, safety, and cost-effectiveness of AEDs in the home.

References

1. Centers for Disease Control and Prevention (CDC). State-specific mortality from sudden cardiac death—United States, 1999. *MMWR* 2002;51(6):123–126.
2. Becker L, Eisenberg M, Fahrenbruch C, et al. Public locations of cardiac arrest. Implications for public access defibrillation. *Circulation* 1998;97(21):2106–2109.
3. Bayes de Luna A, Coumel P, Leclercq JF. Ambulatory sudden cardiac death: mechanisms of production of fatal arrhythmia on the basis of data from 157 cases. *Am Heart J* 1989;117:151–159.
4. Weisfeldt ML, Becker LB. Resuscitation after cardiac arrest: a 3-phase time-sensitive model. *JAMA* 2002;288(23):3035–3058.
5. Cummins RO, Ornato JP, Thies WH, et al. Improving survival from sudden cardiac arrest: the "chain of survival" concept. A statement for health professionals from the Advanced Cardiac Life Support Subcommittee and the Emergency Cardiac Care Committee, American Heart Association. *Circulation* 1991;83(5):1832–1847.
6. Caffrey SL, Willoughby PJ, Pepe PE, et al. Public use of automated external defibrillators. *N Engl J Med* 2002;347(16):1242–1247.
7. White RD, Asplin BR, Bugliosi TF, et al. High discharge survival rate after out-of-hospital ventricular fibrillation with rapid defibrillation by police and paramedics. *Ann Emerg Med* 1996;28(5):480–485.
8. Cummins RO, Eisenberg MS, Hallstrom AP, et al. Survival of out-of-hospital cardiac arrest with early initiation of cardiopulmonary resuscitation. *Am J Emerg Med* 1985;3(2):114–119.
9. Eisenberg MS, Hallstrom AP, Carter WB, et al. Emergency CPR instruction via telephone. *Am J Public Health* 1985;75(1):47–50.
10. Kellermann AL, Hackman BB, Somes G. Dispatcher-assisted cardiopulmonary resuscitation. Validation of efficacy. *Circulation* 1989;80(5):1231–1239.
11. Valenzuela TD, Spaite DW, Meislin HW, et al. Emergency vehicle intervals versus collapse to CPR and collapse to defibrillation intervals: monitoring emergency medical services system performance in sudden cardiac arrest. *Ann Emerg Med* 1993;22(11):1678–1683.
12. Van Hoeyweghen RJ, Bossaert LL, Mullie A, et al. Quality and efficiency of bystander CPR. Belgian Cerebral Resuscitation Study Group. *Resuscitation* 1993;26(1):47–52.
13. Ornato JP. Should bystanders perform mouth-to-mouth ventilation during resuscitation? *Chest* 1994;106(6):1641–1642.
14. Ornato JP, Hallagan LF, McMahon SB, et al. Attitudes of BCLS instructors about mouth-to-mouth resuscitation during the AIDS epidemic. 1990(19):151–156.
15. Wik L, Kramer-Johansen J, Myklebust H, et al. Quality of cardiopulmonary resuscitation during out-of-hospital cardiac arrest. *JAMA* 2005;293(3):299–304.
16. Kern KB, Hilwig RW, Berg RA, et al. Importance of continuous chest compressions during cardiopulmonary resuscitation: improved outcome during a simulated single lay-rescuer scenario. *Circulation* 2002;105(5):645–9.
17. Hallstrom A, Cobb L, Johnson E, et al. Cardiopulmonary resuscitation by chest compression alone or with mouth-to-mouth ventilation. *N Engl J Med* 2000;342(21):1546–1553.
18. Berg RA, Kern KB, Sanders AB, et al. Bystander cardiopulmonary resuscitation. Is ventilation necessary? *Circulation* 1993;88(4 Pt 1):1907–1915.
19. Myerburg RJ, Fenster J, Velez M, et al. Impact of community-wide police car deployment of automated external defibrillators on survival from out-of-hospital cardiac arrest. *Circulation* 2002;106(9):1058–1064.
20. American Heart Association Emergency Cardiac Care Committee. Guidelines for cardiopulmonary resuscitation (CPR) and emergency cardiac care (ECC). *JAMA* 1992; 268: 2171–2295.
21. Weisfeldt ML, Kerber RE, McGoldrick RP, et al. American Heart Association Report on the Public Access Defibrillation Conference December 8–10, 1994. *Circulation* 1995;92:2740–2747.
22. Weisfeldt ML, Kerber RE, McGoldrick RP, et al. Public access defibrillation: a statement for healthcare professionals from the American Heart Association Task Force on Automatic External Defibrillation. *Circulation* 1995;92:2763.
23. Nichol G, Hallstrom AP, Kerber R, et al. American Heart Association Report on the Second Public Access Defibrillation Conference, April 17–19, 1997. *Circulation* 1998;97(13):1309–1314.
24. White RD, Hankins DG, Bugliosi TF. Seven years' experience with early defibrillation by police and paramedics in an emergency medical services system. *Resuscitation* 1998;39(3):145–151.
25. Mosesso VN, Jr., Davis EA, Auble TE, et al. Use of automated external defibrillators by police officers for treatment of out-of-hospital cardiac arrest. *Ann Emerg Med* 1998;32(2):200–207.
26. Page RL, Joglar JA, Kowal RC, et al. Use of automated external defibrillators by a U.S. airline. *N Engl J Med* 2000;343(17):1210–1216.
27. Valenzuela TD, Roe DJ, Nichol G, et al. Outcomes of rapid defibrillation by security officers after cardiac arrest in casinos. *N Engl J Med* 2000;343(17):1206–1209.
28. Cummins RO, Chapman PJ, Chamberlain DA, et al. In-flight deaths during commercial air travel. How big is the problem? *JAMA* 1988;259(13):1983–1988.
29. O'Rourke MF, Donaldson E, Geddes JS. An airline cardiac arrest program. *Circulation* 1997;96(9):2849–2853.
30. Donaldson E, Pearn J. First aid in the air. *Aust New Zealand J Surg* 1996;66(7):431–434.
31. Glazer I. Airline use of automatic external defibrillator: shocking developments. *Aviat Space Environ Med* 2000;71(5):556.
32. Valenzuela TD, Roe DJ, Nichol G, et al. Outcomes of rapid defibrillation by security officers after cardiac arrest in casinos. *N Engl J Med* 2000;343(17):1206–1209.
33. Ornato JP, McBurnie MA, Nichol G, et al. The Public Access Defibrillation (PAD) trial: study design and rationale. *Resuscitation* 2003;56(2):135–47.
34. Hallstrom AP, Ornato JP, Weisfeldt M, et al. Public-access defibrillation and survival after out-of-hospital cardiac arrest. *N Engl J Med* 2004;351(7):637–646.
35. Pell JP, Sirel JM, Marsden AK, et al. Potential impact of public access defibrillators on survival after out of hospital cardiopulmonary arrest: retrospective cohort study. *BMJ* 2002;325(7363):515.
36. Nichol G, Hallstrom AP, Ornato JP, et al. Potential cost-effectiveness of public access defibrillation in the United States. *Circulation* 1998;97(13):1315–1320.
37. Nichol G, Wells GA, Kuntz K, et al. Methodological design for economic evaluation in Public Access Defibrillation (PAD) trial. *Am Heart J* 2005;150(2):202–208.
38. Eisenberg MS, Moore J, Cummins RO, et al. Use of the automatic external defibrillator in homes of survivors of out-of-hospital ventricular fibrillation. *Am J Cardiol* 1989;63(7):443–436.
39. Swenson RD, Hill DL, Martin JS, et al. Automatic external defibrillators used by family members to treat cardiac arrest. *Circulation* 1987;76(suppl IV):IV-463.

PART II ■ CRITICAL PATHWAYS IN THE EMERGENCY DEPARTMENT

CHAPTER 5 ■ NON-ST ELEVATION ACS IN THE EMERGENCY DEPARTMENT

RICHARD J. RYAN, CHRISTOPHER P. CANNON, AND W. BRIAN GIBLER

Why do we need a pathway for patients presenting to the emergency department (ED) with chest pain? Emergency physicians (EPs) encounter this chief complaint on a daily or hourly basis and thus the workup, diagnosis, and treatment should be "routine." But it is not. For EPs and cardiologists alike, these patients represent an enormous challenge to accurately diagnose and appropriately treat. In particular, the ability to risk stratify non-ST-segment elevation myocardial infarction (NSTEMI) patients and initiate appropriate therapy is particularly difficult.

In the United States each year, approximately 5.3 million patients present to EDs with chest discomfort and related symptoms. Ultimately, nearly 1.4 million individuals are hospitalized for unstable angina (UA) and NSTEMI (1,2).

The 2002 American College of Cardiology/American Heart Association (ACC/AHA) UA/NSTEMI guidelines represent an evidence-based approach to the care of patients with ACS (3,4). From these guidelines a clinical pathway can be developed for the ED setting. A clinical pathway for NSTEMI initiated in the ED will allow EPs to standardize the diagnosis and treatment of patients with NSTEMI across the United States. Several summaries of the guidelines emphasizing emergency care have been published (5,6). Despite the 2002 guidelines and the recent 2005 AHA scientific statement on NSTEMI (7,8) adoption of these guidelines into routine emergency practice remains variable (9). The purpose of a clinical pathway for NSTEMI is to provide the EP and cardiologist at any hospital with a practical approach to treating patients with this condition. Basing medical therapy on a well-established clinical pathway will also allow for clinical quality improvement and real-time feedback to the entire hospital health care team.

The EP treating patients that arrive with chest pain must be able to succinctly incorporate the diagnostic elements such as electrocardiography and cardiac biomarker testing, as well as treatment regimens including nitrates, morphine, beta-blockers, calcium channel blockers, angiotensin-converting enzyme inhibitors (ACEIs), antiplatelet agents, and antithrombin drugs for acute coronary syndrome (ACS) for the care of the individual patient. After this, the EP must risk stratify these patients. Those patients with the highest risk can then be identified for guideline-directed pharmacological therapy and early invasive therapy for revascularization. A clinical pathway for NSTEMI patients will help EPs and cardiologists integrate care in an evidence-based, consistent approach for their patients. This will ultimately improve multidisciplinary communication, standardize care, and improve patient outcomes.

A clinical pathway for NSTEMI must be based on guidelines that provide extensive evidence for diagnostic and treatment regimens that provide substantial benefit in the early period after the patient with ACS presents to the ED. The 2002 ACC/AHA UA/NSTEMI guidelines use recommendation classes that rapidly allow one to make choices regarding diagnostic and treatment strategies. A Class I recommendation is generally considered to be useful and effective. Aspirin serves as an excellent example of a Class I treatment. Designation of a regimen as Class IIa identifies a treatment as generally considered effective, but some controversy may be present about the usefulness of a treatment. A Class IIb recommendation suggests that a treatment is controversial but leans toward efficacy. A therapy or diagnostic strategy that is Class III is not useful and may actually be harmful in some cases. Weighting of evidence for these Class I, II, and III recommendations is straightforward. If data from multiple large, randomized trials support a recommendation, then the weight of evidence is A. An evidence grade of B for a therapy is provided if fewer, smaller randomized trials, analyses of nonrandomized studies, or observational registries support a recommendation. Expert consensus provides an evidence grade of C (Table 5-1) (3).

Once an EP identifies a patient with potential ACS, it is critical to quickly risk stratify this patient and promptly deliver guideline-directed therapy. Risk stratification is based on the patient's history, physical examination, 12-lead electrocardiogram (ECG), and cardiac biomarkers such as troponin and creatinine kinase-MB (CK-MB). The risk stratification process includes (a) determining if the symptoms the patient is having are the result of ACS, and (b) among patients with probable/definite ACS, identifying patients who are at higher or lower risk of death and myocardial infarction (MI) as a complication of their ACS event.

In patients with ACS the history usually includes chest discomfort as a central feature. Less-typical symptoms may occur in older adults, patients with diabetes, patients with chronic renal failure, and women. Despite the absence of classic symptoms, these patients are at significant risk for complications with ACS. The characterization of this discomfort, location, severity, frequency, and possible radiation of pain help to identify the patient with ACS. The patient's age, sex, family history of coronary artery disease (CAD), smoking, dyslipidemia, hypertension, diabetes, previous CAD, and cocaine use also tend to increase the pretest likelihood of ACS in the individual presenting to the ED. The differential diagnosis for patients with potential ACS should include pulmonary embolism, aortic dissection, parenchymal lung disease, esophageal reflux, biliary disease, psychiatric illnesses including depression and panic disorder, musculoskeletal pain, and trauma. Part of the patient's history should assess for underlying illnesses such as intracranial tumor, gastrointestinal or other major bleeding, aortic dissection, and hemorrhagic stroke or a major surgery in the previous 2 weeks that can make antithrombotic or antiplatelet therapy potentially dangerous.

The physical examination for patients suspected of having ACS must focus on features associated with high risk for nonfatal myocardial infarction or death. Evidence of cardiogenic failure increases the likelihood that ACS is the cause of the pa-

TABLE 5-1

ACC/AHA CLASSIFICATION OF RECOMMENDATIONS AND LEVELS OF EVIDENCE

Class I:	Conditions for which there is evidence and/or general agreement that a given procedure or treatment is useful and effective.
Class II:	Conditions for which there is conflicting evidence and/or a divergence of opinion about the usefulness/efficacy of a procedure or treatment. IIa. Weight of evidence/opinion is in favor of usefulness/efficacy IIb. Usefulness/efficacy is less well established by evidence/opinion.
Class III:	Conditions for which there is evidence and/or general agreement that the procedure/treatment is not useful/ effective, and in some cases may be harmful.
Level of Evidence A	Data derived from multiple randomized clinical trials
Level of Evidence B	Data derived from a single randomized trial, or nonrandomized studies
Level of Evidence C	Consensus opinion of experts

Adapted from Braunwald E, Antman EM, Beasley JW et al. ACC/ AHA guideline update for the management of patients with unstable angina and non-ST-segment elevation myocardial infarction—002: Summary Article: A Report of the American College of Cardiology/ American Heart Associate Task Force on Practice Guidelines (Committee on the Management of Patients with Unstable Angina). *Circulation* 2002;106:1893–1900.

tient's symptoms. These symptoms may include jugular venous distension, rales, cardiac murmurs, S_3 or S_4 gallops, peripheral edema, a new mitral regurgitation murmur, hypotension (systolic blood pressure <100 mm Hg), tachycardia (pulse >100 bpm), and bradycardia (pulse <60 bpm). An important aspect of the physical examination that must not be minimized is the thorough evaluation for evidence of gross gastrointestinal bleeding or other reasons for contraindications to administering antithrombotic or antiplatelet therapy (Fig. 5-1).

In the assessment of the potential ACS patient, the 12-lead ECG is one of the most important pieces of information the physician will obtain. The ECG is often, and should be, obtained very early in the patient's presentation to the ED, ideally within 10 minutes after the patient's arrival. Many EDs have protocols in place in which the ECG may be obtained prior to a physician's assessment based on the patient's presenting symptoms. ST-segment depression has been shown to be a significant risk indicator for mortality and MI (10). Approximately half of the patients with ST-segment depression will develop MI within hours after presentation to the ED. Transient ST-segment elevation also portends high risk for the patient, likely signifying transient coronary artery occlusion by thrombus. Patients with new T-wave inversion on the initial 12-lead ECG have a less-adverse prognosis in patients with

ACS as compared to ST-segment depression. Approximately 5% of these patients will have an MI or die within 30 days. Bundle-branch blocks that are new or presumed to be new can indicate a high-risk presentation in the emergency setting. A new bundle-branch block, which serves as a criterion for STEMI in the appropriate clinical setting such as prolonged ischemic chest pain, indicates a need for rapid reperfusion therapy. Old bundle-branch blocks are more challenging to interpret in the setting of patients with suspected ACS. The old bundle-branch blocks may suggest underlying coronary disease; however, they also may indicate primary conduction system disease. Finally, patients with a paced rhythm can be a challenge when it comes to diagnosing ACS. The paced rhythm may mask underlying electrocardiographic high-risk features. A normal 12-lead ECG on presentation to the ED does not rule out ACS. Although a normal ECG represents the lowest risk for a given patient, up to a 6% rate of NSTEMI still exists for these patients. The initial ECG results, therefore, provide the clinician with substantial risk stratification information. The ACC/AHA guidelines support obtaining serial 12-lead ECGs in the ED to improve sensitivity for detecting ACS if the initial ECG is nondiagnostic (3).

After the ECG is obtained, blood is obtained from the patient. A complete blood count, renal profile with creatinine, PT/INR, PTT, and cardiac biomarkers are the standard labs ordered. The cardiac biomarkers troponin (I and T) and CK-MB represent the second principal method for identifying patients with ACS at risk for significant complications. Although CK-MB has been the predominant marker of myocardial necrosis used in the past, the troponins I and T in many centers have replaced this traditional marker in accordance with the recent criteria for the redefinition of acute MI promulgated by the European Society of Cardiology and the ACC (11–15). During the last decade, numerous studies have demonstrated that any detectable elevation of troponin identifies patients at high risk for ischemic complications, including patients with renal failure (16,17). Elevated troponin in the setting of ischemic symptoms indicates that the patient has experienced the myocardial necrosis of MI. Elevation of troponin is associated with increased risk of death, and the risk of this complication increases proportionally with the absolute level (18). Like the 12-lead ECG, troponin serves as an independent predictor of substantial patient risk. Studies also have confirmed that patients with ACS and elevated troponins derive greater benefit from treatment with platelet glycoprotein (GP) IIb/ IIIa inhibitors, low-molecular-weight heparin, and early percutaneous coronary intervention (PCI) than those not having elevated troponin levels. It should be emphasized that a normal level of troponin (or CK-MB) on ED presentation, particularly within 6 hours of chest pain onset, does not exclude MI. Serial testing in the ED at 0, 3, and 6 hours and at an interval of 6 to 10 hours once in hospital is necessary to exclude myocardial injury. It should also be noted that an elevated troponin is indicative of cardiac injury but not necessarily ischemic cardiac injury (19). If the clinical presentation is not one of acute ischemic heart disease, then a careful search for alternative causes of cardiac injury is essential, such as congestive heart failure or pulmonary embolus.

Point-of-care testing (POCT) of cardiac markers is becoming more popular in the emergency setting. The benefits of POCT are both speed to diagnosis and to therapy. Point-of-care testing typically accelerates decision making in the ED by providing CK-MB and troponin levels within 15 to 20 minutes after presentation (20). An added benefit is that these results are often directly handed to the treating physician, thus eliminating postlaboratory analysis delays. Many point-of-care devices, however, are less sensitive than are central laboratory analyzers, and thus some patients with minor and/or modest

Demographics: Patient Name, Age, Sex, Race, Date/Time Seen

History of Present Illness:
  1) Time of chest pain onset/symptom onset; duration of longest episode of pain prompting visit
  2) Other locations of pain: Neck, Left shoulder/arm, Right shoulder/arm, Left hand, Right hand, Abdomen, Back, Other _____
  3) Quality of Pain: Pressing/Crushing/Tightness, Sharp/Stabbing, Burning, Ache, Indigestion/Gas, Numbness, Indescribable, Other _____
  4) Pain is reproduced by: Deep breathing, Palpation, Change in position, Other _____
  5) Associated Symptoms: Diaphoresis, Nausea, Vomiting, Dyspnea, Dizziness, Other _____
  6) Diagnosis of most similar chest pain: MI, Angina, Other _____
  7) Recent pain compared with previously diagnosed angina: Worse, Similar, Better, No previous diagnosis of angina, Different

Cardiac Risk Factors: Family history of Coronary Artery disease, Elevated Cholesterol (>200 or taking medication), hypertension (systolic blood pressure >150, diastolic blood pressure >95 or taking medication), diabetes mellitus, smoking (current, past, never)

Past Medical History: MI, Angina, Cardiac Catheterization, Percutaneous Coronary Intervention, Coronary Artery Bypass Grafting

Medications

Allergies

Physical Examination: Vital signs including O_2 saturation

    General: Distress - None; Mild; Moderate; Severe; Diaphoresis

    HEENT: JVD; Carotid Bruits

    Pulmonary: Clear; Rales (bibasilar or less); Rales (>bibasilar), Other _____

    Heart: Mitral regurgitation murmur S_3; S_4

    Abdomen: Abdominal Aortic Aneurysm; Renal/Femoral Artery Bruits; Rectal Examination/Guaiac results: positive/negative

    Extremities: Decreased Peripheral Pulses/ Decreased Perfusion

Laboratory

    Electrocardiogram: Normal; Probable new ST-segment elevation MI ($\geq$ 1.0 mm ST-segment elevation in $\geq$ 2 leads) or new bundle branch block (left or right); New ischemia (> 1.0 mm ST-segment depression in $\geq$ 2 leads); Transient ST-segment elevation or ST-segment elevation not reaching 1.0 mm (0.5 mm < ST-segment elevation < 1.0 mm); Other new ST-segment or T-wave changes of ischemia; Old infarction, old ischemia; non-specific ST-segment or T-wave abnormality

    Cardiac Biomarkers: Troponin T or I Level
                               CK/CK-MB Level

    Adapted from: Emergency Department Chest Pain/ACS Evaluation template, Brigham & Women's Hospital, Boston, Massachusetts and the University Hospital, Cincinnati, Ohio.

FIGURE 5-1. Template for emergency department record, which includes acute coronary syndrome risk assessment. (From Gibler WB, Cannon CP, Blomkalns AL, et al. Practical implementation of the guidelines for unstable angina/non-ST-segment elevation myocardial infarction in the emergency department. *Circulation* 2005;111:2699–2710; *Ann Emerg Med* 2005;46:185–197, with permission.)

elevations in troponin may be missed (21). When central laboratory testing is used, the turnaround time for laboratory results should not exceed 1 hour (3). This 1-hour time period refers to the time the blood is drawn to the time the physician is aware of the results. This time interval has been referred to as "vein-to-brain." This information for ED evaluation is summarized in Figure 5-1.

For the patient with suspected ACS that has a nondiagnostic ECG and normal levels of cardiac biomarkers, what other diagnostic modalities are available to the treating physician for help in the risk stratification of the patient? Tests such as echocardiography for wall motion abnormality, contrast echocardiographic perfusion imaging, and radionuclide perfusion imaging with agents such as sestamibi can be performed at rest, providing compelling risk stratification information for patients presenting to the ED. When performed while the patient is complaining of chest pain or within several hours after discomfort has ceased, these studies can provide excellent negative predictive value for acute myocardial ischemia. Patients with chronic ECG changes such as bundle-branch block or ST-segment/T-wave abnormalities also can be evaluated more extensively using these modalities. The routine use of these diagnostic techniques at a given hospital depends on the availability of cardiologists or nuclear radiologists at the hospital and the particular interests and expertise of the cardiologists or nuclear radiologists at the institution. Standard graded exercise testing and stress echocardiography can be performed in patients with nondiagnostic ECGs, negative cardiac biomarkers, and no recent (<6 hours) pain at rest; however, exercise testing is contraindicated in patients with acute ischemia. Discharge of a patient from the ED may be appropriate for patients without high-risk features presenting to the ED, negative serial cardiac biomarkers, no evidence of ST-segment or T-wave changes, and a negative perfusion imaging test at rest. Careful follow-up by cardiology as an outpatient is necessary so that provocative testing can be performed to rule out a fixed coronary lesion causing crucial stenosis.

The practical implementation of the 2002 ACC/AHA UA/NSTEMI guidelines approach provides an algorithm for the evaluation and management of patients suspected of having an ACS in the ED (Fig. 5-2) (7,8). This information should provide the foundation for any critical pathway developed for ACS/NSTEMI patients. In addition to routine therapy, such as continuous cardiac monitoring, oxygen if needed, and intravenous access, the following therapies are recommended by the 2002 ACC/AHA guidelines: nitrates, morphine, beta-blockers, nondihydropyridine calcium channel blockers (verapamil or diltiazem), ACEIs, antiplatelet agents, and antithrombin agents. Each of these will be reviewed later.

Nitrates, a Class IC recommendation, should be given first by the sublingual route followed by intravenous administration for the relief of ischemia and its associated symptoms. Although there are no randomized, placebo-controlled clinical trials of nitrate use in unstable angina, there are small studies from the prethrombolytic era that suggest a reduction in mortality rate of approximately 35%. As a result of no adequate studies for the use of nitrates in NSTEMI, the recommendations are largely extrapolated from pathophysiological principles and uncontrolled observations (22).

Like the nitrates, morphine is a Class IC recommendation and has no randomized, placebo-controlled clinical trials to support its use. Morphine sulfate remains a recommendation because of its venodilation properties and modest reductions in heart rate. It also may be used to help relieve a patient's anxiety or when acute pulmonary congestion is also present.

The intravenous administration of beta-blockers, a Class IB recommendation, should be used when there is ongoing chest-pain without contraindications to beta-blockade and the pa-

tient is not already taking beta-blockers before presentation. An overview of double-blind, randomized, controlled trials in patients with threatening or evolving MI suggests an approximately 13% reduction in risk of progression to MI for patients. There are no trials with sufficient power to evaluate beta-blockade in patients with unstable angina; however, the proven efficacy of beta-blockers in patients with acute MI, recent acute MI, congestive heart failure, and angina led to their use as being recommended in unstable angina (23). Nondihydropyridine calcium channel blockers, a Class IB recommendation, are recommended in patients with continuing or frequently recurring ischemia when beta-blockers are contraindicated and there is no left ventricular (LV) dysfunction, hypotension, or other contraindication to their use. When administered to patients with LV dysfunction, there is strong evidence that they are detrimental (Class III) (24–26).

ACEIs are a Class IB recommendation. ACEIs are recommended when hypertension persists despite treatment with nitroglycerin and beta-blockers in patients with LV systolic dysfunction or congestive heart failure. They are also recommended for patients with ACS and diabetes. Initiation of ACEIs in the ED is appropriate in the preceding circumstances; however, it is not necessary that this agent be started in this setting. Angiotensin renin blockers can be substituted if the patient is ACEI intolerant (27–29).

Antiplatelet agents that inhibit the aggregation of platelets play an important role in the prevention of thrombosis in the 2002 ACC/AHA UA/NSTEMI guidelines. Three different classes of agents have distinct and separate mechanisms of action: aspirin, clopidogrel, and the GP IIb/IIIa receptor inhibitors. Each will be discussed separately because of these important different mechanisms of action.

Aspirin, an inexpensive and effective antiplatelet agent, acts by blocking the thromboxane A2 pathway. Aspirin is a Class IA recommendation and should be administered to the ACS patient as soon as possible. It is now common practice for prehospital care providers to administer this drug prior to the patient's arrival in the ED. Several studies have shown aspirin to be beneficial in the setting of ACS, showing an approximately 50% reduction in death and MI in patients receiving this therapy (3,30,31).

The thienopyridine clopidogrel is an antiplatelet agent that blocks adenosine diphosphate–stimulated platelet aggregation. The Clopidogrel in Unstable Angina to prevent Recurrent Events (CURE) trial confirmed the additional benefit of clopidogrel with aspirin for UA/NSTEMI. There was a 20% reduction in the primary outcome of cardiac death, MI, or stroke in the CURE trial. This agent was incorporated into the 2002 ACC/AHA UA/NSTEMI guidelines as a Class IA recommendation (32).

The third class of antiplatelet agents that is an important therapy in the 2002 ACC/AHA UA/NSTEMI guidelines is the GP IIb/IIIa receptor inhibitors. Activated platelets express surface GP IIb/IIIa receptors, which bind fibrinogen to allow aggregation. Eptifibatide and tirofiban (small-molecule agents) and abciximab (a monoclonal antibody fragment) are approved for use in patients with ACS and are recommended for patients undergoing early invasive therapy based on the CAPTURE, PURSUIT, PRISM-PLUS, and TACTICS-TIMI 18 (c7E3 Antiplatelet Therapy in Unstable Refractory Angina, Platelet glycoprotein IIb/ IIIa in Unstable angina: Receptor Suppression Using Integrilin™ Therapy, Platelet Receptor Inhibition for ischemic Syndrome Management in Patients Limited to very Unstable Signs and symptoms, and Treat angina with Aggrastat® and determine Costs of Therapy with Invasive or Conservative Strategies-Thrombolysis In Myocardial Infarction 18, respectively) trials (Class IA). The two small-molecule agents eptifibatide and tirofiban provide reversible inhibition of the GP IIb/IIIa receptor and are indicated for patients receiv-

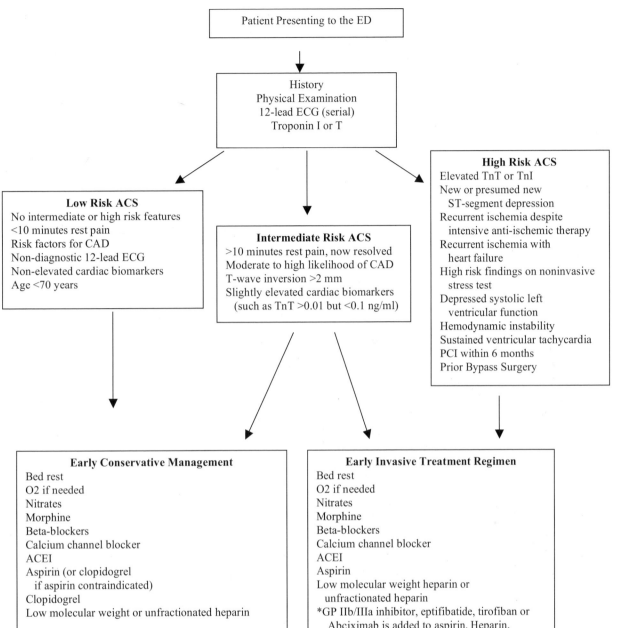

FIGURE 5-2. Integration of the 2002 ACC/AHA guidelines for diagnostic and treatment strategies in the emergency department for patients with acute coronary syndrome (ACS). (From Gibler WB, Cannon CP, Blomkalns AL, et al. Practical implementation of the guidelines for unstable angina/non-ST-segment elevation myocardial infarction in the emergency department. *Circulation* 2005;111:2699–2710; *Ann Emerg Med* 2005;46:185–197, with permission.)

ing conservative therapy or early invasive therapy for ACS (Class IIaA) (1,33–37). It is important to note that abciximab is not indicated for patients receiving only medical management without cardiac catheterization. It is indicated for use in patients in whom early PCI is planned (38). This is a Class IIIA recommendation based on the GUSTO-IV (Global Utilization of Streptokinase and tPA for Occluded arteries) ACS trial (38).

The final therapy to be discussed are the antithrombin agents. Heparin, when given intravenously, blocks thrombin formation by accelerating the action of antithrombin. Heparin is essential to the treatment of patients with ACS. Unfractionated heparin binds to a variety of proteins, which reduces the heparin available to affect antithrombin, resulting in variable anticoagulant responses in patients. Intravenous heparin, however, is considered a fundamental therapy for treating ACS and is a Class IA therapy when given in conjunction with antiplatelet agents (3,39–41). In a number of clinical trials, LMWH has been found to have improved efficacy as compared with unfractionated heparin. The LMWH enoxaparin has been shown to be superior to unfractionated heparin in two large clinical trials, ESSENCE (Efficacy and Safety of Subcutaneous Enoxaparin in Non-Q-wave Coronary Events) and TIMI-11-B, but was equivalent in the most recent study, SYNERGY (Superior Yield of the New strategy of Enoxaparin, Revascularization, and Glycoprotein IIb/IIIa inhibitors) (42,43). The guidelines suggest enoxaparin, but not the other LMWH, is preferred over unfractionated heparin unless coronary artery bypass grafting (CABG) surgery is planned within 24 hours (Class IIaA) (44). Patients with elevated troponin values are most likely to benefit from LMWH therapy. It is important to consider that the use of LMWH should be coordinated with the cardiac catheterization team before PCI. Some cardiac catheterization laboratories prefer not to perform these procedures on patients who have received LMWH. Figure 5-2 is an algorithm that depicts the integration of the 2002 ACC/AHA UA/NSTEMI guidelines for these diagnostic and treatment strategies in the ED.

Fondaparinux (Arixtra), currently used for deep venous thrombosis prophylaxis in orthopedic surgery, is a once daily, subcutaneous, factor Xa inhibitor that has shown encouraging results in the use in patients with UA/NSTEMI. The OASIS-5 trial, that comprised over 20,000 patients with NSTEMI, randomized patients to receive enoxaparin or fondaparinux. The OASIS-5 trial showed that enoxaparin and fondaparinux were clinically equivalent for efficacy (essentially identical rates for cardiovascular death, MI, or recurrent ischemia at 9 days); however, the risk of major bleeding in the fondaparinux arm was reduced by nearly 50%. Interestingly, at later time points, there was emergence of a significant reduction in death alone with the fondaparinux arm, both at 30 days and 6 months, and there was also improvement in the rate of MI (45). Thus, this study brings to the forefront a new goal in the management of patients with ACS, namely to avoid major bleeding, in addition to optimizing antithrombotic therapy.

As previously mentioned, the EP must be able to diagnose, risk stratify, and then treat the patient with ACS. The 2002 ACC/AHA UA/NSTEMI guidelines help in the risk stratification process by defining high, intermediate, and low risk for death or nonfatal MI (Table 5-2) (3). Patients with ACS at low risk for ischemic complications, including death and MI, should be admitted and treated with early conservative management, as shown in Figure 5-2. Early invasive therapy should be considered for all patients with ACS who are deemed at high risk for ischemic complications. Patients at intermediate risk for death or nonfatal MI should receive appropriate therapy for ACS and be considered for possible intervention by a cardiologist.

Patients can evolve in the emergency setting from low to intermediate to high risk. Patients suspected of having ACS but with an initial nondiagnostic ECG and initially negative cardiac biomarkers should have serial cardiac biomarkers and ECGs performed.

The role of the chest pain center should be reserved for low-risk ACS patients. Low-risk ACS patients are those with nondiagnostic 12-lead ECGs and an initial set of nonelevated cardiac biomarkers. Once a patient has completed a normal series of ECGs and cardiac biomarkers through 6 hours, and a test for rest ischemia such as a sestamibi radionuclide perfusion scan is also negative, then the patient can be discharged home from the ED for further follow-up by a cardiologist. This follow-up must include provocative testing to evaluate the patient for a fixed coronary lesion.

The management of patients with ACS can be divided into either early conservative management or early invasive management as mentioned earlier and noted in Figure 5-2. Both strategies include the use of bed rest, oxygen if needed, nitrates, morphine, beta-blockers, calcium channel blockers if beta-blockers are contraindicated and there is no left ventricular dysfunction, and ACEIs.

Patients at low risk for ischemic complications should be treated with an early conservative management strategy. In addition to the preceding therapies, this strategy includes aspirin (Class IA), clopidogrel, unfractionated heparin or enoxaparin (Class IA), and eptifibatide or tirofiban. Because patients in the early conservative therapy arm are not expected to go immediately to the cardiac catheterization lab, clopidogrel should be given to the ACS patient while in the ED. Clopidogrel should be continued for at least 1 month (Class IA) and for up to 9 months (Class IB). Eptifibatide or tirofiban should be administered in patients when continuing ischemia (Class IIaA), elevated cardiac troponins (Class IIaA), and other high-risk features are present (Class IIaA). Abciximab should not be used unless PCI is planned (Class IIIA) (39).

Patients at high risk for ACS should undergo the early invasive treatment strategy. Any patient at high risk for UA/NSTEMI should undergo coronary angiography and revascularization within 12 to 48 hours after presentation to the ED (35,36,46). As noted in Table 5-2 (3), the following criteria are indicative of the high-risk patient:

1. New or presumed new ST-segment depression
2. Elevated troponin I or T
3. Recurrent angina/ischemia at rest or with low levels of activity despite intensive anti-ischemic treatment
4. Recurrent ischemia with associated heart failure (S$_3$ gallop, pulmonary edema, worsening rales, or new or worsening mitral regurgitation)
5. High-risk findings on noninvasive stress testing
6. Depressed systolic LV function (EF ~0.40 on noninvasive study)
7. Hemodynamic instability
8. Sustained ventricular tachycardia
9. PCI within the last 6 months
10. Previous coronary artery bypass surgery

In the high-risk patients, oxygen (if needed), nitrates, morphine, beta-blockers, calcium channel blockers, and ACEI should be administered. In addition, aspirin (Class IA), LMWH or unfractionated heparin (Class IA), and GP IIb-IIIa inhibitors (Class IA) should be administered. It was previously believed that clopidogrel therapy should be postponed in the early invasive treatment strategy until after the patient had undergone cardiac catheterization to determine coronary anatomy. Some cardiologists, however, prefer the initial use of clopidogrel even if cardiac catheterization/PCI is planned as the likelihood of the patient needing emergent coronary artery bypass grafting (CABG) is low.

TABLE 5-2

SHORT-TERM RISK OF DEATH OR NONFATAL MI IN PATIENTS WITH UA/NSTEMI*

Feature	High Risk At least 1 of the following features must be present:	Intermediate Risk No high-risk feature but must have 1 of the following:	Low Risk No high- or intermediate-risk features but may have any of the following features:
History	Accelerating tempo of ischemic symptoms in preceding 48 h	Prior MI, peripheral or cerebrovascular disease, or CABG, prior aspirin use	
Character of pain	Prolonged ongoing (>20 minutes) rest pain	Prolonged (>20 min) rest angina, now resolved, with moderate or high likelihood of CAD Rest angina (>20 min) or relieved with rest or sublingual NTG	New-onset or progressive CCS Class III or IV angina the past 2 weeks without prolonged (>20 min) rest pain but with moderate or high likelihood of CAD
Clinical findings	Pulmonary edema, most likely due to ischemia New or worsening MR murmur S_3 or new/worsening rales Hypotension, bradycardia, tachycardia Age >75 years	Age >70 years	
ECG	Angina at rest with transient ST-segment changes >0.05 mV Bundle-branch block, new or presumed new Sustained ventricular tachycardia	T-wave inversions >0.2 mV Pathological Q waves	Normal or unchanged ECG during an episode of chest discomfort
Cardiac markers	Elevated (e.g., TnT or TnI >0.1 ng/mL)	Slightly elevated (e.g., TnT >0.01 but <0.1 ng/mL)	Normal

* Estimation of the short-term risks of death and nonfatal cardiac ischemic events in UA is a complex multivariable problem that cannot be fully specified in a table such as this; therefore, this table is meant to offer general guidance and illustration rather than rigid algorithms.
Adapted from: Braunwald E, Antman EM, Beasley JW, et al. ACC/AHA guideline update for the management of patients with unstable angina and non-ST-segment elevation myocardial infarction—2002: summary article: a report of the American College of Cardiology/American Heart Association Task Force on Practice Guidelines (Committee on the Management of Patients with Unstable Angina). *J Am Coll Cardiol* 2002;40(7): 1366–1374.

Recent trials have shown a clear benefit of pretreatment with clopidogrel in high-risk patients (47). The PCI-CLARITY trial was an analysis of patients who underwent PCI within the CLARITY-TIMI 28 trial, where patients underwent thrombolysis for ST-elevation MI, and found improved infarct-related artery patency and a reduction in ischemic complications with the addition of clopidogrel (48). PCI-CLARITY prespecified substudy focused on PCI procedures that were performed on average 3.5 days following the patient's MI.

The study looked at the benefit of prior treatment with clopidogrel as compared with receiving clopidogrel as a loading dose in the cath lab at the time of the procedure. The results were impressive, with a 46% reduction in the odds of cardiovascular death, MI, or stroke through 30 days following the procedure in the patients who had been randomized to pretreatment before the procedure, compared to those who received clopidogrel in the cath lab. In addition, a 38% reduction in MI or stroke was observed prior to PCI. Thus, early therapy with clopidogrel prior to PCI had an absolute reduction of 4.5% of cardiovascular death, MI, or stroke. This means that four deaths, MIs, or strokes are prevented for every 100 patients who are pretreated for their PCI. This new data, combined with a meta-analysis involving two other pretreatment trials, PCI-CURE and CREDO, should encourage the wider use of this early pretreatment strategy.

If clopidogrel is administered and the patient requires a revascularization procedure, it is suggested that CABG be delayed for 5 to 7 days because of the risk of bleeding and the potential need for platelet transfusion. Finally, if the patient has a contraindication to aspirin, clopidogrel should be given (Class IA) but with the same caution as noted earlier.

When it comes to choosing LMWH or unfractionated heparin in the early invasive therapy regimen, LMWH is preferred unless bypass surgery is planned within 24 hours (Class IIaA). Because the EP is not aware if CABG will be needed while treating the patient in the ED, unfractionated heparin is mainly used. As for GP IIb-IIIa inhibitor use, the 2002 ACC/AHA UA/NSTEMI guidelines recommend that this therapy be given immediately before PCI in patients receiving early invasive therapy for non-ST-segment elevation ACS.

Figures 5-3 and 5-4 are examples of critical pathways developed for UA/NSTEMI patients that present to an acute care setting. Figure 5-3 (7,8) is based on the CRUSADE quality im-provement initiative order set, whereas Figure 5-4 demonstrates adaptation of the guidelines for a community hospital

MEDICATION ALLERGIES

☐ **Specify:** _____

DIAGNOSTIC STUDIES

☐ 12-lead ECG: Now _____ : In AM _____ Date: _____
☐ 12-lead ECG for recurrent chest pain
☐ Cardiac markers → **Specify:**
  ☐ Troponin I **OR**
  ☐ Troponin T   } 0, 3, 6, 12, 24 hours
  ☐ CK **AND**   } 0, 3, 6, 12, 24 hours
  ☐ CK-MB

LABS

☐ Fasting lipid profile in AM   ☐ CBC q AM
☐ Chemistry Panels in ED and q AM   ☐ Other labs: _____

INITIAL TREATMENT

Oral Antiplatelet Therapies:

☐ Aspirin → **Specify:**   ☐ Enteric-coated ASA
   160-325 mg   **OR**   } _____ mg per day
                           ☐ Non-enteric coated ASA

☐ If aspirin intolerant, clopidogrel: 300 mg loading dose followed by 75 mg po QD

Nitrates and Morphine:

☐ SL NTG 0.4 mg as needed for recurrent chest pain
☐ NTG paste: _____ inches q 6 hours, off from midnight-6 AM
☐ IV NTG: Start at 10 mcg/min if pain not relieved by SL or transdermal NTG and titrate (up to 200 mg/min) for relief of chest pain (keep SBP > 90 mmHg)
☐ **Morphine Sulfate** 1-2 mg every _____ hours as needed for recurrent chest pain

Beta Blockers:

☐ Metoprolol → **Specify:**   ☐ IV: _____ mg q 5 min X _____ doses **OR**
                               ☐ po: _____ mg q _____ hours **OR**

☐ Atenolol → **Specify:**   ☐ IV: _____ mg q 5 min X _____ doses **OR**
                               ☐ po: _____ mg qd

☐ Other → **Specify:** _____

Non-Dihydropyridine Calcium Antagonist (If Beta-blocker contraindicated):

☐ Diltiazem → **Specify:**   ☐ **po:** _____ mg q 8 hours **OR**
                              ☐ **Diltiazem CD/XR:** _____ mg po qd

☐ Verapamil → **Specify:**   ☐ **po:** _____ mg q 8 hours **OR**
                              ☐ **Verapamil SR:** _____ mg po qd

ACE Inhibitor (Angiotensin receptor blocker can be substituted if ACE intolerant):

☐ Enalapril   ☐ **po:** _____ mg q 12 hours

☐ Lisinopril   ☐ **po:** _____ mg qd

FIGURE 5-3. UA/Non-ST-segment elevation (NSTE) initial management standing orders. (From Gibler WB, Cannon CP, Blomkalns AL, et al. Practical implementation of the guidelines for unstable angina/non-ST-segment elevation myocardial infarction in the emergency department. *Circulation* 2005;111: 2699–2710; *Ann Emerg Med* 2005;46:185–197, with permission.) (*continues*)

MANAGEMENT STRATEGY

- NSTE ACS patients with high-risk features should be managed according to the Early Invasive Protocol.

- Patients with moderate-risk features can be managed with either Protocol.

- Patients with low-risk features should be managed according to the Early Conservative Protocol.

High-risk: Elevated Cardiac Markers, ST depression, Transient ST elevation, > 20 min rest pain, Hemodynamic instability, signs of CHF

Moderate-risk: No high-risk features, Prior MI, Prior CABG, T-wave inversions, Rest angina (< 20 min) relieved promptly with NTG, Age > 70 years

Low-risk: No high- or moderate-risk features, progressive angina without prolonged rest pain, Normal cardiac markers, Normal ECG with pain

■ EARLY INVASIVE PROTOCOL

Intravenous Anti-thrombotic Therapies:

☐ **IV unfractionated heparin →**
Initial bolus of 60-70 U/kg bolus (not to exceed 5000 U) + 12-15 U/kg/hr infusion (not to exceed 1000 U/hr) to target aPTT range of 50-70 sec, or 1.5-2.5 times control

☐ **Low-molecular-weight heparin → Specify:**
  ☐ **Enoxaparin:** 1 mg/kg SC q 12 hrs

Intravenous Antiplatelet Therapies:
GP IIb-IIIa Inhibitor → Specify:

☐ **Abciximab:** 0.25 mg/kg IV bolus + 0.125 mcg/kg/min infusion (only for patients planned to undergo PCI within 12-24 hrs) **OR**

☐ **Eptifibatide:** 180 mcg/kg IV bolus + 2.0 mcg/kg/min infusion* **OR**

☐ **Tirofiban:** 0.4 mcg/kg/min IV bolus for 30 min + 0.1 mcg/kg/min infusion*
* For patients with **renal impairment**, administer 1/2 the rate of infusion for eptifibatide and tirofiban

☐ **Schedule for Early Cardiac Catheterization**
Date: _ _/_ _/_ _ _ _
      day month   year

Oral Antiplatelet Therapies:

NOTE: *Add clopidogrel after diagnostic catheterization unless CABG is planned.*

☐ **Clopidogrel:** 300 mg loading dose   75 mg po QD

■ EARLY CONSERVATIVE PROTOCOL

Intravenous Anti-thrombotic Therapies:

☐ **IV unfractionated heparin →**
Initial bolus of 60-70 U/kg bolus (not to exceed 5000 U) + 12-15 U/kg/hr infusion (not to exceed 1000 U/hr) to target aPTT range of 50-70 sec, or 1.5-2.5 times control

☐ **Low-molecular-weight heparin → Specify:**
  ☐ **Enoxaparin:** 1 mg/kg SC q 12 hrs

Oral Antiplatelet Therapies:

☐ **Clopidogrel:** 300 mg loading dose   75 mg po QD

Intravenous Antiplatelet Therapies:

NOTE: *Eptifibatide or tirofiban are indicated for patients with high-risk features who are managed conservatively.*

GP IIb-IIIa Inhibitor → Specify:

☐ **Eptifibatide:** 180 mcg/kg IV bolus + 2.0 mcg/kg/min infusion* **OR**

☐ **Tirofiban:** 0.4 mcg/kg/min IV bolus for 30 min + 0.1 mcg/kg/min infusion*
* For patients with **renal impairment**, administer 1/2 the rate of infusion for eptifibatide and tirofiban

☐ **Schedule for assessment of left ventricular function → Type(s):**

☐ Echocardiogram

☐ Nuclear ventriculogram

☐ **Schedule for stress test → Type(s):**
  ☐ Exercise treadmill test
  ☐ Exercise nuclear perfusion study
  ☐ Dobutamine nuclear perfusion study
  ☐ Persantine nuclear perfusion study
  ☐ Exercise stress echocardiography
  ☐ Dobutamine echocardiography

☐ **Lipid-lowering agent:** Name and dose of drug prescribed: _____

Name of Physician: _____ **Date:** _____ **Time:** _____
Signature: _____

Adapted from: CRUSADE Quality Improvement Initiative tool (http://www.crusadeqi.com)

FIGURE 5-3. *(continued)*

environment. They are based on the 2002 ACC/AHA UA/NSTEMI guidelines.

The development of expert-prepared strategies such as the 2002 ACC/AHA UA/NSTEMI guidelines presents enormous opportunities for EDs to establish evidence-based clinical pathways to allow for standardized, best-practice care for these patients. Developing an evidence-based, best-practice clinical pathway is only part of the challenge. Getting physicians to understand the concept of clinical pathways, to use the path-

way consistently, and to track compliance of physician use of the guidelines is equally challenging. Overcoming the daily barriers to guideline implementation is a constant struggle. Delays in lab turnaround times, high patient volume, and a lack of standardized diagnostic and treatment approaches are just some additional barriers that can inhibit the provision of appropriate care to patients.

The patient with ACS will not only be cared for by the EP, but also a cardiologist and/or internist, family physician, and

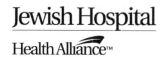

Non-ST Segment Elevation Myocardial Infarction

ALLERGIES_____

HEIGHT_____ WEIGHT _____

NO.	PHYSICIAN ORDERS	HUC /RN
	ORDERS WITH CHECK BOXES MUST BE SELECTED. ALL OTHER ORDERS WILL BE AUTOMATICALLY INITIATED.	
	Inclusion Criteria: Transient ST-Elevation, <u>and/or</u> Persistent ST-Depression, <u>and/or</u> Positive Cardiac Markers	
	DATE/TIME:	
1.	12 Lead EKG (also Right-sided EKG if ST-Segment Elevation in Leads II, III, AVF)	
2.	Portable Chest X-Ray	
3.	Continuous EKG Monitoring	
4.	Pulse Oximetry	
5.	IV Access (x 2 if possible)	
6.	Aspirin 325mg Orally x 1	
7.	☐ Nitroglycerin (NitroStat®) 0.4 mg sublingually x 1; may repeat x 2 for CP at 5-minute intervals for total of 3 doses	
8.	☐ Nitroglycerin 50 mg in 5% Dextrose 250 mL IV infusion, starting at 10 mcg/min = 3 mL/hour; Titrate to Chest Pain free or SBP equal to 90mmHg	
9.	☐ Morphine sulfate_____ mg IVP; may repeat every 10 minutes to a maximum of ____ mg. Maintain SBP greater than 90mmHg	
10.	Metoprolol (Lopressor®) 5mg IVP every 5 minutes x 3 doses HOLD for SBP less than 90 mmHg, Symptoms of Heart Failure, Heart rate less than 60 beats per minute, or History of Asthma/COPD	
11.	Begin Cardiac Heparin Weight Based Protocol	
12.	☐ Enalaprilat (Vasotec®) 1.25mg IVP if SBP is greater than 140mmHg after Beta Blocker and Nitroglycerin	
13.	☐ Lisinopril (Prinivil®) 10mg Orally if SBP is between 100-140mmHg after Beta Blocker and Nitroglycerin	
14.	Draw the following Labs: ☐ CBC ☐ EP1 ☐ CK ☐ CK-MB ☐ Troponin –T STAT, 90 min, 180 min, and 360 min ☐ PT (includes INR/PTT) ☐ Type and Screen ☐ Other labs:	
15.	**Contraindications for GP IIb/IIIa Inhibitors:** • History of bleeding diathesis • Severe Hypertension (SBP greater than 200mmHg; DBP greater than 110mmHg) not adequately controlled on anti-hypertension therapy • Major surgery within preceding 6 weeks • History of Stroke within 30 days or *any* hemorrhagic Stroke • Current or planned administration of another parental GP IIb/IIIa Inhibitor • Dependency on Renal Dialysis (relative contraindications)	
16.	Choose one of the following regimens and treatment strategies, if <u>no contraindications</u> to the use of GP IIb/IIIa Inhibitors **Contact Pharmacy to calculate Patients Creatinine Clearance. Provide the following patient data to pharmacy:** Age: _____ Sex: _____ Weight: _____ Height: _____ Serum Creatinine: _____ **Creatinine Clearance =_____mL/min - Calculated by Pharmacist (name)_____**	
	Invasive Strategy Planned: Eptifibatide (Integrilin®) 180 mcg/kg IV Bolus = _____ mg, followed by an infusion at 2 mcg/kg/min = _____ mL/hour * <u>Renal dosing</u> **required for Creatinine Clearance of less than 50mL/min, start infusion at 1 mcg/kg/min = _____ mL/hour** Consider Clopidogrel: 300 mg loading dose → 75 mg po QD unless CABG is planned	
	Conservative Strategy Planned: Eptifibatide (Integrilin®) 180 mcg/kg IV Bolus = _____ mg, followed by an infusion at 2 mcg/kg/min = _____ mL/hour * <u>Renal dosing</u> **required for Creatinine Clearance of less than 50mL/min, start infusion at 1 mcg/kg/min = _____ mL/hour** AND Clopidogrel (Plavix®) 300mg Orally x 1	
17.	Additional Orders:	
	Physician's Signature: _____ Pager #_____	

FIGURE 5-4. NSTEMI ED Pathway; Jewish Hospital, Cincinnati, Ohio.

hospitalist. These physicians must also be aware of these evidenced-based UA/NSTEMI guidelines for them to be completely effective. Making all physicians who care for these patients aware of the 2002 ACC/AHA UA/NSTEMI guidelines is a significant challenge in any hospital setting. Finally, multiple cardiology groups at an institution can make agreement on specific diagnostic and treatment regimens for patients with ACS difficult to achieve.

Several quality improvement initiatives have been developed to demonstrate methods for changing physician behavior and improving patient outcomes for patients with ACS (49–64). The CRUSADE Quality Improvement Initiative is an ongoing effort to track adherence to the 2002 ACC/AHA UA/NSTEMI guidelines and to provide mechanisms to improve performance. This initiative is a partnership of academicians, industry, and EPs and cardiologists at hospitals throughout the United States. The objectives of CRUSADE include the following:

1. Determine the current awareness and adherence to the 2002 ACC/AHA UA/NSTEMI guidelines for ACS.
2. Implement quality improvement initiatives at site hospitals to promote ACC/AHA diagnostic and treatment recommendations for high-risk ACS patients.
3. Improve clinical outcomes through early guideline implementation, for example, in the ED.

Early evidence with approximately 175,000 patients enrolled suggests that this effort has been successful in increasing awareness and adherence to the 2002 ACC/AHA UA/NSTEMI guidelines. Since October 2003, data have been collected on ED guideline adherence for UA/NSTEMI that provide information that EPs and cardiologists can use to improve the care of these patients (65,66). A structured order set provides specific guideline-based therapy for patients with ACS enrolled in the CRUSADE Quality Improvement Initiative (Fig. 5-3).

There are some strong predictors for successful guideline implementation. Education and communication are the key elements. Strong clinical champions in emergency medicine and cardiology who have effective communication with other EPs, cardiologists, internists, and family physicians at their institutions can develop consensus on clear diagnostic and treatment pathways that incorporate guideline directives. Physicians must demonstrate a clear willingness to partner with other hospital health care specialists. Also essential is the support from the laboratory and hospital administration. Working with the lab to decrease cardiac biomarker turnaround times is essential. Hospital administration can help provide the needed resources and provide support for interdepartmental cooperation. Having the significant involvement of nursing, administration, laboratory, and pharmacy is essential to reaching agreement on a pathway. Aligning the incentives of all parties to provide guideline-directed care is extremely important.

A benefit of guideline directed therapy through the use of clinical pathways is the ability to collect data from a standard source. Data obtained from the pathway can be analyzed, with the results being communicated to the physicians and nurses of the ED, cardiac care unit, and other appropriate units. These data can then serve as a stimulus for continued quality improvement. Data collected for NSTEMI can be compared to both local and national benchmarks, as is being done for AMI as part of JCAHO's (Joint Commission on Accreditation of Healthcare Organizations) CORE measures for AMI (67). Sharing data with multiple physician groups across the hospital (emergency medicine, cardiology, internal medicine, family medicine, and cardiac surgery) and non-physician members of the health care team can help identify areas of success and potential improvement.

Finally, the use of quality improvement tools such as standard diagnostic evaluations for the ED that readily identify high-risk criteria in ED patients as well as standardized medication order sets also can increase adherence to guidelines. Early identification of high-risk patients with ACS in the emergency setting can decrease time to cardiac catheterization and revascularization. The combination of improved communication between all members of the care team involved with ACS patients, the collection of high-quality data on these patients, and the use of quality improvement tools can provide improved, more consistent care for these patients.

Thus, the 2002 ACC/AHA UA/NSTEMI guidelines represent an evidence-based approach to the care of patients with ACS. Adherence to the guidelines can be improved by (a) implementation of a NSTEMI critical pathway in the ED setting, (b) enhanced communication between EPs and cardiologists, and (c) the implementation of quality improvement initiatives. Through this approach, better, more consistent care can be provided and can lead to improved outcomes for those patients with ACS.

References

1. Nourjah P. *National hospital ambulatory medical care survey: 1997 emergency department summary*. Hyattsville, MD: National Center for Health Statistics; 1999:304. Advance data from Vital and Health Statistics.
2. National Center for Health Statistics. *Detailed diagnosis and procedures: national hospital discharge survey, 1996*. Hyattsville, MD: National Center for Health Statistics; 1998:13. Data from Vital and Health Statistics.
3. Braunwald E, Antman EM, Beasley JW, et al. ACC/AHA 2002 guideline update for the management of patients with unstable angina and non-ST-segment elevation myocardial infarction—summary article: a report of the American College of Cardiology/American Heart Association task force on practice guidelines (Committee on the Management of Patients With Unstable Angina). *J Am Coll Cardiol* 2002;40:1366–1374.
4. Braunwald E, Mark DB, Jones RH, et al. *Unstable Angina: Diagnosis and Management*. Rockville, MD: Agency for Health Care Policy and Research and the National Heart, Lung, and Blood Institute, US Public Health Service, US Department of Health and Human Services. 1994:1. AHCPR publication No. 94–0602.
5. Pollack CV Jr, Gibler WB. 2000 ACC/AHA guidelines for the management of patients with unstable angina and non-ST-segment elevation myocardial infarction: a practical summary for emergency physicians. *Ann Emerg Med* 2001;38:229–240.
6. Pollack CV Jr, Roe MT, Peterson ED. 2002 Update to the ACC/AHA guidelines for the management of patients with unstable angina and non-ST-segment elevation myocardial infarction: implications for emergency department practice. *Ann Emerg Med* 2003;41:355–369.
7. Gibler WB, Cannon CP, Blomkalns AL, et al. Practical implementation of the guidelines for unstable angina/non-ST-segment elevation myocardial infarction in the emergency department. *Circulation* 2005;111:2699–2710.
8. Gibler WB, Cannon CP, Blomkalns AL, et al. Practical implementation of the guidelines for unstable angina/non-ST-segment elevation myocardial infarction in the emergency department. *Ann Emerg Med* 2005;46:185–197.
9. McGlynn EA, Asch SM, Adams J, et al. The quality of health care delivered to adults in the United States. *N Engl J Med* 2003;348:2635–2645.
10. Savonitto S, Ardissino D, Granger CB, et al. Prognostic value of the admission electrocardiogram in acute coronary syndromes. *JAMA* 1999;28(1):707–713.
11. Apple FS, Wu AHB, Jaffe AS. European Society of Cardiology and American College of Cardiology guidelines for redefinition of myocardial infarction: how to use existing assays clinically and for clinical trials. *Am Heart J* 2002;144:981–986.
12. Jaffe AS, Ravkilde J, Roberts R, et al. It's time for a change to a troponin standard. *Circulation* 2000;102:1216–1220.
13. Heidenreich PA, Alloggiamento T, Melsop K, et al. The prognostic value of troponin in patients with non-ST elevation acute coronary syndromes: a meta-analysis. *J Am Coll Cardiol* 2001;38:478–485.
14. Newby LK, Christenson RH, Ohman EM, et al. Value of serial troponin T measures for early and late risk stratification in patients with acute coronary syndromes. The GUSTO-IIa Investigators. *Circulation* 1998;98:1853–1859.
15. Alpert JS, Thygesen K, Antman E, et al. Myocardial infarction redefined—a consensus document of The Joint European Society of Cardiology/American College of Cardiology Committee for the redefinition of myocardial infarction. *J Am Coll Cardiol* 2000;36:959–969.
16. Aviles RJ, Askari AT, Lindahl B, et al. Troponin T levels in patients with acute coronary syndromes, with or without renal dysfunction. *N Engl J Med* 2002;346:2047–2052.

17. Han JH, Lindsell CJ, Ryan RJ, et al. Changes in cardiac troponin T measurements are associated with adverse cardiac events in patients with chronic kidney disease. *Am J Emerg Med* 2005;23(4):468–473.
18. James S, Armstrong P, Califf R, et al. Troponin T levels and risk of 30-day outcomes in patients with the acute coronary syndrome: prospective verification in the GUSTO-IV trial. *Am J Med* 2003;115:178–184.
19. Jaffe AS. Elevations in cardiac troponin measurements: false false-positives: the real truth. *Cardiovasc Toxicol* 2001;1:87–92.
20. Novis DA, Jones BA, Dale JC, et al. Biochemical markers of myocardial injury test turnaround time: a College of American Pathologists Q-Probes study of 7020 troponin and 4368 creatine kinase-MB determinations in 159 institutions. *Arch Pathol Lab Med* 2004;128:158–164.
21. James SK, Lindahl B, Armstrong P, et al. A rapid troponin I assay is not optimal for determination of troponin status and prediction of subsequent events at suspicion of unstable coronary syndromes. *Int J Cardiol* 2004;93:113–120.
22. Yusuf S, Collins R, MacMahon S, et al. Effect of intravenous nitrates on mortality in acute myocardial infarction: an overview of the randomised trials. *Lancet* 1988;1:1088–1092.
23. Armstrong P. Stable ischemic syndromes: section 2: clinical cardiology (Califf RM, section ed). In: Topol EJ, ed. *Textbook of cardiovascular medicine.* Philadelphia: Lippincott-Raven; 1998:351–353.
24. White HD. Unstable angina: ischemic syndromes. In: Topol EJ, ed. *Textbook of cardiovascular medicine.* Philadelphia: Lippincott-Raven; 1998:365–394.
25. Gibson RS, Boden WE, Theroux P, et al. Diltiazem and re-infarction in patients with non-Q-wave myocardial infarction. Results of a double-blind, randomized, multicenter trial. *N Engl J Med* 1986;315:423–429.
26. Lubsen J, Tijssen JG. Efficacy of nifedipine and metoprolol in the early treatment of unstable angina in the coronary care unit: findings from the Holland Interuniversity Nifedipine/Metoprolol Trial (HINT). *Am J Cardiol* 1987;60:18A–25A.
27. Indications for ACE inhibitors in the early treatment of acute myocardial infarction: systematic overview of individual data from 100000 patients in randomized trials. ACE Inhibitor Myocardial Infarction Collaborative Group. *Circulation* 1998;97:2202–2212.
28. Flather M, Yusuf S, Kober L, et al. Long-term ACE-inhibitor therapy in patients with heart failure or left-ventricular dysfunction: a systematic overview of data from individual patients. ACE-Inhibitor Myocardial Infarction Collaborative Group. *Lancet* 2000;355:1575–1581.
29. Pfeffer MA, McMurray J, Leizorovicz A, et al. Valsartan in acute myocardial infarction trial (VALIANT): rationale and design [trial results presented at: American Heart Association Scientific Sessions; November 2003; Orlando, FL.] *Am Heart J* 2000;140:727–750.
30. Yusuf S, Wittes J, Friedman L. Overview of results of randomized clinical trials in heart disease. II. Unstable angina, heart failure, primary prevention with aspirin and risk factor modification. *JAMA* 1988;260:2259–2263.
31. Collaborative overview of randomized trials of antiplatelet therapy, I: prevention of death, myocardial infarction, and stroke by prolonged antiplatelet therapy in various categories of patients. Antiplatelet Trialists' Collaboration. *BMJ* 1994;308:81–106.
32. Yusuf S, Zhao F, Mehta SR, et al. Effects of clopidogrel in addition to aspirin in patients with acute coronary syndromes without ST-segment elevation. *N Engl J Med* 2001; 345:494–502.
33. Antman EM. Glycoprotein IIb/IIIa inhibitors in patients with unstable angina/non-ST-segment elevation myocardial infarction: appropriate interpretation of the guidelines. *Am Heart J* 2003;146:S18–S22.
34. Cannon CP, Weintraub WS, Demopoulos LA, et al. TACTICS Comparison of early invasive and conservative strategies in patients with unstable coronary syndromes treated with the glycoprotein IIb/IIIa inhibitor tirofiban. *N Engl J Med* 2001;344:1879–1887.
35. Boersma E, Akkerhuis KM, Theroux P, et al. Platelet glycoprotein IIb-IIIa receptor inhibition in non-ST-elevation acute coronary syndromes: early benefit during medical treatment only, with additional protection during percutaneous coronary intervention. *Circulation* 1999;100:2045–2048.
36. Kong DF, Califf RM, Miller DP, et al. Clinical outcomes of therapeutic agents that block the platelet glycoprotein IIb/IIIa integrin in ischemic heart disease. *Circulation* 1998;98:2829–2835.
37. Inhibition of platelet glycoprotein IIb-IIIa with eptifibatide in patients with acute coronary syndromes. The PURSUIT Trial Investigators. Platelet Glycoprotein IIb/IIIa in Unstable Angina: Receptor Suppression Using Integrilin Therapy. *N Engl J Med* 1998;339:436–443.
38. Simoons ML. GUSTO IV-ACS Investigators. Effect of glycoprotein IIb/IIIa receptor blocker abciximab on outcome in patients with acute coronary syndromes without early coronary revascularization: the GUSTO IV-ACS randomised trial. *Lancet* 2001;357:1915–1924.
39. Lincoff AM. Direct thrombin inhibitors for non-ST-segment elevation acute coronary syndromes: what, when and where? *Am Heart J* 2003;146:S23–S30.
40. Oler A, Whooley MA, Oler J, et al. Adding heparin to aspirin reduces the incidence of myocardial infarction and death in patients with unstable angina. A meta-analysis. *JAMA* 1996;276:811–815.
41. Antman EM. Hirudin in acute myocardial infarction. Thrombolysis and Thrombin Inhibition in Myocardial Infarction (TIMI) 9B trial. *Circulation* 1996;94:911–921.
42. Antman EM, Cohen M, Radley D, et al. Assessment of the treatment effect of enoxaparin for unstable angina/non-Q-wave myocardial infarction. TIMI 11 B-ESSENCE meta-analysis. *Circulation* 1999;100:1602–1608.
43. Ferguson J, Califf R, Antman E, et al. Enoxaparin vs unfractionated heparin in high-risk patients with non-ST-segment elevation acute coronary syndromes managed with an intended early invasive strategy: primary results of the SYNERGY randomized trial. *JAMA* 2004;292:45–54.
44. Petersen JL, Mahaffey KW, Hasselblad V, et al. Efficacy and bleeding complications among patients randomized to enoxaparin or unfractionated heparin for antithrombin therapy in non-ST-segment elevation acute coronary syndromes: a systematic overview. *JAMA* 2004;292:89–96.
45. MICHELANGELO OASIS 5 Steering Committee. An international randomized double-blind study evaluating the efficacy and safety of fondaparinux versus enoxaparin in the acute treatment of unstable angina/non ST-segment elevation MI acute coronary syndromes. *Am Heart J* 2005;150(6):1107.
46. Kleiman NS, Lincoff AM, Flaker GC, et al. Early percutaneous coronary intervention, platelet inhibition with eptifibatide, and clinical outcomes in patients with acute coronary syndromes. PURSUIT Investigators. *Circulation* 2000;101:751–757.
47. Sabatine MS, Cannon CP, Gibson CM, et al. Effect of clopidogrel pretreatment before percutaneous coronary intervention in patients with ST-elevation myocardial infarction treated with fibrinolytics: The PCI-CLARITY Study. *JAMA* 2005;294:1224–1232.
48. Sabatine MS, Cannon CP, Gibson CM, et al. Addition of clopidogrel to aspirin and fibrinolytic therapy for myocardial infarction with ST-segment elevation. *N Engl J Med* 2005;352:1179–1189.
49. Allison JJ, Kiefe CI, Weissman NW, et al. Relationship of hospital teaching status with quality of care and mortality for Medicare patients with acute MI. *JAMA* 2000;284:1256–1262.
50. Alexander KP, Peterson ED, Granger CB, et al. Potential impact of evidence-based medicine in acute coronary syndromes: insights from GUSTO-IIb. Global use of strategies to open occluded arteries in acute coronary syndromes trial. *J Am Coll Cardiol* 1998;32:2023–2030.
51. Cabana MD, Rand CS, Powe NR, et al. Why don't physicians follow clinical practice guidelines? A framework for improvement. *JAMA* 1999;282:1458–1465.
52. Califf RM, Faxon DP. Need for centers to care for patients with acute coronary syndromes. *Circulation* 2003;107:1467–1470.
53. Fuster V, Badimon L, Badimon JJ, et al. The pathogenesis of coronary artery disease and the acute coronary syndromes. *N Engl J Med* 1992;326:242–250.
54. Gibbons RJ, Smith S, Antman E, et al. American College of Cardiology/ American Heart Association clinical practice guidelines, part I: where do they come from? *Circulation* 2003;107:2979–2986.
55. Gibbons RJ, Smith SC, Antman E, et al. American College of Cardiology/ American Heart Association clinical practice guidelines, part II: evolutionary changes in a continuous quality improvement project. *Circulation* 2003; 107:3101–3107.
56. Grilli R, Magrini N, Penna A, et al. Practice guidelines developed by specialty societies: the need for a critical appraisal. *Lancet* 2000;355:103–106.
57. Hamm CW, Bertrand M, Braunwald E. Acute coronary syndrome without ST elevation: implementation of new guidelines. *Lancet* 2001;358:1533–1538.
58. Leape LL, Weissman JS, Schneider EC, et al. Adherence to practice guidelines: the role of specialty society guidelines. *Am Heart J* 2003;145:19–26.
59. Boden WE, Pepine CJ. Introduction to "optimizing management of non-ST-segment elevation acute coronary syndromes." Harmonizing advances in mechanical and pharmacologic intervention. *J Am Coll Cardiol* 2003;41:1S–6S.
60. Prevention of cardiovascular events and death with pravastatin in patients with coronary heart disease and a broad range of initial cholesterol levels. The Long-Term Intervention with Pravastatin in Ischemic Disease (LIPID) Study Group. *N Engl J Med* 1998;339:1349–1357.
61. Biviano AB, Rabbani LE, Paultre F, et al. Usefulness of an acute coronary syndrome pathway to improve adherence to secondary prevention guidelines. *Am J Cardiol* 2003;91:1248–1250.
62. Mehta RH, Montoye CK, Gallogly M, et al. Improving quality of care for acute myocardial infarction: The Guidelines Applied in Practice (GAP) Initiative. *JAMA* 2002;287:1269–1276.
63. Fonarow GC, Gawlinski A, Moughrabi S, et al. Improved treatment of coronary heart disease by implementation of a cardiac hospitalization atherosclerosis management program (CHAMP). *Am J Cardiol* 2001;87:819–822.
64. Fonarow GC, Gawlinski A. Rationale and design of the Cardiac Hospitalization Atherosclerosis Management Program at the University of California Los Angeles. *Am J Cardiol* 2000;85:10A–17A.
65. Hoekstra J, Pollack CV Jr, Roe MT, et al. Improving the care of patients with non-ST-elevation acute coronary syndromes in the emergency department: the CRUSADE initiative. *Acad Emerg Med* 2002;9:1146–1155.
66. Staman KL, Roe MR, Fraulo ES, et al. Quality improvement tools designed to improve adherence to the ACC/AHA guidelines for the care of patients with non-ST-segment acute coronary syndromes: the CRUSADE quality improvement initiative. *Crit Pathways Cardiol* 2003;2:34–40.
67. JCAHO. Specification Manual for National Hospital Quality Measures. Oakbrook, IL: Author; 2005.

CHAPTER 6 ■ THROMBOLYSIS FOR ST-ELEVATION MYOCARDIAL INFARCTION IN THE EMERGENCY DEPARTMENT

JOSHUA M. KOSOWKSY

OVERVIEW
INITIAL ED EVALUATION
THROMBOLYSIS VERSUS PCI
CHOICE OF THROMBOLYTIC AGENT
ADJUNCTIVE THERAPY FOR PATIENTS UNDERGOING
    THROMBOLYSIS
RESCUE PCI
INTRACRANIAL HEMORRHAGE
SUMMARY

OVERVIEW

Patients with acute ST-segment elevation myocardial infarction (STEMI) comprise the population at highest risk among patients with chest pain who present to the emergency department (ED). These patients require not only prompt diagnosis and treatment, but also often need immediate stabilization. The advent of highly effective, time-dependent treatment for STEMI makes the application of critical pathways to this population especially appropriate.

INITIAL ED EVALUATION

All patients presenting with symptoms suggestive of STEMI should undergo rapid evaluation for possible reperfusion therapy (Fig. 6-1 and Table 6-1). Among patients with suspected STEMI and without contraindications, the prompt use of reperfusion therapy is associated with improved survival (1).

The delay from patient arrival at the ED to initiation of thrombolytic therapy should be less than 30 minutes; alternatively, if percutaneous coronary intervention (PCI) is chosen, the delay from patient arrival at the ED to balloon inflation should be less than 90 minutes (2). Because there is not an interval considered to be a threshold effect for the benefit of shorter times to reperfusion, these goals should not be understood as "ideal" times, but rather as the longest times considered acceptable. On the other hand, these goals may not be relevant for patients with an appropriate reason for delay, such as uncertainty about the diagnosis, need for evaluation and treatment of other life-threatening conditions, or delays associated with the patient's informed choice to have more time to consider the decision.

The history taken in the ED must be thorough enough to establish the likelihood of STEMI, but should be obtained expeditiously so as not to delay implementation of reperfusion

therapy. It is important to consider that the differential diagnosis may include conditions that can be exacerbated by thrombolysis and anticoagulation. For example, severe tearing pain radiating directly to the back should raise the suspicion of aortic dissection, and appropriate studies should be undertaken.

Patients should be questioned about previous bleeding problems, history of ulcer disease, cerebral vascular accidents, unexplained anemia, or melena. In addition, patients should be asked about previous ischemic stroke, intracerebral hemorrhage, or subarachnoid hemorrhage. The use of antiplatelet, antithrombin, and thrombolytic agents as part of the treatment for STEMI will exacerbate any underlying bleeding risks. Hypertension should be assessed, because chronic, severe, poorly controlled hypertension and severe uncontrolled hypertension on presentation are relative contraindications to thrombolytic therapy (Table 6-2).

The 12-lead electrocardiogram (ECG) is critical to the decision pathway because of strong evidence that ST-segment elevation identifies patients who benefit from reperfusion therapy (3). A 12-lead ECG should be performed and shown to an experienced emergency physician within 10 minutes of ED arrival on all patients with symptoms suggestive of STEMI. If the initial ECG is not diagnostic, the patient remains symptomatic, and there is a high clinical suspicion for STEMI, serial ECGs at 5- to 10-minute intervals should be performed. For patients with left bundle branch block (LBBB) not known to be new, bedside echocardiography may be helpful in clarifying the diagnosis of STEMI. If the diagnosis remains in doubt, PCI may, in fact, be preferable to thrombolytic therapy (see later discussion).

Most clinical trials have demonstrated the potential for functional, clinical, and mortality benefits only when thrombolytic therapy is given *within 12 hours*. However, it is reasonable to administer therapy to patients with 12 to 24 hours of continuing symptoms who meet ECG criteria for thrombolysis.

THROMBOLYSIS VERSUS PCI

Controversy remains about which form of reperfusion therapy is superior in particular clinical settings. Part of the uncertainty derives from the continual introduction of new agents, devices, and strategies, which quickly make previous studies less relevant to contemporary practice. As a result, the evidence base regarding the best approach to reperfusion therapy is somewhat dynamic.

The availability of interventional cardiology facilities is a key determinant of whether PCI can be provided. For facilities that can offer PCI, the literature generally suggests that this approach is superior to pharmacological reperfusion (4) (although many of the trials comparing pharmacological and PCI

39

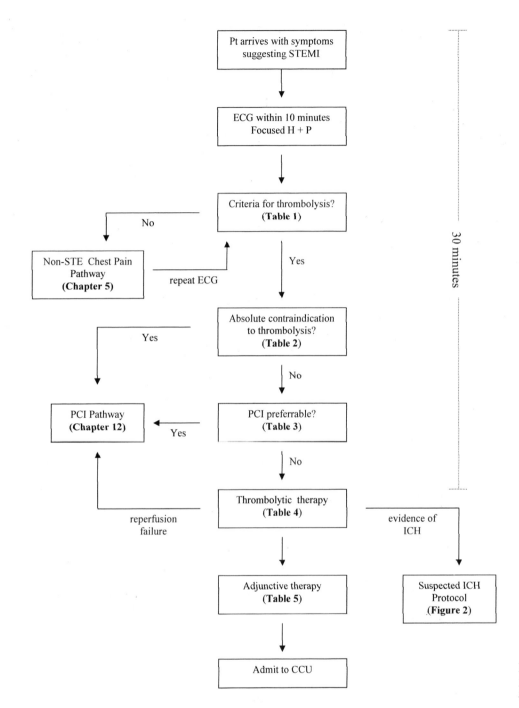

FIGURE 6-1. Thrombolysis pathway for STEMI in the emergency department.

strategies were conducted before the advent of more recent strategies). Still, not all laboratories can provide prompt, high-quality primary PCI with the staffing required for 24-hour coverage. Even when round-the-clock coverage is available, the volume of cases in the laboratory may be insufficient for the team to acquire and maintain skills required for rapid PCI reperfusion strategies.

Patient-specific factors also come into play. For example, longer duration of symptoms at presentation tends to favor a PCI strategy, because the ability to produce a patent infarct artery is much less dependent on symptom duration in patients undergoing PCI than in patients undergoing thrombolysis (5). Also, when estimated mortality is extremely high, as is the case in patients with cardiogenic shock, the evidence clearly favors a PCI strategy (6).

The option of transferring patients to another facility for PCI raises additional considerations. Delays in door-to-balloon time versus door-to-needle time of more than 60 minutes because of interhospital transfer appear to negate any mortality benefit of primary PCI over immediate thrombolysis (7,8). At the same time, the DANAMI-2 trial found that patients had better composite outcomes when transferred for PCI within 2 hours of presentation than when treated with thrombolytics at local hospitals without PCI capabilities (9). On the basis of these and other studies, the 2004 American College of Cardiology/American Heart Association (ACC/AHA) Guidelines recommend that if PCI capability is not accessible within 90 minutes, STEMI patients should undergo thrombolysis unless contraindicated.

Facilitated PCI refers to a strategy of initiating thrombolytic

TABLE 6-1

CRITERIA FOR THROMBOLYSIS IN STEMI

Clinical Criteria	ECG Criteria
Onset of ischemic symptoms within 12 hours	ST elevation greater than 0.1 mV in at least 2 contiguous precordial leads
	OR
	ST elevation greater than 0.1 mV in at least 2 contiguous precordial leads
	OR
	New or presumably new LBBB

Adapted from 2004 ACC/AHA Practice Guidelines.

therapy prior to PCI, particularly when a delay to PCI is anticipated. Theoretical advantages include earlier time to reperfusion, improved patient stability, greater procedural success rates, and higher thrombosis in myocardial infarction flow rates. Unfortunately, recent studies have not demonstrated any benefit in reducing infarct size or improving patient outcomes (10–12).

Given the current state of the literature, one cannot state definitively that a particular reperfusion approach is superior for all patients, in all clinical settings, at all times of day (Table 6-3). What is most important is that some type of reperfusion therapy be selected for every appropriate patient with STEMI.

Case-by-case determinations run the risk of delaying reperfusion by unnecessarily confounding the decision-making process. Instead, the choice of strategy is typically made on the basis of a predetermined, institution-specific protocol that represents a collaborative effort from cardiologists, emergency physicians, nurses, and other appropriate personnel. For non-interventional hospitals, this may entail formal agreements allowing the expeditious transfer of patients to the nearest appropriate interventional facility. In truly complex cases that are not covered directly by an agreed-on protocol, immediate cardiology consultation is advisable.

CHOICE OF THROMBOLYTIC AGENT

Over the past two decades, various thrombolytic regimens have been approved for use in STEMI, and each has its strengths and weaknesses (Table 6-4). On the whole, however, the differences among regimens are relatively minor. The literature suggests that accelerated-dose alteplase with intravenous heparin provides a mortality advantage over streptokinase, although it is substantially more expensive and confers a slightly greater risk of intracranial hemorrhage (ICH) (13). Single-bolus, weight-based TNK (tenecteplase) and double-bolus reteplase are associated with virtually identical rates of mortality and similar rates of ICH to accelerated-dose alteplase (14). TNK has been shown to have a 20% lower risk of non-ICH major bleeding. Combination therapy with abciximab and half-dose reteplase or tenecteplase can be considered for prevention of reinfarction and other complications of STEMI in selected patients: anterior location of MI, age less than 75 years, and no risk factors for bleeding (15,16). However, this regimen is associated with a

TABLE 6-2

CONTRAINDICATIONS TO THROMBOLYSIS IN STEMI

Absolute Contraindications	Relative Contraindications
Any prior ICH HTN	History of chronic, severe, poorly controlled HTN
Known structural cerebral vascular lesion (e.g., arteriovenous malformation)	Severe uncontrolled HTN on presentation (SBP >180 mm Hg or DBP >100 mm HG)
Known malignant intracranial neoplasm (primary or metastatic)	History of prior ischemic stroke greater than 3 months, dementia, or other known intracranial pathology
Ischemic stroke within 3 months **EXCEPT** acute ischemic stroke within 3 hours	Traumatic or prolonged (>10 min) CPR or major surgery (<3 weeks)
Suspected aortic dissection	Recent internal bleeding (<2–4 weeks)
Active bleeding or bleeding diathesis (excluding menses)	Noncompressible vascular punctures
Significant closed-head or facial trauma within 3 months	Pregnancy
	Active peptic ulcer
	Current use of anticoagulants: the higher the INR, the higher the risk of bleeding
	For streptokinase: prior exposure (>5 days)
	or
	prior allergic reaction to these agents

Adapted from 2004 ACC/AHA Practice Guidelines.

TABLE 6-3

ASSESSMENT OF REPERFUSION OPTIONS FOR PATIENTS WITH STEMI

PCI Generally Preferred	Thrombolysis Generally Preferred
Skilled PCI lab available with surgical backup and time to balloon up to <90 min	Early presentation <3 hours from symptom onset and delay to PCI
High-risk STEMI patient Cardiogenic shock Killip class ≥3	Invasive strategy not an option Cath lab occupied/not available No vascular access Lack of access to a skilled PCI lab
Relative contraindication to thrombolysis (including increased bleeding risk)	Delay to PCI Prolonged transport
Late presentation >3 hours from symptom onset	Door-to-balloon >90 min (Door-to-balloon)–(door-to-needle) >1 hr
Diagnosis of STEMI in doubt (e.g., LBBB not known to be new)	

Adapted from 2004 ACC/AHA Practice Guidelines.

doubling in the risk of major bleeding and is more complicated, hence it is not widely used. Once again, making the appropriate decision to administer a thrombolytic without delay is generally more important than which regimen is chosen. Therefore, the choice of thrombolytic regimen is often determined by protocol at the institutional level.

ADJUNCTIVE THERAPY FOR PATIENTS UNDERGOING THROMBOLYSIS

Adjunctive therapy plays a key role in the overall management of patients undergoing thrombolysis for STEMI, facilitat-

ing and maintaining coronary reperfusion, limiting the consequences of myocardial ischemia, and reducing the likelihood of recurrent events (Table 6-5).

Standard therapies such as oxygen, nitrates, and morphine are important in terms of maximizing myocardial oxygen delivery and relieving ischemic discomfort and/or pulmonary congestion. Aspirin, at an initial dose of 162 to 325 mg, should be chewed by patients who have not taken aspirin before presentation (17). Unlike thrombolytic agents, there is little evidence of a time-dependent effect of aspirin on early mortality. However, data do support the contention that a chewable aspirin is absorbed more quickly than one swallowed. Aspirin suppositories (300 mg) can be used safely and are the recommended route of administration for patients with severe nausea and vomiting or known upper-gastrointestinal disorders. In

TABLE 6-4

COMPARISON OF APPROVED FIBRINOLYTIC AGENTS

	Streptokinase	Alteplase	Reteplase	Tenecteplase—tPA
Dose	1.5 MU over 30–69 min	Up to 100 mg in 90 min[1]	10 U over 2 min, repeated at 30 min[2]	<60 kg: 30 mg 60–69 kg: 35 mg 70–79 kg: 40 mg 80–90 kg: 45 mg >90 kg: 50 mg[3]
Bolus administration	No	No	Yes	Yes
Antigenic	Yes	No	No	No
Systemic fibrinogen depletion	Marked	Mild	Moderate	Minimal
90-min patency rates	50%	75%	7%	75%
TIMI grade 3 flow	32%	54%	60%	63%
Cost per dose	$613	$2,974	$2,750	$2,833 for 50 mg

[1] Bolus 15 mg, then infusion 0.75 mg/kg over 30 minutes (max 50 mg), then 0.5 mg/kg over 60 min (max 35 mg).
[2] If given as combination therapy with abciximab, administer first dose only.
[3] If given as combination therapy with abciximab, administer half of weight-based dose.

TABLE 6-5

ADJUNCTIVE THERAPY FOR STEMI PATIENTS UNDERGOING THROMBOLYSIS

Adjunctive therapy to thrombolysis
Oxygen, nitroglycerin (SL and/or IV), morphine
ASA, 162–325 mg chewed (if not already administered)
Clopidogrel, 300 mg PO
Metoprolol, 5–15 mg IV, if no contraindications
UFH, bolus of 60 U/kg (maximum 4,000 U) followed by infusion of 12 U/kg/hr (maximum 1,000 U)*

*Enoxaparin (30-mg IV bolus followed by 1.0 mg/kg SC every 12 hours) is a reasonable option in patients <75 years of age and without significant renal dysfunction.

patients with true aspirin allergy, clopidogrel should be administered.

Evidence from two recent large trials suggests that the addition of clopidogrel 75 mg daily (with a 300-mg loading dose in one trial of patients <75 years old) to aspirin and standard thrombolytic therapy reduces morbidity and mortality (18,19). Clopidogrel should not be withheld because of concerns about a potential future need for surgical revascularization, as fewer than 5% of STEMI patients require urgent coronary artery bypass grafting (CABG).

It is reasonable to administer intravenous beta-blocker therapy promptly to STEMI patients who do not have contraindications, especially if tachycardia or hypertension is present. However, data on the early use of intravenous beta-blockade in STEMI are inconclusive, and patterns of use vary (20). Relative contraindications to beta-blocker therapy include bradycardia, hypotension, moderate or severe left ventricular failure, signs of peripheral hypoperfusion or shock, second- or third-degree atrioventricular block, and active asthma. Beta-blockers should not be administered to patients with STEMI precipitated by cocaine use because of the risk of exacerbating coronary spasm (21).

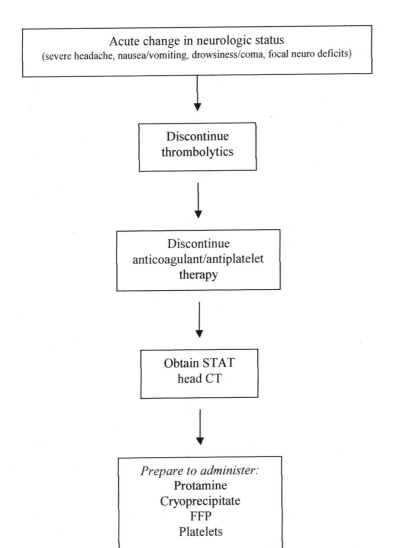

FIGURE 6-2. Suspected intracranial hemorrhage protocol

Unfractionated heparin (UFH) should be given intravenously to patients undergoing reperfusion therapy with alteplase, reteplase, or tenecteplase according to weight-based dosing. A bolus of 60 U/kg (maximum 4,000 U) is administered, followed by an infusion of 12 U/kg/hr (maximum 1,000 U). It may also be reasonable to administer UFH intravenously to patients undergoing reperfusion therapy with streptokinase. Low-molecular-weight heparin is an acceptable alternative to UFH for patients younger than 75 years of age who are receiving thrombolytic therapy, provided that significant renal dysfunction (serum creatinine greater than 2.5 mg/dL in men or 2.0 mg/dL in women) is not present. Enoxaparin (30-mg IV bolus followed by 1.0 mg/kg SC every 12 hours until hospital discharge) used in combination with full-dose tenecteplase is the most comprehensively studied regimen (16).

RESCUE PCI

Intravenous thrombolytic therapy successfully restores coronary TIMI 2/3 flow at 90 minutes in only 50% to 85% of patients with STEMI (22). Nevertheless, multiple randomized, prospective trials have failed to show benefit to performing *routine PCI* of the infarct-related artery immediately following thrombolytic therapy (23–25). In contrast, *rescue PCI* (or *salvage PCI*)—defined as PCI performed within 12 hours after *failed thrombolysis*—is associated with reductions in morbidity that are maintained up to 1 year (26).

Persistence of unrelenting ischemic chest pain, absence of resolution of ST-segment elevation (by 50% or more), and hemodynamic or electrical instability generally indicate failed pharmacological reperfusion and the need to consider rescue PCI. Unfortunately, these clinical markers of reperfusion have limited predictive value (27). If failure of thrombolysis is not recognized and corrected quickly (within 3 to 6 hours of onset of symptoms), salvage of ischemic myocardium is unlikely.

INTRACRANIAL HEMORRHAGE

Intracranial hemorrhage represents the most important risk of thrombolytic therapy and may be fatal in one-half to two-thirds of patients. Fortunately, the risk of ICH using any of the standard thrombolytic regimens falls below 1% (2). Nevertheless, the occurrence of a change in neurological status during or after reperfusion therapy, particularly within the first 24 hours after initiation of treatment, should be considered to be due to ICH until proven otherwise. Thrombolytic, antiplatelet, and anticoagulant therapies should be discontinued until brain imaging has ruled this out (Fig. 6-2).

SUMMARY

Few areas in medicine have evolved as dramatically over the past 30 years as the approach to the patient with STEMI. Large, randomized clinical trials have proven the efficacy of multiple thrombolytic regimens, alone and in conjunction with various antiplatelet and antithrombotic therapies, in reducing infarct size, recurrent events, and mortality. The proliferation of therapies adds to the complexity of treating STEMI in the ED and inserts additional time pressures, not to mention increasing the opportunity for error. A well-designed critical pathway, supported by the literature and agreed on by cardiologists and emergency physicians, represents the best approach to incorporating these crucial interventions safely into daily clinical use.

REFERENCES

1. Thrombolytic Therapy Trialists' (FTT) Collaborative Group. Indications for thrombolytic therapy in suspected acute myocardial infarction: collaborative overview of early mortality and major morbidity results from all randomised trials of more than 1000 patients. *Lancet* 1994;343:311–322.
2. ACC/AHA guidelines for the management of patients with ST-elevation myocardial infarction—executive summary: a report of the American College of Cardiology/American Heart Association Task Force on Practice Guidelines. *Circulation* 2004;110:588–636
3. Menown IB, Mackenzie G, Adgey AA. Optimizing the initial 12-lead electrocardiographic diagnosis of acute myocardial infarction. *Eur Heart J* 2000; 21:275–283.
4. Keeley EC, Boura JA, Grines CL. Primary angioplasty versus intravenous thrombolytic therapy for acute myocardial infarction: a quantitative review of 23 randomised trials. *Lancet* 2003;361:13–20.
5. Zeymer U, Tebbe U, Essen R, Haarmann W, Neuhaus KL, for the ALKK-Study Group. Influence of time to treatment on early infarct-related artery patency after different thrombolytic regimens. *Am Heart J* 1999;137:34–38.
6. Wu AH, Parsons L, Every NR, Bates ER, for the Second National Registry of Myocardial Infarction. Hospital outcomes in patients presenting with congestive heart failure complicating acute myocardial infarction: a report from the Second National Registry of Myocardial Infarction (NRMI-2). *J Am Coll Cardiol* 2002;40:1389–1394.
7. Gore JM, Granger CB, Simoons ML, et al. Stroke after thrombolysis: mortality and functional outcomes in the GUSTO-I trial. Global Use of Strategies to Open Occluded Arteries. *Circulation* 1995;92:2794–2795.
8. Nallamothu BK, Bates ER. Percutaneous coronary intervention versus thrombolytic therapy in acute myocardial infarction: is timing (almost) everything? *Am J Cardiol* 2003;92:824–826.
9. Andersen HR, Nielsen TT, Rasmussen K, et al, for the DANAMI- 2 Investigators. A comparison of coronary angioplasty with thrombolytic therapy in acute myocardial infarction. *N Engl J Med* 2003;349:733–742.
10. Kastrati A, Mehilli J, Schlotterbeck K, et al. Early administration of reteplase plus abciximab vs abciximab alone in patients with acute myocardial infarction referred for percutaneous coronary intervention: a randomized controlled trial. *JAMA* 2004;291:947–954.
11. Facilitated percutaneous coronary intervention for acute ST-segment elevation myocardial infarction: Results from the prematurely terminated ADdressing the Value of facilitated Angioplasty after Combination therapy or Eptifibatide monotherapy in acute Myocardial Infarction (ADVANCE MI) trial. *Am Heart J* 2005;150:116–122.
12. ASSENT-4: Assessment of the Safety and Efficacy of a New Thrombolytic Regimen - 4. European Society of Cardiology Congress, Stockholm, Sweden, September 2005.
13. The GUSTO investigators. An international randomized trial comparing four thrombolytic strategies for acute myocardial infarction. *N Engl J Med* 1993;329:673–682.
14. Single-bolus tenecteplase compared with front-loaded alteplase in acute myocardial infarction: the ASSENT-2 double-blind randomized trial. Assessment of the Safety and Efficacy of a New Thrombolytic Investigators. *Lancet* 1999;354:716–722.
15. Topol EJ, for the GUSTO V Investigators. Reperfusion therapy or acute myocardial infarction with thrombolytic therapy or combination reduced thrombolytic therapy and platelet glycoprotein IIb/IIIa inhibition: the GUSTO V randomised trial. *Lancet* 2001;357:1905–1914.
16. Assessment of the Safety and Efficacy of a New Thrombolytic Regimen (ASSENT)-3 Investigators. Efficacy and safety of tenecteplase in combination with enoxaparin, abciximab, or unfractionated heparin: the ASSENT-3 randomised trial in acute myocardial infarction. *Lancet* 2001;358:605–613.
17. Antithrombotic Trialists' Collaboration. Collaborative metaanalysis of randomised trials of antiplatelet therapy for prevention of death, myocardial infarction, and stroke in high-risk patients. *BMJ* 2002;324:71–86.
18. Sabatine MS, Cannon CP, Gibson CM, et al. Addition of clopidogrel to aspirin and thrombolytic therapy for myocardial infarction with ST elevation. *N Engl J M* 2005;352:1179–1189.
19. COMMIT/CCS-2: Clopidogrel and Metoprolol in Myocardial Infarction Trial/Second Chinese Cardiac Study. European Society of Cardiology Congress, Stockholm, Sweden, September 2005.
20. Freemantle N, Cleland J, Young P, Mason J, Harrison J. Beta blockade after myocardial infarction: systematic review and meta regression analysis. *BMJ* 1999;318:1730–1737.
21. Kloner RA, Hale S. Unraveling the complex effects of cocaine on the heart. *Circulation* 1993;87:1046–1047.
22. Granger CB, White HD, Bates ER, Ohman EM, Califf RM. A pooled analysis of coronary arterial patency and left ventricular function after intravenous thrombolysis for acute myocardial infarction. *Am J Cardiol* 1994;74: 1220–1228.
23. The TIMI Research Group. Immediate vs delayed catheterization and angioplasty following thrombolytic therapy for acute myocardial infarction: TIMI II A results. *JAMA* 1988;260:2849–2858.
24. Topol EJ, Califf RM, George BS, et al. A randomized trial of immediate

versus delayed elective angioplasty after intravenous tissue plasminogen activator in acute myocardial infarction. *N Engl J Med* 1987;317:581–588.

25. Simoons ML, Arnold AE, Betriu A, et al. Thrombolysis with tissue plasminogen activator in acute myocardial infarction: no additional benefit from immediate percutaneous coronary angioplasty. *Lancet* 1988;1:197–203.

26. Ellis SG, da Silva ER, Heyndrickx G, et al. Randomized comparison of rescue angioplasty with conservative management of patients with early failure of thrombolysis for acute anterior myocardial infarction. *Circulation* 1994;90:2280–2284.

27. Goldman LE, Eisenberg MJ. Identification and management of patients with failed thrombolysis after acute myocardial infarction. *Ann Intern Med* 2000; 132:556–565.

CHAPTER 7 ■ HEART FAILURE IN THE EMERGENCY DEPARTMENT

W. FRANK PEACOCK

DEMOGRAPHICS
DISEASE MANAGEMENT
OBSERVATIONS FROM ADHERE-EM
CHEST RADIOGRAPHY
DIAGNOSIS WITH NATRIURETIC PEPTIDES
CLINICAL TRIALS USING NATRIURETIC PEPTIDES FOR
    ED DECISION MAKING
PHYSIOLOGY: HEMODYNAMIC MISMATCH, NOT
    VOLUME OVERLOAD
RISK STRATIFICATION
EARLY USE OF VASOACTIVE THERAPY: IMPLICATIONS
    OF RISK STRATIFICATION
ADHERE-EM DISEASE MANAGEMENT
CONCLUSIONS

DEMOGRAPHICS

Heart failure (HF) is the most common reason for hospitalization in patients older than age 65 and is the most common reason for rehospitalization in the same group. It accounts for more costs to Medicare than any other single disease entity. The money spent annually on HF in the United States exceeds the gross domestic product of Kuwait.

The prevalence of HF has risen sharply, resulting in part from the rapid growth of the elderly population, improved survival following acute myocardial infarction and treatment of chronic hypertension (1). As expected, the number of HF hospitalizations has also risen. In 2004, there were over 1 million HF hospitalizations in the United States and another 1 million in Europe. It is estimated that these hospitalizations account for more than 75% of the 46 billion dollars spent each year on the care of HF patients (2).

Our understanding of the demographics of HF has evolved significantly over the last decade. If clinical trials were to define the HF population, the typical patient might be described as outlined in Table 7-1. However, large databases show that clinical trials do not reflect the true HF population. The Acute Decompensated Heart Failure National Registry (ADHERE) has contributed importantly to our current understanding of HF. This registry includes hospitalization information on patients discharged with a diagnosis of, or primary treatment for, acute decompensated heart failure (ADHF) (Diagnostic Related Group 127). The registry contains information on greater than 200,000 ADHF hospitalizations and can be examined to determine current patient demographics and treatment regimens for ADHF. Evaluation of this data set indicates that the average ADHF patient is much older, more often female, and burdened by more coexistent disease than previously appreciated (see Table 7-1).

The ADHERE registry has also provided important information regarding the process of care. Most patients ultimately diagnosed with ADHF present to the emergency department (ED). Of the overall inpatient ADHF population, 78% were admitted through the ED. In the hospitalized population, the chief complaint is remarkably consistent, with 89% reporting shortness of breath. Once admitted to the hospital, 79% of ADHF patients are placed in either a telemetry bed (66%) or an intensive care unit (ICU) (13%). These admission destinations represent some of the greatest costs for the U.S. hospital system and suggest opportunities for improved management strategies. As a consequence, in an effort to decrease the cost associated with inpatient admission, reimbursement strategies to encourage short stay observation unit treatment have been structured. Usually managed as part of an emergency visit, observation unit admissions increased approximately 100% between 2003 and 2004. Finally, even in the patient destined for hospitalization, because most admissions arise following an ED visit, appropriate ED evaluation and intervention are required to initiate quality care.

TABLE 7-1

PATIENTS IN RANDOMIZED CONTROLLED TRIALS

Age:	50–60 years old
Sex:	70% to 80% men
Comorbidities:	Diabetes 20% to 25%
Renal insufficiency:	Infrequent (mean Cr 1.1 to 1.3)
Ventricular function:	75% to 80% systolic dysfunction (LVEF<0.40)
PAC use:	30% to 40%
In hospital mortality:	1.5% to 2.5%

Patients from ADHERE Database

Median age	75 years
Female gender	52%
Race White	72%
Black	20%
History of HF	75%
Ejection fraction <40%	59%
Hospitalized within 6 months	23%
Chronic renal insufficiency (creatinine >1.5 mg/dL)	30%
Systolic BP >90 mm Hg at presentation	98%
Initial BNP	667 pg/mL

Recently a second iteration of the ADHERE registry was begun. Specifically designated as an emergency module (ADHERE-EM), this registry records data on the emergency medicine encounter and will ultimately track outcomes for 60,000 ED ADHF patients. Additional features have been added to the ADHERE-EM registry. One of the most important improvements is the ability to track visits longitudinally, so that the long-term impact of diagnostic and treatment interventions can be evaluated. Also unique to the ADHERE-EM registry is the requirement that participating institutions implement a disease management strategy at the beginning of data collection. Participating centers are required to implement at least three of the first five disease management strategies listed in Table 7-2.

DISEASE MANAGEMENT

Historically, hospitals have approached the financial aspects of their medical operations by utilizing a departmental framework. In this manner the hospital is divided into units, with each being responsible for its own costs and profits. Although this is an attractive model for management of a chain of independent gas stations, the application to a medical facility, where reimbursements do not necessarily return equally to all participants involved in a patient's outcome, can result in impediments to quality care. For example, the department of cardiology may wish to use an expensive therapy because it is able to shorten cardiology care unit (CCU) length of stay by 1 day and improve their DRG remuneration margin. However, the pharmacy may be less than enthusiastic due to the fact that they must provide this medication at increased costs to their budget, but not receive any direct pharmacy department value from a shorter CCU admission.

Disease management is therefore the principle of removing artificial barriers to improved patient outcomes so that all the participants involved in ADHF care are similarly invested and rewarded based on the final clinical outcome, rather than their individual departmental financial result. This approach is particularly attractive in chronic disease management, such as ADHF, where a number of studies have demonstrated shorter length of hospitalization, a lower revisit frequency (3,4), and a decreased mortality when disease management has been applied to HF (3). In a recent meta-analysis of 29 trials that included over 5,000 HF patients, they demonstrated that when multidisciplinary team follow-up was used, there was a reduction of both mortality and HF hospitalizations by approximately 25%; mortality RR 0.75 (95% CI 0.59 to 0.96), HF hospitalizations RR 0.74 (95% CI 0.63 to 0.87) (5). One of the important parameters of disease management is that no specific therapy or device is mandated. It is merely the provision of care across departmental lines, with the shared goals of increasing quality patient outcomes.

OBSERVATIONS FROM ADHERE-EM

Initial data from the ADHERE-EM registry has already identified trends in ADHF patients that were not readily apparent from historical data. First, as would be suspected intuitively, ED patients appear to have greater severity of illness than the hospitalized cohort. Although patients admitted to the hospital by the ED constitute nearly 80% of the inpatient cohort, this population has a severity of illness that is diluted by the 20% of patients representing direct admissions from a non–acute care environment (e.g., a physician's office). Increased severity of illness in the ED ADHF population is manifest by greater rates of renal insufficiency, higher mean blood urea nitrogen (BUN) and creatinine, higher B-type natriuretic peptide (BNP) levels, and importantly, increased troponin levels. The median troponin in the ED patient with ADHF has been reported to be 0.06 ng/mL for troponin I, and 0.03 ng/mL for troponin T. Although controversial, these findings have clear outcome implications in the ED ADHF population.

In an analysis of 70,000 ADHF patients from the ADHERE data set, only 6.3% had an elevated troponin. However those with increased troponin had markedly worsened acute adverse outcomes that included longer hospitalization, longer ICU time, an increased rate of the composite of endotracheal intubation, intra-aortic balloon counterpulsation, and coronary artery bypass grafting, as well as a fourfold increase in acute mortality (Table 7-3) (6). In a separate analysis of 14,000 ADHF patients (7) with elevated troponin, those receiving vasodilator therapy had in-hospital mortality rates of only 5%, compared to 22% when inotropic therapy was used, despite risk adjustment for systolic and diastolic blood pressure, BUN, creatinine, sodium, heart rate, dyspnea at rest, and age. An elevated troponin is clearly a marker of near-term serious adverse outcomes in ED patients with ADHF.

The ADHERE-EM registry has also provided insight into the challenge of diagnosis in the ED environment. If the initial ED admitting diagnosis is compared to the diagnosis obtained following the complete hospitalization, when all testing and patient responses to therapy can be considered, the diagnosis

TABLE 7-2

COMPONENTS OF A DISEASE MANAGEMENT PROGRAM

Participating Sites in ADHERE-EM were required to implement at least 3 of the first 5 following processes:

1. Treatment algorithms
2. Order sets
3. Physician/RN education
4. Patient education
5. Discharge instructions
6. Feedback loop (data-monitoring tools)

TABLE 7-3

ACUTE ADVERSE OUTCOMES ASSOCIATED WITH ELEVATED TROPONIN IN ACUTE DECOMPENSATED HEART FAILURE

	Troponin (−) N = 65,590	Troponin (+) N = 4,410
CABG, IABCP, ET Intubation	6%	18%
Hospital LOS	4.1 days	5.1 days
ICU LOS	2.3 days	2.9 days
Mortality	2.7%	8.1%

CABG, coronary artery bypass grafting; IABCP, intra-aortic balloon counter pulsation; ET intubation, endotracheal intubation; LOS, length of stay.

is concordant in only 83% of patients. This suggests that the ED misdiagnosis rate in patients ultimately determined to have ADHF is 17%. This has clear implications for the selection of therapies and interventions.

This misdiagnosis rate is consistent with other literature. In the Breathing Not Properly trial (8), the correct diagnosis of HF, based on history and physical in over 1,500 patients presenting to the ED with acute dyspnea, was 75%. When BNP results were considered, the correct diagnosis rate increased to 81.5%. Their suggested misdiagnosis rate of 18.5% is consistent with the error rate as determined by the ADHERE-EM registry.

Thus, the potential for misdiagnosis must be considered in the setting of adverse outcomes. The VMAC trial (9) was a double-blind, randomized, standard therapy controlled study of 489 ADHF patients receiving either nitroglycerin or nesiritide. Of these, 1% of the nitroglycerin group and 0.5% of the nesiritide cohort sustained symptomatic hypotension within 3 hours. This low rate of symptomatic hypotension has clinical outcomes in the ED. If, after an intravenous vasodilator is administered to a patient with suspected ADHF, symptomatic hypotension occurs, the possibility of misdiagnosis must be considered. Vasodilator-induced hypotension occurs in 1 of 100 ADHF patients, whereas misdiagnosis is seen in nearly one in five patients ultimately found to have ADHF. Additionally, although the rate of symptomatic hypotension from a vasodilator being given to patients with an ADHF mimic is unknown (e.g., pulmonary embolus, pneumonia), this cohort could reasonably be expected to sustain symptomatic hypotension. Therefore, when faced with symptomatic hypotension, the clinician must first consider that misdiagnosis is numerically much more likely than a primary drug effect. In this situation the drug should be terminated immediately and the differential diagnosis reconsidered.

A number of challenges exist that result in ED misdiagnosis. This is the consequence of the lack of sensitivity and specificity of history and physical exam findings, an elderly patient population with numerous coexistent pathologies (e.g., chronic obstructive pulmonary disease [COPD] and HF), environmental factors (a loud and sometimes chaotic ED), limits to testing in the ED, and the compressed time course of an ED visit.

As has been demonstrated by the ADHERE registry, approximately three-quarters of patients with ADHF represent repeat visits of previously established disease. However, because the ADHF population has a median age of approximately 75 years, concurrent disease can represent a significant challenge in determining which pathology has prompted the current presentation. In one study, the sensitivities and specificities of common physical findings were determined (Table 7-4) (10), and none have sufficient accuracy to be considered definitive.

Furthermore, testing in the ED is limited to those interventions that can be performed rapidly and that have limited invasiveness. Consequently, workups are limited to electrocardiogram (ECG), blood testing, and radiologic studies. An ECG should be performed in all ED-suspected ADHF patients. Although it is of value to diagnose acute ischemia in the breathless patient, it is so insensitive for the detection of ADHF as to be functionally useless.

CHEST RADIOGRAPHY

A chest radiograph should be obtained in all suspected ADHF patients. It has better accuracy than the ECG, but must be interpreted with caution. X-rays cannot exclude abnormal left ventricular (LV) function, but can eliminate other diagnoses (e.g., pneumonia). The x-ray findings of HF are, in descending order of frequency: dilated upper lobe vessels, cardiomegaly,

TABLE 7-4

SENSITIVITY OF HISTORY AND PHYSICAL FINDINGS FOR AN ADHF DIAGNOSIS

Variable	Sensitivity	Specificity	Accuracy
Hx of HF	62	94	80
Dyspnea	56	53	54
Orthopnea	47	88	72
Rales	56	80	70
S₃	20	99	66
JVD	39	94	72
Edema	67	68	68

From Dao Q, Krishnaswamy P, Kazanegra R, et al. Utility of B-type natriuretic peptide in the diagnosis of congestive heart failure in an urgent-care setting. *JACC* 2001;37(2):379–385.

interstitial edema, enlarged pulmonary artery, pleural effusion, alveolar edema, prominent superior vena cava, and Kerley lines (11). Because abnormalities lag the clinical appearance by hours, therapy is not withheld pending a film.

In chronic HF patients, which is the common ED presentation, the chest x-ray (CXR) signs of congestion have unreliable sensitivity, specificity, and predictive value in identifying patients with high pulmonary capillary wedge pressure (PCWP) (12). In one analysis, radiographic pulmonary congestion was absent in 53% of patients with mild to moderately elevated PCWP (16 to 29 mm Hg) and in 39% of those with markedly elevated PCWP (>30 mm Hg).

Cardiomegaly can suggest an HF diagnosis, and a cardiothoracic ratio >60% correlates with increased 5-year mortality (13), but this cannot help in the compressed time frame of ED decision making. Ultimately, the CXR has poor sensitivity for cardiomegaly (14). In fact, in patients with echocardiographically proven cardiomegaly, 22% had cardiothoracic ratios <50% (14). The poor detection of cardiomegaly by the CXR has been explained by intrathoracic cardiac rotation.

Pleural effusions are missed by CXR, especially if the patient has undergone endotracheal intubation because the film will be obtained while the patient is supine. In patients with pleural effusions, the sensitivity, specificity, and accuracy of the supine CXR was reported to be 67%, 70%, and 67%, respectively (15). Likewise the sensitivity for HF findings with a portable CXR is poor, and it is precisely in the patient who is the most unstable that the portable CXR is most commonly performed. In mild HF, only dilated upper lobe vessels were found in greater than 60% of patients. The frequency that CXR HF parameters are found increases with the severity of HF. With severe HF, x-ray findings occurred in at least two-thirds of patients, except for Kerley lines, which occurred in only 11%, and a prominent vena cava, which occurred in 44% (11).

DIAGNOSIS WITH NATRIURETIC PEPTIDES

B-type natriuretic peptide, discovered approximately 20 years ago and available for less than 5 years as an assay, has become the one of the most common tests performed in the ED for the evaluation of suspected ADHF. Initially released as point-of-care test, lab-based platforms driven by the need to decrease cost and improve accuracy have been developed by at least three different companies. Furthermore, the biologically inactive fragment that is released during BNP synthesis, NT-pro BNP, is also available for use as an assay. Differences between these two assays are found in Table 7-5.

BNP is first synthesized as pre-pro BNP, but the molecule is subsequently cleaved into several protein fragments. Stored in membrane granules (16) and released due to an increased ventricular pressure or volume stimulus, BNP is cleared by a C receptor, neutral endopeptidases (17), and to some extent by the kidney (18). Biologically, natriuretic peptides constitute a group of signalling proteins used to facilitate communication between various feedback loops (19). As such, BNP functions as a cardiac telephone. In response to cardiac stress (20,21), via a number of neurohormonal interactions, BNP causes rapid vasodilation (22), increases cardiac lusitropy, and causes the kidney to increase urinary volume and sodium excretion (22).

BNP levels correlate fairly well ($r = 0.7$) with PCWP (10). BNP levels increase in proportion to HF severity and to other conditions associated with elevated intracardiac pressures (e.g., myocardial infarction, primary pulmonary hypertension, pulmonary embolus). Furthermore, the half-life of exogenously administered BNP is 22 minutes, which provides the opportunity for additional applications of BNP measurement. With effective treatment for decompensated HF, PCWP declines accompanied by a similar decline in BNP levels (10).

Although BNP is frequently regarded as an HF test, a number of pathologic events are associated with non-HF elevations. Median BNP levels can be increased approximately twofold in medically treated essential hypertension with coexistent left ventricular hypertrophy (23,24), threefold in hepatic cirrhosis, and 25-fold in dialysis patients (18), although all these estimates include significant ranges around the median (25). In

HF, BNP levels are proportional to illness severity and may be elevated as much as 25 times baseline. Other confounders included advanced age (23,26), where there is good correlation between BNP, age, and LV mass index (27). BNP is also a strong predictor of the future development of post-MI HF (28).

Other conditions may confound the results of BNP testing. BNP has a negative correlation with obesity (29,30). Consequently, in the morbidly obese, heart failure must be considered likely based on symptoms at presentation and at levels of BNP not usually reflective of severe HF.

Summaries of several studies (20,31,32) indicate the sensitivity of BNP for diagnosing HF ranges from 85% to 97%, with a specificity of 84% to 92%. The positive predictive value is reported at 70% to 95% (10,20), whereas negative predictive value is consistently in excess of 95% (10,33). Several reports have detailed potential confounders and have reported asymptomatic HF clinic patients with BNP as high as 572 and symptomatic HF patients with BNP <100 pg/mL. Per this analysis, patients with a falsely negative BNP were more likely to be younger, female, have a nonischemic HF etiology, have better preserved cardiac and renal function, and be less likely to have atrial fibrillation (34).

CLINICAL TRIALS USING NATRIURETIC PEPTIDES FOR ED DECISION MAKING

In the largest analysis to evaluate BNP in a blinded fashion, the Breathing Not Properly trial (35) had physicians estimate the diagnostic probability of HF in 1,586 patients presenting to the ED with dyspnea. The final diagnosis was determined by two cardiologists blinded to the BNP level. When emergency physicians documented their certainty of the presence or absence of congestive heart failure (CHF) in dyspneic patients, 43% were rated as being uncertain. If BNP was added, the number of patients that would have been rated as having an uncertain diagnosis decreased to only 11%. This suggests that BNP testing helps medical decision making in the cohort of patients for whom the diagnosis is not readily apparent.

The PRIDE study (36) evaluated NT pro-BNP levels in 600 ED patients presenting with acute dyspnea and found similar results to BNP for the diagnosis of CHF. In patients ultimately diagnosed with acute CHF, median NT pro-BNP levels were 4,054 pg/mL, as compared to patients without acute CHF, whose median NT pro-BNP levels were 131 pg/mL. In this analysis, NT pro-BNP levels also had a direct correlation with New York Heart Association Class.

The Basel trial evaluated the clinical impact of the availability of BNP testing during an ED visit. By their methodology, the availability of BNP testing was randomized. When BNP testing was not utilized, the length of hospitalization was 13.7 days, compared to only 10.6 days when BNP testing was available. As would be expected by the large difference in hospitalization time, there was a significant savings by having BNP testing available in the ED. Although this was a European study with a different medical economic climate, the Basel trial demonstrated that performance of an ED BNP level decreases both cost and length of hospitalization (37).

It is well established that indices of cardiac filling pressure (e.g., elevated PCWPs, cardiac S_3) are the best predictors of HF outcomes. Unfortunately, this data is difficult to obtain in the ED. Consequently, emergency physicians must rely on notoriously less accurate history and physical data to make disposition decisions. In the REDHOT trial (Rapid Emergency Department Heart Failure Outpatient Trial) (38), a blinded BNP was obtained on 464 patients presenting to the ED with

---

TABLE 7-5

DIFFERENCES BETWEEN BNP AND NT-PROBNP

Characteristic	BNP	NT-proBNP
Components	BNP molecule	NT fragment (1–76)
Molecular weight	4 kilodaltons	8.5 kilodaltons
Synthesis	Cleavage from proBNP	Cleavage from proBNP
Half-life	20 minutes	120 minutes
Clearance mechanism	Neutral endopeptidase Clearance receptors	Renal clearance
Increased levels with normal aging	+	+ + + +
Estimated GFR correlation	− 0.20	− 0.60
Approved cutoff(s) for CHF diagnosis	100 pg/mL	Age <75: 125 pg/mL Age ≥75: 450 pg/mL
Entry on U.S. market	November 2000	December 2002

dyspnea. They reported that 30-day survivors had much lower BNP concentrations compared to those who died during the same period (764 vs. 2,096 pg/mL, respectively). Unfortunately, in this study using ED physicians blinded to BNP levels, the discharged cohort had a mean BNP of 976 pg/mL, whereas those that were hospitalized had a mean BNP of 767 pg/mL. This study clearly suggested that clinical grounds alone were insufficient to effect an accurate disposition decision.

The greatest utility for BNP is in the ED patient presenting with features suggesting HF. In this cohort, a level less than 100 pg/mL may support the exclusion of HF from the differential diagnosis. Alternatively, in patients with markedly elevated BNP, greater than 500 pg/mL, HF is likely, although confirmatory testing is suggested. In the remaining "gray zone" of levels between 100 and 500 pg/mL, further evaluation is necessary to determine the primary cause of the patient's symptoms.

PHYSIOLOGY: HEMODYNAMIC MISMATCH IS NOT VOLUME OVERLOAD

Some consideration must be given to the concept that ADHF is not a homogenous ED presentation. Although there is little literature describing physiology in patients presenting to the ED, clinically there are two distinct syndromes. These can be characterized by the nature of their presentation. It is important to realize that these may occur to varying degrees in the same patient; however, for the sake of this discussion the presentations are addressed as either that of volume overload or hemodynamic mismatch. These two presentations are easily distinguished by the acuity of their symptoms and their response to vasodilation.

In the volume overload cohort, the acuity of presentation is of only moderate respiratory distress; complaints predominately are driven by exertional limitations or discomfort from excessive volume. These patients may have tremendous volumes removed by diuretics, and although they may have some initial improvement with vasodilation, their symptoms only gradually improve by volume removal.

This is in contradistinction to the group with hemodynamic mismatch. In this cohort, patients function relatively near their baseline until suffering a precipitous decompensation and presenting to the ED with severe respiratory distress. With unimpressive or baseline levels of fluid overload, this cohort undergoes a remarkable improvement with vasodilation. They may return to being nearly asymptomatic within 30 minutes of treatment, although the volume removed in this time frame is less than 100 milliliters. The underlying pathophysiology in this presentation is hypothesized to be excessive systemic vascular resistance resulting in diminishing cardiac output that can be reversed by vasodilator therapy.

RISK STRATIFICATION

Risk stratification is a well-known process in the setting of suspected acute coronary syndromes, and proper interventions in response to positive investigation have reasonably well defined responses that should be instituted. ADHF does not have the extensive data set like acute coronary syndrome for risk stratification, although a number of definitive measures exist.

ADHF risk stratification occurs across a spectrum of disease and can be divided into low- and high-risk predictors of adverse outcomes. Patients with low risk of adverse outcomes will receive less-aggressive therapy and may be considered for shorter hospitalizations, possibly in the observation unit. Patients at high risk for adverse events should get aggressive therapy consistent with their risk of adverse events.

Two studies have evaluated the low-risk population. The first, by Diercks (39), evaluated a number of parameters available at ED presentation to determine the best markers of successful therapy. Low risk was defined as discharge within 24 hours and no death or repeat hospitalization within 30 days. Parameters predicting low risk were a negative troponin and an initial systolic blood pressure (BP) exceeding 160 mm Hg. Burkhardt (40), using similar methodology, identified predictors of short stay failure. They reported that a BUN at ED presentation that exceeded 30 mg/dL was associated with an increased probability of hospitalization for longer than 24 hours. Thus, this marker can be used to assist in the selection of patients appropriate for a short stay unit.

At the other extreme of risk stratification are parameters identifying the risk of acute mortality. In an analysis of over 80,000 patients (41) from the ADHERE registry, a BUN exceeding 43 mg/dL was the single greatest acute mortality predictor. Patients with a BUN higher than 43 mg/dL have a risk of mortality of nearly 9%, compared to only 2.8% when the BUN was below 43 mg/dL. Systolic BP below 115 mm Hg was the next most powerful mortality predictor, and when combined with a high BUN, mortality rose to over 15%. Finally, when the creatinine exceeded 2.75 mg/dL, in combination with a BUN above 43 mg/dL and BP below 115 mm Hg, in-hospital mortality was higher than 22%.

Using this data, a simple risk stratification tool can be developed to assist in determining which patients are appropriate candidates for a short stay unit and which patients have a mortality risk of sufficient magnitude that aggressive care is warranted (Fig. 7-1).

EARLY USE OF VASOACTIVE THERAPY: IMPLICATIONS OF RISK STRATIFICATION

Once an ED patient is identified as having increased risk of mortality, what interventions may alter that outcome are poorly described. The ADHERE registry has provided some information to guide ED therapy in patients at high risk for adverse outcomes. Outcomes based on the early use of intravenous vasoactive therapy, defined as any agent administered to obtain a hemodynamic effect (e.g., nitroglycerin, nesiritide, nitroprusside, dobutamine, dopamine), have been evaluated. In this report (42), data from 46,599 patient visits was analyzed to determine vasoactive usage. Of this cohort, 7,500 received an intravenous vasoactive agent and were then stratified based on the location of where their therapy occurred. The ED group of 4,096 patients received intravenous (IV) vasoactive therapy a mean of 1.1 hours from presentation, as compared the group of 3,499 patients, who received their vasoactive in the hospital, a mean of 22.2 hours after presentation. Examination of outcomes associated with in-hospital therapy identified profound differences between the two groups. ED therapy was favored both statistically and clinically in every parameter, including mortality, ICU and overall length of stay, and the use of invasive procedures.

This report has been followed with a similar analysis examining the difference in outcomes associated with the timing of nesiritide administration (43). As before, this analysis used location of administration as an indicator of time to therapy, but excluded patients with systolic blood pressure below 90 mm Hg (because vasodilators would be inappropriate in this cohort). In this analysis, average time to ED administration was 2.8 hours in 1,613 patients, as compared to an average time of 15.5 hours after presentation in the 2,687 patients from

Shortness of Breath in the ED

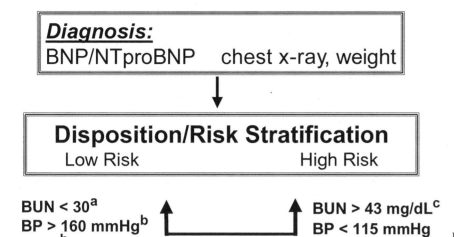

FIGURE 7-1. Risk stratification tool developed to assist in determining which patients are appropriate candidates for a short stay unit and which patients have a mortality risk of sufficient magnitude that aggressive care is warranted.

the hospitalized cohort. Outcomes favored ED initiation and found that the ED nesiritide was associated with decreased length of stay (5.4 vs. 4.2 days, $P = 0.0001$) and lower ICU transfer rate (2% vs. 7%, $P = 0.0001$) compared to therapy delayed until arrival on the inpatient unit. There was also a trend to improved mortality with early nesiritide, but this was statistically limited due to its sample size (3.1% vs. 3.9%, $P = 0.15$).

These analyses (42,43) have been reported in terms of hazard ratios (Fig. 7-2), all of which clearly demonstrate (in terms of mortality, hospital length of stay exceeding 4 day, and ICU length of stay exceeding 4 days) that early therapy is associated with important clinical outcome benefits.

ADHERE-EM DISEASE MANAGEMENT

The ADHERE-EM registry has collected data at each enrolling institution relative to when a disease management program was instituted. As described earlier, to participate in the registry, three of the five disease management strategies listed in Table 7-2 were required to be implemented at the time the registry was begun. Consequently, data can be analyzed before and after a hospital's disease management strategy was put in place. Of the patients enrolled in ADHERE-EM prior to disease-management implementation, 88% received IV diuretics a median of 7.0 hours after admission to the ED. After the disease management program was initiated, the overall rate of diuretic therapy in ADHF improved to 92%. This suggests not only decreased time to treatment, but diagnostic accuracy improvement as well. Furthermore, patients treated with diuretics received their therapy nearly 1 hour sooner, at a median of 6.1 hours after presentation. Similar trends were noted in other therapies. Before disease management implementation, vasoactive agents were administered in only 32% of patients, at a median of 14.7 hours after ED presentation. Putting a disease management program into place increased vasoactive use so that 42% of ADHF patients received their therapy while still in the ED. Postdisease management includes vasoactive

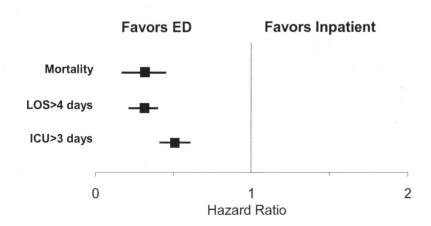

FIGURE 7-2. Hazard ratios that demonstrate that (in terms of mortality, hospital length of stay exceeding 4 days, and ICU length of stay exceeding 4 days) early therapy is associated with important clinical outcome benefits.

TABLE 7-6

IMPACT OF DISEASE MANAGEMENT ON CLINICAL OUTCOMES

Outcome	Before DM	After DM
Number in cohort	N = 2,405	N = 1,326
Death	3.6%	2.3%
Mechanical ventilation	3.6%	3.1%
ICU length of stay	3 days	2.5 days

therapy given a median of 8.7 hours after arrival. Remarkably, the consequence of these interventions resulted in significant out-come improvements, with decreased mortality, lower rates of mechanical ventilation, and shorter ICU length of hospitalization (Table 7-6). It is readily apparent that early ED therapy results in significant outcome benefit in ADHF.

CONCLUSIONS

An accurate diagnosis of ADHF is the first step required for effective therapy in this common ED presentation. Both disposition and therapy are then driven by the results of risk stratification, which is used to identify patients at both low and high risk of adverse outcomes. Low-risk patients may be appropriate for observation unit therapy. Importantly, because delays are associated with increased morbidity and mortality, those with high-risk features should be considered for early vasoactive therapy. Finally, a disease management program provides improved outcomes, including mortality reduction, for the ED management of ADHF.

References

1. American Heart Association. Heart disease and stroke statistics—2005 update. Dallas, TX: American Heart Association; 2005.
2. O'Connell JB. The economic burden of heart failure. *Clin Cardiol* 2000;23: III6–10.
3. Kahn KL, Rogers WH, Rubenstein LV, et al. Measuring quality of care with explicit process criteria before and after implementation of the DRG-based prospective payment system. *JAMA* 1990;264(15):1969–1973.
4. Ashton CM, Kuykendall DH, Johnson ML, et al. The association between the quality of inpatient care and early readmission. *Ann Intern Med* 1995 Mar 15;122(6):415–421.
5. McAlister FA, Stewart S, Ferrua S, et al. Multidisciplinary strategies for the management of heart failure patients at high risk for admission: a systematic review of randomized trials. *J Am Coll Cardiol* 2004;44(4):810–819.
6. Peacock WF, DeMarco T, Emerman CL, et al. Heart failure with an elevated troponin is associated with increased morbidity and mortality: an ADHERE registry analysis. *Ann Emerg Med* 2004;44(4):S72.
7. DeMarco T, Peacock WF, Emerman CL, et al. Effect of initial troponin status on outcomes after treatment with inotropes vs vasodilators for acutely decompensated heart failure: an ADHERE registry analysis. *Circulation* 2004;110(17)(Suppl):1745.
8. Maisel AS, Krishnaswamy P, Nowak RM, et al. Rapid measurement of B-type natriuretic peptide in the emergency diagnosis of heart failure. *N Engl J Med* 2002;18;347(3):161–167.
9. Publication committee for the VMAC Investigators. Intravenous nesiritide versus nitroglycerin for treatment of decompensated congestive heart failure: the VMAC trial. *JAMA* 2002;287:1531–1540.
10. Dao Q, Krishnaswamy P, Kazanegra R, et al. Utility of B-type natriuretic peptide in the diagnosis of congestive heart failure in an urgent-care setting. *JACC* 2001;37(2):379–385.
11. Chait A, Cohen HE, Meltzer LE, et al. The bedside chest radiograph in the evaluation of incipient heart failure. *Radiology* 1972;105:563–566.
12. Chakko S, Woska D, Marinez H, et al. Clinical, radiographic, and hemodynamic correlations in chronic congestive heart failure: conflicting results may lead to inappropriate care. *Am J Med* 1991;90:353–359.
13. Koga Y, Wada T, Toshima H, et al. Prognostic significance of electrocardiographic findings in patients with dilated cardiomyopathy. *Heart Ves* 1993; 8:37–41.
14. Kono T, Suwa M, Hanada H, et al. Clinical significance of normal cardiac silhouette in dilated cardiomyopathy—evaluation based upon echocardiography and magnetic resonance imaging. *Japanese Circulation Journal* 1992; 56(4):359–365. 92;56(4):359–365.
15. Ruskin JA, Gurney JW, Thorsen MK, et al. Detection of pleural effusions on supine chest radiographs. *AJR* 1987;148:681–683.
16. Nakao K, Mukoyama M, Hosoda K, et al. Biosynthesis, secretion, and receptor selectivity of human brain natriuretic peptide. *Can J Physiol Pharmacol* 1991;59:1500–1506.
17. Lainchbury JG, Richards AM, Nicholls MG, et al. Brain natriuretic peptide and neutral endopeptidase inhibition in left ventricular impairment. *J Clin Endo Metab* 1999;84:723–729.
18. Mair J, Thomas S, Puschendorf B. Natriuretic peptides in assessment of left-ventricular dysfunction. *Scan J Clin Invest* 1999;59(suppl 230):132–42.
19. Stevens TL, Rasmussen TE, Wei CM, et al. Renal role of the endogenous natriuretic peptide system in acute congestive heart failure. *J Card Fail* 1996; 2:119–125.
20. Cowie MR, Struthers AD, Wood DA, et al. Value of natriuretic peptides in assessment of patients with possible new heart failure in primary care. *Lancet* 1997;350:1349–1353.
21. Packer M, Carver JR, Rodeheffer RJ, et al. Effect of oral milrinone on mortality in severe chronic heart failure. *NEJM* 1991;325:1468–75.
22. Struthers AD: Ten years of natriuretic peptide research: a new dawn for their diagnostic and therapeutic use? *BMJ* 1994;308(6944):1615–1619.
23. Wallen T, Landahl T, Herner T, et al. Brain natriuretic peptide in an elderly population. *J Int Med* 1997;242:307–311.
24. Buckley MG. Plasma concentrations and comparisons of brain and atrial natriuretic peptide in normal subjects and in patients with essential hypertension. *J Hum Hyperten* 1993;7(3):345–50.
25. Jensen KT, Carstens J, Ivarsen P, et al. A new, fast and reliable radioimmunoassay of brain natriuretic peptide in human plasma. Reference values in healthy subjects and in patients with different diseases. *Scand. J Clin Lab Invest* 1997;57:529–540.
26. Lernfelt B. Aging and left ventricular function in elderly healthy people. *Am J Card* 1991;68:547–549.
27. Sayama H, Nakamura Y, Saito N, et al. Relationship between left ventricular geometry and brain natriuretic peptide levels in elderly subjects. *Geron* 2000;46(2):71–77.
28. Bettencourt P, Ferreira A, Pardal-Oliveira N, et al. Clinical significance of brain natriuretic peptide in patients with postmyocardial infarction. *Clin Card* 2000;23(12):921–927.
29. Mehra MR, Uber PA, Park M, et al. Obesity and suppressed B-type natriuretic peptide levels in heart failure. *JACC* 2004;43(9):1590–1595.
30. McCord J, Mundy BJ, Hudson MP, et al. The relationship between obesity and B-type natriuretic peptide levels. *Arch Int Med* 2004;164(20):2247–2252.
31. Niinuma H, Nakamura M, Hirarnori K. Plasma B-type natriuretic peptide measurement in a multiphasic health screening program. *Cardiology* 1998; 90:89–94.
32. Davis M, Espiner E, Richards G, et al. Plasma brain natriuretic peptide in assessment of acute dyspnea. *Lancet* 1994;343:440–444.
33. McDonagh TA, Robb, SD, Morton, JJ, et al. Biochemical detection of left ventricular systolic dysfunction. *Lancet* 1998;351:9–13.
34. Tang WHW, Girod JP, Lee MJ, et al. Plasma B-type natriuretic peptide levels in ambulatory patients with established chronic symptomatic systolic heart failure. *Circulation* 2003;108:2964–2966.
35. Maisel AS, McCord JM, Nowak RM, et al. Bedside B-type natriuretic peptide in the emergency diagnosis of heart failure: with reduced or preserved ejection fraction: results from the Breathing Not Properly (BNP) multinational study. *J Am Coll Cardiol* 2003;410(11):2010–2017.
36. Januzzi JL, Camargo CA, Anwaruddin S, et al. The N-Terminal Pro-BNP Investigation of Dyspnea in the Emergency Department (PRIDE) Study. *Am J Cardiol* 2005;95:948–954.
37. Mueller C, Scholer A, Laule-Kilian K, et al. Use of b-type natriuretic peptide in the evaluation and management of acute dyspnea. *N Engl J Med* 2004; 350:647–654.
38. Maisel A, Hollander JE, Guss D, et al. Primary Results of the Rapid Emergency Department Heart Failure Outpatient Trial (REDHOT). A multicenter study of B-type natriuretic peptide levels, emergency department decision making, and outcomes in patients presenting with shortness of breath. *JACC* 2004;44(6):1328–1333.
39. Diercks DB, Kirk JD, Peacock WF, et al. Identification of emergency department patients with decompensated heart failure at low risk for adverse events and prolonged hospitalization. *J Card Fail* 2004;10(Suppl)(4):S118.
40. Burkhardt J, Peacock WF, Emerman CL. Elevation in blood urea nitrogen predicts a lower discharge rate from the observation unit. *Ann Emerg Med* 2004;44(Suppl)(4):S99.
41. Fonarow GC, Adams KF Jr, Abraham WT, et al. Risk stratification for in-hospital mortality in acutely decompensated heart failure: classification and regression tree analysis. *JAMA* 2005;293(5):572–580.
42. Peacock WF, Emerman CL, Costanzo MR, et al. Early initiation of intravenous therapy improves heart failure outcomes: an analysis from the ADHERE Registry Database. *Ann of Emerg Med* 2003;42(4):S26.
43. Peacock WF, DeMarco T, Emerman CL, et al. Early use of nesiritide in the emergency department is associated with improved outcome: an ADHERE registry analysis. *Ann Emerg Med* 2004;44(Suppl)(4):S78.

CHAPTER 8 ■ ATRIAL FIBRILLATION IN THE EMERGENCY DEPARTMENT

MICHAEL A. ROSS AND ANTONIO X. BONFIGLIO

EPIDEMIOLOGY
CLASSIFICATION
PATHOPHYSIOLOGY
MANAGEMENT OF ATRIAL FIBRILLATION
INITIAL EVALUATION
TREATMENT OF ATRIAL FIBRILLATION
Emergent Electrical Cardioversion of Unstable Atrial Fibrillation
   Patients
Medical Management of Atrial Fibrillation—Medications to
   Control Heart Rate
Treatment Protocols for Acute Onset Atrial Fibrillation
Treatment Protocols for Uncomplicated Acute Onset Atrial
   Fibrillation—Electrical Therapy Protocols
Treatment Protocols for Uncomplicated Acute Onset Atrial
   Fibrillation—Drug and Electrical Protocols (the Role of the
   Observation Unit)
Antithrombotic Therapy for Patients with Atrial Fibrillation

EPIDEMIOLOGY

The most common clinically important disturbance in cardiac rhythm seen in the emergency department (ED) is atrial fibrillation (AF) (1). An estimated 2.2 million Americans have paroxysmal or persistent AF. AF affects approximately 2% of the U.S. population in the sixth decade of life, and its prevalence increases with advancing age. In patients over 75 years old, greater than 10% have experienced AF. AF is also associated with other conditions corresponding with advanced age such as coronary artery disease, hypertension, congestive heart failure, valvular heart disease, hyperthyroidism, and diabetes (2,3).

Because of its higher prevalence in the elderly and the growth of that age group, AF has become a rising cause of hospitalization. AF accounts for 34.5% of admissions for a cardiac rhythm disturbance. Complications of AF range from cardiac decompensation to thromboembolic events such as an acute ischemic stroke. The relative risk of death in patients with AF is one and a half times greater in men and almost two times greater in women (3,4).

CLASSIFICATION

Several terms used in reference to AF must first be understood. Acute onset AF is defined as having been present for less than 48 hours. This distinction is important because it will direct therapy in selected cases. Paroxysmal, or recurrent, AF is that which has occurred at least twice and terminated. Persistent AF is that which does not terminate. Subsequent termination of AF does not change the designation as persistent. If AF persists for more than 1 year, then it is classified as long standing. Lone AF is defined as that occurring in a patient who is under 60 years of age and without echocardiographic or clinical evidence of cardiovascular disease. It is estimated that lone AF represents between 12% and 30% of all AF patients. These classifications do not apply to AFs that last less than 30 seconds or are secondary to precipitating conditions such as cardiac surgery, myocarditis, acute myocardial infarction (MI), hyperthyroidism, or acute pulmonary disease (4).

PATHOPHYSIOLOGY

Histological analysis of atrial tissue in patients in chronic AF shows changes beyond those expected by the underlying disease process itself. There is often a mixture of patchy fibrosis or inflammation and normal atrial tissue accounting for nonhomogeneity of atrial refractoriness. Histological changes of myocarditis have been found in atrial biopsy specimens of 66% of patients with lone AF. Atrial fiber hypertrophy and atrial dilation can be demonstrated by biopsy or echocardiography in patients with long-standing AF (4). Selected toxic and metabolic conditions may also contribute to AF.

The causes of AF are many and can be both intrinsic to the heart itself or extrinsic, secondary to other conditions. Two useful pneumonics regarding causes of AF divide causes into noncardiac causes and cardiac causes. Noncardiac causes can be summarized by the pneumonic TRAPS and include Thyrotoxicosis, Recreational drug use (sympathomimetics and endogenous catecholamines), Alcohol, Pulmonary disease (including pulmonary embolus), and Sepsis, or infection. Cardiac causes can be summarized by the pneumonic CATCH WAVE and include Congestive heart failure, Acute coronary syndromes, TaChy-brady syndrome (sick sinus syndrome), Hypertension, Wolff-Parkinson-White syndrome, After cardiac surgery, Valvular heart disease, and mEdical noncompliance (Table 8-1) (5–8).

In terms of atrial electrical activity, AF occurs through two processes—enhanced depolarization of one or several foci and re-entry involving one or several circuits. Usually AF starts when a trigger, often a premature atrial contraction or repetitive depolarization, finds its way into an aberrant circuit where it does not encounter refractory myocardium (4,9). Electrophysiological mapping studies have found that AF often originates in the muscular sleeve of the pulmonary veins and then propagates through the atrial tissue. A re-entrant impulse is one that travels repetitively along an abnormal electrical circuit. If the propagation of the atrial depolarization is along one re-entrant pathway, this can result in regular arrhythmic depolarizations and atrial flutter. However, more chaotic and irregular electrical activity along multiple circuits is usually the case and leads to AF. These depolarizations compete for the atrioven-

TABLE 8-1

CAUSES OF ATRIAL FIBRILLATION

CATCH WAVE: Cardiac causes of atrial fibrillation	• **C**ongestive heart failure • **A**cute coronary syndromes and myocarditis • Ta**Ch**y-brady syndrome (sick sinus syndrome) • **H**ypertension • **W**olff-Parkinson-White (pre-excitation) syndrome • **A**fter cardiac surgery • **V**alvular heart disease • m**E**dical noncompliance
TRAPS: Noncardiac causes of atrial fibrillation	• **T**hyrotoxicosis • **R**ecreational drug use (sympathomimetics and endogenous catecholamines) • **A**lcohol • **P**ulmonary disease (including pulmonary embolus) • **S**epsis or infection

tricular (AV) node and, depending on their magnitude and time of arrival, may be propagated through the AV node and into the ventricle causing a ventricular contraction (4,10). Often, in a healthy nodal conduction system, the ventricular response is fast producing an irregular tachycardia. On a cellular level, AF has been found to essentially propagate itself. Actual atrial electrical remodeling occurs with continued AF. This involves the down regulation of calcium channels, shortening action potential duration, thus decreasing the refractory period of the myocardial tissue (4,9). A regular ventricular response in light of the chaos in atrial conduction can also be indicative of AV nodal dissociation.

On the electrocardiogram (ECG) AF is characterized by a lack of defined and regular atrial depolarization resulting in an absence of discernible P-waves and chaotic and irregular undulations in their place, often called f-waves. These f-waves occur at rates often between 400 and 600 beats per minute. With atrial flutter, the rates range from 250 to 350 beats per minute. Induction through the AV node is variable, often leading to an irregular depolarization and contraction by the ventricle. The gross appearance on the ECG is the absence of P-waves with varying ventricular contractions that are often irregular. This can be seen with or without other conduction disturbances like bundle branch blocks or accessory pathways and is independent of the morphology of the tracing (6,11). In atrial flutter the typical rate of the atrial flutter waves is roughly 240 to 320 beats per minute. When patients in atrial flutter experience AV nodal conduction rates of 2:1, then the resulting rhythm is a regular tachycardia of roughly 150 beats per minute. Often the nonconducted flutter wave is buried in the preceding T-wave, giving the appearance of a sinus tachycardia with a rate of 150. Atrial flutter with 2:1 conduction should be suspected in any patient with a tachycardia of 150 beats per minute, especially if it is a narrow complex (11).

Once the heart's intrinsic rhythm is altered by AF, then its function and blood flow are also altered. Cardiac output and stroke volume decline from a lack of adequate preload filling of the ventricle by the contributions of the atrial contraction (12). This results in the loss of the "atrial kick" that would otherwise be provided with normal filling times as well as the loss of organized and rhythmic atrial activity. The irregularity

of the ventricular response as well as the tachycardia of the ventricle can also lead to decreased cardiac output. Poor cardiac output in the presence of underlying coronary artery disease or cardiomyopathy will precipitate or exacerbate congestive heart failure (CHF) or exacerbate acute cardiac ischemia. On the other hand, CHF can cause AF, making this a rhythm disturbance that can become self-propagating in congestive heart failure patients. The turbulence of blood in the atria that occurs in AF can cause blood to pool and clot, particularly in the left atrial appendage. Because of this, patients are at a substantial thromboembolic risk and require anticoagulation based on their risk profile (see Table 8-6) (12,13).

MANAGEMENT OF ATRIAL FIBRILLATION

There are four primary issues in the management of AF: (a) ventricular rate control, (b) restoration of sinus rhythm, (c) anticoagulation issues, and (d) treatable causes of AF. Underlying treatable causes were described earlier and will not be discussed in this chapter. See Figure 8-1 for a general outline of the treatment of AF (12).

INITIAL EVALUATION

Several issues need to be addressed in the initial evaluation of patients with AF. These include the hemodynamic stability of the patient, whether the symptoms have been present for more or less than 48 hours, and what may have caused the AF to occur. AF of more than 48 hours duration is more likely to form an intracardiac thrombus, which may subsequently embolize if conversion to sinus rhythm occurs. As such, it is important to determine if the onset of symptoms is less than 48 hours (14–16). If the symptom onset cannot be clearly determined, then it may be prudent to consider the onset to be greater than 48 hours and focus on rate control rather conversion to sinus rhythm. It is also important to characterize whether the symptoms are an isolated event or a paroxysmal recurrent event because this may affect long-term treatment decisions. The history should also focus on identifying potential causes that may have triggered AF and to focus appropriate testing (14).

The clinical presentation of AF in the ED ranges from the asymptomatic patient in whom it is an incidental finding, to those with an uncomplicated acute onset of symptoms, and to those suffering an acute end organ compromise by hypoperfusion or thromboembolization (17). Symptomatically, AF may or may not produce symptoms that allow the patient to identify the exact time of onset. Patients may describe the onset as a sudden feeling of palpitation, weakness, dizziness, syncope, or dyspnea. The examination of patients in AF will usually suggest the arrhythmia by the classical irregularly irregular pulse, irregular venous pulsations, and variation in the loudness of the first heart sound (4,12,14). The patient's blood pressure is critically important in the identification of patients that are in hypotensive shock and may require urgent cardioversion (12,18). The temperature can point to sepsis, or thyrotoxicosis, as an etiology. Physical examination findings can also point to etiologies such as CHF, pulmonary disease, thyroid disease, or recent cardiac surgery.

All patients with palpitations or symptoms suggestive of AF should have an initial ECG performed to confirm the rhythm, as well as identify confounding issues such as evidence of an acute coronary syndrome, Wolff-Parkinson-White (WPW) syndrome, or electrolyte disturbances such as hypokalemia (4). These confounders may have an impact on selecting therapies. Additionally, patients should have an intravenous line placed,

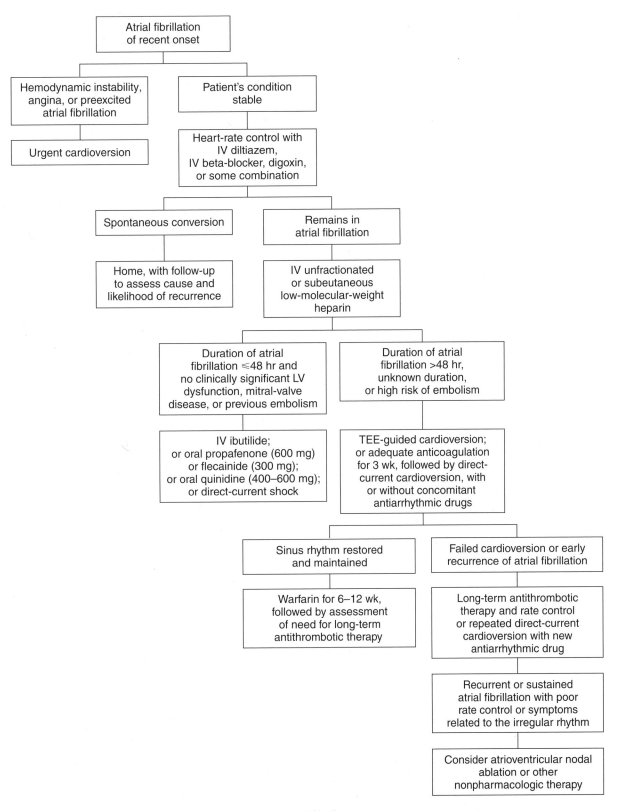

FIGURE 8-1. Management of recent onset atrial fibrillation.
(From Falk RH. Atrial fibrillation. *N Engl J Med* 2001;344:1067–1078, with permission.)

receive supplemental oxygen if they are hypoxic or symptomatic, and be placed on a cardiac monitor to follow their heart rate. This will help determine if and when a patient returns to a normal sinus rhythm. Cardiac monitors may not provide an accurate measure of the patient's heart rate because most cardiac monitoring equipment determines the heart rate by measuring the R to R interval, and this is irregular in AF (7). When in doubt, it is most accurate to count the number of complexes on a rhythm strip over a fixed time interval, such as 6 seconds, which is then multiplied by ten, to determine the patient's heart rate. Following conversion to sinus rhythm patients should have an ECG repeated and remain on the monitor for at least a brief period of time because some will continue to go in and out of AF (7,10).

Given the multiple causes of AF, selected testing can be performed to determine the cause. Specifically, if an acute coronary syndrome is suspected, then cardiac markers such as creatine kinase-MB (CK-MB) or cardiac troponins may be ordered. Pulse oximetry should be considered to help identify patients that are hypoxic from CHF or pulmonary embolism (PE). Brain natriuretic peptide (BNP) may be used as a screening tool to identify patients with CHF as a cause, or result, of AF. Electrolytes and renal function labs may be of value in these patients. Coagulation studies and a complete blood count with platelets may be indicated for patients taking warfarin or heparin, or for patients at risk of bleeding such as those with liver or bone marrow failure. Thyroid function testing or toxicology screening can be ordered as needed as well. A chest x-ray may be useful to identify CHF or pneumonia in the dyspneic patient. If clinically indicated, then imaging for a pulmonary embolus may be needed. An ECG may help identify if a patient is in CHF (4,7,14,18,19). Transesophageal echocardiography may be useful in identifying a clot in the left atrial appendage; however, this study is usually performed in settings other than the ED (15,16).

TREATMENT OF ATRIAL FIBRILLATION

Emergent Electrical Cardioversion of Unstable Atrial Fibrillation Patients

For patients with unstable AF, cardioversion is the treatment of choice. This would include patients that are hypotensive or with other signs of shock, such as acute mental status changes due to cerebral hypoperfusion, and ongoing severe ischemic chest pain. These symptoms often only occur when the heart rate exceeds 150 beats per minute. Patients with acute MI and AF with a rapid ventricular response should be electrically cardioverted if they do not promptly respond to medical therapy. Cardioversion is also often the preferred method for AF patients with pre-excitation syndromes such as WPW (7,12,18).

The electrical cardioversion of AF or flutter should be done in the synchronized mode to avoid shock during the relative refractory period, which can lead to ventricular fibrillation. If synchronized shocks are not possible because of the patient's rhythm or condition, then a higher energy shock should be used (defibrillation doses). When cardioverting AF in a monophasic mode, a setting of 100 to 200 joules (J) is often needed. However, when using a biphasic synchronized cardioverting waveform, a setting of 100 to 120 J is usually adequate to convert the patient. When cardioverting atrial flutter, a lower monophasic setting of 50 to 100 J is usually sufficient (18).

Medical Management of Atrial Fibrillation—Medications to Control Heart Rate

The heart rate in AF with a rapid ventricular response may be controlled using a number of medications that include beta-blockers, calcium channel blockers, and magnesium. These drugs work by blocking conduction at the AV node. Doses and major side effects are listed in Table 8-2. Because of its very short duration of action, adenosine should not be used to manage AF or flutter. Because of its late onset of action and marginal efficacy, digoxin is only listed as a class IIb medication in the setting of CHF. In the ED, rate control should be achieved if the patients' ventricular response is greater than 120 beats per minute. In outpatients, the heart rate is considered controlled when it is between 60 to 80 at rest and 90 to 115 during moderate exercise. Therapy requires careful titration and bradycardia may occur, though often only transiently. In general, for patients with good left ventricular (LV) function, beta-blockers or calcium channel blockers may be used. For patients with CHF, diltiazem, amiodarone, and digoxin may be used. For patients with pre-excitation conditions (i.e., WPW) and AF, rate control may be achieved with amiodarone, propafenone, procainamide, flecainide, or sotalol. In pre-excitation conditions, beta-blockers, calcium channel blockers, digoxin, and adenosine are contraindicated. For patients with chronic AF, control of a rapid ventricular response is a common clinical presentation. Medications to control the ventricular rate are often the mainstay of their treatment in the ED (4,7,12,18,19).

Medical Management of Atrial Fibrillation—Medications to Control Heart Rhythm

Restoration of sinus rhythm offers physiological benefits. Atrial mechanical systole is responsible for 5% to 30% of cardiac output and may be of particular importance in patients with underlying cardiac disease (20). Additionally, otherwise healthy patients find the palpitation symptoms of AF to be particularly unsettling. Several medications are used to pharmacologically cardiovert patients to a sinus rhythm. These are listed in Table 8-3 (4,18,19). Although it has long been believed that there was a long-term benefit of maintaining sinus rhythm as much as possible, versus simply controlling rate, the results of two studies have indicated that this is not necessarily true (21,22). The American AFFIRM trial and a separate European study both found that the incidence of death and complications of AF (stroke) was the same whether rate or rhythm control strategies were chosen. Although not statistically significant, the 5-year mortality favored the rate control group over the rhythm control group at 21.3% versus 23.8%. The incidence of stroke was roughly equal in both groups and largely occurred after anticoagulants had been stopped. The study population tended to be older patients, roughly 68 years old, with persistent or recurrent AF. In fact, more rhythm control patients were hospitalized and had adverse drug effects than the rate control group. This study did not adequately address the management of acute AF, particularly in younger patients (23).

Treatment Protocols for Acute Onset Atrial Fibrillation

Because prolonged AF leads to changes within the heart, which in fact perpetuate further AF, cardioversion to sinus rhythm is

TABLE 8-2

INTRAVENOUS PHARMACOLOGICAL AGENTS FOR HEART RATE IN PATIENTS WITH ATRIAL FIBRILLATION

Drug[a]	Loading Doses	Onset	Maintenance Dose	Major Side Effects	Class Recommendation
Diltiazem	0.25 mg/kg IV over 2 min	2–7 min	5–15 mg/hr infusion	Hypotension, heart block, HF	I[c]
Esmolol[d]	0.5 mg/kg over 1 min	5 min	0.05–0.2 mg/kg/^{1}min^{-1}	Hypotension, heart block, bradycardia, asthma, HF	I
Metoprolol[d]	2.5–5 mg IV bolus over 2 min; up to 3 doses	5 min	N/A	Hypotension, heart block, bradycardia, asthma, HF	I[c]
Propranollol[d]	0.15 mg/kg IV	5 min	N/A	Hypotension, heart block, bradycardia, asthma, HF	I[c]
Verapamil	0.075–0.15 mg/kg IV over 2 min	3–5 min	N/A	Hypotension, heart block, HF	I[c]
Digoxin	0.25 mg IV each 2 h, up to 1.5 mg	2 h	0.125–0.25 mg daily	Digitalis toxicity, heart block, bradycardia	IIb[b]
Magnesium[e]	2.5 grams over 20 minutes	<30 min	N/A	Hypotension, bradycardia	

HF, Heart failure.
[a] Drugs are listed alphabetically within each class of recommendation.
[b] Type 1 in congestive HF.
[c] IIb in congestive HF.
[d] Only representative members of the type of beta-adrenergic antagonist drugs are included in the table, but other, similar agents could be used for this indication in appropriate doses.
[e] Part 7.3 Management of symptomatic bradycardia and tachycardia. In 2005 AHA guidelines for CPR and ECC. *Circulation* 2005;112:IV-67–IV-77; Davey MJ, Teubner. A randomized controlled trial of magnesium sulfate, in addition to usual care, for rate control in atrial fibrillation. *Ann Emerg Med* 2005;45:347–353.

more likely to be successful the sooner it is conducted. Thus, patients presenting to the ED with acute-onset AF benefit from timely restoration of sinus rhythm. The management of AF was detailed in the GEFAUR-1 study, a prospective multicenter observational study of 1,178 patients in 12 EDs in Spain. Although rate and rhythm control are considered to be the mainstay of care for these patients in the ED, pharmacological rate control was used in only 68% of patients with a pulse over 100 beats per minute, and it was effective in only 48% of cases. Of patients whose AF onset was less than 48 hours, only 42% had rhythm control attempted, and it was successful in only 65% of cases in the ED. These results suggest that a standardized approach, such as treatment protocols for AF, is needed (17).

Treatment Protocols for Uncomplicated Acute Onset Atrial Fibrillation—Electrical Therapy Protocols

If the patient with AF is stable, then the management is based on whether AF has been present for more or less than 48 hours' duration. Due to the thromboembolic risks involved, it is ideal to limit cardioversion to patients whose AF has been present for less than 48 hours or where the absence of a left atrial thrombus has been documented by transesophageal echocardiography. However, this should not preclude the cardioversion of an unstable patient. Patients with greater than 48 hours of symptoms require a minimum of 3 weeks of anticoagulation before conversion to sinus rhythm and 4 weeks of anticoagulation after conversion to minimize the risk of thromboembolic events (4,7,12,19). If the onset of AF cannot be determined by

history, then it is safest to assume that the onset is greater than 48 hours and treat accordingly (4). The issues regarding the management of AF less than 48 hours are primarily that of rate control and restoration of sinus rhythm.

Electrical cardioversion to convert AF patients that are stable, less than 48 hours' duration and uncomplicated, has been reported in two studies. The first, by Michael et al, involved a retrospective chart review of 655 ED patients with AF. Patients were excluded if their primary treatment condition was not related to AF, if their symptoms resolved before an ECG was obtained, if they were clinically unstable requiring emergent cardioversion, if they had cardiac complications such as acute CHF or Acute Coronary Syndrome (ACS), or if other medical conditions warranted admission. Of the 331 eligible study patients, 71 (22%) were managed by heart rate control alone, 180 (54%) by chemical cardioversion, and 80 (24%) by electrical cardioversion. Patients spent an average of 5 hours in the ED. There were more patients with greater than 48 hours of symptoms in the rate control group (39%) and chemical treatment group (20%) than the electrical treatment group (8%). Conversion occurred in 75% of rate control patients, 50% of chemical cardioversion patients, and 89% of electrical cardioversion patients. Minor complications occurred in 3% of rate control patients, 9% of chemical cardioversion patients, and no electrical cardioversion patients. Eighty-three percent of electrical cardioversion patients had failed chemical cardioversion prior to electrical cardioversion. Overall, 10% of patients returned within 7 days, with no treatment complications identified (1).

Another retrospective chart review of 388 uncomplicated AF by Burton had similar results. In this study 99% had fewer than 48 hours of symptoms, and all were treated with electrical cardioversion in the ED. Of electrically cardioverted patients,

TABLE 8-3

RECOMMENDED DOSES OF DRUGS PROVEN EFFECTIVE FOR PHARMACOLOGICAL CARDIOVERSION OF ATRIAL FIBRILLATION

Drug[a]	Route of Administration	Dosage[b]	Potential Adverse Effects
Amiodarone	Oral	Inpatient: 1.2–1.8 g per day in divided dose until 10 g total, then 200–400 mg per day maintenance or 30 mg/kg as single dose	Hypotension, bradycardia, QT prolongation, torsades de pointes (rare), GI upset, constipation, phlebitis (IV)
	Intravenous / Oral	5–7 mg/kg over 30–60 min, then 1.2–1.8 g per day continuous IV or in divided oral doses until 10 g total, then 200–400 mg per day maintenance	
Dofetilide	Oral	Creatinine clearance (mL/min) Dose (mcg BID) greater than 60 500 40–60 250 20–40 125 less than 20 Contraindicated	QT prolongation, torsades de pointes; adjust dose for renal function, body size, and age
Flecainide	Oral	200–300 mg[c]	Hypotension, rapidly conducting atrial flutter
	Intravenous	1.5–3.0 mg per kg over 10–20 min[c]	
Ibutilide	Intravenous	1 mg over 10 min; repeat 1 mg when necessary	QT prolongation, torsades de pointes
Propafenone	Oral	450–600mg	Hypotension, rapidly conducting atrial flutter
Quinidine[d]	Intravenous	1.5–2.0 mg per kg over 10–20 min[c]	QT prolongation, torsades de pointes, GI upset, hypotension
	Oral	0.75–1.5 g in divided doses over 6–12 h, usually with a rate-slowing drug	GI upset, hypotension

GI, gastrointestinal; IV, intravenous; BID, twice a day.
[a] Drugs are listed alphabetically.
[b] Dosages given in the table may differ from those recommended by the manufacturers.
[c] Insufficient data are available on which to base specific recommendations for the use of one loading regimen over another for patients with ischemic heart disease or impaired left ventricular function, and these drugs should be used cautiously or not at all in such patients.
[d] The use of quinidine loading to achieve pharmacological conversion of atrial fibrillation is controversial, and safer methods are available with the alternative agents listed in the table. Quinidine should be used with caution.
From Fuster V, Rydén LE, Asinger RW, et al. ACC/AHA/ESC guidelines for the management of patients with atrial fibrillation. *Circulation* 2001; 104:2118–2150, with permission.

37% received rate control medications, and 29% received chemical cardioversion drugs prior to electrical therapy. Cardioversion was successful in 86% of patients; however, 9% of cardioverted patients were still admitted for evaluation. Overall, 6.4% of patients had complications of the procedure, of which 79% were attributable to procedural sedation and analgesia, and the rest attributable to cardioversion. Overall, 86% of patients were discharged home from the ED, 78% following successful cardioversion and 9% following failed cardioversion. On follow-up 10% of patients returned to the ED within 7 days, and 6% of patients that were successfully cardioverted patients returned because of a relapse of AF (24).

In a smaller prospective study of biphasic cardioversion of 34 patients with acute uncomplicated AF by Lo, 88% of attempts were successful. Complications occurred in 9% of patients and were all related to sedation; 22% of patients experienced recurrent AF on follow-up. A setting of 100 J was effective in 91% of patients using biphasic cardioversion. The mean length of stay was 5.6 hours in the ED and 15 hours in the hospital (25).

Treatment Protocols for Uncomplicated Acute Onset Atrial Fibrillation—Drug and Electrical Protocols (the Role of the Observation Unit)

Traditionally when initial conversion to sinus rhythm fails, these patients are admitted to the hospital to achieve rate control, restore sinus rhythm, and test for comorbidities or complications such as MI or embolic events. The incidence of serious cardiovascular complications within this group may be as high as 20% (26). It has been reported that hospital length of stay for AF is markedly greater than for any other arrhythmia (27,28). However, a subset of acute-onset AF patients that may not require inpatient admission has also been described. A study by Mulcahy suggests that approximately one-third of admitted patients with acute-onset AF may not have required inpatient admission (29). Falk has proposed a management algorithm for stable patients with recent-onset AF that may avoid hospitalization by using a combination of initial rate control and various therapies to encourage conversion to sinus rhythm (12) (see Fig. 8-1).

In the United States there has been growing interest in the ED observation unit (EDOU) as an alternative to inpatient admission. In the United States it is estimated that more than one fourth of metropolitan EDs have an EDOU. In this setting patients with other conditions are aggressively managed using accelerated treatment or diagnostic protocols, with high discharge rates, lower costs, and improved satisfaction (30–34). The EDOU offers an ideal alternative to inpatient admission for the management of stable patients with AF presenting to the ED, that have failed initial attempts at conversion in the ED (20,35).

Koenig reported an EDOU protocol that was essentially a derivation of the algorithm described by Falk (Table 8-4). In his study, 67 patients were identified as uncomplicated AF, had achieved initial rate control in the ED, yet had failed to convert to sinus rhythm after 4.7 hours in the ED. Of these patients, 73% received medications to control rate and 73% received medications to convert rhythm. The average heart rate on ED arrival was 137 and on EDOU admission was 92 beats per minute. The EDOU management protocol (Fig. 8-1) includes continued rate control, testing for comorbidities, discretionary use of cardioverting drugs, and if this failed, then discretionary electrical cardioversion. While in the EDOU, 82% of patients converted to sinus rhythm and 81% of patients were discharged following 11.8 hours in the EDOU. Of the 23% of patients that did convert following medications in the EDOU, 31% were electrically cardioverted with 4 of 5 (80%)

TABLE 8-4

ED OBSERVATION UNIT PROTOCOL FOR THE TREATMENT OF AAF

EDOU inclusion criteria

Systolic BP >100 mm Hg, PR under 110 beats/min for 1 h (with treatment)

No chest pain with rate controlled

No evidence of acute comorbidities: MI, CHF, PE, CVA, etc.

Onset known to be less than 48 h

Cardiologist and emergency physician agree with plan to observe

EDOU interventions

Cardiac and ST-segment monitoring

Vital signs every 2 hours

Anticoagulation: aspirin, discretionary heparin (SC or IV)

Rate control as needed with calcium channel blockers, β-blockers, or digoxin

Testing: CK-MB and myoglobin at 0 and 4 hours from arrival in ED

Repeat ECG when patient converts and/or at 4 hours from arrival in the ED

Educate patient on cardioversion (medical or electrical) if treatment fails within 12 h

NPO at 12 h for electrical cardioversion to occur outside EDOU

EDOU disposition parameters

Home from the EDOU

    Patient converts and remains in sinus rhythm for 1 h

    Negative CK-MB rule-out

    Stable condition

    Discuss home medication therapy with cardiologist

Admit (inpatient) from the EDOU

    Failure to maintain rate control

    Positive CK-MB test results

    Unstable condition

Time frame

Less than 18 h

BP, blood pressure; PR, pulse rate; MI, myocardial infarction; CHF, congestive heart failure; PE, pulmonary embolism; CVA, cerebral vascular accident (stroke); NPO, nothing by mouth.
From Koenig BO, Ross MA, Jackson RE. An emergency department observation unit protocol for acute-onset atrial fibrillation is feasible. *Ann Emerg Med* 2002;39:374–381, with permission.

TABLE 8-5

RISK FACTORS FOR ISCHEMIC STROKE AND SYSTEMIC EMBOLISM IN PATIENTS WITH NONVALVULAR ATRIAL FIBRILLATION

Risk Factors (Control Groups)	Relative Risk
Previous stroke or TIA	2.5
History of hypertension	1.6
Congestive heart failure	1.4
Advanced age (continuous, per decade)	1.4
Diabetes mellitus	1.7
Coronary artery disease	1.5

TIA indicates transient ischemic attack. Relative risk refers to comparison with atrial fibrillation patients without these risk factors. As a group, patients with nonvalvular atrial fibrillation have about a sixfold increased risk of thromboembolism compared with patients in normal sinus rhythm. Data from collaborative analysis of five primary prevention trials.
From Fuster V, Rydén LE, Asinger RW, et al. ACC/AHA/ESC guidelines for the management of patients with atrial fibrillation. *Circulation* 2001;104:2118–2150, with permission.

returning to sinus rhythm and being discharged. Interestingly, serial testing and evaluations was positive for acute pathology in 7% of patients, including some patients that converted to sinus rhythm. Complications included MI (2), sepsis (2), and ventricular tachycardia (1). Seven-day return visits occurred in 4.5% with no major complications (36,37).

Decker reported preliminary results of a prospective randomized study of an 8-hour EDOU protocol for uncomplicated acute onset AF. Following care in the ED, patients were randomized to the EDOU or to an inpatient bed. The rate of conversion to NSR between groups was similar (88% vs. 95%), but the median length of stay was shorter for patients in the EDOU group (10 vs. 24 hours), and 80% of EDOU patients were discharged from the EDOU. The rate of recurrent AF was also not significantly different between groups (26% vs. 34%) (38).

Antithrombotic Therapy for Patients with Atrial Fibrillation

Although up to one-quarter of ischemic strokes in patients with a history of AF occur from sources outside the heart, intracardiac thrombus remains a major risk. Turbulence from AF and the resulting decreased laminar flow leads to clot formation, most commonly in the left atrial appendage. Unfortunately, transthoracic echocardiography cannot reliably detect this clot.

TABLE 8-6

RECOMMENDATIONS FOR ANTITHROMBOTIC THERAPY IN PATIENTS WITH ATRIAL FIBRILLATION BASED ON THROMBOEMBOLIC RISK STRATIFICATION

Patient Features	Antithrombotic Therapy	Grade of Recommendation
Age less than 60 yrs • No heart disease (lone AF)	Aspirin (325 mg daily) or no therapy	I
Age less than 60 yrs • Heart disease but no risk factors[a]	Aspirin (325 mg daily)	I
Age greater than or equal to 60 yrs • No risk factors[a]	Aspirin (325 mg daily)	I
Age greater than or equal to 60 yrs • With diabetes mellitus or CAD	Oral anticoagulation (INR 2.0–3.0) Addition of aspirin, 81–162 mg daily is optional	IIb
Age greater than or equal to 75 yrs • Especially women	Oral anticoagulation (INR ~2.0)	I
HF LV ejection fraction less than or equal to 0.35 Thyrotoxicosis Hypertension	Oral anticoagulation (INR 2.0–3.0)	I
Rheumatic heart disease (mitral stenosis) Prosthetic heart valves Prior thromboembolism Persistent atrial thrombus on TEE	Oral anticoagulation (INR 2.5–3.5 or higher may be appropriate)	I

[a]Risk factors for thromboembolism include HF, LV ejection fraction less than 0.35, and history of hypertension.
AF, atrial fibrillation; CAD, coronary artery disease; HF, heart failure; INR, international normalized ratio; LV, left ventricular; TEE, transesophageal echo.
From Fuster V, Rydén LE, Asinger RW, et al. ACC/AHA/ESC guidelines for the management of patients with atrial fibrillation. *Circulation* 2001;104:2118–2150, with permission.

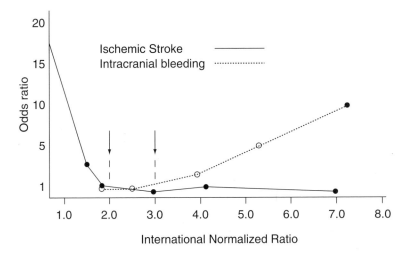

FIGURE 8-2. Adjusted odds ratios for ischemic stroke and intracranial bleeding in relation to intensity of anticoagulation in randomized trials of antithrombotic therapy for patients with AF. (From Fuster V, Rydén LE, Asinger RW, et al. ACC/AHA/ESC guidelines for the management of patients with atrial fibrillation. *Circulation* 2001;104: 2118–2150, with permission.)

However, transesophageal echo is capable of detecting left atrial appendage clots (13,15). The long-term risk of stroke in patients with AF is dependent on the number of underlying risk factors present (Table 8-5) (4). The annualized risk of thrombotic complications in the absence of anticoagulation for AF patients is 1% for lone AF, 5% for an average risk AF patient, and 12% for a high-risk patient (39). The decision to place a patient on long-term anticoagulation is dependent on their risk profile. A summary of American College of Cardiology/American Heart Association (ACC/AHA) recommendations for antithrombotic therapy based on thromboembolic risk are shown in Table 8-6 (4). The target INR is based on a balance between the bleeding risk and the thrombotic risk depending on underlying risk factors present. This is displayed in Figure 8-2. For most emergency physicians anticoagulation remains an issue that is managed in coordination with the patient's primary care physician or cardiologist. As stated earlier, full anticoagulation should not delay emergent cardioversion of patients with AF that is complicated by symptoms or signs of hemodynamic instability resulting in angina pectoris, MI, shock, or pulmonary edema. This is a class I ACC/AHA recommendation for the management of AF (4,18).

A more common issue is facing the emergency physician is a patient presenting in AF that is less than 72 hours' duration. A study by Stoddard reported that left atrial thrombi have been identified by transesophageal echo even in AF of less than 72 hours' duration (15). However, despite this finding, many treatment guidelines still allow for the cardioversion of AF known to be of less than 48 hours in duration without anticoagulation (12,14). This recommendation is made because despite the presence of thrombi, the incidence of clinically significant thromboembolism in AF less than 48 hours' duration is similar to the incidence of thromboembolism in patients treated with anticoagulation and delayed cardioversion (15,16). The decision to anticoagulate patients with less than 48 hours of AF before and after cardioversion may be made based on an assessment of the patient's risk (4,18).

In conclusion, AF represents one of the most significant cardiac arrhythmias that emergency physicians will manage. There are many important risk factors to consider—such as the duration of symptoms, complications, and comorbidities. There are also many treatment options available to the emergency physician, each with their own risks and benefits.

References

1. Michael JA, Stiell IG, Agarwal S, et al. Cardioversion of paroxysmal atrial fibrillation in the emergency department. *Ann Emerg Med* 1994;33: 379–387.
2. Noble J. *Textbook of primary care medicine.* 3rd ed. St. Louis, MO: Mosby; 2001.
3. Go AS, Hylek EM, Phillips KA, et al. Prevalence of diagnosed atrial fibrillation in adults: national implications for rhythm management and stroke prevention: the AnTicoagulation and Risk Factors In Atrial Fibrillation (ATIA) study. *JAMA* 2001;285:2370–2375.
4. Fuster V, Rydén LE, Asinger RW, et al. ACC/AHA/ESC guidelines for the management of patients with atrial fibrillation: executive summary—a report of the American College of Cardiology/American Heart Association Task Force on Practice Guidelines and the European Society of Cardiology Committee for Practice Guidelines and Policy Conferences. *Circulation* 2001;104:2118–2150.
5. Herzog E, Fischer A, Steinberg J. The rate control, anticoagulation therapy, and electrophysiology/antiarrhythmic medication pathway for the management of atrial fibrillation and atrial flutter. *Crit Pathways in Cardiol* 2005; 4:121–126.
6. Goldberger, AL. *Clinical electrocardiography: a simplified approach.* 6th ed. St. Louis, MO: Mosby; 1999.
7. Yealy DM, Delbridge TR. Dysrhythmias. In: Marx JA, Hockberger RS, Walls RM. *Rosen's emergency medicine: concepts & clinical practice.* 5th ed. St. Louis, MO: Mosby; 2002:1053–1065.
8. Zipes DP, Braunwald E, Libby P, et al. *Braunwald's heart disease: a textbook of cardiovascular medicine.* 7th ed. Philadelphia: Saunders; 2005.
9. Veenhuyzen GD, Simpson CS, Abodllah H. Review: atrial fibrillation. *CMAJ* 2004;171:755–760.
10. Everett TH, Olgin JE. Basic mechanism of atrial fibrillation. *Cardiol Clin* 2004;22:9–20.
11. Wagner GS. Atrial flutter/fibrillation spectrum. In: Wagner GS, Marriott HJL. *Marriott's practical electrocardiography.* 9th ed. Baltimore: Williams & Wilkins; 1994:269–295.
12. Falk RH. Atrial fibrillation. *N Engl J Med* 2001;344:1067–1078.
13. Klein AL, Grimm RA, Murray RD, et al. Use of transesophageal echocardiography to guide cardioversion in patients with atrial fibrillation. *N Engl J Med* 2001;344:1411–1420.
14. Huguai L, Easly A, Barrington W, et al. Evaluation and management of atrial fibrillation in the emergency department. *Emerg Med Clin North Am* 1998;16:289–303.
15. Stoddard MF, Dawkins PR, Prince CR, et al. Left atrial appendage thrombus is not uncommon in patients with acute atrial fibrillation and a recent embolic event: a transesophageal echocardiographic study. *J Am Coll Cardiol* 1995;25:453–459.
16. Weigner MJ, Caulfield TA. Risk of clinical thromboembolism associated with conversion to sinus rhythm in patients with atrial fibrillation lasting less than 48 hours. *Ann Intern Med* 1997;126:615–620.
17. del Arco C, Martin A, Laguna P, et al. Analysis of current management of atrial fibrillation in the acute setting: GEFAUR-1 study. *Ann Emerg Med* 205;46:424–430.
18. Part 7.3 Management of symptomatic bradycardia and tachycardia. In 2005 AHA guidelines for CPR and ECC. *Circulation* 2005;112:IV-67–IV-77.
19. Atkins DL, Dorian P, Gonzalez ER, et al. Treatment of tachyarrhythmias. *Ann Emerg Med* 2001;37:S91–S109.
20. Radford MJ Atrial fibrillation. In: Graff LG. *Observation medicine.* Boston: Andover Medical; 1993:125–132.
21. The Atrial Fibrillation Follow-up Investigation of Rhythm Management (AFFIRM) Investigators. A comparison of rate control and rhythm control in patients with atrial fibrillation. *N Engl J Med* 2002;347:1825–1833.
22. Van Gelder IC, Hagens VE, Bosker HA, et al. A comparison of rate control and rhythm control in patients with recurrent persistent atrial fibrillation. *N Engl J Med* 2002;347:1834–1840.

23. Falk RL. Editorial: management of atrial fibrillation—radical reform or modest modification? *N Engl J Med* 2002;347:1883–1884.

24. Burton JH, Vinson DR, Drummond K, et al. Electrical cardioversion of emergency department patients with atrial fibrillation. *Ann Emerg Med* 2004;44:20–30.

25. Lo GK, Fatovich DM, Haig AD. Biphasic cardioversion of acute atrial fibrillation in the emergency department. *Emerg Med J* 2006;23:51–53.

26. Friedman HZ, Scot FG, Bonema JD, et al. Acute complications associated with new-onset atrial fibrillation. *Am J Cardiol* 1991;67:437–439.

27. Prystowsky EN, Benson DW, Fuster V, et al. Management of patients with atrial fibrillation; a statement for healthcare professionals from the Subcommittee on Electrocardiography and Electrophysiology, American Heart Association. *Circulation* 1996;93:1262–1277.

28. Bialy D, Lehmann MH, Schumacher DN, et al. Hospitalization for arrhythmias in the United States: importance of atrial fibrillation [abstract]. *J Am Coll Cardiol* 1992;19:41A.

29. Mulcahy B, Coates WC, Hennerman PL, et al. New-onset atrial fibrillation: When is admission medically justified? *Acad Emerg Med* 1996;3:114–119.

30. Rydman RJ, Isola MI, Roberts RR, et al. Emergency department observation unit versus hospital inpatient care for a chronic asthmatic population: a randomized trial of health status outcome and cost. *Med Care* 1998;36:599–609.

31. Rydman RJ, Roberts RR, Albrecht GL, et al. Patient satisfaction with an emergency department asthma observation unit. *Acad Emerg Med* 1999;6:178–183.

32. Gomez MA, Jefferey LA, Karagounis LA, et al. An emergency department based protocol for rapidly ruling myocardial ischemia reduces hospital time and expense: results of a randomized study (ROMIO). *J Am Coll Cardiol* 1996;28:25–33.

33. Farkouh ME, Smars PA, Reeder GS, et al. A clinical trial of a chest-pain observation unit for patients with unstable angina. *N Engl J Med* 1998;339:1882–1888.

34. Rydman RJ, Zalenski RJ, Roberts RR, et al. Patient satisfaction with an emergency department chest pain observation unit. *Ann Emerg Med* 1997;29:109–116.

35. Cunningham R, Mikhail MG. Management of patients with syncope and cardiac arrhythmias in an emergency department observation unit. *Emerg Med Clin N Am* 2001;19:1:105–122.

36. Koenig BO, Ross MA, Jackson RE. An emergency department observation unit protocol for acute-onset atrial fibrillation is feasible. *Ann Emerg Med* 2002;39:374–381.

37. Ross MA, Davis B, Dresselhouse A. The role of an emergency department observation unit in a clinical pathway for atrial fibrillation. *Crit Pathways in Cardiol* 2004;3:8–12.

38. Decker WW, Goyal DG, Boie ET, et al. A prospective, randomized trial of an emergency department observation unit for acute onset atrial fibrillation. [abstract]. *Acad Emerg Med* 2003;10:543–544.

39. Ansell J, Hirsh J, Poller L, et al. The pharmacology and management of vitamin K antagonists, the seventh ACCP conference on antithrombotic and thrombolytic therapy. *Chest* 2004;126:204S–233S.

40. Davey MJ, Teubner. A randomized controlled trial of magnesium sulfate, in addition to usual care, for rate control in atrial fibrillation. *Ann Emerg Med* 2005;45:347–353.

CHAPTER 9 ■ STROKE AND TRANSIENT ISCHEMIC ATTACK

ABDUL ABDULLAH AND LEE H. SCHWAMM

CLINICAL DIAGNOSIS OF STROKE AND TIA
CURRENT RECOMMENDED TREATMENTS
Thrombolysis in Acute Ischemic Stroke (AIS)
MERCI for AIS
Antithrombotics for AIS
Emergent Carotid Endarterectomy (CEA) for AIS/TIA
Evidence-Based Interventions in Hemorrhagic Stroke
Role of Blood Pressure (BP) Control in the Acute Stage of AIS
NEUROIMAGING PATHWAYS IN THE EMERGENCY
  DEPARTMENT (ED) FOR ACUTE STROKE
VARIABILITY IN STROKE CARE
RATIONALE FOR DEVELOPING CRITICAL CARE
  PATHWAYS FOR STROKE AND TIA
MULTI- OR INTERDISCIPLINARY TEAM SELECTION FOR
  CRITICAL PATHWAY DEVELOPMENT AND
  EXECUTION: STROKE QUALITY IMPROVEMENT AT
  MGH
Stroke Quality Improvement Infrastructure
PATHWAYS ORGANIZATION INTO THE CHAIN OF
  STROKE SURVIVAL
Community Education
The Role of Telemedicine in Connecting Providers
Effective Communication with Prehospital Providers
Prevention of Complications Due to Stroke
SUMMARY

classify a transient syndrome with evidence of infarction as an ischemic stroke rather than a TIA. This has led to some attempts at reclassification and to emphasize the importance of treating ischemic stroke and TIA in a similar manner.

Neuroimaging techniques, including CT (computed tomography), MRI (magnetic resonance imaging), and PET (positron emission tomography), have revolutionized our concepts of temporal events that occur in relation to brain ischemia (2). This technology allows neurologists to detect ischemic episodes more accurately and quickly. Efficient discovery of brain infarction is valuable in initiating secondary prevention strategies that will reduce the risk of subsequent debilitating events.

In a study of patients diagnosed with TIA in an emergency department (ED), 10.5% of the patients suffered an ischemic stroke within 90 days of the diagnosed TIA, and of those, 50% had an ischemic stroke within a 24- to 48-hour time period. Increased risk was associated with advanced age, diabetes mellitus, hypertension, and a history of vascular disease (3). Thus, clinicians have proposed a new definition of TIA that takes into consideration the fact that a TIA can result in permanent damage to the brain. The definition is targeted at facilitating brain imaging and rapid intervention (2).

In light of these findings, it is apparent that the urgent evaluation of an ischemic stroke or TIA should not be significantly divergent because both have the potential for substantial short-term deleterious consequences.

CLINICAL DIAGNOSIS OF STROKE AND TIA

Stroke is a major cause of morbidity and mortality in the United States. It is the third leading cause of death and continues to be a primary cause of long-term disability in the United States. About 700,000 Americans have a new or recurrent stroke each year: 88% of all strokes are ischemic, 9% are due to intracerebral hemorrhage, and 3% are due to subarachnoid hemorrhage (1). Because treatment is available for acute ischemic stroke (AIS), it is critical to have methods for rapidly identifying the stroke, subtype and initiating treatment protocols. An example of such an algorithm can be seen in Figure 9-1 and is also available in a hyperlinked version on our stroke management internet resource at http://www.acutestroke.com.

Although it is important to distinguish ischemic stroke from transient ischemic attack (TIA) because they reflect different clinical syndromes, it is also important to recognize that they frequently reflect the same underlying pathophysiology, namely atherosclerosis or thromboembolism. TIA, sometimes called a "ministroke" in common parlance, is defined as "a sudden, focal neurological deficit that lasts for less than 24 hours (and) is confined to an area of the brain or eye perfused by a specific artery," whereas ischemic stroke lasts more than 24 hours. Although both of these are clinical syndromes and do not require evidence of brain infarction by neuroimaging, many physicians would

CURRENT RECOMMENDED TREATMENTS

Thrombolysis in Acute Ischemic Stroke

IV tPA (Intravenous recombinant tissue plasminogen activator-rtPA)

The efficacy of tPA has been evaluated by two major studies: the NINDS tPA trial and the ECASS study (4,5). The NINDS tPA trial was a randomized, double-blind, placebo-controlled trial that demonstrated that patients treated within 3 hours of symptom onset for ischemic stroke had a better clinical outcome at 3 months. This benefit was measured as a 12% absolute and 30% relative greater chance of having minimal or no disability at 3 months in all four outcome measures (NIH Stroke Scale, Barthel Index, Modified Rankin Scale, Glasgow Outcome Scale) as compared with placebo-treated patients. Secondary analysis of the NINDS trial showed statistically significant improvement in the median National Institute of Heath Stroke Scale (NIHSS) score at 24 hours in the tPA group (8 versus 12; $P <0.02$). All the stroke subtypes benefited consistently from tPA treatment. Rates of symptomatic intracerebral hemorrhage within 36 hours after the onset of stroke were 6.4% in patients who received tPA versus 0.6% for patients who received placebo ($P <0.001$) (4).

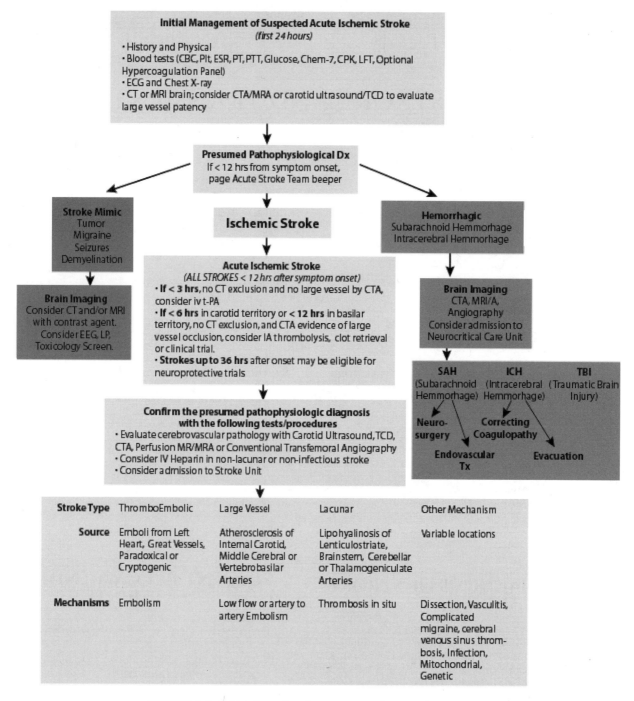

FIGURE 9-1. Initial diagnosis and management of suspected acute stroke.

The ECASS trials (ECASS 1, ECASS 2) attempted to increase the time window of treatment with the administration of tPA within 6 hours of symptom onset. The ECASS trials did not meet their primary efficacy endpoints, but meta-analyses confirm the benefit of tPA in the first 3 hours after stroke onset and suggest that tPA may be beneficial between 3 and 5 hours after stroke onset in a subset of patients with preserved brain parenchyma on imaging (5,6).

The major consensus organizations and evidence-based guidelines recommend administering tPA for carefully selected AIS patients within the 3-hour window of established symptom onset time (7,8). In addition, pooled data analysis of three large trials (ATLANTIS [Alteplase thrombolysis for acute noninter-

ventional therapy in ischemic stroke], ECASS, and NINDS) using an adjusted multiple regression model demonstrated that earlier treatment is strongly linked to a larger benefit, and patients should be treated as rapidly as possible (9).

The development of a critical care pathway for thrombolysis in acute stroke treatment attempts to ensure the efficient and equitable delivery of tPA to appropriate patients. Critical care protocols aid in rapid identification and treatment of ischemic strokes, thereby increasing the rates of IV tPA use and decreasing the practice deviations (10–12). Our Massachusetts General Hospital (MGH) acute stroke critical pathway for thrombolytic therapy is shown in Figure 9-2. This algorithm is placed

(*Text continues on page 71*)

?Acute Stroke?

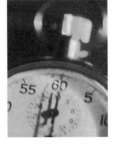

Chief Complaint at Triage Sudden Onset of Any of the Following:
- **Sudden numbness/weakness of face, arm, leg (especially unilateral)**
- **Confusion, difficulty speaking or understanding**
- **Facial droop**
- **Loss of coordination, difficulty walking or unexplained falls**
- **Visual disturbances**

Symptom onset within 6 hours of arrival in ED?
PAGE ACUTE STROKE BEEPER
<u>Message</u>: "Acute stroke, (pt name) in ED now, (Trauma attending name)"

<u>**Triage Nurse Action**</u>:

Identification of potential acute stroke w/in 6 hours of onset of symptoms
Page Acute Stroke beeper
Document VS & time of onset of symptoms
Assess for:
- o Contrast allergy
- o Medication history:
  - Coumadin (date/time of last dose?)
  - Aspirin (date/time of last dose?)

Triage to Trauma/Acute & notify Attending Physician
- o Request coordinator page Neuro Resident on call for ED
- o If no response from Acute Stroke Team, page again or call Neuro ICU fellow

---

<u>**Trauma/Acute Primary Nurse Actions**</u>:

12-lead ECG then initiate patient monitoring using Travel Monitor
Record VS q 15 minutes
Place 18g angio in forearm (preferably antecubital)
Anticipate order for oxygen at 2-10 lpm to maintain SpO2 at ≥ 95%
Serum labs per Acute Stroke protocol
Anticipate order to travel on monitor with RN
Frequent neuro reassessment and documentation of findings
MAINTAIN STRICT NPO STATUS including medications
If ordered for tPA, see attached preparation and administration protocol

FIGURE 9-2. MGH acute stroke critical pathway for thrombolytic therapy. (*continues*)

MGH Emergency Department
ACUTE STROKE PROTOCOL
FOR THROMBOLYSIS (IV/IA)

Eligible Patients: Onset of Symptoms or Last Seen Well <6 Hr before ED Arrival
Location: Emergency Department

Major responsibilities for the urgent evaluation and treatment of acute stroke patients who present to the ED. Please refer to other guidelines for the management of inpatients with acute stroke symptoms, or those who present between 6 to 12 hrs after onset of symptoms. Refer to the on-line detailed protocols at www.acutestroke.com. This document is divided into Pre-Treatment, Treatment and Post-Treatment phases:

PRE-TREATMENT PHASE

ED Triage Nurse Responsibilities (Check as complete when appropriate):

- ❑ Identifies patients with symptoms of acute stroke based on clinical presentation or entry notification from prehospital EMS personnel
- ❑ If the patient was last seen normal (or at baseline level of functioning) < 6 hours before ED arrival, immediately page the Acute Stroke Team with message "Acute stroke, (state patient name), in ED now; (state Trauma attending name)"
- ❑ Obtain Acute Stroke Protocol packet and review responsibilities as outlined on cover:
  - Document vital signs
  - Document time of onset of symptoms
  - Specifically assess for exclusion criteria for t-PA as outlined on packet cover including:
    - Past medical/surgical history
    - Allergies
    - Medications (if on Coumadin or aspirin, note time of last dose)
- ❑ Send to Trauma/Acute and notify ED Attending

Coordinator in Trauma/Acute:

- ❑ Notify Neurology Resident on call for ED and immediately page Acute Stroke Team if not already notified by Triage RN

Primary Nurse in Trauma/Acute:

- ❑ Acquire 12-lead ECG and immediately prepare for patient to travel to CT with portable monitor and oxygen
- ❑ Document vital signs every 15 minutes
- ❑ Place 18 gauge angiocatheter in large vein, preferably antecubital, saline lock
- ❑ Anticipate order for oxygen at 2-10 liters/minute to maintain $SpO_2 \geq 95\%$
- ❑ Anticipate orders for labs as follows:
  - CBC, platelets, ESR
  - Blood bank specimen for type & screen
  - PT/PTT/INR
  - Na/K/Cl/CO2/BUN/Cr/Glucose
  - SGOT, SGPT, alk phos
  - CPK, troponin
  - If the patient's age is <55 years, add hypercoagulation screen
- ❑ Travel with patient to CT (bring IV tPA to CT if indicated and ordered)

FIGURE 9-2. *(continues)*

- ❑ Document hourly neurologic reassessment (more frequently if changes occur)
- ❑ Maintain strictly NPO (including meds) until swallowing screen performed and passed
- ❑ Anticipate order for IV tPA to be started in CT
- ❑ Do not insert NG tube or foley unless ordered by MD

ED Physician Responsibilities:
- ❑ Ensure that Stroke Team has been paged
- ❑ Notify CT of Acute Stroke Patient for urgent CT/CTA
- ❑ If accepting request for transfer of acute stroke patient inform the referring facility that the Stroke Team will contact them and immediately page the Acute Stroke Team with message, "Acute stroke (state name of patient) at (state name of referring facility and telephone number), (state ED attending name)."
- ❑ Rapid evaluation of patient to rule out acute MI, aortic dissection, other co-morbid condition or non-stroke etiology (i.e., stroke mimic) and medical contraindications to tPA. Identify severity of neurologic deficit and potential contraindications to IV tPA.
- ❑ Obtain CXR before Brain CT **only** if clinically indicated for respiratory compromise or to exclude underlying aortic or cardiac injury
- ❑ Unless airway compromise requires immediate need for intubation, facilitate rapid assessment of NIH Stroke Scale by Stroke Team prior to intubation
- ❑ Review treatment plan with Acute Stroke Team and any potential contraindications

Neurologist Responsibilities (includes Resident, Fellow or Attending):
- ❑ Respond within 5 minutes to Acute Stroke Pager contact
- ❑ Examine patient, document NIHSS, and establish time of onset, review inclusion and exclusion criteria and document reasons for non-treatment if contraindicated
- ❑ Review non-contrast CT or MR brain imaging with radiologist and order CTA-CTP unless contraindicated. Do not delay initiation of tPA for further imaging (e.g. MRI) unless diagnosis is uncertain
- ❑ Discuss risks and benefits of tPA and other treatment options with family/patient from standard tPA information sheet and obtain written consent when appropriate

Radiologist Responsibilities:
- ❑ Report to CT immediately upon start of non-contrast CT, and provide immediate interpretation upon completion of imaging.
- ❑ Supervise the administration of IV contrast for CTA/CTP.
- ❑ Provide immediate access to the 16 slice CT scanner for any acute stroke patient who is a thrombolysis candidate, including removing a patient from the scanner if necessary.

Radiology Technologist Responsibilities:
- ❑ Facilitate the immediate access of acute stroke patients into the scanner
- ❑ Assist in obtaining IV access for contrast if none present
- ❑ Page the emergency neuroradiologist as soon as notified of the acute stroke patient and upon patient arrival in the scanner area
- ❑ Execute the standard acute stroke CT/CTA protocols in collaboration with the neuroradiologist and Acute Stroke Team

TREATMENT PHASE: IV tPA Administration for Patients Arriving Within 3 Hours

ED Nurse Responsibilities:
- ❑ Mix and draw up tPA per protocol:

FIGURE 9-2. (*continues*)

- o Provide physician with the 10% bolus dose, either in CT area or ED bay
- o Prepare the infusion
- o If tPA is mixed but patient does not receive drug, initiate rebate and restocking procedures
- ❑ Once infusion begins monitor vital signs as follows:
    - o Every 15 min for 2 hours, then:
    - o Every 30 minutes for 6 hours, then:
    - o Every 60 minutes for 16 hours
- ❑ Notify physician immediately if SBP/DBP > 175/100
- ❑ Do not insert Foley catheter or nasogastric tube unless ordered
- ❑ Document hourly neurologic reassessment (more frequently if changes occur)

Neurologist Responsibilities (includes Resident, Fellow or Attending):
- ❑ Calculate IV tPA dose based on weight estimate and tPA dosing table:
    - o Document estimated weight
    - o Review with nursing staff to ensure accuracy
    - o Write order for tPA total dose as a bolus plus infusion
    - o Administer the 10% bolus over 1 minute and document time on ED medication order sheet
- ❑ Repeat NIHSS evaluation if patient exam has changed significantly
- ❑ Strict control of blood pressure for 24 hours per protocol
- ❑ Request an Acute Stroke admission bed to the CMF Service. The patient remains under the care of the Acute Stroke Team until officially transferred to the CMF Attending
- ❑ Coordinate the post tPA care with the ED attending to ensure continuity until the patient can be transferred out of the ED

POST-TREATMENT PHASE: after IV tPA Administration

ED Nurse Responsibilities:
- ❑ Document neurologic assessment hourly or more frequently if changes occur
- ❑ Vital sign monitoring as described above under "Treatment Phase"
- ❑ Verify the patency of IV and completion of the tPA dose
- ❑ Provide nursing report to the accepting nurse
- ❑ Provide family/patient with appropriate resource materials about stroke

Neurologist Responsibilities (includes Resident, Fellow or Attending):
- ❑ ICU/Acute Stroke Unit admission for monitoring during first 24 hours
- ❑ Modify the standard POE order set for stroke post tPA as indicated
- ❑ Vital signs every 15 minutes for 2 hours, then every 30 minutes for 6 hours, then every 1 hour for 16 hours
- ❑ Strict control of blood pressure for 24 hours per protocol
- ❑ Restrict patient intake to strict NPO including meds until swallowing screen performed and passed
- ❑ Continuous pulse oximetry monitoring, order oxygen by nasal cannula or mask to maintain O2 sat > 95%
- ❑ Tylenol 650 mg po/pr every 4 hours prn T > 99.4; consider cooling for T > 102
- ❑ No antiplatelet agents or anticoagulants (including heparins for DVT prophylaxis) in first 24 hours
- ❑ No Foley catheter, nasogastric tube, arterial catheter or central venous catheter for 24 hr, unless absolutely necessary
- ❑ For any worsening of neurologic condition, STAT HEAD CT, and initiate the post-tPA ICH protocol if significant hemorrhage is detected.
- ❑ Coordinate care with accepting CMF team resident.

FIGURE 9-2. (*continues*)

MASSACHUSETTS GENERAL HOSPITAL
Department of Nursing

TITLE: EMERGENCY DEPARTMENT ADMINISTRATION OF INTRAVENOUS TISSUE PLASMINOGEN ACTIVATOR FOR ACUTE ISCHEMIC STROKE

GENERIC NAME: Alteplase

TRADE NAME: Activase

APPLICABLE UNIT: EMERGENCY DEPARTMENT

ACTION: Tissue plasminogen activator (tPA) for thrombolysis

INDICATION: Treatment of acute ischemic stroke

CRITICAL ELEMENTS:
1. Usual Dosage Range and Route:
   a. 0.9 mg/kg to a maximum of 90 mg:
      - First 10% of calculated dose GIVEN BY PHYSICIAN as intravenous bolus dose
      - Remaining 90% of calculated dose given in infusion over 1 hour
2. Verify that the Stroke Neurologist has reviewed the inclusion/exclusion criteria and discussed the plan with the patient and/or family if available
3. Verify that administration will start within three hours of symptom onset or time last known well
4. Document neurologic assessment findings at least hourly or more frequently if neurologic changes occur
5. If the patient's neurologic status declines during tPA infusion the following actions should be taken:
   a. Stop the infusion
   b. Page the Stroke Neurologist
   c. Draw and send PT/PTT, D-Dimer and fibrinogen
   d. Prepare for emergent CT

EQUIPMENT:
- 1 vial of Activase (tPA) 100 mg <u>or</u> two vials of Activase (tPA) 50 mg each
- One 10 ml syringe
- Two 19-gauge needles
- One blunt canula
- Standard pump tubing
- Intravenous infusion pump
- 100 cc bag of 0.9% NS
- Alcohol wipes
- Two red medication labels

ADMINISTRATION PROTOCOL: It is appropriate to mix tPA prior to CT even if it is not used: See below procedure for returning tPA that is mixed but not administered.
1. Verify the bolus dose, infusion dose and discard dose with the Stroke Neurologist
2. Reconstitute the vial of t-PA with the supplied preservative-free water:
   a. Direct stream of water into lypophilized cake
   b. Swirl but DO NOT SHAKE (slight foaming is common)
   c. Let stand several minutes to allow large bubbles to dissipate
   d. Final concentration is 1 mg/ml

FIGURE 9-2. (*continues*)

3. Using a 10 ml syringe, withdraw the bolus dose directly from the Activase bottle (see dosing sheet for bolus dose based on patient weight*). Fill out red medication label with all required information (patient name, medication, dosage, time, date, RN signature). Write "BOLUS DOSE" and affix label to syringe.
4. Hand the bolus dose syringe to the Stroke Neurologist and verify again the bolus dose, infusion dose and rate and discard dose
5. Stroke Neurologist will administer bolus dose via intravenous push method over one minute
    a. Stroke Neurologist will document administration of bolus dose on ED Medication Administration record including time, dose, route, initials and signature
6. Fill out red medication label with all required information (patient name, medication, dosage, time, date, RN signature). Write "INFUSION DOSE" and affix label to Activase bottle
7. Draw waste dose from bottle and verify waste amount by showing to the Stroke Neurologist and another nurse.
8. Connect Activase bottle to IV pump tubing, carefully priming to avoid discarding any medication.
9. Verify patency of IV site and tubing connections
10. Verify that all blood work has been drawn and sent
11. Attach noninvasive blood pressure cuff to other arm
12. Set infusion pump rate according to dosing sheet and start infusion with a total infusion time of 1 hour. Document infusion start time and name of Stroke Neurologist.
13. When pump alarms "no flow above", there is still some tPA left in the tubing which must be infused. Remove the IV tubing connector from the Activase bottle and attach it to a newly spiked 100 cc bag of 0.9% NS. Continue the infusion at the current setting to deliver the remainder of the original tPA volume over the remaining time. Continue the infusion until the preset volume is completed.
14. Document end time of infusion. Expect to see significant volume remaining in 100 cc 0.9% NS bag.

PRECAUTIONS AND SIDE EFFECTS:
- Hemorrhage (GI, GU, catheter puncture site, intracranial, retroperitoneal, pericardial, gingival, epistaxis)
- New ischemic stroke
- Bruising
- Anaphylaxis
- Laryngeal edema
- Rash, urticaria

PROTOCOL FOR RETURNING UNUSED MEDICATION:
When tPA is mixed but not administered or the packaging is damaged, the reconstituted and unused tPA should be returned for pharmacy credit:
1. If tPA is removed from Omnicell but not reconstituted and the packaging is intact, return to Omnicell under the patient's name
2. If tPA is reconstituted or the packaging is not intact and the medication was not used, place a patient identification label on any container holding reconstituted drug _ tPA bottle, syringe or IV bag. (Remove blunt canula or needles from syringes.) Place containers in a plastic bag if necessary to prevent spillage
3. Place all containers in the blue bin in the Trauma/Acute med room (bin is labeled "tPA return")
4. Do not place any IV administration equipment (tubing, etc.) in the blue bin

rt-PA Dosing Converter Sheet

- Total Dose to be given not to exceed **90 mg**
- Bolus dose is 10% of total dose

FIGURE 9-2. (*continues*)

Estimated Weight (lbs)	Conversion to Kilograms (Kg)	Total iv t-PA Dose (mg) at 0.9 mg/kg	t-PA Bolus (mg) *10% of total *	t-PA Bolus (ml)	Discard Dose t-PA (Not for infusion)	Infusion Dose (mg)	Infusion Rate (ml/hr)
220+	100	90	9	9	10	81	81
210	95.5	85.9	8.6	8.6	14.1	77.3	77.3
200	90.9	81.8	8.2	8.2	18.2	73.6	73.6
190	86.4	77.7	7.8	7.8	22.3	70	70
180	81.8	73.6	7.4	7.4	26.4	66.3	66.3
170	77.3	69.5	7	7	30.5	62.6	62.6
160	72.7	65.5	6.5	6.5	34.5	58.9	58.9
150	68.2	61.4	6.1	6.1	38.6	55.2	55.2
140	63.6	57.3	5.7	5.7	42.7	51.5	51.5
130	59.1	53.2	5.3	5.3	46.8	47.9	47.9
120	54.5	49.1	4.9	4.9	50.9	44.2	44.2
110	50	45	4.5	4.5	55	40.5	40.5
100	45.5	40.9	4.1	4.1	59.1	36.8	36.8

For more information about stroke, please see www.strokeassociation.org

Provider Feedback Sheet

The MGH Acute Stroke Quality Taskforce (ASQT) values your feedback about the acute stroke care process and about how we might improve. In our effort to make this packet as informative and helpful to you as possible, we would welcome any comments or suggestions you might have.

e-mail us at ASQT@partners.org, or to write your feedback on the *back of this sheet.*

FIGURE 9-2. (continued)

in the context of catheter-based and nonreperfusion strategies in our acute stroke algorithms, as shown in Figure 9-3.

IA Thrombolysis for AIS

PROACT II (Prolyse in Acute Cerebral Thromboembolism II) was the first randomized multicenter trial to show the clinical efficacy of IA thrombolysis in patients with acute stroke of less than 6 hours' duration caused by middle cerebral artery (MCA) occlusion. The study demonstrated a 15% absolute benefit with 40% of the r-proUK treated group ($P = 0.04$) achieving independence (Modified Rankin score of 2 or less) at 90 days, compared to only 25% of the control patients. The recanalization rate at the end of treatment was 66% for the r-proUK group and 18% for the control group ($P <0.001$) (13).

Clinical trials assessing the use of combined IV and IA-tPA are underway. One such pilot study demonstrated that combined IV/IA treatment was feasible and provided better results with respect to recanalization, even though it was not coupled with improved clinical outcomes (14). The latest guidelines suggest that even though IA thrombolysis alone or in combination with IV tPA (also called bridging therapy) is promising, the applicability of this intervention still needs to be validated by randomized studies and should only be performed at centers with dedicated personnel and experienced operators (8).

MERCI for AIS

Previously the only Food and Drug Administration (FDA)-approved treatment for AISs was IV rtPA. However, the FDA recently approved a mechanical embolectomy device (MERCI [Mechanical Embolus Removal in Cerebral Ischemia]) for clot removal within 8 hours of symptom onset. It is a treatment option for patients who do not qualify for r-tPA administration. The primary study outcome for the unblinded, single-arm MERCI trial was the rate of recanalization of the basilar artery, terminal internal carotid artery, or the main middle cerebral artery branches versus control subjects from the PROACT 2 trial (46% versus 18% in an intention to treat analysis). At 90 days, patients with recanalization were more likely to be alive and independent (Modified Rankin score of ≤2) than those without recanalization (15).

Antithrombotics for AIS

Aspirin is the only antiplatelet agent that has been thoroughly evaluated for AIS (7). A placebo-controlled trial of aspirin (325 mg/dL) reported no major decline in rate of neurological deterioration. Patients were enrolled within 48 hours of onset of stroke symptoms and treated for 5 days (16). Administration

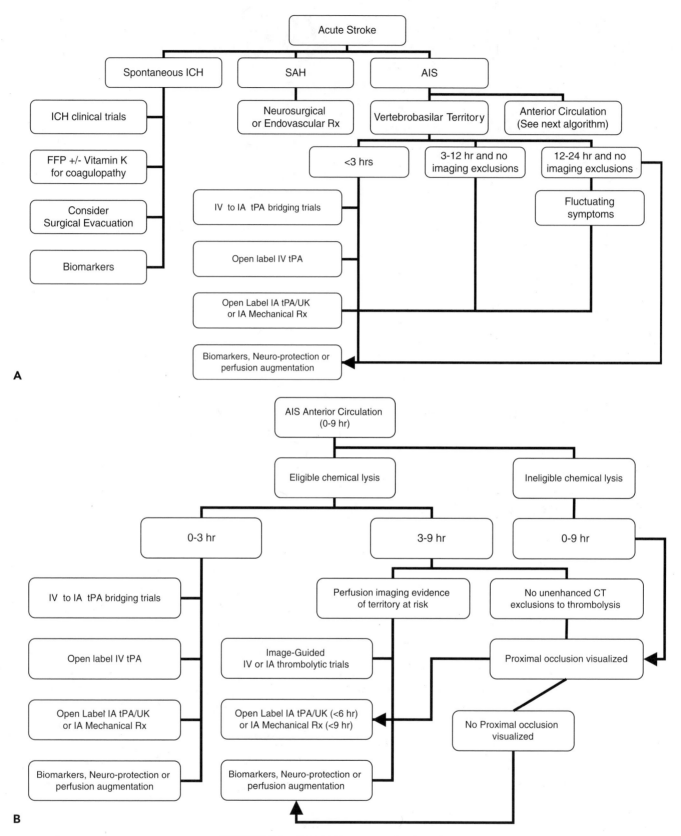

FIGURE 9-3. (A,B) MGH acute stroke algorithms.

of abciximab, an intravenous chimeric mouse–human monoclonal antibody directed against the platelet glycoprotein IIb/IIIa receptor, has shown promising results when given within 6 hours of stroke onset and is under study (8).

The meta-analysis of eight trials provides more detailed data regarding the efficacy of antiplatelet agents (17). It essentially shows that, for every 1,000 acute strokes treated with aspirin, there are approximately 7 fewer early recurrent strokes and 13 fewer deaths and/or dependencies (7). Based on these data, current recommendations endorse the use of aspirin within 48 hours of onset of stroke symptoms because the benefits, though small, are significant, particularly in light of safety and cost considerations. However, aspirin and other antithrombotics should not be used within 24 hours of the use of thrombolytic therapies (7,8).

Emergent Carotid Endarterectomy (CEA) for AIS/TIA

The efficacy of emergent CEA for acute ischemic strokes and TIA (18,19) remains unproven, though some studies have shown promising results. One retrospective study of 21 patients for CEA performed within 24 hours of diagnostic workup for TIA or AIS showed the survival rates at 1 and 5 years to be 90% and 62%, respectively (20). In another study of 67 patients (58% strokes, 42% TIA), flow through the internal carotid artery was re-established in 93% of patients (21). Diffusion or perfusion mismatch criteria for the selection of candidates for CEA may lead to improved patient selection (22).

Evidence-Based Interventions in Hemorrhagic Stroke

Surgery or Endovascular Therapy for Aneurysmal SAH (Followed by Nimodipine for Vasospasm)

Incidence of subarachnoid hemorrhage (SAH) from an intracranial aneurysm rupture occurs at a frequency of 6 or 8 per 100,000 person-years (23). The International Subarachnoid Aneurysm Trial (ISAT) compared the safety and efficacy of endovascular treatment of ruptured intracranial aneurysms and conventional neurosurgical treatment (craniotomy and clipping of the ruptured intracranial aneurysm). A total number of 2,143 patients with ruptured intracranial aneurysms were enrolled and randomly assigned to neurosurgical clipping ($n = 1,070$) or endovascular treatment by detachable platinum coils ($n = 1,073$). At 1 year, endovascular coiling reduced the relative risk of death and dependence by 22.6% with an absolute risk reduction of 6.9% (24).

SAH may result in cerebral vasospasm, which is the delayed narrowing of large-volume arteries at the base of the brain. Cerebral vasospasm is often coupled with radiographic or cerebral blood flow evidence of reduced perfusion in the distal territory of the affected artery. A number of prospective, randomized trials for the oral agent nimodipine demonstrate that it consistently reduces poor outcome due to vasospasm in all grades of patients (25).

Correcting Coagulopathy in Intracerebral Hemorrhage

Spontaneous intracerebral hemorrhage (SICH) is the most fatal form of stroke with a mortality rate between 30% and 55%, increasing to as high as 67% in patients receiving oral anticoagulant therapy (OAT). There are currently no standardized guidelines for reversal of the anticoagulant effect in the patients with OAT-ICH. Administering 10 mg vitamin K with every treatment to support the supply of prothrombin-dependent clotting factors has been recommended. Other treatment options include fresh frozen plasma (FFP), prothrombin complex concentrates (PCC), and recombinant activated factor VIIa (rFVIIa) (26). Rapid correction of the abnormal International Normalized Ratio (INR) is associated with successful reversal at 24 hours; compared to patients who were not successfully reversed at 24 hours, patients whose INR was successfully reversed within 24 hours had a shorter median time from diagnosis to first dose of FFP (90 minutes versus 210 minutes; $P = 0.02$). In a multivariate model, shorter time to vitamin K as well as FFP predicted INR correction (27). An example of a clinical protocol for reversal of anticoagulation is presented in the following extract.

MGH Strategy for Correcting Coagulopathy in Intracerebral Hemorrhage

a) Warfarin

If the patient is on warfarin and the INR is elevated or if the prothrombin time (PT) is elevated in the absence of warfarin therapy physicians at MGH administer vitamin K 10 mg IV over 10 minutes followed by FFP 10 mL/kg over 90 minutes. Vitamin K and FFP must be dosed at once and the team must designate a single physician to take personal responsibility for ensuring that these therapies are administered as fast as possible. Vitamin K should be administered within 5 minutes of the order.

As soon as FFP is ordered, a "runner" should be dispatched to the blood bank to collect FFP, which should be administered as soon as possible.

b) Standard (Unfractionated) Heparin

The preferred immediate therapy at MGH to correct coagulopathy is to administer Protamine 10 to 50 mg IVP over 1 to 3 minutes.

c) Low-Molecular-Weight Heparin

Protamine sulfate reverses only about 60% of the antifactor Xa activity of low-molecular-weight heparin and has negligible effects on danaparoid (a mixture of anticoagulant glycosaminoglycans used to treat heparin-induced thrombocytopenia) and fondaparinux (a synthetic antithrombin-binding pentasaccharide with exclusive antifactor Xa activity). Therefore more research is needed to develop a more effective treatment.

d) Direct Thrombin Inhibitors (Argatroban, Lepirudin, Bivalirudin, Ximelagatran)

There is no specific antidote for these drugs at this time. At MGH, antifibrinolytic agents such as Amicar (EACA) are used at the attending physician's discretion.

e) Platelet Disorders

In the cases of thrombocytopenia (platelet count $<100,000/\mu L$), platelets are transfused until the platelet count exceeds $100,000/\mu L$. For Von Willebrand syndromes, 0.3 μg/kg DDAVP is administered intravenously over a period of 30 minutes. Phone consult is initiated with a staff member of hematology or transfusion medicine for dosing of VWF factor concentrate. DDAVP is also of benefit in patients with:
-Uremic platelet dysfunction.
-Congenital platelet function disorders
-Recent ingestion of combinations of antiplatelet agents such (e.g., ASA and clopidogrel).
(See http://www.stopstroke.org for more details)

Role of Blood Pressure (BP) Control in the Acute Stage of AIS

In the acute stage of AIS, the role of BP control and the appropriate target of BP have not been defined. Lowering BP acutely with antihypertensive agents has been shown to worsen tissue perfusion and clinical outcomes and is not recommended. Induced hypertension from vasoactive agents may augment tissue perfusion and preserve oligemic brain tissue, but this approach remains unproven. The main risks of induced hypertension are cardiac morbidity, brain edema, hypertensive encephalopathy, and hemorrhagic conversion of infarction. The current recommendations in patients not eligible for IV tPA are to leave blood pressure untreated in the acute setting unless it is associated with end-organ injury such as myocardial ischemia or exceeds 220/120; for tPA eligible patients, BP control is required to reduce hemorrhagic risk (8).

NEUROIMAGING PATHWAYS IN THE EMERGENCY DEPARTMENT FOR ACUTE STROKE

Neuroimaging technology plays a pivotal role in identifying pathophysiologic mechanisms of stroke and supports the triage of patients into the various clinical pathways that stroke patients may require. Several modalities are available, and research is ongoing to identify the optimal imaging devices and characteristics.

An unenhanced brain CT (noncontrast CT) is the most important and extensively available imaging technique to exclude hemorrhagic stroke and stroke mimics and is quite sensitive for identifying subacute strokes. To be eligible for fibrinolytic (thrombolytic) treatment, a patient must have an acute unenhanced CT scan without evidence of hemorrhage or well-established acute stroke (i.e., no signs of hemorrhage, major mass effect, or visible newly hypodense areas) (28). The presence of at least one of the clinical parameters such as coma on arrival, vomiting, severe headache, current warfarin therapy, systolic blood pressure >220 mm Hg, or a high glucose level >170 mg/dL in a nondiabetic patient doubles the chance of intracranial hemorrhage (29). Brain imaging is compulsory to differentiate ischemic stroke from hemorrhage or other anatomic brain lesions in an emergency setting (30). CT angiography (CTA) in the setting of acute stroke can reliably show the site of vascular occlusion, show length of stenosed vascular segment, and help assess the collateral circulation. Occlusion at the level of the Circle of Willis (internal carotid artery, basilar artery, and middle cerebral artery trunk) can be detected with high sensitivity and specificity (31). A study has shown that the combination of non-contrast-enhanced CT (NECT), perfusion CT (PCT), and CTA can deliver important diagnostic information within 15 minutes regarding the extent of the infarct and the perfusion deficit. This can aid in therapeutic decision making, especially if both diffusion-weighted imaging (DWI) and perfusion-weighted imaging (PWI) are not available or cannot be performed (32). The three-dimensional computer generated reconstructions provide amazing vascular details from CTA.

MRI is highly sensitive and accurate (100% sensitivity, 100% accuracy) in detecting intracranial bleeding (33,34). DWI visualizes acute ischemic brain tissue when the energy metabolism is impaired in the tissue. It can show ischemic changes within minutes of the onset of stroke symptoms (35–37). It also allows for the assessment of a tissue signature that helps date the temporal evolution of stroke in the first few weeks after stroke and easily quantify the volume of infarcted tissue (38). Diffusion restriction (DWI) with low apparent diffusion coefficients (ADC) is considered the best diagnostic factor to identify acute cerebral ischemia and infarction (39).

Perfusion disturbance on PWI without a corresponding DWI abnormality delineates a "penumbra" or at-risk tissue (19). This PWI > DWI mismatch may identify individuals who will respond to reperfusion therapy beyond the strict windows of opportunity established for IV tPA based on time of onset of ischemic symptoms. A PWI < DWI pattern may indicate that reperfusion has already occurred and thus there is no need for thrombolysis. As DWI hyperintensity does not necessarily signify irreversible ischemic infarction, there remains a chance that a patient with a matched lesion PWI = DWI is still a reasonable candidate for thrombolysis, if CT does not also show a hypointensity that matches perfusion abnormality (40).

Presently, no evidence is available to show that MRI is superior to CT for selecting patients for intravenous recombinant tissue plasminogen activator (r-tPA) (8).

VARIABILITY IN STROKE CARE

The Paul Coverdell National Acute Stroke Registry (PCNASR) is being developed to improve the quality of acute stroke care consistently throughout the United States. Recently, results from four pilot prototype registries were published. The Coverdell data exposed wide variations in care. The researchers noted that optimal treatments are provided infrequently, and only a small number of acute stroke patients receive interventions according to recognized guidelines. Less than 10% of acute strokes arrived at the hospital within 1 hour of stroke onset, and less than 25% of total strokes arrived within 3 hours of stroke symptoms. Rates of administration of r-tPA were between 3% and 8.5% of all AIS, and only 20% of the patients who received tPA received it within 60 minutes of arrival. Stroke onset time was very poorly documented (41).

There is a substantial disconnect in the U.S. health care system between care for the patient and the documentation of that care. The use of multidisciplinary charting tools and the development of critical pathways may be able to ameliorate this gap in quality of stroke care.

After an updated Cochrane systematic review for assessing implications of using care pathways in stroke, no evidence was found that indicated that the pathways provide significant additional benefits over standard medical care in terms of mortality or discharge destination. In fact, there was some evidence that patients in the care pathway group were more functionally dependent on discharge. There is weak evidence that a care pathway might be associated with fewer urinary tract infections and readmissions and more wide-ranging use of CT brain scans. There is still inadequate published randomized controlled data to support the routine execution of care pathways for acute stroke or stroke rehabilitation (42).

Nevertheless, there are sound reasons to believe that care pathways may result in better treatment of stroke. California Acute Stroke Pilot Registry (CASPR) investigators showed that implementation of standard stroke orders in six participating hospitals in California resulted in high adherence rates in two-thirds of the selected measures of stroke care. These preprinted order forms even helped academic hospitals increase tPA utilization (43). Randomized controlled trials comparing routine care to care supported by stroke clinical pathways need to be undertaken.

RATIONALE FOR DEVELOPING CRITICAL CARE PATHWAYS FOR STROKE AND TIA

In 2005, the anticipated direct costs (including hospital, nursing home, physicians or other professionals, drugs, and home health care) and indirect costs (comprising morbidity and mortality [lost future earnings]) of stroke will be $56.8 billion in the United States (1). At MGH, over 500 patients with ischemic stroke or TIA are admitted every year, with approximately 60% of these cases presenting via the ED. Due to such a huge volume, the development of critical pathways for stroke and TIAs is a cornerstone for ensuring optimal quality of care at MGH. In circumstances of high patient volume and costs, critical care pathways help ensure the initiation of best practices, streamline patient care, reduce unnecessary variations in care delivery, and decrease resource utilization (44). To ensure high-quality acute stroke care, current recommendations endorse the development of a stroke system of care model that supports the development of clinical pathways consisting of protocols customized to each institution based on national guidelines (45).

MULTI- OR INTERDISCIPLINARY TEAM SELECTION FOR CRITICAL PATHWAY DEVELOPMENT AND EXECUTION: STROKE QUALITY IMPROVEMENT AT MGH

Stroke Quality Improvement Infrastructure

Continuous quality improvement (CQI) initiatives are a critical component of a systems approach to stroke care. CQI strategies are helpful in monitoring and improving performance on various quality indicators as well as improving the performance of the system of care itself and determining the extent of success for various QI initiatives (46). Prospective case ascertainment combined with retrospective case review are critical to identify acute stroke patients in a timely manner that will permit real-time intervention to comply with national recommendations (47). Several large organizations have developed stroke quality improvement programs, the largest of which are the American Heart Association Get With The Guidelines GWTG–Stroke program and the Centers for Disease Control PCNSR. GWTG–Stroke is a rapid-cycle, continuous QI initiative developed to monitor acute stroke treatment and secondary prevention measures. We at MGH use an internally developed intranet acute stroke log (Fig. 9-4) that helps concurrently identify all acute stroke patients and track key quality variables that are subsequently entered into the GWTG–Stroke database. In addition, standard admit order templates (Fig. 9-5) are also available to our physicians via the electronic medical record and computerized physician order entry systems that prompt clinicians to initiate key acute and secondary prevention interventions for patients starting in the ED.

Experience at MGH has shown that stroke neurologists need to champion QI initiatives to achieve success in stroke pathways. Evidence has shown that lack of physician participation and leadership is a major contributor to the failure of a critical pathway (46,48). At the same time, the cooperation and collaboration with nurses is essential. In September 2004, we formed an Acute Stroke Quality Taskforce (ASQT) to address key aspects of acute stroke care at MGH, according to the requirements outlined in the new Massachusetts Department of Public Health (DPH) regulations for Primary Stroke Service licensure. Previously most of the efforts for QI/QA were carried out only by the acute stroke service in isolation. The organizational charts for our QI effort are presented in Figure 9-6.

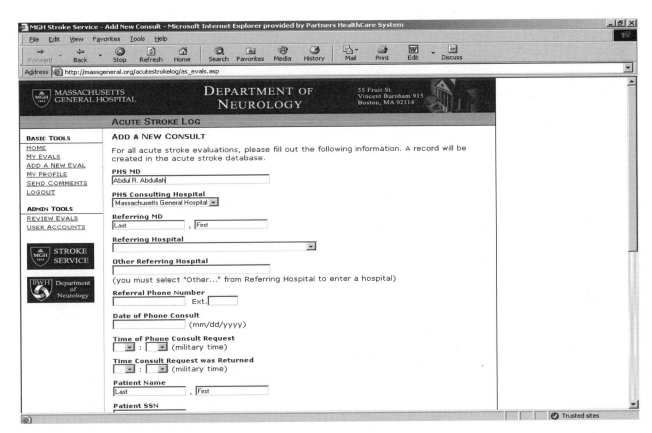

FIGURE 9-4. Intranet acute stroke log at MGH.

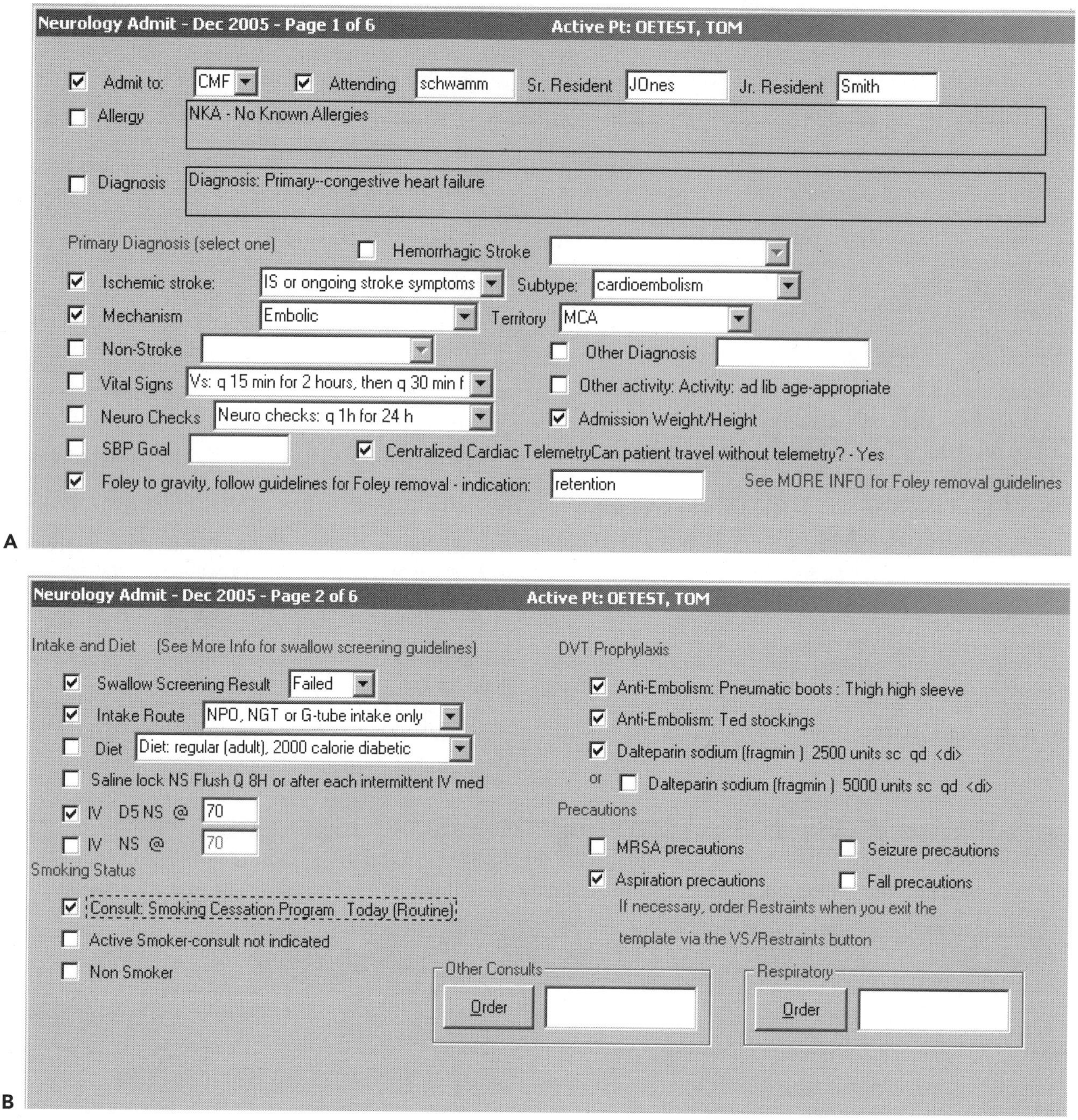

FIGURE 9-5. (A–C) Standard neurology admit order templates and computerized physician order entry systems at MGH. (*continues*)

The ASQT has taken a multidisciplinary approach to increase the number of eligible acute stroke patients arriving at MGH within 2 hours of symptom onset who receive IV tPA, with an emphasis on a door-to-tPA-needle time of less than 60 minutes. To facilitate and expedite the notification of both the ED and the acute stroke team, the ASQT has worked with the MGH Communications Service to develop an acute stroke code designation, which is being integrated into all new MGH emergency contact information. For an internal stroke education plan, the task force updated the hospital and nursing orientation materials and implemented a standard curriculum for all nurses within the many practice areas at MGH. To provide education to the general public

and others within the MGH community, a stroke poster has been developed on stroke signs and symptoms and the appropriate emergency response. This poster is part of the public education approach of the hospital's larger educational mission and was included in an employee education initiative cosponsored by the hospital regulatory compliance office. To identify opportunities for improvement, the ASQT uses rapid-cycle feedback through real-time case reviews to learn from and prevent delays in care of any particular acute stroke patient. This has been accomplished through a collaborative data collection model between compliance-based nurse abstractors and neurology-based clinical research fellows and coordinators.

Neurology Admit - Dec 2005 - Page 3 of 6   **Active Pt: OETEST, TOM**

Medications

- [ ] Acetylsalicylic acid (asa) 81 mg po qd
- or [x] Acetylsalicylic acid (asa) 325 mg po qd
- [ ] Acetaminophen (tylenol) 325-650 mg po q4h <di> prn:<r>
- [x] Thiamine hcl 100 mg po qd
- or [ ] Thiamine hcl 100 mg iv qd
- [ ] Ranitidine hcl (zantac) 150 mg po bid
- or [ ] Ranitidine hcl (zantac) 50 mg iv q8h
- or [ ] Esomeprazole (nexium) 20 mg po qd <di>
- [ ] Bisacodyl (dulcolax suppositories) 10 mg pr qd prn:<r>
- [ ] Aluminum/magnesium hydroxide+simethicone ii (mylanta ii) 15 ml po qid (ac + hs) prn:<r>
- [x] Insulin regular human sliding scale if bs <= 200 give 0 units ; for bs from 201 to 250 give 4
- [ ] Oxycodone 5 mg/acetaminophen 325 mg 1-2 tab po [Q4H ▼] PRN:<R>

- [ ] Dexamethasone (decadron) 4 mg po q4h
- or [ ] Dexamethasone (decadron) 4 mg iv q6h
- [ ] Folic acid (folate) 1 mg po qd
- [ ] Maalox susp 15 ml po qid prn:<r>
- [ ] Phenytoin (dilantin) 100 mg po tid <di> <fdi>
- or [ ] Fosphenytoin 100 mg_pe iv tid <di>
- [ ] Magnesium sulfate 2 gm iv q4h prn:<r>
- [ ] Multivitamins (mvi) 1 tab po qd
- [ ] Senna tablets 2 tab po bid
- [ ] Docusate sodium (colace) 100 mg po bid

C

FIGURE 9-5. (*continued*)

PATHWAYS ORGANIZATION INTO THE CHAIN OF STROKE SURVIVAL

Recent efforts have emphasized the importance of developing "stroke systems of care" that integrate discrete components of treatment and prevention into a continuum of care (45). Previously, there was an emphasis on improving individual components of stroke care such as hospital-based acute care or secondary prevention. The Primary Stroke Center recommendations formulated by the Brain Attack Coalition reflect competencies based largely in this single domain of stroke care (49). The Institute of Medicine (IOM) has explored the implementation of a systems approach for executing a change in health care delivery and closing the quality gap among patients. Taking into consideration that health systems are complex entities, IOM has proposed the establishment of a coordinated structure of care that amalgamates preventive care with treatment services and also encourages patient access to evidence-based care (50).

Community Education

Educating the public about the recognition of risk factors, signs, and symptoms of stroke is vital in improving quality of care for stroke patients. Increased awareness may augment the appropriate use of emergency response numbers such as 911 and earlier presentation at the ED (51,52). It has been reported that more rapid patient activation of 911 is associated with a higher rate of thrombolysis (53).

The Role of Telemedicine in Connecting Providers

The spectrum of telemedicine for stroke can range from straightforward technology such as telephone conversations

or teleradiology to sophisticated methods such as real-time videoconferencing for patient examination and evaluation ("TeleStroke"). Telemedicine and interfacility transport systems play a critical role in linking providers at community hospitals to more comprehensive stroke centers within a specific stroke system of care (45). Several groups have convincingly demonstrated the interrater reliability of performing the NIHSS over TeleStroke systems with excellent correlation coefficients and statistical significance (54,55). TeleStroke brings stroke neurologist expertise to the patient's bedside in remote hospital facilities without access to stroke expertise. TeleStroke systems need to capture data from multiple different sources and integrate them into clinical decision making and documentation. An example of a software tool to support this activity at the MGH and Partners TeleStroke Center is provided in Figure 9-7.

Effective Communication with Prehospital Providers

Emergency medical technicians and paramedics can be trained to recognize symptoms of stroke or TIA (28). Several prehospital stroke scales have been developed to improve identification of strokes at dispatch and first responder for emergency medical services (EMS) personnel, thus minimizing the amount of delay from symptom onset to the ED arrival. The Cincinnati Stroke Scale (CSS) identifies acute stroke patients by assessment of facial droop, arm drift, and speech difficulties only. The Los Angles Prehospital Stroke Screen (LAPSS) includes added demographic and medical history factors such as age, history of seizures, symptom duration, blood glucose levels, and pre-existing ambulatory status. In Massachusetts, the Boston Operation Stroke Scale (BOSS) was developed as the prehospital assessment tool and includes elements and strategies drawn from both the LAPSS and CSS.

Critical Pathways Committee (Acute Stroke Quality Taskforce [ASQT]) – Structure and Projects

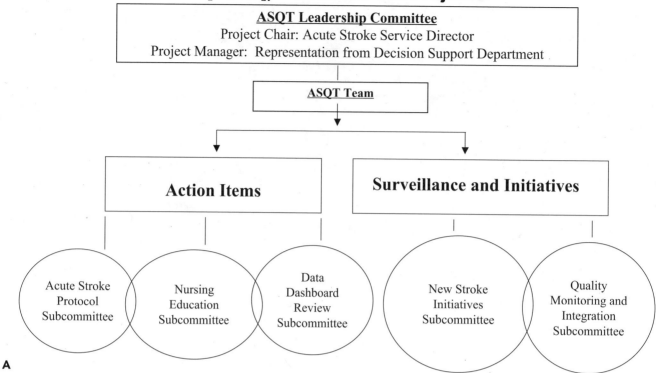

ASQT Membership at MGH:

Stroke Neurology: Stroke Service Director 1; Stroke Neurologists 2

Stroke Clinical Research: Research Fellows 2

Neuroradiology: Neuroradiologist 1

Interventional Neurology: Interventional Neurologist 1

Anesthesiology: Anesthesiologist 1

Emergency Medicine: Director 1

Neurology Nurses: 3

Emergency Medicine Nursing: 1

Speech and Language Pathologists: 2

Hospital Management Representation: Associate Chief Nurse 1; Vice President Neurosciences 1

Case Management Department: 3

FIGURE 9-6. (A,B) Critical Pathways Committee at MGH: Structure, Projects, and Membership.

A systems approach can identify and implement measures that decrease the time between the receipt of an emergency call for a possible stroke and the dispatch of EMS personnel (45). Proper identification of stroke by EMS personnel not only guides transport of the patient to the most suitable facility but also allows the use of stroke-specific basic or advanced life support interventions prior to the patient's arrival to the hospital (56,57).

Prehospital notification and the implementation of a stroke code system can shorten door-to-CT time and increased rates of thrombolysis (58). For instance, MGH utilizes a software system to digitally archive all prehospital notification calls (ASC Marathon Software, Inc.; Acorn Recording Solutions, Inc.), which can be useful in analyzing the impact of prehospital notification and for providing feedback to EMS providers on dispatch and field diagnostic accuracy.

Prevention of Complications Due to Stroke

According to national recommendations, "a stroke system should make certain that clinical pathways are used consistently to ensure the organized application of interventions to prevent or limit stroke progression or secondary complications" (45). Many of the steps necessary to avoid medical complications, including deep vein thrombosis (DVT), pulmonary embolism, and aspiration pneumonia, should be initiated in the ED (45).

Prevention of Aspiration Pneumonia by Evaluation of Swallowing Ability

Pneumonia is a major complication occurring in the setting of AIS. Deaths due to pneumonia comprise approximately 35%

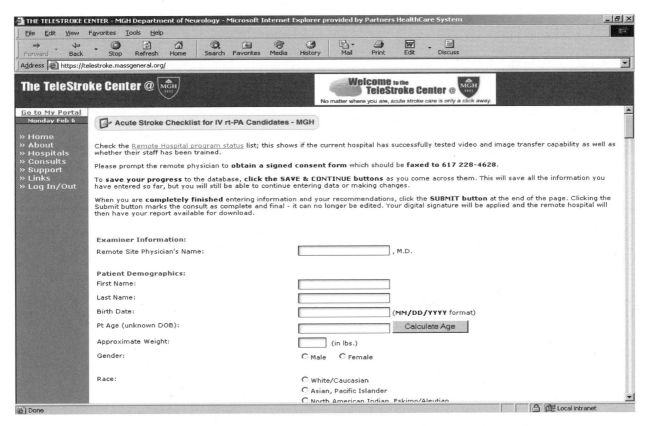

FIGURE 9-7. Internally developed MGH and Partners TeleStroke Center software tool.

of the deaths that happen after AIS. Aspiration pneumonia due to AIS causes a threefold increase in mortality rates (59). Within the first 3 days of stroke onset, dysphagia can become clinically apparent in 42% to 67% of patients (60,61).

The Stroke Practice Improvement Network registry conducted a prospective study for the collection of data involving 15 health care institutions in North America. The study demonstrated that the use of a formal dysphagia screening protocol produced a threefold reduction in the incidence of pneumonia in patients hospitalized with ischemic strokes (62). The American Stroke Association consensus guidelines recommend that a swallow evaluation be performed in all stroke patients before any oral intake of medications, food, or fluid (19).

Prevention of Deep Vein Thrombosis (DVT) and Pulmonary Embolism (PE)

DVT and PE are frequent complications after stroke. About 5% of early deaths can be attributed to PE (63). Low-molecular-weight heparins (LMWH) have been found to be equivalent or better than unfractionated heparins in preventing DVT (7). A systematic review of 10 randomized controlled trials for LMWH demonstrated a significant decrease in the risk of DVT and PE but raised the likelihood of extracranial bleeding that can normally be treated with blood transfusion (64). If the patients have contraindications to anticoagulants, pneumatic compression devices or elastic stockings should be initiated in the ED (7).

Summary

In summary, though stroke and TIA reflect a relatively small number of ED admissions, the ED remains a critical location for implementation of evidence-based acute stroke therapy. Be-

yond the obvious need for a highly organized response to permit the delivery of thrombolytic therapy, key subacute intervention designed to prevent in-hospital complications and recurrent stroke can be effectively implemented in the ED using critical pathways incorporating standing orders and templates. Focused applications of these principles and critical pathways will likely translate into improved patient outcomes.

References

1. American Heart Association. *Heart disease and stroke statistics—2005 update.* Dallas, TX: American Heart Association; 2005.
2. Albers GW, Caplan LR, Easton JD, et al. Transient ischemic attack—proposal for a new definition. *N Engl J Med* 2002;347(21):1713–1716.
3. Johnston SC, Gress DR, Browner WS, et al. Short-term prognosis after emergency department diagnosis of TIA. *JAMA* 2000;284(22):2901–2906.
4. National Institute of Neurological Disorders and Stroke rt-PA Stroke Study Group. Tissue plasminogen activator for acute ischemic stroke. *N Engl J Med* 1995;333(24):1581–1587.
5. Hacke W, Kaste M, Fieschi C, et al. Intravenous thrombolysis with recombinant tissue plasminogen activator for acute hemispheric stroke. The European Cooperative Acute Stroke Study (ECASS). *JAMA* 1995;274(13): 1017–1025.
6. Hacke W, Kaste M, Fieschi C, et al. Randomised double-blind placebo-controlled trial of thrombolytic therapy with intravenous alteplase in acute ischaemic stroke (ECASS II). Second European-Australasian Acute Stroke Study Investigators. *Lancet* 1998;352(9136):1245–1251.
7. Albers GW, Amarenco P, Easton JD, et al. Antithrombotic and thrombolytic therapy for ischemic stroke: the Seventh ACCP Conference on Antithrombotic and Thrombolytic Therapy. *Chest* 2004;126(3 Suppl):483S–512S.
8. Adams H, Adams R, Del Zoppo G, et al. Guidelines for the early management of patients with ischemic stroke: 2005 guidelines update a scientific statement from the Stroke Council of the American Heart Association/American Stroke Association. *Stroke* 2005;36(4):916–923.
9. Hacke W, Donnan G, Fieschi C, et al. Association of outcome with early stroke treatment: pooled analysis of ATLANTIS, ECASS, and NINDS rt-PA stroke trials. *Lancet* 2004;363(9411):768–774.
10. Katzan IL, Hammer MD, Furlan AJ, et al. Quality improvement and tissue-

type plasminogen activator for acute ischemic stroke: a Cleveland update. *Stroke* 2003;34(3):799–800.

11. Smith RW, Scott PA, Grant RJ, et al. Emergency physician treatment of acute stroke with recombinant tissue plasminogen activator: a retrospective analysis. *Acad Emerg Med* 1999;6(6):618–625.
12. Chiu D, Krieger D, Villar-Cordova C, et al. Intravenous tissue plasminogen activator for acute ischemic stroke: feasibility, safety, and efficacy in the first year of clinical practice. *Stroke* 1998;29(1):18–22.
13. Furlan A, Higashida R, Wechsler L, et al. Intra-arterial prourokinase for acute ischemic stroke. The PROACT II study: a randomized controlled trial. Prolyse in Acute Cerebral Thromboembolism. *JAMA* 1999;282(21):2003–2011.
14. Lewandowski CA, Frankel M, Tomsick TA, et al. Combined intravenous and intra-arterial r-TPA versus intra-arterial therapy of acute ischemic stroke: Emergency Management of Stroke (EMS) Bridging Trial. *Stroke* 1999;30(12):2598–2605.
15. Smith WS, Sung G, Starkman S, et al. Safety and efficacy of mechanical embolectomy in acute ischemic stroke: results of the MERCI trial. *Stroke* 2005;36(7):1432–1438.
16. Roden-Jullig A, Britton M, Malmkvist K, et al. Aspirin in the prevention of progressing stroke: a randomized controlled study. *J Intern Med* 2003;254(6):584–590.
17. Gubitz G, Sandercock P, Counsell C. Antiplatelet therapy for acute ischaemic stroke. *Cochrane Database Syst Rev* 2000;(2):CD000029.
18. Alberts MJ, Latchaw RE, Selman RW, et al. Recommendations for comprehensive stroke centers: a consensus statement from the Brain Attack Coalition. *Stroke* 2005;36(7):1597–1616.
19. Adams H, Adams R, Del Zoppo G, et al. Guidelines for the early management of patients with ischemic stroke: A scientific statement from the Stroke Council of the American Stroke Association. *Stroke* 2003;34(4):1056–1083.
20. Gay JL, Curtil A, Buffiere S, et al. Urgent carotid artery repair: retrospective study of 21 cases. *Ann Vasc Surg* 2002;16(4):401–406.
21. Huber R, Muller BT, Seitz RJ, et al. Carotid surgery in acute symptomatic patients. *Eur J Vasc Endovasc Surg* 2003;25(1):60–67.
22. Krishnamurthy S, Tong D, McNamara KP, et al. Early carotid endarterectomy after ischemic stroke improves diffusion/perfusion mismatch resonance imaging: report of two cases. *Neurosurgery* 2003;52(2):238–242.
23. Linn FH, Rinkel GJ, Algra A, et al. Incidence of subarachnoid hemorrhage: role of region, year, and rate of computed tomography: a meta-analysis. *Stroke* 1996;27(4):625–629.
24. Molyneux A, Kerr RS, Yu LM, et al. International Subarachnoid Aneurysm Trial (ISAT) of neurosurgical clipping versus endovascular coiling in 2143 patients with ruptured intracranial aneurysms: a randomised trial. *Lancet* 2002;360(9342):1267–1274.
25. Mayberg MR, Batjer HH, Dacey R, et al. Guidelines for the management of aneurysmal subarachnoid hemorrhage. A statement for healthcare professionals from a special writing group of the Stroke Council, American Heart Association. *Stroke* 1994;25(11):2315–2328.
26. Steiner T, Rosand J, Diringer M. Intracerebral hemorrhage associated with oral anticoagulant therapy: current practices and unresolved questions. *Stroke* 2006;37(1):256–262.
27. Goldstein JN, Thomas SH, Frontiero V, et al. Timing of fresh frozen plasma administration and rapid correction of coagulopathy in warfarin-related intracerebral hemorrhage. *Stroke* 2006;37(1):151–155.
28. Acute Ischemic Stroke 2003 Update. In: Cummings RO, ed. *ACLS provider manual.* Dallas, TX: American Heart Association; 2003.
29. Panzer RJ, Feibel JH, Barker WH, et al. Predicting the likelihood of hemorrhage in patients with stroke. *Arch Intern Med* 1985;145(10):1800–1803.
30. Britton M, Hindmarsh T, Murray V, et al. Diagnostic errors discovered by CT in patients with suspected stroke. *Neurology* 1984;34(11):1504–1507.
31. Knauth M, Von Kummer JR, Jansen O, et al. Potential of CT angiography in acute ischemic stroke. *AJNR Am J Neuroradiol* 1997;18(6):1001–1010.
32. Schramm P, Schellinger PD, Klotz E, et al. Comparison of perfusion computed tomography and computed tomography angiography source images with perfusion-weighted imaging and diffusion-weighted imaging in patients with acute stroke of less than 6 hours' duration. *Stroke* 2004;35(7):1652–1658.
33. Kidwell CS, Chalea JA, Saver JL, et al. Hemorrhage early MRI evaluation (HEME) study: preliminary results of a multicenter trial of neuroimaging in patients with acute stroke symptoms within 6 hours of onset. Hemorrhage early MRI evaluation (HEME) study. *Stroke* 2003;34(2):239.
34. Chalea JA, Latour LL, Jeggeries N, et al. Hemorrhage and early MRI evaluation from the emergency room (HEME-ER): a prospective, single center comparison of MRI to CT for the emergency diagnosis of intracerebral hemorrhage in patients with suspected cerebrovascular disease. *Stroke* 2003;34(2):239–240.
35. Busza AL, Allen KL, King MD, et al. Diffusion-weighted imaging studies

36. of cerebral ischemia in gerbils. Potential relevance to energy failure. *Stroke* 1992;23(11):1602–1612.
36. Warach S, Gaa J, Siewert B, et al. Acute human stroke studied by whole brain echo planar diffusion-weighted magnetic resonance imaging. *Ann Neurol* 1995;37(2):231–241.
37. Warach S, Chien D, Li W, et al. Fast magnetic resonance diffusion-weighted imaging of acute human stroke. *Neurology* 1992;42(9):1717–1723.
38. Schwamm LH, Koroshetz WJ, Sorensen AG, et al. Time course of lesion development in patients with acute stroke: serial diffusion- and hemodynamic-weighted magnetic resonance imaging. *Stroke* 1998;29(11):2268–2276.
39. Hamilton BE. Acute cerebral ischemia-infarction. In: Osborn AG, Blaser S, Salzman KL, eds. *Diagnostic imaging: brain.* Philadelphia: WB Saunders; 2004:76–79.
40. Greer D, Oliveira-Filho J, Koroshetz WJ. The role of neuroimaging in selecting treatments for patients with acute stroke. *Curr Neurol Neurosci Rep* 2001;1(1):26–32.
41. Reeves MJ, Arora S, Broderick JP, et al. Acute stroke care in the US: results from 4 pilot prototypes of the Paul Coverdell National Acute Stroke Registry. *Stroke* 2005;36(6):1232–1240.
42. Kwan J, Sandercock P. In-hospital care pathways for stroke: a Cochrane systematic review. *Stroke* 2003;34(2):587–588.
43. CASPRC Investigators. The impact of standardized stroke orders on adherence to best practices. *Neurology* 2005;65(3):360–365.
44. Every NR, Hochman J, Becker R, et al. Critical pathways: a review. Committee on Acute Cardiac Care, Council on Clinical Cardiology, American Heart Association. *Circulation* 2000;101(4):461–465.
45. Schwamm LH, Pancioli A, Acker JE 3rd, et al. Recommendations for the establishment of stroke systems of care: recommendations from the American Stroke Association's Task Force on the Development of Stroke Systems. *Stroke* 2005;36(3):690–703.
46. Yandell B. Critical paths at Alliant Health System. *Qual Manag Health Care* 1995;3(2):55–64.
47. Broderick JP. Logistics in acute stroke management. *Drugs* 1997;54(Suppl 3):109–117.
48. Hampton DC. Implementing a managed care framework through care maps. *J Nurs Adm* 1993;23(5):21–27.
49. Alberts MJ, Hademenos G, Latchaw RE, et al. Recommendations for the establishment of primary stroke centers. Brain Attack Coalition. *JAMA* 2000;283(23):3102–3109.
50. Institute of Medicine. *Crossing the quality chasm: a new health system for the 21st century.* Washington DC: National Academies Press; 2001.
51. Becker K, Fruin M, Gooding T, et al. Community-based education improves stroke knowledge. *Cerebrovasc Dis* 2001;11(1):34–43.
52. Harraf F, Sharma AK, Brown MM, et al. A multicentre observational study of presentation and early assessment of acute stroke. *BMJ* 2002;325(7354):17.
53. CASPRC Investigators. Prioritizing interventions to improve rates of thrombolysis for ischemic stroke. *Neurology* 2005;64(4):654–659.
54. Wang Y, Lee SB, Pardue C, et al. Remote evaluation of acute ischemic stroke: reliability of National Institutes of Health Stroke Scale via telestroke. *Stroke* 2003;34(10):e188–e191.
55. Shafqat S, Kvedar JC, Guanci MM, et al. Role for telemedicine in acute stroke. Feasibility and reliability of remote administration of the NIH stroke scale. *Stroke* 1999;30(10):2141–2145.
56. Suyama J, Crocco T. Prehospital care of the stroke patient. *Emerg Med Clin North Am* 2002;20(3):537–552.
57. Sahni R. Acute stroke: implications for prehospital care. National Association of EMS Physicians Standards and Clinical Practice Committee. *Prehosp Emerg Care* 2000;4(3):270–272.
58. Belvis R, Cocho D, Marti-Fabregas J, et al. Benefits of a prehospital stroke code system. Feasibility and efficacy in the first year of clinical practice in Barcelona, Spain. *Cerebrovasc Dis* 2005;19(2):96–101.
59. Katzan IL, Cebul RD, Husak SH, et al. The effect of pneumonia on mortality among patients hospitalized for acute stroke. *Neurology* 2003;60(4):620–625.
60. Perry L, Love CP. Screening for dysphagia and aspiration in acute stroke: a systematic review. *Dysphagia* 2001;16(1):7–18.
61. Kidd D, Lawson J, Nesbitt R, et al. The natural history and clinical consequences of aspiration in acute stroke. *QJM* 1995;88(6):409–413.
62. Hinchey JA, Shephard T, Furie K, et al. Formal dysphagia screening protocols prevent pneumonia. *Stroke* 2005;36(9):1972–1976.
63. Collaboration AT. Collaborative overview of randomised trials of antiplatelet therapy—III: Reduction in venous thrombosis and pulmonary embolism by antiplatelet prophylaxis among surgical and medical patients. *BMJ* 1994;308(6923):235–246.
64. Bath PM, Iddenden R, Bath FJ. Low-molecular-weight heparins and heparinoids in acute ischemic stroke: a meta-analysis of randomized controlled trials. *Stroke* 2000;31(7):1770–1778.

CHAPTER 10 ■ THE ROLE OF EXERCISE TESTING IN CHEST PAIN UNITS: EVOLUTION, APPLICATION, RESULTS

EZRA A. AMSTERDAM, J. DOUGLAS KIRK, DEBORAH B. DIERCKS, WILLIAM R. LEWIS, AND SAMUEL D. TURNIPSEED

IDENTIFICATION OF LOW CLINICAL RISK
CHEST PAIN UNIT CONCEPT
Accelerated Diagnostic Protocols
Evolution of Early Exercise Testing
Early Exercise Testing in an Accelerated Diagnostic Protocol
EXERCISE TESTING IN CHEST PAIN UNITS
Method of UC Davis: Immediate Exercise Testing
COMPARISON OF EXERCISE TESTING AND
  MYOCARDIAL STRESS SCINTIGRAPHY
Immediate Exercise Testing in Special Populations
Further Issues
SUMMARY

Despite advances in the management of low-risk patients presenting to the emergency department (ED) with chest pain, this syndrome remains a major clinical challenge (1), accounting for over 8 million ED visits and more than two million hospital admissions annually in the United States for presumed acute coronary syndrome (ACS) at a cost of cost of $8 billion (2). However, a coronary event is confirmed in only a minority of these patients (3) who pose a dilemma to the clinician because of inadvertent discharge of those with a life-threatening condition versus unnecessary admission for a benign process with associated expense. The continuum of risk for this population is depicted in Figure 10-1 and the single largest group is the one with noncardiac chest pain. The early era of coronary care units (CCUs) had a low threshold for admission of these patients, as reflected in the recommendation that "Patients should be admitted to the CCU solely on suspicion of having a myocardial infarction" (4). To the degree that this concept has persisted, it reflects a focus on patient welfare as well as the litigation potential of missed ACS (5). Although appropriate alternative approaches have subsequently evolved, inadvertent discharge of patients with ACS remains a challenge. Indeed, recent data suggest that this problem persists at a rate of up to 5% and accounts for a substantial morbidity and mortality (6). However, a consequence of the low threshold for admission has been large numbers of unnecessary hospitalizations and inefficient resource utilization.

Chest pain units (CPU) have been developed to provide safe, accurate and cost-effective management of low-risk patients presenting with possible ACS. Their original purpose was to facilitate rapid coronary reperfusion therapy, but these units have subsequently evolved into centers for management of the lower risk population that comprises the majority of patients presenting with chest pain. The latter include those without objective evidence of myocardial ischemia or injury on presentation in whom accelerated risk stratification can identify those requiring admission and those who can be safely discharged with outpatient follow-up (7–14). Basic to this approach is the accelerated diagnostic protocol (ADP) culminating in stress testing after a negative initial assessment for ACS. The primary stress test has been exercise electrocardiography (ECG). The ADP is predicated on initial recognition of patients with low clinical risk on presentation.

IDENTIFICATION OF LOW CLINICAL RISK

Multiple studies have demonstrated that low clinical risk can be recognized on presentation and that this finding identifies a group that neither requires nor benefits from traditional intensive care. Lee et al reported that in patients admitted to rule out a coronary event, those with <5% probability of acute myocardial infarction (MI) could be identified by type of chest pain, past history, and initial ECG (15). Extension of this approach to over 4,600 patients demonstrated that the initial clinical assessment could distinguish those with less than <1% probability of major complications (16). The prognostic importance of the initial ECG in patients admitted to rule out MI was demonstrated by Brush et al (7), who found that a negative ECG on admission was associated with a 0.6% rate of serious complications during hospitalization compared with a 14% incidence in those with an abnormal ECG. An earlier study indicated that in patients admitted for preinfarction angina, a normal ECG predicted benign early and late outcomes in contrast to ECG evidence of ischemia, which correlated with markedly increased cardiac morbidity and mortality (18). These findings were confirmed by Schroeder and colleagues in their report that in patients in whom MI was ruled out, ECG evidence of ischemia was associated with a 1-year mortality similar to that of post-MI patients (19). An important concept to emerge from these studies was that, although the etiology of chest pain is frequently elusive, basic clinical tools provide powerful estimates of cardiac risk.

Recognition of low clinical risk stimulated alternative approaches to conventional coronary care, such as reduced time in the CCU (20,21), direct admission to a step-down unit (22), and observation in a short stay unit (23). Recent innovations in the management of low-risk patients include guidelines, critical pathways, new serum markers of cardiac injury, novel ECG monitoring systems, early treadmill testing or noninvasive cardiac imaging, coronary calcium screening in the ED, noninvasive coronary angiography by computed tomography, and conventional coronary angiography (7–14,20).

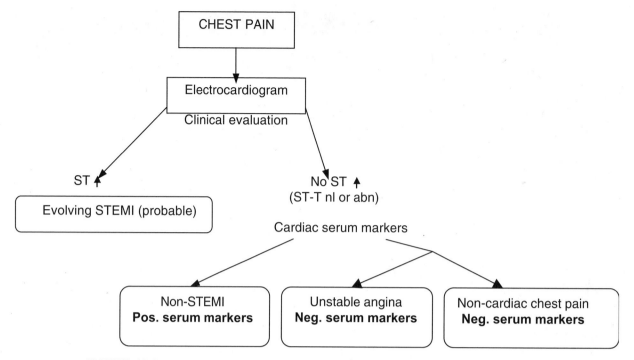

FIGURE 10-1. Spectrum of patients presenting to the emergency department with chest pain. Hx, history; PE, physical examination; MI, myocardial infarction; nl, normal; abn, abnormal; pos., positive; neg., negative; STEMI, ST segment elevation MI. (From Lewis WR, Amsterdam EA. Observation units, clinical decision units and chest pain centers. In: Becker RC, Alpert JS, eds. *Cardiovascular medicine: practice and management.* London: Arnold; 2001:85–103, with permission.)

CHEST PAIN UNIT CONCEPT

Risk is low but not negligible in patients selected for CPU evaluation. CPUs provide an integrated approach to management of these patients that affords (a) early identification of clinical risk and (b) further stratification of low-risk patients to identify those who require admission and those who can be discharged (7–14,20). CPUs vary in form and may either occupy a designated structural area or function as virtual units comprising primarily personnel and process. Close coordination between ED physicians and cardiologists is an essential element for successful functioning of the unit. The strategy is based on a protocol-driven process that employs current standards of care for efficient and timely treatment in conformity with the guidelines of the American College of Cardiology (ACC) and American Heart Association (AHA) (24).

Accelerated Diagnostic Protocols

Accelerated dignostic protocols (ADPs) have been increasingly utilized in low-risk patients with the final step comprising one of the cardiac stress tests methods if the ACS is excluded. The most commonly used ADPs usually entail 6 to 12 hours of clinical observation, serial 12-lead ECGs, continuous ECG monitoring, and measurement of serial serum cardiac injury markers (10,12,14,20,24). Positive findings indicate ACS (usually non-ST elevation [non-STE] ACS, rarely ST elevation MI) and mandate admission for further management. Negative findings are consistent with the absence of MI and ischemia at rest. In these cases, a stress test is performed to detect inducible ischemia. Patients with a positive test are admitted, and those with a negative result are discharged to outpatient follow-up. Multiple methods are currently available to detect stress-induced ischemia, the most widely available and readily appli-cable of which is treadmill exercise testing. The utility of this test in conjunction with ADPs has been has been well demon-strated, as indicated by its safety and predictive accuracy in this setting.

Evolution of Early Exercise Testing

Until it was validated by recent studies, there were strong admonitions against early exercise testing even in low-risk patients presenting with symptoms suggestive of ACS (9,25). The evolution of this approach is reflected in The 31st Bethesda Conference on Emergency Cardiac Care (1999) that "ADPs, including exercise testing as a key element, have been associated with reduced hospital stay and lower costs" (10). The absence of adverse effects and the accurate identification of low clinical risk were also recognized. A subsequent Science Advisory of the AHA concluded that contemporary studies "confirmed the safety of symptom-limited treadmill exercise ECG testing after 8 to 12 hours of evaluation in patients who have been identified as being at low to intermediate risk by a clinical algorithm that uses serum markers of myocardial necrosis and resting ECGs" (26). This strategy is incorporated in the 2002 guidelines of the ACC/AHA for management of patients with non-ST-elevation ACS in which it is recommended that exercise testing can be performed in stable, low-risk patients if "a follow-up 12-lead ECG and cardiac marker measurements after 6 to 8 hours of observation are normal" (23). Recent exercise testing guidelines are in accord with these recommendations (27,28). It is noteworthy that these recent recommendations reflect evolution from earlier versions, which advised exercise testing only after patients had been symptom free for a "minimum of 48 hours" (29).

All studies of early exercise testing in patients presenting with chest pain have required that patients are clinically stable with no ECG evidence of ischemia/injury. The criteria for a positive test for myocardial ischemia are the standard indicators: ≥1.0 mm horizontal or downsloping ST segment shift 60 to 80 msec after the J point. Other exercise-induced alterations that indicate an abnormal test and the need for further evaluation include angina, arrhythmias, and exercise-induced fall in blood pressure. The first two investigations of this method included only small numbers of patients, but they demonstrated its safety in low-risk patients in the ED setting (30,31), and its utility was confirmed in multiple subsequent publications (Table 10-1). Of note, there have been no reports of adverse events in any study of early exercise testing of low-risk patients.

Early Exercise Testing in an Accelerated Diagnostic Protocol

The first study of exercise testing in patients with the clinical profile of those currently included in ADPs was published from our institution in 1994. In this investigational protocol, selected patients presenting with chest pain who were designated for admission by ED physicians to rule out ACS underwent immediate treadmill testing (32) (Table 10-1). The study group comprised 93 patients in whom ED symptom-limited exercise testing was performed by a cardiologist using a modified Bruce protocol without prior measurement of any markers. The test was performed within a median time of less than 1 hour from the decision to admit. Positive tests occurred in 13% of patients, negative in 64%, and nondiagnostic (no ischemia but peak heart rate <85% of age-predicted maximum) in 13%. Ischemic ECG changes occurred at a significantly lower percentage of age-predicted maximal heart rate (70%) in patients with true-positive tests compared to those with false-positives (>90%) (Fig. 10-2). No complications were associated with exercise testing. Coronary angiography revealed significant coronary artery disease (CAD) in 6 of the 13 patients with

positive tests, 5 of whom had multivessel involvement. A majority (54%) of the 81 patients with negative or nondiagnostic results was discharged immediately after the exercise test. At 6-month follow-up, there were no coronary events in patients with negative or nondiagnostic exercise tests. There are several unique aspects of this study, which demonstrated the utility of early exercise testing in low-risk patients and provided the basis for our current approach of "immediate" exercise testing in low-risk patients without excluding MI by a traditional series of negative cardiac serum markers. In contrast to the preceding studies, it included only patients who were assigned to admission for a traditional rule-out MI protocol. In these patients, exercise testing was performed prior to the latter process, there were no adverse effects of testing, true- and false-positive tests were related to the heart rate at ST-segment depression, the majority of patients were discharged immediately following a negative or nondiagnostic test, and there were no coronary events during the posthospital course. Of note, one patient with a positive test was found to have non-ST-elevation MI by subsequent serial serum enzymes. Coronary angiography revealed right coronary artery stenosis, coronary angioplasty was performed, and the clinical course was uncomplicated.

Gibler and associates demonstrated the utility of early exercise testing in 782 patients in whom low risk was indicated by an ADP (33) (Table 10-1). Their protocol included serial ECGs and serum CK-MB, 9 hours of continuous ST-segment monitoring, and a resting ECG followed by symptom-limited exercise testing in those with negative findings. There were no adverse effects and no mortality at 30-day follow-up in the patients with negative tests. The negative predictive value of the exercise test was 99%. Although the positive predictive value was less than 50%, only 9 of 782 patients (<2%) had positive exercise tests, which was lower than in our initial investigation (32).

TABLE 10-1

STUDIES OF EXERCISE ECG TESTING IN CHEST PAIN CENTERS[a]

Author	No. Pts	Percent Positive Tests[b]	Negative Predictive Value[c]	Positive Predictive Value[c]	Adverse Exercise Test Events
Tsakonis	28	17.8	100%		0
Kerns et al	32	0	100%		0
Lewis and Amsterdam	93	13.0	100%	46%	0
Gibler et al	782	1.2	99%	44%	0
Gomez et al	100	7	100%	0%	0
Zalenski	224	8	98%	16%	0
Polanczyk	276	24	98%	15%	0
Kirk et al	212	12.5	100%	57%	0
Amsterdam et al	1000[d]	13	88.7%	33%	0

[a]Includes studies in which results of exercise ECG tests could be distinguished from those of other forms of stress testing.
[b] Positive exercise ECG.
[c] Based on clinical follow-up or further cardiac evaluation.
[d] Includes a small number of patients in Kirk et al.
Adapted from Amsterdam EA, Kirk JD, Diercks DB, et al. Early exercise testing in the management of low risk patients in chest pain centers. *Prog Cardiovasc Dis* 2004;46:438–452.

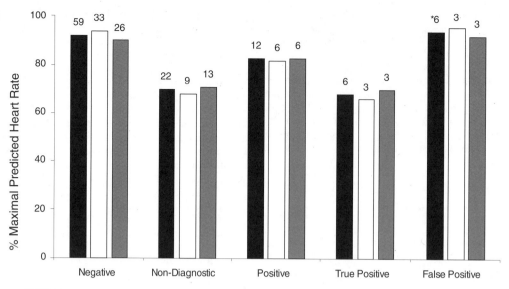

FIGURE 10-2. Treadmill exercise results. Percent maximal predicted heart rate attained versus exercise electrocardiographic result for all patients (black bars), men (open bars), women (gray bars). Numbers above bars represent number of patients. *Percent maximal predicted heart rate for patients with true-positive tests vs. false-positive tests, $P < 0.01$. (From Lewis WL, Amsterdam EA. Utility and safety of immediate exercise testing of low-risk patients admitted to the hospital for suspected acute myocardial infarction. *Am J Cardiol* 1994;74:987–990, with permission.)

EXERCISE TESTING IN CHEST PAIN UNITS

The foregoing studies (30–33) supported the safety and excellent predictive value of negative exercise tests in patients identified as low risk (Table 10-1). Further, a large majority of patients selected for exercise testing by an ADP had negative findings, and although the positive predictive value was modest, positive tests were infrequent and resulted in the need for further evaluation in only small numbers of patients (Table 10-1). The utility of this strategy was confirmed in its ability to safely and efficiently reduce unnecessary admissions in low-risk patients. Interestingly, the relative frequency of patients with true- and false-positive exercise tests in this setting is actually similar to that seen in asymptomatic individuals (34), confirming the value of clinical indicators in identifying the probability of disease in patients presenting to the ED with chest pain (10,14,15,19,32,33).

The Rapid Rule-Out of Myocardial Ischemia Observation (ROMIO) study of Gomez and coworkers was the first prospective, controlled investigation of ADP-exercise testing (35) (Table 10-1). It evaluated 100 patients with chest pain, half of whom were randomly assigned to admission for regular care and half to a chest pain center protocol consisting of a 12-hour observation period with standard ECGs, continuous ST-segment monitoring, and serial CK-MBs. Observation and monitoring were negative in 44 patients in the accelerated protocol in whom symptom-limited exercise testing was performed without adverse effects, demonstrating normal tests in 93% and positive results in 7%. The latter were all false positives, based on coronary angiography. All patients with negative tests were discharged after the exercise evaluation, and there were no coronary events at 30-day follow-up. However, compared to regular care, the observation protocol was associated with substantial reductions in length of stay (11.0 vs. 22.8 hours) (Fig. 10-3) and total cost ($624 per patient at 30 days). This was the first study to document the anticipated cost savings by an observation unit protocol.

Although the potential for cost savings by the ADP-exercise testing strategy was apparent, this advantage had not been firmly established. Additionally, there was also the possibility, as suggested by Roberts and coworkers, that this approach could actually lead to higher costs by capturing very low risk patients who would previously have been discharged directly from the ED (36). Their prospective, randomized trial, in which the primary outcomes were length of stay and total cost, demonstrated that both variables were significantly less for ADP patients than those receiving standard care (33 vs. 45 hours, $P < 0.01$; and $1528 vs. $2095, $P < 0.001$) (36). Extrapolation of the cost benefit indicated a potential annual national savings of over $238 million.

In a prospective, cross-sectional study, Zalenski et al evaluated 317 patients by a 12-hour ADP followed by exercise testing (37) (Table 10-1). A unique aspect of this trial was admission of all patients to obtain a diagnosis to which the ADP evaluation could be compared. Exercise testing was performed in 224 patients with negative observation data and was negative in 66%, positive in 8%, and inconclusive in 26% because of failure of patients to reach 85% of age-predicted maximal heart rate. In this study, the accuracy of the ADP-exercise strategy was based solely on comparison with admission diagnosis. In combination with the CK-MB data and serial ECGs, the exercise test had a high sensitivity (90%) and excellent negative predictive value (98%); as in prior studies, specificity and positive predictive value were low (51% and 16%, respectively). Cost analysis demonstrated a savings of $567 per patient managed by the ADP-exercise test strategy.

Polanczyk et al evaluated the prognostic significance of the exercise test performed within 48 hours of presentation in 276 low-risk patients admitted for chest pain (38) (Table 10-1). Twenty-six percent of these patients had a history of CAD. The test was performed within 12 hours in 7% of patients, at 12 to 24 hours in 45%, and after 24 hours in 48%. The Bruce treadmill protocol was used in 84% of the patients, and the modified version was used in 12%. A negative test was defined by achievement of at least one stage on the Bruce protocol without evidence of ischemia. Positive tests were "those in which the results were interpreted as highly predictive of significant coronary disease or strongly positive" and "inconclusive

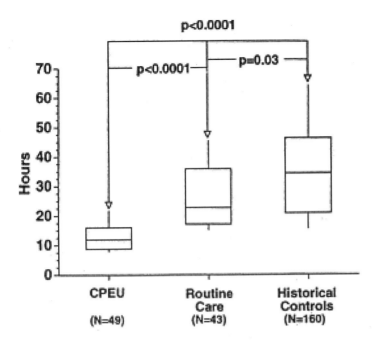

FIGURE 10-3. Length of hospital stay after randomization among patients in the rapid rule-out (chest pain evaluation unit [CPEU]), routine care, and historical control groups for whom acute myocardial infarction or unstable angina was ruled out. The top, bottom, and middle lines of the boxes correspond to the 75th, 25th, and 50th percentiles, respectively. (From Gomez MA, Anderson JL, Labros AK, et al. An emergency department-based protocol for rapidly ruling out myocardial ischemia reduces hospital time and expense: results of randomized study (ROMIO). *J Am Coll Cardiol* 1996;28:25–33, with permission.)

tests were those consistent with but not diagnostic of ischemia" or without evidence of ischemia but at a peak work of <3 METs. The test was negative in 71% of patients, positive in 24%, and inconclusive in 5%. Outcome data were available at 6 months for 92% of the study group. Events during the follow-up period were defined as cardiac death, MI, or myocardial revascularization. During this interval, there was no mortality, and the event rate in the negative exercise test cohort was 2% compared to 15% in those with positive or equivocal tests. In the negative test group, compared to those with positive or equivocal tests, there were also fewer repeat ED visits (17% vs. 21%, P <0.05) and fewer readmissions (12% vs. 17%, P <0.01). The negative predictive value of the exercise test was 98%; sensitivity and specificity were 73% and 74%, respectively. In addition to the documented prognostic utility of the exercise test, this study afforded other noteworthy features. The investigators demonstrated the safety of the early exercise test in patients with a history of CAD, and their definition of test results yielded a low rate of inconclusive diagnoses, increasing the clinical utility of the test in clinical decision making.

Mandatory stress testing in a CPU was evaluated by Mikhail and coworkers for its safety, utility and cost-effectiveness (39). After negative findings for myocardial ischemia or infarction, a total of 424 patients underwent cardiac stress evaluation, which included 247 exercise treadmill tests. The remainder of the tests were stress imaging studies; no data are given for the results of the different test modalities. The tests were negative in 392 (92.6%) patients, and average stay in the chest pain unit was 12.8 hours. At 5-month follow-up, there was no mortality or MI in any of the patients discharged after a negative evaluation. A final diagnosis of ischemic heart disease was made in 44 patients admitted from the chest pain center, 24 (55%) of whom were identified only on stress testing. Evaluation in the CPU with mandatory stress testing was associated with a cost-per-case saving of 62% for each patient who would otherwise have been admitted to the inpatient service.

The largest prospective, randomized trial comparing management by an ADP-stress test with regular inpatient care is that of Farkouh et al (40). They studied 424 patients with a diagnosis of unstable angina based on symptoms who had negative ECGs and were considered to be at intermediate risk. The observation protocol, which included ECGs, ST-segment monitoring, and serial serum creatine kinase-MB measurements, differed from prior studies in its duration of only 6 hours. Patients with negative ADP findings underwent either exercise testing or pharmacologic stress imaging, depending on their ability to exercise. Patients with negative tests were discharged, and those with positive or equivocal results were admitted. Forty-six percent of patients in the ADP-stress test group had a negative overall evaluation and were directly discharged after a median stay of 9.2 hours. At 6 months, there was no significant difference in cardiac events in the ADP-stress test group versus the regular care patients (6.6% vs. 8.5%, respectively) (Fig. 10-4). Events were broadly defined (primary: death, MI, heart failure, stroke, cardiac arrest; secondary: any revisit to the ED or hospitalization for cardiac diagnosis or care). There were no primary events in the ADP-stress test patients with negative evaluations and early discharge. The authors emphasized that this group represented 46% of patients who ordinarily would have been admitted but in whom the accelerated protocol avoided admission. Finally, the use of cardiac procedures and hospitalization for cardiac care during the follow-up period was significantly higher in the hospital admission patients ($P = 0.003$), amounting to an estimated 61% increase in costs.

The foregoing studies of the last decade reflect the parallel and interdependent development of CPUs, ADPs, and early exercise testing in low-risk patients presenting to the ED with chest pain. Integration of these methods into a protocol-driven process has firmly established the contemporary CPU as safe, accurate, and efficient. After a negative observation period of 12 hours or less to exclude MI and ischemia at rest, exercise testing has been feasible to detect or exclude inducible ischemia. The negative predictive value of this strategy is very high (~98%), and the low positive predictive accuracy is not problematical because the frequency of positive exercise tests is low, resulting in a small number of patients requiring admission for further inpatient evaluation. Additionally, the exercise test avoids inappropriate discharge of patients not identified by the observation process. Estimates of cost-effectiveness indicate the potential for substantial savings by chest pain centers through reduction of unnecessary admissions and decrease of inadvertent discharges of ACS patients. The CPU is a relatively recent development and investigation is ongoing to determine optimal implementation of this concept, which will vary with

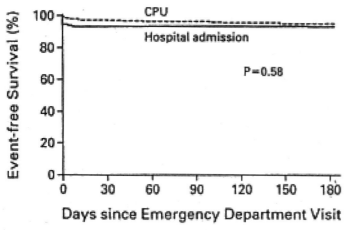

NO. AT RISK					
CPU	203	200	200	198	197
Hospital admission	194	194	194	194	194

FIGURE 10-4. Kaplan Meier curves for survival free of a primary cardiovascular event in the hospital-admission group and the chest pain unit group. Primary outcome: myocardial infarction, death, acute congestive heart failure, stroke, out-of-hospital cardiac arrest. (From Farkouh MI, Smars PA, Reeder GS, et al. A clinical trial of a chest-pain observation unit for patients with unstable angina. *N Engl J Med* 1998;339:1882–1888, with permission.)

the resources of individual institutions and the expertise and experience of the responsible physicians. In this regard, as previously noted (10–14), we have employed a unique approach to the management of low-risk patients at our institution.

Method of UC Davis: Immediate Exercise Testing

Our evaluation of low-risk patients in the University of California (Davis) CPU differs from that of the previous studies in that we apply exercise testing "immediately" after identification of low-risk patients on presentation. Serial cardiac injury markers are not obtained in this selected group, as described in our first study 10 years ago (32). Since then, over ~5,000 patients have been assessed by this strategy with no adverse effects. Our current approach embodies several modifications based on our continuing experience, as documented in our second study (41) (Table 10-1). In this investigation of 212 patients, those with a history of CAD were not excluded, exercise testing was performed by internists trained in this technique, who serve as attending physicians on the CPU, and cardiac injury markers were not obtained prior to testing. Strict selection criteria for exercise testing were, as before, absence of hemodynamic dysfunction or cardiac arrhythmias, normal or near-normal ECGs, and no evidence of a noncardiac cause of chest pain on screening examination (Table 10-2). Symptom-limited treadmill exercise was performed by a modified Bruce protocol with the

following endpoints: ischemic ST-segment shift (1.00 mm horizontal or downsloping depression 60 to 80 msec after the J point), symptoms, or arrhythmias, any of which is an indication for immediate termination of the test (Table 10-3). Negative exercise tests were obtained in 59% of patients, positive in 13%, and nondiagnostic in 28% (negative exercise ECG but failure to reach ≥85% of age-predicted maximum heart rate). Patients with positive tests were admitted, and all patients with negative exercise tests and 93% with nondiagnostic results were discharged directly from the ED. In the latter group, the decision to discharge was based on achievement of adequate functional capacity (e.g., ≥2 stages of the Bruce protocol or ≥75% of maximum predicted heart rate). Further evaluation demonstrated CAD in 57% of those with a positive test, and 30-day follow-up revealed no mortality or morbidity in the negative or nondiagnostic groups. This study demonstrated the safety of proceeding to exercise testing in carefully selected patients on the basis of the initial presentation without serial ECGs or cardiac injury markers. However, its limited numbers required a larger patient population for confirmation of the feasibility of this strategy.

TABLE 10-2

SELECTION CRITERIA FOR IMMEDIATE EXERCISE TEST

Chest pain suspicious for myocardial ischemia
Able to exercise
ECG normal, minor ST-T changes, or no change from previous abnormal ECG
Hemodynamically stable, no arrhythmia
A single negative serum marker is measured in selected patients

TABLE 10-3

IMMEDIATE EXERCISE TEST PROCEDURE AND END POINTS

Modified Bruce treadmill protocol[a]
Symptom-limited
Other end points
  Ischemia (≥1.0 mm ST segment shift for 80 msec after the J point)
  ↓Blood pressure (≥10 mm Hg systolic)
  Significant arrhythmia (sustained supraventricular tachyarrhythmia; high-grade ventricular ectopy [≥2consecutive beats, sustained bigeminy])
Positive result: ≥1.0 mm horizontal ST segment shift
Nondiagnostic result: <85% maximum predicted heart rate with no ST shift

[a]Includes two initial 3-minute states (1.7 mph, 0% grade and 1.7 mph, 5% grade) before the standard Bruce protocol.

In the largest single-center study of exercise testing in low-risk patients, we reported our results in 1,000 patients (42) (Table 10-1). This study incorporated our current approach, which includes confirmation of a single negative cardiac injury marker prior to exercise testing. As depicted in Figure 10.5, almost two-thirds of the patients had negative immediate exercise tests, approximately 13% were positive, and less than 25% were nondiagnostic. There was no mortality during the 30-day follow-up interval. The negative predictive value for a cardiac event was 99.7% at 30 days. In the nondiagnostic group, all events were accounted for by revascularization in 32% of the 79 patients who had further evaluation. The positive predictive value of the exercise test was 33% for a cardiac event (four non-Q MIs detected after admission, 12 myocardial revascularizations) or a confirmatory imaging test for CAD (two patients). These results extended our previous findings to a large, heterogeneous population in that testing was uncomplicated, the bulk of patients had negative tests and could be released directly from the ED, negative predictive value was excellent, and the low positive predictive value involved a relatively small group with positive exercise tests. We have confirmed the safety and accuracy of our method in patients with known CAD by a specific study of immediate exercise testing of 100 consecutive patients (43). Although exercise testing is considered to have limited value in women, our experience has confirmed the reliability of a negative immediate exercise test in this group. The negative predictive value of the test was 99% in 661 women with a mean age of 54 years studied in our CPU (44).

COMPARISON OF EXERCISE TESTING AND MYOCARDIAL STRESS SCINTIGRAPHY

The utility of myocardial scintigraphy has been well established in patients presenting with chest pain (45). However, the cost and logistics of this method are prohibitive for many institutions. In this regard, we have shown that >70% of low-risk patients presenting with chest pain qualify for immediate exercise testing and that more complex and expensive stress imaging techniques can be appropriately reserved for the remainder of patients (46). Moreover, a comparative study of 239 low-risk patients by Senaratne et al revealed that early treadmill testing was as informative as and more cost-effective than scintigraphy in identifying low-risk patients who did not require hospitalization (47). In this study, in which the follow-up period was 20 months, exercise testing was applicable in all but 9.6% of patients. These investigators report that, compared to scintigraphy as the initial cardiac study, exercise testing yielded a savings of over $86,000 in this group of patients. In contrast to our strategy in which noncardiologists assess patients and perform immediate exercise testing, with cardiology consultation available as required, Senaratne et al emphasize the essential role of cardiologists in these processes. In this regard, the expertise of our noncardiology CPU physicians in performing exercise testing has been confirmed by their accuracy in test interpretation and the complete absence of complications (48). Analysis of 645 immediate exercise ECGs revealed a concordance of greater than 98% between the interpretations of these physicians and our staff cardiologists.

Investigators at the Mayo Clinic have recently noted that the rate of positive pharmacologic stress imaging studies is so high in patients who are not candidates for exercise testing as part of an ADP that they recommend direct admission of the latter group (49). They also advocate that community hospitals developing CPUs apply their resources to exercise testing rather than more costly and logistically complex scintigraphy. Although we support the latter recommendation for smaller institutions, we have not found a prohibitive rate of positive stress imaging results in the group unable to perform exercise testing and the method is an integral component of our ADP in the latter group (50).

Immediate Exercise Testing in Special Populations

We have recently explored a number of other issues presented by early exercise testing in patients presenting with chest pain.

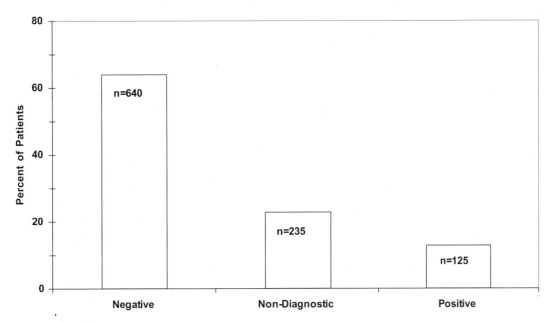

FIGURE 10-5. Proportion of 1,000 patients with negative, positive, and nondiagnostic immediate exercise tests. Numbers in bars indicate number of patients. (From Amsterdam EA, Kirk JD, Diercks DB, et al. Immediate exercise testing to evaluate low-risk patients presenting to the emergency department with chest pain. *J Am Coll Cardiol* 2002;40:251–256, with permission.)

The use of beta-blockers or rate-limiting calcium channel blockers often precludes diagnostic exercise testing because of attenuation of exertional heart rate by these agents. As anticipated, we have found that these drugs are associated with reduction of peak exercise heart rate and rate-pressure product, resulting in an increased frequency of nondiagnostic tests compared to patients not receiving these agents (51). However, a majority (>60%) of patients taking these medications did have a diagnostic test. Therefore, it is our experience that use of these drugs should not preclude early exercise testing.

Recent trials of non-STE ACS have demonstrated the prognostic importance of risk scores based on multiple clinical factors in patients presenting with this diagnosis, including elevated cardiac injury markers, ST-segment deviation, older than 65 years of age, more than three coronary risk factors, known CAD, two or more anginal episodes in the previous 24 hours, and aspirin use in the previous 7 days. These factors comprise the thrombosis in myocardial infarction (TIMI) risk score for prediction of fatal and nonfatal coronary events, which increase directly with the number of these risk factors (52). However, in patients presenting to our CPU, we have found that, with the exception of elevated cardiac injury markers and ST-segment deviation, both of which preclude exercise testing, the test can be safely performed for reliable risk stratification regardless of the presence of the other TIMI risk factors (53). Because it has been reported that augmenting the standard exercise ECG with additional leads enhances its sensitivity for detecting ischemia (54), we evaluated this innovation in our CPU patients. In this setting, the addition of four leads (two posterior and two right-sided) to the standard 12-lead ECG enhanced the sensitivity of the test without altering specificity (55): sensitivity rose only minimally from 7.6% to 8.0% based on detection of two patients who were positive only in the additional leads compared to 37 patients with positive findings in the standard exercise ECG. These additional leads were also not useful in detecting ischemia or injury in the resting ECG in patients admitted to our CPU (56). Interestingly, in our study of 2,021 patients referred for elective outpatient treadmill testing, we also found that the 16-lead exercise ECG did not afford increased sensitivity in this setting (57), thereby failing to confirm the prior report of Michaelides (54).

A notable aspect of our CPU experience has been the high recidivism rate of patients discharged from our unit with a negative evaluation. During a 7.5-year period, 13% of 1,960 patients had two or more negative immediate exercise tests and accounted for 26% of the CPU visits (58). Further, of the latter group, almost 10% had 4 or more negative exercise tests during this period. The multiexercise test patients were relatively young (mean age 52 years), and a majority were women. In this regard, it is essential to emphasize that beyond the traditional differential diagnosis of multiple somatic etiologies of chest pain (59), common and underdiagnosed conditions responsible for this symptom include anxiety syndromes and somatoform disorders (10,59–61).

Further Issues

Several aspects of our application of immediate exercise testing in CPU patients warrant comment. As previously noted, patients in whom this method is utilized are carefully screened to confirm their low-risk status, as outlined in Table 10-2. The test is terminated at the initial appearance of any abnormality (Table 10-3). Although noncardiologists perform the clinical assessment and exercise tests in CPU patients, these specially trained physicians have ready availability of consultation by staff cardiologists. In regard to the relatively large proportion (>20%) of patients with nondiagnostic tests (negative but peak heart rate <85% of predicted maximum), we have found that those with negative tests at ≥80% of maximum predicted heart rate had uneventful outcomes on follow-up (42). Therefore, utilization of this lower heart rate for a diagnostic test for the purpose of risk stratification appears prudent and would reduce the nondiagnostic group by 25% (43). Although our follow-up is only 30 days, the purpose of our approach is to determine short-term risk. This strategy is predicated on timely follow-up and further outpatient evaluation. Finally, although clinical assessment is basically reliable in identifying low-risk patients, it is imperfect and can result in inadvertent exercise testing in patients with ACS. This possibility is minimized by physician expertise and experience together with continued caution in the selection of patients for testing and in the indications for test termination.

A recurrent question concerns the necessity of performing exercise testing prior to discharge after a negative ADP, rather than a short time after discharge. The former approach provides the most efficient completion of the evaluation and obviates concern regarding lack of return of patients for the outpatient test, which would contribute to the hazard of incomplete assessment and missed ACS (6). However, where testing is not feasible and the system and patient characteristics are conducive to early return for testing (within 48 hours), it is reasonable to consider this approach. In this regard, we have discharged selected very low risk patients from our CPU without a predischarge exercise test. We have specifically studied this approach in a group of very low risk women presenting to the ED with chest pain who were fewer than 50 years old, nondiabetic, and nonsmokers (62). Of the entire group of 346 women, 175 were discharged from the CPU without exercise testing. At 30-day follow-up, none of these patients had confirmatory evidence of CAD or ACS. Our results suggest that the risk of ACS is minimal in women with low-risk profiles who present with chest pain and that stress testing in the CPU may not be necessary to determine disposition in these patients. These findings have implications for optimal utilization of limited resources.

SUMMARY

CPUs are not established for assessment of low-risk patients presenting to the ED with symptoms suggestive of ACS. ADPs, of which treadmill testing is a key component, have been developed within these units to enhance clinical evaluation. Studies of the last decade have established the utility of early exercise testing, which has been safe, accurate, and cost-effective in this setting. Specific protocols for ADPs vary but most require 6 to 12 hours of observation by serial ECGs and cardiac injury markers to exclude infarction and high-risk unstable angina before proceeding to exercise testing. However, in the CPU at UC Davis Medical Center, our approach includes "immediate" treadmill testing without a traditional process to rule out MI. Extensive experience has validated this strategy in a large, heterogeneous population. It can be anticipated that the optimal strategy for evaluating low-risk patients presenting to the ED with chest pain will continue to evolve based on current research and the development of new methods.

References

1. Gibler WB, CP Cannon, AL Blomkains, et al. Practical implementation of the guidelines for unstable angina/non-ST-segment elevation myocardial infarction in the emergency department. *Ann Emerg Med* 2005;46:185–197.
2. Pozen MW, D'Agostino RB, Selker HP, et al. Predictive instrument to improve coronary-care-unit admission practices in acute ischemic heart dis-

ease: a prospective multicenter clinical trial. *N Engl J Med* 1984;310: 1273–1278.

3. Karlson, BW, Herlitz J, Wiklund O, et al. Early prediction of acute myocardial infarction from clinical history, examination and electrocardiogram in the emergency room. *Am J Cardiol* 1991;68:171–175

4. Lown B, Vassaux C, Hood WB, et al. Unresolved problems in coronary care. *Am J Cardiol* 1967;20:494–508.

5. Karcz A, Holbrook J, Burke MC, et al. Massachusetts emergency medicine closed malpractice claims: 1988–1990. *Ann Emerg Med* 1993;22:553–559.

6. Pope JH, Aufderheide TP, Ruthazer R, et al. Missed diagnoses of acute cardiac ischemia in the emergency department. *N Engl J Med* 2000;342: 1163–1170.

7. Graff L, Joseph T, Andelman R, et al. American College of Emergency Physicians Information Paper: Chest pain units in emergency departments—a report from the short-term observation services section. American College of Emergency Physicians. *Am J Cardiol* 1995;76(14):1036–1039.

8. Jesse RL, Kontos MC, Roberts CS. Evaluation of chest pain in the emergency department. *Curr Prob Cardiol* 1997;22:151–236.

9. Selker HP, Zalenski RJ, Antman EM, et al. An evaluation of technologies for identifying acute cardiac ischemia in the emergency department. Executive summary of a National Heart Attack Alert Program Working Group report. *Ann Emerg Med* 1997;29:164–166.

10. Hutter AM, Amsterdam EA, Jaffe AS. Task force 2: Acute coronary syndromes: Section 2B-Chest discomfort evaluation in the hospital, 31st Bethesda Conference. *J Am Coll Cardiol* 2000;35:853–862.

11. Lewis WR, Amsterdam EA. Chest pain emergency units. *Curr Opin Cardiol* 1999;14:32.

12. Kirk JD, Diercks DB, Turnipseed SD, et al. Evaluation of chest pain suspicious for acute coronary syndrome: use of an accelerated diagnostic protocol in a chest pain evaluation unit. *Am J Cardiol* 2000;85(5A):40B–48B.

13. Lewis WR, Amsterdam EA. Observation units, clinical decision units and chest pain centers. In: Becker RC, Alpert JS, eds. *Cardiovascular medicine: practice and management.* London: Arnold; 2001:85–103.

14. Amsterdam EA, Lewis WR, Kirk JD, et al. Acute ischemic syndromes: Chest pain center concept. *Cardiol Clin* 2002;20:117–136.

15. Lee TH, Cook EF, Weisberg M, et al. Acute chest pain in the emergency room: identification and examination of low-risk patients. *Arch Intern Med* 1985;145:65–69.

16. Goldman L, Cook F, Johnson PA, et al. Prediction of the need for intensive care in patients who come to emergency departments with acute chest pain. *N Engl J Med* 1996;334:1498–1504.

17. Brush JE, Jr, Brand DA, Acampora D, et al. Use of the initial electrocardiogram to predict in-hospital complications of acute myocardial infarction. *N Engl J Med* 1980;312:1137–1141.

18. Gazes PC, Mobley EM, Jr, Faris HM, et al. Preinfarctional (unstable) angina—a prospective study—a ten year follow-up. Prognostic significance of electrocardiographic changes. *Circulation* 1973;48:331–337.

19. Schroeder J, Lamb IH, Hu M. Do patients in whom myocardial infarction has been ruled out have a better prognosis after hospitalization than those surviving infarction? *N Engl J Med* 1980;303:1–5.

20. Lee TH, Goldman L. Evaluation of the patient with acute chest pain. *N Engl J Med* 2000;342:1187–1195.

21. Mulley AG, Thibault GE, Hughes RA, et al. The course of patients with suspected myocardial infarction: The identification of low-risk patients for early transfer from intensive care. *N Engl J Med* 1980;302:943–948.

22. Fineberg HV, Scadden D, Goldman L. Care of patients with a low probability of acute myocardial infarction: cost effectiveness of alternatives to coronary-care-unit admission. *N Engl J Med* 1984;310:1301–1307.

23. Gaspoz JM, Lee TH, Weinstein MC, et al. Cost-effectiveness of a new short-stay unit to "rule out" acute myocardial infarction in low risk patients. *J Am Coll Cardiol* 1994;24:1249.

24. Braunwald E, Antman EM, Beasley JW, et al. ACC/AHA 2002 guideline update for the management of patients with unstable angina and non-ST-segment elevation myocardial infarction. Available at http://www.acc.org/clincal/guidelines/unstable/unstable.pdf. Accessed May 19, 2006.

25. Braunwald E, Mark DB, Jones RH, et al. Unstable angina: diagnosis and management. Agency for Health Care Policy and Research Publication No. 94-06062, Rockville, MD; 1994.

26. Stein RA, Chaitman BR, Balady GJ, et al. Safety and utility of exercise testing in emergency room chest pain centers. An advisory from the Committee on Exercise, Rehabilitation, and Prevention, Council on Clinical Cardiology, American Heart Association. *Circulation* 2000;102:1463–1467.

27. Fletcher GF, Balady GJ, Amsterdam EA, et al. Exercise standards for testing and training. A statement for healthcare professionals from the American Heart Association. *Circulation* 2001;104:1694–1740.

28. Gibbons RJ, Balady GJ, Bricker JT, et al. ACC/AHA 2002 guideline update for exercise testing: summary article. A report of the American College of Cardiology/American Heart Association task force on practice guidelines (committee to update the 1997 exercise testing guidelines). *J Am Coll Cardiol* 2002;40:1531–1540.

29. Gibbons RJ, Balady GJ, Beasley JW, et al. ACC/AHA guidelines for exercise testing. A report of the American College of Cardiology/American Heart Association task force on practice guidelines (committee on exercise testing). *J Am Coll Cardiol* 1997;30:260–315.

30. Tsakonis JS, Shesser R, Rosenthal R, et al. Safety of immediate treadmill testing in selected emergency department patients with chest pain: a preliminary report. *Am J Emerg Med* 1991; 9:557–559.

31. Kerns JR, Shaub TF, Fontanarosa PB. Emergency cardiac stress testing in the evaluation of emergency department patients with atypical chest pain. *Ann Emerg Med* 1993;22:794–798.

32. Lewis WL, Amsterdam EA. Utility and safety of immediate exercise testing of low-risk patients admitted to the hospital for suspected acute myocardial infarction. *Am J Cardiol* 1994;74:987–990.

33. Gibler WB, Runyon JP, Levy RC, et al. A rapid diagnostic and treatment center for patients with chest pain in the emergency department. *Ann Emerg Med* 1995;25:1–8.

34. Laslett LJ, Amsterdam EA. Management of the asymptomatic patient with an abnormal exercise ECG. *J Am Med Assoc* 1984;252:1744–1746.

35. Gomez MA, Anderson JL, Labros AK, et al. An emergency department-based protocol for rapidly ruling out myocardial ischemia reduces hospital time and expense: results of randomized study (ROMIO). *J Am Coll Cardiol* 1996;28:25–33.

36. Roberts RR, Zalenski, RJ, Mensah EK. Costs of an emergency department-based accelerated diagnostic protocol vs hospitalization in patients with chest pain. *J Am Med Assoc* 1997;278:1670–1676.

37. Zalenski RJ, McCarren M, Roberts, et al. An evaluation of a chest pain diagnostic protocol to exclude acute cardiac ischemia in the emergency department. *Arch Int Med* 1997;157:1085–1091.

38. Polanczyk CA, Johnson PA, Hartley LH, et al. Clinical correlates and prognostic significance of early negative exercise tolerance test in patients with acute chest pain seen in the hospital emergency department. *Am J Cardiol* 1998;81:288–292.

39. Mikhail MG, Smith FA, Gray M, et al. Cost-effectiveness of mandatory stress testing in chest pain center patients. *Ann Emerg Med* 1997;29;88–98.

40. Farkouh MI, Smars PA, Reeder GS, et al. A clinical trial of a chest-pain observation unit for patients with unstable angina. *N Engl J Med* 1998; 339:1882–1888.

41. Kirk JD, Turnipseed S, Lewis WR, et al. Evaluation of chest pain in low-risk patients presenting to the emergency department: the role of immediate exercise testing. *Ann Emerg Med* 1998;32:1–7.

42. Amsterdam EA, Kirk JD, Diercks DB, et al. Immediate exercise testing to evaluate low-risk patients presenting to the emergency department with chest pain. *J Am Coll Cardiol* 2002;40:251–256.

43. Lewis WL, Amsterdam EA, Turnipseed S, et al. Immediate exercise testing of low risk patients with known coronary artery disease presenting to the emergency department with chest pain. *J Am Coll Cardiol* 1999;33: 1843–1847.

44. Diercks DB, Kirk JD, Turnipseed S, et al. Exercise treadmill testing in women evaluated in a chest pain unit. *Acad Emerg Med* 2001;8:565 (abstract).

45. Kontos MC, Jesse RL, Schmidt KL, et al. Value of acute rest sestamibi perfusion imaging for evaluation of patients admitted to the emergency department with chest pain. *J Am Coll Cardiol* 1997;30:976–982.

46. Amsterdam EA, Kirk JD, Diercks DB, et al. Assessment of low risk patients presenting to the emergency department with chest pain: immediate treadmill test or cardiac stress imaging? *J Am Coll Cardiol* 2001;37:149A (abstract).

47. Senaratne MJ, Carter D, Irwin M. Adequacy of an exercise test in excluding angina on patients presenting to the emergency department with chest pain. *Ann Noninvas Electrocardiol* 1999;4:408–415.

48. Kirk JD, Turnipseed S, Diercks DB, et al. Interpretation of immediate exercise treadmill test: interreader reliability between cardiologist and noncardiologist in a chest pain evaluation unit. *Ann Emerg Med* 2000;36:10–14.

49. Ramakrishna G, Milavetz JJ, Zinsmeister AR, et al. Effect of exercise treadmill testing and stress imaging on the triage of patients with chest pain: CHEER substudy. *Mayo Clin Proc* 2005;80:322–329.

50. Amsterdam EA, WR Lewis. Stress imaging in chest pain units: is less more? *Mayo Clin Proc* 2005;80(3):317–319.

51. Diercks DB, Kirk JD, Turnipseed S, et al. Utility of immediate exercise treadmill testing in patients taking beta blockers or calcium channel blockers. *Am J Cardiol* 2002;90:882–885.

52. Antman EM, Cohn M, Bernin PJLM, et al. The TIMI risk score for unstable angina/non-ST elevation MI, *JAMA* 2000;284:835–842.

53. Amsterdam EA, Diercks DB, Kirk JD, et al. Multiple clinical risk factors do not preclude immediate exercise testing in a chest pain evaluation unit. *J Am Coll Cardiol* 2005;41:349A.

54. Michaelides AN, Psomdaki ZD, Dilaveris PE, et al. Improved detection of coronary artery disease by exercise electrocardiography with the use of right precordial leads. *N Engl J Med* 1999;340:340–345.

55. Diercks DB, Kirk JD, Turnipseed S, et al. Use of additional electrocardiographic leads in low-risk patients undergoing exercise treadmill testing. *Acad Emerg Med* 2001;8:564 (abstract).

56. Ganim RP, Lewis WR, Diercks DB, et al. Right precordial and posterior electrocardiographic leads do not increase detection of ischemia in low risk patients presenting with chest pain. *Cardiology* 2004;102:100–103.

57. Sabapathy R, Bloom HL, Lewis WR, et al. Right precordial and posterior chest leads do not increase detection of positive response in electrocardiogram during exercise treadmill testing. *Am J Cardiol* 2003;91:75–77.

58. Amsterdam EA, Kirk JD, Diercks DB, et al. Coronary artery disease in

patients with multiple emergency department visits and negative immediate exercise tests for chest pain: an important minority in a total cohort of over 3,000 low risk patients presenting with chest pain. *J Am Coll Cardiol* 2004; 43:225A (abstract).

59. Lewis WR, Amsterdam EA. Chest pain. In: Gershwin ME, Hamilton ME, eds. *The pain management handbook: a concise guide to diagnosis and treatment*. Totowa, NJ: Humana Press; 1998:79–115.

60. Carter C, Maddock R, Amsterdam EA, et al. Panic disorder and chest pain in the coronary care unit. *Psychosomatics* 1992;33:302–309.
61. Thurston RC, Keefe FJ, Bradley L, et al. Chest pain in the absence of coronary artery disease: a biopsychosocial perspective. *Pain* 2001;93:95–100.
62. Amsterdam EA, Diercks D, Kirk JD, et al. Evaluation of low risk women presenting to the emergency department with chest pain: is early stress testing necessary for risk stratification? *Circulation* 2005;112:II-647.

PART III ■ CRITICAL PATHWAYS
IN THE HOSPITAL

CHAPTER 11 ■ CRITICAL PATHWAYS FOLLOWING THROMBOLYSIS

CHRISTOPHER P. CANNON AND PATRICK T. O'GARA

ASSESSMENT OF EARLY REPERFUSION
Rescue PCI
CARDIOGENIC SHOCK
FACILITATED PCI
Full-Dose Fibrinolytic Therapy Alone
Combination of Fibrinolytic therapy and GP IIb/IIIa Inhibition
GP IIb/IIIa Inhibitor Alone
ROUTINE INVASIVE VERSUS CONSERVATIVE STRATEGY
Conservative Strategy
Reducing Other Cardiac Testing
REDUCING HOSPITAL (AND ICU) LENGTH OF STAY
Identification of Low-Risk Patients
Strategy of Early Discharge following Thrombolysis
SECONDARY PREVENTION AND FOLLOW-UP
CONCLUSION

The use of fibrinolytic therapy for acute ST-segment elevation myocardial infarction (MI) has dramatically reduced mortality (1). As discussed in chapter 6, an emergency department (ED) pathway for thrombolysis focuses on several components of immediate treatment: (a) rapid time to treatment—both overall time to treatment as well as the door-to-drug time; (b) accurate dosing (i.e., avoiding medication errors); and (c) adjunctive therapy with antiplatelet, antithrombin, and anti-ischemic medications (1). A second component of therapy, however, is the appropriate use of cardiac procedures (i.e., what revascularization strategies are needed following the start of thrombolysis). In addition, hospital length of stay is an area where cost savings can likely be achieved without compromising patient safety.

There are four broad categories of strategies for revascularization: (a) rescue percutaneous coronary intervention (PCI) for patients with evidence of failed thrombolysis (or early reocclusion) where PCI is used to reopen the persistently occluded coronary artery; (b) facilitated PCI, in which a thrombolytic drug (or other pharmacologic agents) is given prior to planned immediate PCI; (c) routine invasive strategy PCI, in which PCI is performed within a few days after thrombolysis; and (d) conservative strategy, where angiography and PCI are performed only if the patient has recurrent ischemia at rest or has evidence of ischemia on stress testing.

ASSESSMENT OF EARLY REPERFUSION

A key factor in prognosis is the success of early reperfusion. The "open artery theory" notes that if early reperfusion is achieved, the infarct size is reduced, left ventricular (LV) dysfunction is reduced, and survival is improved. One way of quantifying early reperfusion is with angiography, which has been assessed 60 to 90 minutes after thrombolysis in many clinical trials of thrombolysis. Mortality after fibrinolytic therapy is closely related to the degree to which flow has been restored in the infarct-related artery, and the thrombolysis in myocardial infarction (TIMI) flow grading system has been well validated for assessing reperfusion (Table 11-1). In angiographic trials, improved mortality has been seen with patent arteries (TIMI grade 2 or 3 flow), with the lowest mortality among those with TIMI grade 3 flow, which has established this as the ideal goal for early therapy (2).

For clinical care, however, a noninvasive technique is needed; one that may be more useful for evaluating myocardial perfusion is electrocardiogram (ECG) assessment of ST-segment resolution. More than 50% resolution of ST-segment elevation at 60 to 90 minutes has been shown to be a good indicator of enhanced myocardial perfusion and recovery of LV function, reduced infarct size, and improved prognosis (3–5). In the TIMI-14 study, ST-segment resolution of more than 70% was a stronger indicator of better survival than TIMI grade 3 flow (5). Other techniques used to assess reperfusion include myocardial contrast echocardiography (6) and myocardial angiographic perfusion with assessment of angiographic blush in the myocardium (7).

The American College of Cardiology/American Heart Association (ACC/AHA) Guidelines suggest that it is reasonable to monitor clinical symptoms, the pattern of ST-segment elevation, and cardiac rhythm over the 60 to 180 minutes after the start of fibrinolytic therapy (1). Noninvasive findings that suggest reperfusion include relief of symptoms, maintenance or restoration of hemodynamic and/or electrical stability, and

TABLE 1-1

THE TIMI FLOW GRADE CLASSIFICATION USED TO ASSESS EARLY REPERFUSION

- TIMI grade 0 flow refers to the absence of any antegrade flow beyond a coronary occlusion.
- TIMI grade 1 flow is faint antegrade coronary flow beyond the occlusion, although filling of the distal coronary bed is incomplete.
- TIMI grade 2 flow is delayed or sluggish antegrade flow with complete filling of the distal territory.
- TIMI grade 3 flow is normal flow that fills the distal coronary bed completely.

Classification from TIMI Study Group. The Thrombolysis in Myocardial Infarction (TIMI) Trial; Phase I findings. *N Engl J Med* 1985;312:932–936.

a reduction of at least 50% of the initial ST-segment elevation on follow-up ECG done at 60 to 90 minutes. In general, indicators of failed reperfusion include persistent ischemic chest pain, no resolution of ST-segment elevation, and hemodynamic or electrical instability. An invasive strategy (rescue PCI) should be considered for patients with one of these indicators.

Rescue PCI

Rescue PCI refers to PCI that is performed early (usually within 12 hours after fibrinolysis) in patients with evidence of failed reperfusion—thus with a goal of opening the persistently occluded infarct-related artery. There is now a good evidence base of randomized trials to support the addition of rescue PCI into standard clinical care.

The first randomized trial was conducted by Ellis and colleagues, which studied anterior MI patients with a documented occluded artery (8). Those randomized to a rescue PCI strategy done within 8 hours after the onset of symptoms in patients had a lower mortality rate and decreased frequency of a composite endpoint of death or CHF (8). This trial, and observational studies supporting these benefits (9,10), led to recommendations that rescue PCI be considered following thrombolysis, but its uptake in clinical practice has been relatively haphazard.

Two more recent studies have lent much clearer support to the routine incorporation of rescue PCI into critical pathways. One trial randomized 181 patients with STEMI and evidence of failed reperfusion who had been referred for coronary angiography and had TIMI flow grade ≤2 (11). Patients were randomize to undergo coronary stenting or balloon angioplasty, with a primary endpoint of myocardial salvage index, defined as the proportion of initial scintigraphic perfusion defect salvaged by rescue intervention, as assessed 7 to 10 days after PCI. Myocardial salvage index was significantly greater in the stenting group (0.35 versus 0.25; P = 0.005). One-year mortality tended to favor the stenting group, 8% versus 12% (relative risk, 0.6; P = 0.35). This study concluded that patients with failed thrombolysis benefit from rescue PCI in terms of myocardial salvage, with greater myocardial salvage with coronary stenting (11).

Most importantly, however, the recent REACT trial has reaffirmed the benefit of rescue PCI. This trial studied 427 acute MI patients within 6 hours of pain onset that had failed thrombolysis (diagnosed by <50% resolution of ST elevation on ECG at 90 minutes) (12). They were randomized to conservative treatment, repeat thrombolysis, or rescue PCI. The rate of death, MI, stroke, or severe heart failure at 6 months was significantly reduced with rescue PCI of 15.3% versus 29.8% and 31.0% for the conservative and repeat thrombolysis groups, respectively (each P <0.002) (Fig. 11-1) (12). Thus, rescue PCI should be a part of standard post-thrombolysis care if there are indications of failed thrombolysis. For timing, although benefit of rescue PCI has been seen in these trials when performed on average 6 to 10 hours following thrombolysis, the earlier reperfusion can be achieved the better, and thus efforts are important to shorten time to intervention, as they are for fibrinolysis and primary PCI.

CARDIOGENIC SHOCK

One related group of patients falls into this category where early intervention is warranted—patients with evidence of hemodynamic instability. An early invasive approach is recommended for patients in cardiogenic shock, and it may improve outcomes in patients with pulmonary edema (Killip class III).

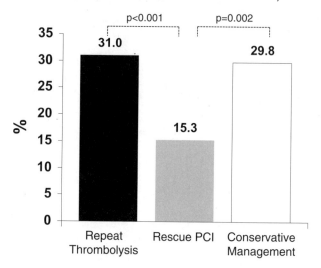

FIGURE 11-1. The benefit of rescue percutaneous coronary intervention following failed thrombolysis. (Data from Gershlick AH, Stephens-Lloyd A, Hughes S, et al. Rescue angioplasty after failed thrombolytic therapy for acute myocardial infarction. *N Engl J Med* 2005;353(26):2758–2768.)

The efficacy of early revascularization in patients in cardiogenic shock following an acute MI was first suggested in an observational study (13) and then demonstrated in the SHOCK trial in patients (14). In the revascularization group, 49% of patients had initially been treated with thrombolytic therapy. The benefit was limited to patients under age 75 in whom 20 lives were saved per 100 treated at 6 months (14). It should be noted, however, that 80% of the patients in this trial had received thrombolysis and/or intra-aortic balloon pumping, and revascularization was carried out 18 to 36 hours following presentation. Thus, this was not a "primary PCI" strategy, but more an early invasive strategy following thrombolysis. According to this strategy, though, critical pathways at hospitals without cardiac catheterization laboratories should include the immediate transfer to a tertiary care center for early revascularization.

FACILITATED PCI

Facilitated PCI is a term that encompasses both the pharmacologic therapy and immediate "primary" PCI. It is an attempt to combine the early achievement of an open infarct-related artery with the pharmacologic therapy and the high rates of TIMI grade 3 flow accomplished with PCI. Several types of pharmacologic regimens have been tested: standard (full-dose) thrombolytic therapy, half-dose thrombolytic therapy with a glycoprotein (GP) IIb/IIIa inhibitor, or a GP IIb/IIIa inhibitor alone.

The rationale came from the importance of early TIMI grade 3 flow. In addition, some evidence supporting the notion of facilitated PCI came from an analysis of several of the primary angioplasty in myocardial infarction (PAMI) trials of primary PCI (15). Of these patients, 16% had TIMI grade 3 flow before PCI, and their 6-month mortality was just 0.5% as compared with 2.8% and 4.4% for patients with TIMI grade 2 and 0/1 flow, respectively, at the time of the start of PCI (15). Thus, it could be reasoned that if you could increase the rates of TIMI 3 flow before PCI, mortality would be improved.

Initial trials performed in the 1980s, such as TAMI-I and

TIMI IIA, compared angioplasty performed immediately after thrombolysis to delayed PCI at 18 hours to 10 days as indicated (16–18). There was no benefit on LV function, the primary endpoint, and trends toward harm on bleeding, recurrent ischemia, need for coronary artery bypass graft (CABG), and even higher mortality (7% versus 3%) in a European trial (16–18). However, since that time there have been many advances in management, including the routine administration of aspirin, GP IIb/IIIa inhibitors and thienopyridines, and stents, and thus many trials were initiated to re-examine this issue. A number of studies, mostly nonrandomized, have suggested that facilitated PCI may be beneficial (19).

Full-Dose Fibrinolytic Therapy Alone

The use of full-dose fibrinolytic therapy as the "facilitating" pharmacologic agent before PCI was tested in several trials, but most definitively in the ASSENT-4 PCI trial (20). A total of 1,667 patients with large STEMIs presenting within 6 hours were randomized to either standard PCI or full-dose tenecteplase (TNK) followed by PCI (that was carried out quickly—on average approximately 1 hour postrandomization). They all received aspirin and unfractionated heparin; GP IIb/IIIa inhibitors were discouraged in the thrombolytic arm, but allowed in the primary PCI arm. The trial was stopped early by the Data and Safety Monitoring Board because of a higher rate of mortality in the pretreatment arm (6% compared with 3%). The primary endpoint—death, congestive heart failure, or shock within 90 days—occurred significantly more frequently in the facilitated PCI arm (18.8% versus 13.7%) (20) (Fig. 11-2). In addition, higher rates of reinfarction (6% versus 4%), repeat target revascularization (7% versus 3%), and stroke (1.8% versus 0%), half of which were intracranial hemorrhages, were seen in the facilitated PCI group. Thus, contrary to the hypothesis, the use of a thrombolytic to open the artery appeared to worsen outcomes, potentially by the known prothrombotic effects of thrombolysis.

Combination of Fibrinolytic Therapy and GP IIb/IIIa Inhibition

A related strategy that might overcome the prothrombotic effects of thrombolysis has also been tested with the use of half-dose fibrinolytic therapy combined with GP IIb/IIIa inhibition before PCI. This unfortunately has not looked promising thus far.

A small randomized trial, the BRAVE study, evaluated whether early administration of the combination of half-dose reteplase plus abciximab produced better results compared

with abciximab alone in patients with acute MI referred for PCI (21). The primary outcome measure was assessment of the final infarct size according to a single-photon emission computed tomography perfusion imaging performed between 5 and 10 days after randomization in the 228 patients studied. As expected, patients who received combination therapy had higher coronary patency rates than those treated with abciximab alone (40% vs. 18%, respectively) at the time of initial angiography. This angiographic advantage, however, did not translate into improved myocardial salvage as measured by nuclear scintigraphy. Moreover, bleeding rates were higher in the group receiving the combination of reteplase and abciximab prior to PCI (21). Nearly identical results were seen in another small trial, the ADVANCE MI trial. This trial of just 151 patients also found higher rates of mortality or heart failure with the combination therapy (half-dose fibrinolytic and GP IIb/IIIa inhibitor) than for treatment with a GPIIb/IIIa inhibitor alone (22). The rate of major bleeding was also substantially increased (22). Additional studies are ongoing, but to date this strategy is not encouraging. Thus, based on current evidence, it appears that one needs to choose a single strategy—thrombolysis or primary PCI, but not both.

GP IIb/IIIa INHIBITOR ALONE

Another possible approach to facilitated PCI is the administration of a GP IIb/IIIa inhibitor alone prior to PCI. In the SPEED and TIMI 14 trials, abciximab alone restored TIMI grade 3 flow in 27% to 32% of patients at 60 to 90 minutes, and up to 50% of patients achieved TIMI grade 2 or 3 flow (19,23). There may be benefit from such therapy in the ED in an attempt to improve epicardial vessel patency and possibly microvascular perfusion prior to PCI without the risk of intracranial hemorrhage (or prothrombotic effects) associated with thrombolytic therapy.

Trials evaluating this approach are in progress. In the TIGER-PA pilot trial, 100 patients with a STEMI who were to be treated with primary PCI were given heparin in the emergency room and then randomly assigned to tirofiban given in the emergency room (an average of 33 minutes before PCI) or later in the catheterization laboratory (24). Starting the GP IIb/IIIa inhibitor in the emergency room led to significant improvements in TIMI grade 3 flow (32% versus 10%) and a greater likelihood of TIMI myocardial perfusion grade 3 flow (32% versus 6%) (24). A meta-analysis of all trials to date, however, failed to show benefit (but no harm was seen either) (25) (Fig. 11-3). Because nearly all patients are treated with this agent starting at the time of PCI, it is reasonable to consider starting it earlier to improve perfusion, although further studies are

ASSENT-4: 90-Day Primary End Point

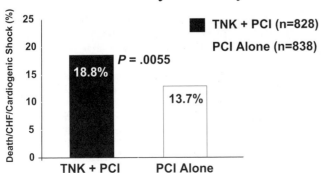

FIGURE 11-2. Primary results of the ASSENT-4PCI trial comparing facilitated PCI using full-dose thrombolytic therapy vs. primary PCI. (Data from ASSENT-4 PCI Investigators. Primary versus tenecteplase-facilitated percutaneous coronary intervention in patients with ST-segment elevation acute myocardial infarction (ASSENT-4 PCI): randomised trial. *Lancet* 2006;367(9510):569–578.)

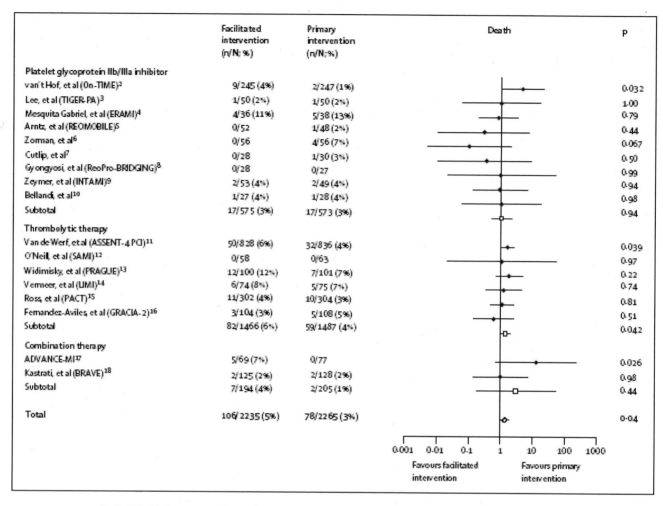

FIGURE 11-3. Meta-analysis of mortality comparing facilitated and primary PCI. (Reproduced with permission from Keeley EC, Boura JA, Grines CL. Comparison of primary and facilitated percutaneous coronary interventions for ST-elevation myocardial infarction: quantitative review of randomised trials. *Lancet* 2006;367(9510):579–588.)

required to determine the clinical benefit of early GP IIb/IIIa inhibitor therapy.

ROUTINE INVASIVE VERSUS CONSERVATIVE STRATEGY

In the TIMI IIB randomized trial, 3,339 patients treated with tissue-type plasminogen activator (t-PA) were randomized to either an invasive strategy consisting of cardiac catheterization 18 to 48 hours later followed by angioplasty or bypass surgery if the anatomy was suitable, or to a conservative strategy in which catheterization and PCI were performed only for recurrent spontaneous ischemia or a positive exercise test (26–28).

Death or MI were similar to 42 days (10.9% for invasive versus 9.7% for conservative; P = NS) (26). Similarly, no difference between the two strategies was observed through 1 year (27) or 3 years of follow-up (28). Similarly the SWIFT trial (29) and other studies (30–36) failed to show benefit of a routine invasive approach. The current AHA/ACC guideline recommendation is to reserve cardiac catheterization after *successful* thrombolytic therapy to patients with spontaneous or inducible ischemia, or those with significantly reduced LV function (with "viable" myocardium).

Of note, however, more recent observational studies have shown a lower rate of mortality in patients undergoing routine PCI after thrombolysis versus those managed conservatively (37,38). The more recent GRACIA randomized trial of 500 patients did see a benefit with significantly lower mortality at 1 year with routine PCI following thrombolysis as compared with standard care (39). Thus, it may be reasonable to perform catheterization in other high-risk patients who may benefit from revascularization, including those with prior MI and those with significant ventricular arrhythmias.

Conservative Strategy

For lower-risk patients, an "early conservative" strategy is recommended, whereby patients are monitored for recurrent angina, or if not, they undergo provocative testing for ischemia with exercise testing or myocardial perfusion imaging. If ischemia is documented, then coronary angiography and revascularization are performed. The benefit of this approach (compared with only medical management) was seen in the DANAMI trial. This trial consisted of 1,008 patients with an acute STEMI who were treated with a thrombolytic agent and had developed either spontaneous symptomatic angina or inducible post-MI ischemia on a predischarge exercise test; the patients were randomly assigned to conservative therapy or to revascularization with PCI or CABG 2 to 10 weeks after the MI. There was a significantly lower rate of the primary endpoint (mortality, reinfarction, or admission for unstable angina) at 1 year (15% vs. 30%), with this benefit largely due to a lower rate of reinfarction or recurrent ischemia requiring hospitalization (40). Thus, patients with acute STEMI who have recurrent angina or ischemia on predischarge stress testing should undergo coronary arteriography, followed by PCI or CABG based on anatomic considerations.

Reducing Other Cardiac Testing

With risk stratification to dictate the judicious use of coronary angiography and PCI, there are other potential areas where testing can be targeted to appropriate patients, notably laboratory tests and echocardiography. During some admissions, multiple measurements of lipid profiles or liver function are ordered, and these may be unnecessary. Our pathway lists what the recommended blood tests are for the house staff. In this fashion, routine ordering of bloods that are not needed may be reduced.

Echocardiography is used widely to assess LV function after MI, the most powerful determinant of subsequent prognosis (41–43). The ACC/AHA Acute MI Guidelines recommend that LV function be assessed in all patients (44). However, one study, now validated by three other groups, has shown that several clinical features (nonanterior MI, no prior Q waves, total CK <1,000 IU, and no evidence of congestive heart failure) can be used to predict normal LV function (ejection fraction >40%) with 97% specificity (45–47). Thus, for patients with small non-Q wave MI, assessment of LV function via echocardiography or ventriculography may not be necessary, a strategy that could have potential implications for more cost-effective care. In our pathway, echocardiography is recommended for most patients, except those with small inferior MIs without complications in whom LV function can be inferred to be normal according to the aforementioned clinical prediction rule (45).

REDUCING HOSPITAL (AND ICU) LENGTH OF STAY

Reduction in hospital length of stay has been the driving force behind the creation of critical pathways. In acute MI, length of stay was quite long just 5 years ago. In GUSTO-I, the median length of stay was 9 days (48). In a follow-up analysis that divided patients into those who had an uncomplicated course (no recurrent ischemia, congestive heart failure, or any other complication) versus any one of these complications, the median length of stay *for both groups* was 9 days. In the TIMI 9 Registry conducted in 1995, for uncomplicated patients with STEMI the median length of stay was 8 days (47,49). Thus, it appears that length of stay has historically been long in patients with acute MI, and opportunities exist to reduce it safely, especially in low-risk patients.

Identification of Low-Risk Patients

With the benefit of aggressive reperfusion therapy in acute MI, it has been possible to identify patients who are at low risk of subsequent mortality or morbidity (50). In the TIMI II trial, a group of patients were prespecified as "low risk" if they had the following characteristics: age <70 years; no prior MI, inferior, or lateral MI; normal sinus rhythm; and Killip class 1 at admission (26). Similar observations have been made in GUSTO-I (48), which led to a more updated risk stratification scheme—the TIMI risk score (51) (Fig. 11-4).

Strategy of Early Discharge following Thrombolysis

Identification of low-risk patients has led to the possibility of early hospital discharge for such uncomplicated patients (48,52). A pilot trial of such a strategy in 80 patients suggested that hospital stay and costs could be significantly reduced without an increase in morbidity and mortality (53). However, it should be noted that all patients who received reperfusion therapy also underwent immediate coronary angiography, the information from which was used in the triage of the patients. Such a strategy is not applicable to standard practice (53). Recently, the cost-effectiveness of early discharge has been subjected to decision analysis, and it was observed that for patients with an uncomplicated MI treated with thrombolytic therapy, the incremental cost of keeping the patient in the hospital beyond 3 days ($624 per day for hospital and physicians' services) and extending the hospital stay to 4 days would cost $105,629 per year of life saved. These data emphasize the cost benefits of early discharge in acute MI. Thus, the strategy of early hospital

TIMI Risk Score for STEMI

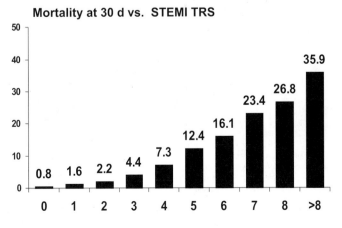

Mortality at 30 d vs. STEMI TRS

Historical		
Age	65-74	2pts
	>75	3pts
DM/HTN/Angina		1pt

Exam	
SBP < 100 mmHg	3pts
HR > 100 bpm	2pts
Killip II – IV	2pts
Weight < 67 kg	1pt

Presentation	
Anterior STE or LBBB	1pt
Time to Rx > 4hr	1pt

Risk Score = Total (0-14)

FIGURE 11-4. TIMI Risk Score for STEMI. (Reproduced with permission from Morrow DA, Antman EM, Charlesworth A, et al. TIMI risk score for ST-elevation myocardial infarction: A convenient, bedside, clinical score for risk assessment at presentation: an intravenous nPA for treatment of infarcting myocardium early II trial substudy. *Circulation* 2000;102:2031–2037.)

discharge looks very promising and feasible, although there are only limited observational data to demonstrate its safety.

It should be noted that data regarding the efficacy and safety of early discharge are available from the PAMI-2 trial, in which 471 low-risk patients were randomized to a strategy of early discharge or to conventional hospital discharge (54). Clinical outcomes at 6 months were similar in both groups: mortality, 0.8% versus 0.4% for early discharge versus standard care ($P = 1.0$); unstable angina, 10.1% versus 12.0% ($P = $ NS); recurrent MI, 0.8% versus 0.4% ($P = $ NS); or the combination of death, unstable angina, MI, congestive heart failure, or stroke, 15.2% versus 17.5% ($P = 0.49$) (54). On the other hand, for the early discharge critical pathway group, hospital length of stay was 3 days shorter (4.2 days versus 7.1 days; $P = 0.0001$), and hospital costs were lower ($\$9,658 \pm \$5,287$ versus $\$11,604 \pm \$6,125$; $P = 0.002$) (54). Thus, in low-risk primary angioplasty patients, early discharge appears to be safe and to result in a substantial reduction in hospital length of stay and cost savings.

All STEMI patients treated with thrombolytic therapy are treated in the ED and admitted to the coronary care unit (CCU). Low-risk patients are transferred out of the CCU after 24 hours, whereas others are transferred when their condition allows. The target hospital length of stay is similar to PAMI II, with 3 days for low-risk patients and 5 days for higher-risk patients. Registry data have shown a steady decline in hospital length of stay over recent years, with current averages in the range of 3 to 5 days.

SECONDARY PREVENTION AND FOLLOW-UP

Because follow-up is critical in the overall management of all acute coronary syndromes, the primary care physician receives a phone call, a fax summary, or the hospital discharge instructions, a letter from the cardiologist, and the hospital discharge summary (the latter three are also sent to other physicians caring for the patient). It provides another opportunity for the cardiologist to ensure that the patient receives long-term treatment with key medications such as aspirin, clopidogrel, beta-blockers, and statins (55,56). Involvement of the patient is also critical, and thus patient education regarding diagnosis, prognosis, and risk factor modification begins in-hospital on the first day. This teaching continues with the patient's primary nurse, as well as dietary consultation if needed.

CONCLUSION

Following thrombolysis, critical pathways are designed to provide an evidence-based approach to revascularization, judicious use of cardiac procedures, and an appropriate, but shortening, length of hospital stay. Then follow-up information on the importance of secondary prevention is critical to the long-term outcomes of patients with STEMI.

References

1. Antman EM, Anbe DT, Armstrong PW, et al. ACC/AHA guidelines for the management of patients with ST-elevation myocardial infarction—executive summary. A report of the American College of Cardiology/American Heart Association Task Force on Practice Guidelines (Writing Committee to revise the 1999 guidelines for the management of patients with acute myocardial infarction). *J Am Coll Cardiol* 2004;44(3):671–719.
2. Anderson JL, Karagounis LA, Becker LC, et al. TIMI perfusion grade 3 but not grade 2 results in improved outcome after thrombolysis for myocardial infarction: ventriculographic, enzymatic and electrocardiographic evidence from the TEAM-3 Study. *Circulation* 1993;87:1829–1839.
3. Schroder R, Dissmann R, Bruggemann T, et al. Extent of early ST segment elevation resolution: a simple but strong predictor of outcome in patients with acute myocardial infarction. *J Am Coll Cardiol* 1994;24:384–391.
4. Schroder R, Wegscheider K, Schroder K, et al. Extent of early ST segment elevation resolution: a strong predictor of outcome in patients with acute myocardial infarction and a sensitive measure to compare thrombolytic regimens. A substudy of the International Joint Efficacy Comparison of Thrombolytics (INJECT) trial. *J Am Coll Cardiol* 1995;26:1657–1664.
5. de Lemos JA, Antman EM, Rifai N, et al. ST-segment resolution and serum myoglobin ratio predict reperfusion after thrombolytic therapy: a TIMI 14 substudy. *J Am Coll Cardiol* 1999;33(Suppl A):391A.
6. Ito H, Okamura A, Isakura K, et al. Myocardial perfusion patterns related to thrombolysis in myocardial infarction perfusion grades after coronary angioplasty in patients with acute anterior wall myocardial infarction. *Circulation* 1996;93:1993–1999.
7. Gibson CM, Cannon CP, Murphy SA, et al. Relationship of the TIMI myocardial perfusion grades, flow grades, frame count, and percutaneous coronary intervention to long-term outcomes after thrombolytic administration in acute myocardial infarction. *Circulation* 2002;105:1909–1913.
8. Ellis SG, Ribeiro da Silva E, et al. Final results of the randomized RESCUE study evaluating PTCA after failed thrombolysis for patients with anterior infarction. *Circulation* 1993;88:I–106.
9. Abbottsmith CW, Topol EJ, George BS, et al. Fate of patients with acute myocardial infarction with patency of the infarct-related artery achieved with successful thrombolysis versus rescue angioplasty. *J Am Coll Cardiol* 1990;16:770–778.
10. Gibson CM, Cannon CP, Greene RM, et al. Rescue angioplasty in the Thrombolysis in Myocardial Infarction (TIMI) 4 trial. *Am J Cardiol* 1997;80:21–26.
11. Schomig A, Ndrepepa G, Mehilli J, et al. A randomized trial of coronary stenting versus balloon angioplasty as a rescue intervention after failed thrombolysis in patients with acute myocardial infarction. *J Am Coll Cardiol* 2004;44(10):2073–2079.
12. Gershlick AH, Stephens-Lloyd A, Hughes S, et al. Rescue angioplasty after failed thrombolytic therapy for acute myocardial infarction. *N Engl J Med* 2005;353(26):2758–2768.
13. Bengston JR, Kaplan AJ, Pieper KS, et al. Prognosis in cardiogenic shock after acute myocardial infarction in the interventional era. *J Am Coll Cardiol* 1992;20:1482–1489.
14. Hochman JS, Sleeper LA, Webb JG, et al. Early revascularization in acute myocardial infarction complicated by cardiogenic shock. *N Engl J Med* 1999;341(9):625–634.
15. Stone GW, Cox D, Garcia E, et al. Normal flow (TIMI-3) before mechanical reperfusion therapy is an independent determinant of survival in acute myocardial infarction: analysis from the primary angioplasty in myocardial infarction trials. *Circulation* 2001;104(6):636–641.
16. Topol EJ, Califf RM, George BS, et al. A randomized trial of immediate versus delayed elective angioplasty after intravenous tissue plasminogen activator in acute myocardial infarction. *N Engl J Med* 1987;317:581–588.
17. TIMI Research Group. Immediate vs delayed catheterization and angioplasty following thrombolytic therapy for acute myocardial infarction. TIMI II A results. *JAMA* 1988;260:2849–2858.
18. Simoons ML, Arnold AER, Betriu A, et al. Thrombolysis with tissue plasminogen activator in acute myocardial infarction: no additional benefit from immediate percutaneous coronary angioplasty. *Lancet* 1988;1:197–203.
19. Herrmann HC, Moliterno DJ, Ohman EM, et al. Facilitation of early percutaneous coronary intervention after reteplase with or without abciximab in acute myocardial infarction: results from the SPEED (GUSTO-4 Pilot) Trial. *J Am Coll Cardiol* 2000;36(5):1489–1496.
20. ASSENT-4 PCI Investigators. Primary versus tenecteplase-facilitated percutaneous coronary intervention in patients with ST-segment elevation acute myocardial infarction (ASSENT-4 PCI): randomised trial. *Lancet* 2006;367(9510):569–578.
21. Kastrati A, Mehilli J, Schlotterbeck K, et al. Early administration of reteplase plus abciximab vs abciximab alone in patients with acute myocardial infarction referred for percutaneous coronary intervention: a randomized controlled trial. *JAMA* 2004;291(8):947–954.
22. Advance MI Investigators. Facilitated percutaneous coronary intervention for acute ST-segment elevation myocardial infarction: results from the prematurely terminated ADdressing the Value of facilitated ANgioplasty after Combination therapy or Eptifibatide monotherapy in acute Myocardial Infarction (ADVANCE MI) trial. *Am Heart J* 2005;150(1):116–122.
23. Antman EM, Giugliano RP, Gibson CM, et al. Abciximab facilitates the rate and extent of thrombolysis: results of TIMI 14 trial. *Circulation* 1999;99:2720–2732.
24. Lee DP, Herity NA, Hiatt BL, et al. Adjunctive platelet glycoprotein IIb/IIIa receptor inhibition with tirofiban before primary angioplasty improves angiographic outcomes: results of the TIrofiban Given in the Emergency Room before Primary Angioplasty (TIGER-PA) pilot trial. *Circulation* 2003;107(11):1497–1501.
25. Keeley EC, Boura JA, Grines CL. Comparison of primary and facilitated percutaneous coronary interventions for ST-elevation myocardial infarction: quantitative review of randomised trials. *Lancet* 2006;367(9510):579–588.
26. TIMI Study Group. Comparison of invasive and conservative strategies after treatment with intravenous tissue plasminogen activator in acute myocardial infarction. Results of the Thrombolysis in Myocardial Infarction (TIMI) Phase II Trial. *N Engl J Med* 1989;320:618–627.

27. Williams DO, Braunwald E, Knatterud G, et al. One-year results of the Thrombolysis in Myocardial Infarction Investigation (TIMI) phase II trial. *Circulation* 1992;85(2):533–542.
28. Terrin ML, Williams DO, Kleiman NS, et al. Two- and three-year results of the Thrombolysis in Myocardial Infarction (TIMI) Phase II clinical trial. *J Am Coll Cardiol* 1993;22:1763–1772.
29. SWIFT (Should We Intervene Following Thrombolysis?) Trial Study Group. SWIFT trial of delayed elective intervention v. conservative treatment after thrombolysis with anistreplase in acute myocardial infarction. *BMJ* 1991;302:555–560.
30. Every NR, Larson EB, Litwin PE, et al. The association between on-site cardiac catheterization facilities and the use of coronary angiography after acute myocardial infarction. *N Engl J Med* 1993;329:546–551.
31. Every NR, Parson LS, Fihn SD, et al. Long-term outcome in acute myocardial infarction patients admitted to hospitals with and without on-site cardiac catheterization facilities. *Circulation* 1997;96:1770–1775.
32. Blustein J. High-technology cardiac procedures. The impact of service availability on service use in New York State. *JAMA* 1993;270:344–349.
33. Rouleau JL, Moye LA, Pfeffer MA, et al. A comparison of management patterns after acute myocardial infarction in Canada and the United States. *N Engl J Med* 1993;328:779–784.
34. Pilote L, Califf RM, Sapp S, et al. Regional variation across the United States in the management of acute myocardial infarction. *N Engl J Med* 1995;333:565–572.
35. Mark DB, Naylor CD, Hlatky MA, et al. Use of medical resources and quality of life after acute myocardial infarction in Canada and the United States. *N Engl J Med* 1994;331:1130–1135.
36. Tu JV, Pashos CL, Naylor D, et al. Use of cardiac procedures and outcomes in elderly patients with myocardial infarction in the United States and Canada. *JAMA* 1997;336:1500–1505.
37. Stenestrand U, Wallentin L. Early revascularisation and 1-year survival in 14-day survivors of acute myocardial infarction: a prospective cohort study. *Lancet* 2002;359(9320):1805–1811.
38. Gibson CM, Karha J, Murphy S, et al. Percutaneous coronary intervention during the index hospitalization is associated with reduced recurrent myocardial infarction and improved survival following thrombolytic administration. *J Am Coll Cardiol* 2003;41:398A.
39. Fernandez-Aviles F, Alonso JJ, Castro-Beiras A, et al. Routine invasive strategy within 24 hours of thrombolysis versus ischaemia-guided conservative approach for acute myocardial infarction with ST-segment elevation (GRACIA-1): a randomised controlled trial. *Lancet* 2004;364(9439):1045–1053.
40. Madsen JK, Grande P, Saunamaki K, et al. Danish multicenter randomized study of invasive versus conservative treatment in patients with inducible ischemia after thrombolysis in acute myocardial infarction (DANAMI). *Circulation* 1997;96:748–755.
41. Multicenter Postinfarction Research Group. Risk stratification and survival after myocardial infarction. *N Engl J Med* 1983;309:331–336.
42. Zaret BL, Wackers FJT, Terrin ML, et al. Value of radionuclide rest and exercise left ventricular ejection fraction in assessing survival of patients after thrombolytic therapy for acute myocardial infarction: results of the Thrombolysis in Myocardial Infarction (TIMI) Phase II study. *J Am Coll Cardiol* 1995;26:73–79.
43. Nicod P, Gilpin E, Dittrich H, et al. Influence on prognosis and morbidity of left ventricular ejection fraction with and without signs of left ventricular failure after acute myocardial infarction. *Am J Cardiol* 1988;61:1165–1171.
44. Ryan TJ, Anderson JL, Antman EM, et al. ACC/AHA guidelines for the management of patients with acute myocardial infarction: a report of the American College of Cardiology/American Heart Association Task Force on Practice Guidelines (Committee on Management of Acute Myocardial Infarction). *J Am Coll Cardiol* 1996;28:1328–1428.
45. Silver MT, Rose GA, Paul SD, et al. A clinical rule to predict preserved left ventricular ejection fraction in patients after myocardial infarction. *Ann Intern Med* 1994;121:750–756.
46. Tobin K, Stomel R, Harber D, et al. Validation of a clinical prediction rule for predicting left ventricular function post acute myocardial infarction in a community hospital setting. *J Am Coll Cardiol* 1996;27(Suppl. A):318A.
47. Bahit MC, Murphy SA, Gibson CM, et al. Critical pathway for acute ST-segment elevation myocardial infarction: estimating its potential impact in the TIMI 9 Registry. *Crit Path Cardiol* 2002;1:107–112.
48. Newby LK, Eisenstein EL, Califf RM, et al. Cost effectiveness of early discharge after uncomplicated acute myocardial infarction. *N Engl J Med* 2000;342(11):749–755.
49. Cannon CP, Antman EM, Gibson CM, et al. Critical pathway for acute ST segment elevation myocardial infarction: evaluation of the potential impact in the TIMI 9 registry. *J Am Coll Cardiol* 1998;31(Suppl. A):192A.
50. Hillis LD, Forman S, Braunwald E, et al. Risk stratification before thrombolytic therapy in patients with acute myocardial infarction. *J Am Coll Cardiol* 1990;16:313–315.
51. Morrow DA, Antman EM, Charlesworth A, et al. TIMI risk score for ST-elevation myocardial infarction: a convenient, bedside, clinical score for risk assessment at presentation: an intravenous nPA for treatment of infarcting myocardium early II trial substudy. *Circulation* 2000;102:2031–2037.
52. Mark DB, Sigmon K, Topol EJ, et al. Identification of acute myocardial infarction patients suitable for early hospital discharge after aggressive interventional therapy. Results from the Thrombolysis and Angioplasty in Acute Myocardial Infarction Registry. *Circulation* 1991;83:1186–1193.
53. Topol EJ, Bure K, O'Neill WW, et al. A randomized controlled trial of hospital discharge three days after myocardial infarction in the era of reperfusion. *N Engl J Med* 1988;318:1083–1088.
54. Grines CL, Marsalese DL, Brodie B, et al. Safety and cost-effectiveness of early discharge after primary angioplasty in low risk patients with acute myocardial infarction. *J Am Coll Cardiol* 1998;31:967–972.
55. Scandinavian Simvastatin Survival Study Group. Randomised trial of cholesterol lowering in 4444 patients with coronary heart disease: the Scandinavian Simvastatin Survival Study (4S). *Lancet* 1994;344:1383–1389.
56. Sacks RM, Pfeffer MA, Moye LA, et al. The effect of pravastatin on coronary events after myocardial infarction in patients with average cholesterol levels. *N Engl J Med* 1996;335:1001–1009.

CHAPTER 12 ■ PRIMARY PCI

AMR E. ABBAS AND CINDY L. GRINES

PREPROCEDURAL PATHWAYS
Comparison to Thrombolytic Therapy
Impact of Time to Reperfusion and Need to Transfer
ADJUNCTIVE PHARMACOLOGY
Aspirin
Heparin
GP IIb/IIIa Inhibitors
Thrombolytic Agents
Clopidogrel
Statins
Beta-Blockers
PROCEDURAL PATHWAYS
Angioplasty versus Stenting
Management of Thrombus
Adjunctive Pharmacology
Use of Intra-Aortic Balloon Pump (IABP)
Use of Percutaneous Left Ventricular Assist Device (p-VAD)
MANAGEMENT OF NO REFLOW
MANAGEMENT OF REPERFUSION INJURY
EMERGENCY CORONARY BYPASS SURGERY
POSTPROCEDURAL PATHWAYS
Admission
Vascular Access Management
Adjunctive Pharmacology
Imaging
Long-Term Follow-up
CONCLUSION

Since the release of the first edition of *Critical Pathways* a tremendous amount of data has been published on primary percutaneous intervention (PCI) for acute myocardial infarction with ST segment elevation (AMI). Percutaneous mechanical reperfusion has proved to be the most effective modality for complete and sustained restoration of coronary flow in patients with AMI compared to thrombolysis (1). Transfer of patients to facilities with primary PCI, within reasonable time, was shown to be superior to thrombolytic therapy (2,3), and even superior to combined lytic and transfer protocols (4). Technically, stenting has become the standard method for managing infarct-related arteries (5,6); early administration of glycoprotein IIb/IIIa inhibitors (GP IIb/IIIa) has been shown to lead to satisfactory clinical and angiographic parameters (7,8). However, the use of distal protection devices (9,10) and thrombectomy devices (11) have failed to show any benefit in randomized controlled trials. Novel techniques that have been developed to prevent damage due to myocardial reperfusion include hypothermia (12,13) and hyperbaric oxygen (14). However, those have only showed modest benefit. For patients with cardiogenic shock, PCI and intra-aortic balloon counterpulsation (IABP) remain the only therapeutic modalities currently recommended.

The American Heart Association/American College of Cardiologists (AHA/ACC) guidelines consider as a class I recommendation PCI within 90 min from diagnosis of infarction in AMI <12 hours and carried out in centers with proven expertise. If symptom duration is <3 hours, PCI is recommended in the event that the procedure is carried out <1 hour from diagnosis. Moreover, PCI is recommended as the treatment of choice if the patient arrives >3 hours from symptom onset. PCI is also recommended in patients with heart failure or pulmonary edema and symptom onset <12 hours. On the other hand, when the onset of AMI symptoms is >12 hours, PTCA is recommended in the case of heart failure, electric or hemodynamic instability, or persistent ischemic symptoms (15). This chapter will divide the primary PCI pathways for AMI into phases: preprocedural, procedural, and postprocedural (Fig. 12-1).

PREPROCEDURAL PATHWAYS

Comparison to Thrombolytic Therapy

In the analysis by Keeley and Grines of 23 randomized studies comparing PCI with thrombolytic therapy in AMI, primary PCI was better than thrombolytic therapy at reducing overall short-term death (7% vs. 9%; $P = 0.0002$), nonfatal reinfarction (3% vs. 7%; $P <0.0001$), stroke (1% vs. 2%; $P = 0.0004$), and the combined endpoint of death, nonfatal reinfarction, and stroke (8% vs. 14%; $P <0.0001$) (1). These results remained in favor of PCI during long-term follow-up and were independent of both the type of thrombolytic agent used and whether or not the patient was transferred for primary PCI. At our institution, all patients with ST-elevation MI (STEMI) <12 hours receive primary PCI.

Impact of Time to Reperfusion and Need to Transfer

Time to Reperfusion

This remains controversial because patency after PCI is the same in both early and late treated patients. Unfortunately, in the NRMI 3 and 4 analyses, the median time for transfer for AMI was 180 minutes with only 4.2% of patients treated within 90 minutes, as the guidelines recommend (16). Brodie et al evaluated patients with AMI of <12 hours' duration, without cardiogenic shock, who were treated with primary PCI in the Stent Primary Angioplasty in Myocardial Infarction (Stent PAMI) Trial ($n = 1,232$) to assess the effect of time to reperfusion on outcomes. Improvement in ejection fraction from baseline to 6 months was substantial with reperfusion at <2 hours but was modest and relatively independent of time to reperfusion after 2 hours. There were no differences in 1- or 6-month mortality by time to reperfusion. There were also

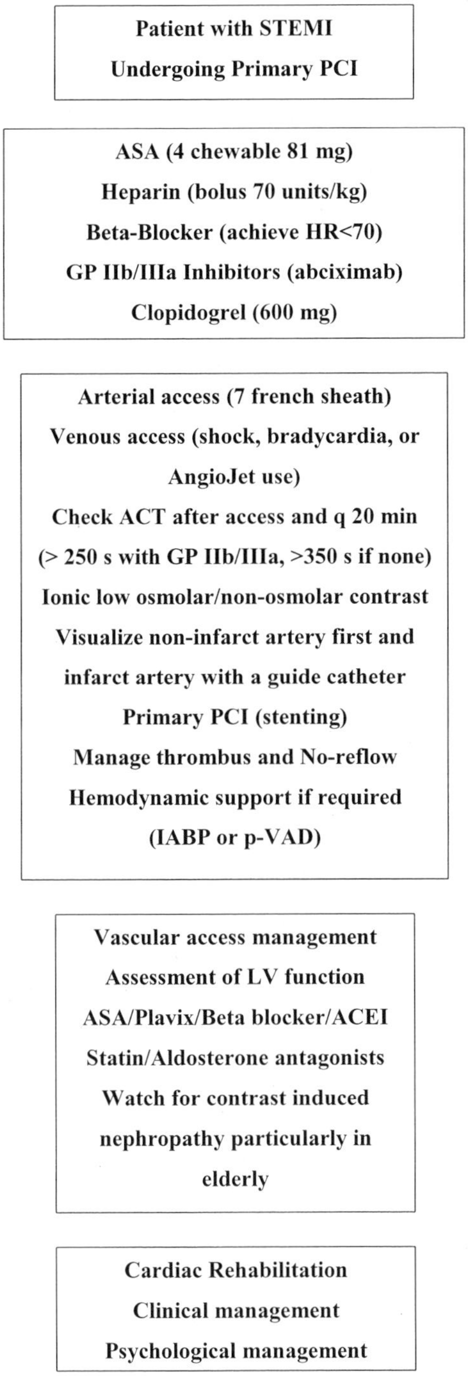

Patient with STEMI
Undergoing Primary PCI

ASA (4 chewable 81 mg)
Heparin (bolus 70 units/kg)
Beta-Blocker (achieve HR<70)
GP IIb/IIIa Inhibitors (abciximab)
Clopidogrel (600 mg)

Arterial access (7 french sheath)
Venous access (shock, bradycardia, or AngioJet use)
Check ACT after access and q 20 min (> 250 s with GP IIb/IIIa, >350 s if none)
Ionic low osmolar/non-osmolar contrast
Visualize non-infarct artery first and infarct artery with a guide catheter
Primary PCI (stenting)
Manage thrombus and No-reflow
Hemodynamic support if required (IABP or p-VAD)

Vascular access management
Assessment of LV function
ASA/Plavix/Beta blocker/ACEI
Statin/Aldosterone antagonists
Watch for contrast induced nephropathy particularly in elderly

---

Cardiac Rehabilitation
Clinical management
Psychological management

FIGURE 12-1. The primary PCI pathways for AMI shown in phases: preprocedural, procedural, and postprocedural.

no differences in other clinical outcomes by time to reperfusion, except that reinfarction and infarct artery reocclusion at 6 months were more frequent with later reperfusion (17). This is different from lytic therapy, where time to reperfusion is inversely related to outcome.

In a more recent analysis of four studies of 1,122 patients with AMI randomized between September 2001 and December 2003, O'Neill et al demonstrated excellent clinical outcomes in patients with AMI receiving primary PCI. The major adverse event rates were 4.5% at 30 days, with a mortality of 2% and no significant difference between anterior and nonanterior

infarctions. On the multivariate analysis, door-to-balloon (P <0.0001) and onset-to-door time (P = 0.025) remained independent predictors of final infarct size (18).

Adding to the controversy, in patients with late presentation, a recent study demonstrated that in patients with AMI without persistent symptoms presenting 12 to 48 hours after symptom onset, primary PCI reduces infarct size compared to usual care (19). This suggests that the window for primary PCI may be extended beyond 12 hours. At our institution, patients with STEMI who have residual chest pain with ST-segment elevation presenting beyond 12 hours are managed by primary PCI.

Transfer

Studies that evaluated transfer to centers where primary PCI could be performed demonstrated superiority of mechanical versus pharmacological reperfusion. To date five trials have randomized STEMI patients to transfer for primary PCI versus lytic therapy. The PRAGUE 1 study (300 patients) compared three strategies in patients with AMI <6 hours from onset: (a) thrombolysis in the hospital, (b) thrombolysis during transfer for facilitated PTCA, and (c) transportation to a center for primary PTCA without thrombolytic treatment. The primary end point of death, reinfarction, and stroke at 30 days was less frequent in the transfer for PCI group (8%) compared to the second (15%) and first (23%; P <0.02). The incidence of reinfarction was significantly reduced by transportation for PCI (4). In the PRAGUE 2 study, 850 patients with AMI <12 hours were randomized to transfer for primary PCI (<120 km) versus on-site thrombolysis in the original hospital. The study ended prematurely due to excess mortality in the subgroup, which presented with ≥3 hours of symptoms, and overall 30-day mortality was 6.8% for the angioplasty group and 10% for thrombolysis group (P = 0.12). Complications only occurred during transfer (1.2%). The combined end point was less frequent in the PCI group (P <0.003), with more stroke in the thrombolysis group (P = 0.03) (3). The DANAMI 2 study compared on-site thrombolytic treatment with transfer to another center for PCI and again was stopped prematurely due to more PCI benefit. There were no deaths during transfer, and there was a 75% reduction in the relative risk of reinfarction (P = 0.0003) and decreased major adverse cardiac events (MACE) at 30 days (P = 0.02) in the PCI group. Primary PCI was of benefit in the different groups, including inferior or anterior infarctions and regardless of the time from symptom onset to intervention (2). Mean time from symptom onset to randomization was 135 minutes. In Figure 12-2, our recommendations to improve transfer and reperfusion time are listed.

ADJUNCTIVE PHARMACOLOGY

Aspirin

The use of aspirin prior to primary PCI is unequivocal and should be given to all patients unless a true allergy exists (20). We provide patients with four tablets of chewable baby aspirin, which is more effective than 81 mg alone, and we avoid the enteric coated form for more rapid delivery of the drug.

Heparin

The HEAP study did not support the use of heparin as pretreatment for angioplasty (21). However, heparin is routinely initiated in the ED intravenously at a dose of 70 units/kg prior to arrival to the cardiac catheterization laboratory.

Pre-hospital ECG

> Direct transfer to PCI center (bypassing closest hospital)

> EMS authority to mobilize cath lab

Hospital without PCI capability

> Ambulance remains at hospital, patient not taken off stretcher

> Avoid IV infusion pumps (delays in switching equipment)

> Authority to transfer patient to tertiary care center without delay of speaking to a

> cardiologist

Tertiary Care Center

> Direct transfer to cath lab (bypassing EC, residents and fellows)

> Phone call to mobilize team, have patient pre-registered, prepare cath lab

> supplies

> Expedited patients prep

> Engage suspected infarct artery with guiding catheter and prompt reperfusion

Primary PCI with no surgery on site

FIGURE 12-2. Recommendations to improve transfer delays and reperfusion time in the United States.

GP IIb/IIIa Inhibitors

A recent meta-analysis of the studies involving GP IIb/IIIa inhibitors in patients with ST segment elevation AMI (11 trials, involving 27,115 patients) demonstrated that when compared with the control group, abciximab was associated with a significant reduction in short-term (30 days) mortality (2.4% vs. 3.4%, $P = 0.047$) and long-term (6 to 12 months) mortality (4.4% vs. 6.2%, $P = 0.01$). This was observed in patients undergoing primary PCI but not in those treated with fibrinolysis or in all trials combined. Abciximab was associated with a significant reduction in 30-day reinfarction, both in all trials combined (2.1% vs. 3.3%, $P <0.001$), in primary angioplasty (1.0% vs. 1.9%, $P = 0.03$), and in fibrinolysis trials (2.3% vs. 3.6%, $P <0.001$). Abciximab did not result in an increased risk of intracranial bleeding (0.61% vs. 0.62%, $P = 0.62$) overall, but was associated with an increased risk of major bleeding complications when combined with fibrinolysis (5.2% vs. 3.1%, $P <0.001$) (22). In our institution, abciximab is frequently given for ST-segment elevation AMI in the absence of contraindications. Some operators administer the abciximab bolus intracoronary. Because few data exist regarding the use of small molecular weight GP IIb/IIIa inhibitor agents in AMI, we do not advocate the use of eptifibatide or tirofiban for STEMI.

Thrombolytic Agents

Thrombolytics are occasionally administered prior to PCI either as a failed primary revascularization protocol (rescue PCI) or as a facilitative modality in an attempt to enhance pre-PCI TIMI flow (facilitated PCI). Three recent trials, MERLIN (23), REACT (24), and STOPAMI (25), suggested greater myocardial salvage and fewer MACE with rescue PCI compared to conservative therapy. Despite multiple recent trials CAPITAL AMI (26), BRAVE (27), ON-TIME (28), and GRACIA-1 (29), to date no trial has shown that facilitated PCI is superior to primary PCI alone. In fact, no trial has shown clinical benefit, and some trials have suggested harm. The largest trial to date, ASSENT-4, was stopped prematurely due to increased deaths, reinfarction, and MACE in the facilitated arm compared to primary PCI. Although, the AHA/ACC guidelines allowed facilitated PCI as a class IIb recommendation in high-risk patients where PCI will be delayed and there is a low risk of complications due to bleeding (15), given the data from recent trials showing harm, we do not recommend facilitation with thrombolytics. The use of GP IIb/IIIa inhibitors does not appear to cause harm, but these should not be used if their administration will delay transfer to the cath lab. This may be particularly a problem with the complex dosing regimens required for eptifibatide.

Clopidogrel

In patients 75 years of age or younger who have AMI with ST-segment elevation and who receive aspirin and a standard fibrinolytic regimen, the addition of clopidogrel was found to improve the patency rate of the infarct-related artery and reduce ischemic complications (30). Moreover, in the recent mega trial (COMMITT) that included over 40,000 patients with STEMI who were randomized to clopidogrel versus placebo, there was a decrease in the incidence of death and the composite incidence of death/MI/stroke with the use of clopidogrel for up to 4 weeks postdischarge. There was no increase in the incidence of major bleeding with the use of clopidogrel (31). However, it should be kept in mind that the preoperative use of clopidogrel in patients undergoing coronary artery bypass graft (CABC) surgery has been shown to be associated with a significantly increased risk of bleeding and blood transfusion (32). Because 90% of patients with STEMI who go to the cath lab will undergo primary PCI and, in our experience, virtually no patients with STEMI will undergo CABG in the first few days, we recommend 600-mg loading dose of clopidogrel in the EC. The higher dose provides more rapid onset of action and more complete platelet inhibition. We usually continue clopidogrel for 9 to 12 months based on the results from the CURE (33) and CREDO trials (34).

Statins

Even though the use of high-dose statin therapy has shown to reduce MACE in patients with acute coronary syndrome (ACS), this benefit has not been tested in patients with AMI with ST-segment elevation in randomized trials. Because the outcomes of these patients are primarily determined by arrhythmias and pump failure, acute statin administration may not affect early outcomes. However, a recent analysis of the NRMI database demonstrated that patients with AMI who continued or newly started on statin therapy within 24 hours had 25% to 30% the in-hospital mortality of patients who discontinued or did not receive statin therapy (35). At our institution we extrapolate the data from the benefit of high-dose statin in patients with ACSs and administer 80 mg of atorvastatin in patients with STEMI.

Beta-Blockers

In the Controlled Abciximab and Device Investigation to Lower Late Angioplasty Complications (CADILLAC) trial, preprocedural intravenous beta-blockade enhanced myocardial recovery and 30-day mortality in patients with AMI undergoing primary PCI. However, these effects were confined to patients untreated with oral beta-blocker medication before admission (36). Beta-blockers should be given to all patients if blood pressure tolerates in the absence of contraindications (Table 12-1). An analysis of the PAMI trials demonstrated that treatment with beta-blockers after successful primary PCI is associated with reduced 6-month mortality, with the greatest benefit in patients with a low ejection fraction or multivessel coronary disease (37). Beta-blockers are given in the ED as sequential 5 mg IV of Lopressor (in the absence of contraindications) until the heart rate is <70 bpm and is continued for at least 1 to 2 years.

PROCEDURAL PATHWAYS

Angioplasty versus Stenting

A 7-french system is almost exclusively used at our institution. This is because of the better support and torque provided by the guiding catheter as well as better visualization during dye injection around the balloon and stent delivery systems. We do not advocate obtaining venous access unless there is hemodynamic instability or a transvenous pacemaker is required.

At our institution all patients receive stenting for primary PCI unless the patient will require CABG, in which case angio-

TABLE 12-1

CONTRAINDICATIONS TO BETA-BLOCKERS

Heart rate <60 beats per minute

Systolic arterial pressure <100 mm Hg

Moderate or severe left ventricular failure

Signs of peripheral hypoperfusion

PR interval >0.24 sec

Second- or third-degree atrioventricular block

Severe chronic obstructive pulmonary disease or history of asthma requiring home oxygen or oral steroids

plasty is performed as a bridge to CABG. Bare metal stenting remains the current primary PCI strategy at our institution.

Initial fears of stenting in patients with AMI due to the theoretical risk of occlusion when implanting it in lesions with high thrombotic content have resolved with the influx of clinical trials (5,6). Obtaining a greater luminal diameter, resolving the residual dissection that may predispose to reocclusion, and a lower incidence of target vessel revascularization with the use of stents has helped establish stents as the current standard of care. However, stenting may be associated with a lower degree of TIMI III flow compared to PTCA, in part due to distal embolization of the thrombus previously fragmented by predilatation with the balloon (38). Direct stenting without predilatation has thus been suggested in patients with AMI in the absence of calcified lesions and when achieving full stent expansion is doubtful (39,40). The role of drug-eluting stents (DES) remains unclear. The roles of sirolimus (41) and paclitaxel-eluting stents (42) in the setting of AMI, were studied in two separate studies and were presented at the American College of Cardiology annual scientific meeting, Atlanta, Georgia, 2006. The first study randomized 712 patients with AMI to either bare metal stents or sirolimus-eluting stents. The composite end point of target vessel failure (target vessel revascularization, AMI, and cardiac death) was twice as common in the bare metal stent group (14.3% vs. 7.3%, $P < 0.0036$). This was driven mainly by the difference in target vessel revascularization (13.4% vs. 5.6%, $P < 0.001$). On the other hand, another study of 619 patients comparing receiving either bare metal stenting or paclitaxel-eluting stents showed no difference in major adverse cardiac events at 1 year (12.6% vs. 8.7%, $P = 0.12$). However, the paclitaxel trial enrolled patients with left main disease, large thrombus burden, and bifurcation lesions that were excluded in the sirolimus trial. Moreover, the bare metal-stent arm patients in the paclitaxel study only received the Express stent, while there was no restriction in the type of bare metal stent in the sirolimus study. The conflicting results of these two studies highlights the ongoing controversy that exists in this manner. At our sirolimus stent use in the setting of AMI has increased.

Management of Thrombus

Despite significant developments in the pharmacology of antiplatelet agents (GP IIb/IIIa inhibitors, clopidogrel) and antithrombotic agents (direct thrombin inhibitors, low-molecular-weight heparin), the persistence of an angiographic thrombus in infarct lesions is strongly associated with a high risk of distal embolization and no-reflow events leading to poor angiographic and clinical outcomes. Approaches that have been developed for mechanical management of thrombi include thrombus aspiration catheters (Export catheter, Diver catheter, and Pronto catheter), rheolytic systems (AngioJet), distal protection devices (balloon occlusions and filter systems), and mechanical Thrombectomy (X-sizer). However, the majority of these agents have not been thoroughly studied or have proven disappointing in multicenter randomized trials. In the enhanced myocardial efficacy and removal by aspiration of liberated debris (EMERALD) study of 501 patients with AMI who underwent primary or rescue PCI with and without the Percu-Surge distal protection device (9), distal protection was no more effective than conventional intervention; neither was it safer nor able to reduce mortality. This was also replicated in the results of the protection devices in PCI Treatment of Myocardial Infarction for Salvage of Endangered Myocardium (PROMISE) in which a filter-based distal protection device failed to improve myocardial perfusion and infarct size in acute-MI patients undergoing primary PCI (10). In another disappointing multicenter randomized study (AngioJet in acute

MANAGEMENT OF THROMBUS

Keep ACT >350 sec, or >250 to 300 if GP IIb/IIIa
  inhibitors are used
Ionic low-osmolar or nonosmolar agents
Perform thrombectomy using aspiration catheters prior to
  balloon inflation
Avoid thrombolytics (may activate platelets)
Stent if any dissection is present, avoid if heavy thrombus
  burden
Consider prolonged, low-pressure inflations with slightly
  oversized balloons
Intracoronary abciximab (bolus dose given)

myocardial infarction, AIMI) (11), the use of rheolytic thrombectomy using the AngioJet system increased the incidence of complications, including infarct size and mortality, compared to conventional interventional therapy. On the other hand, the X-Sizer in AMI patients for negligible embolization and optimal ST resolution (XAMINE) study (43) compared the results of 200 patients in 14 European centers randomized to receive treatment with the X-Sizer system or conventional therapy in the AMI culprit artery, with clear evidence of thrombus and TIMI grade 0 to 1 flow in the initial coronary angiography. The primary end point was the magnitude of postprocedural ST-segment resolution, which was significantly better in the group treated with the X-Sizer system. Thrombectomy was also more effective in reducing the incidence of distal embolization and slow-flow/no-reflow. At our institution, aspiration catheters are quickly prepared and used in the presence of angiographically visible large thrombus to manually aspirate debris in the syringe. This is performed prior to initial balloon dilatation (Table 12-2). The Dethrombosis to Enhance Reperfusion in Myocardial Infarction (DEAR-MI) demonstrated improvement in myocardial blush grade and ST-segment resolution with the use of an aspiration catheter (44).

Adjunctive Pharmacology

Heparin remains the standard antithrombotic agent of choice for primary PCI. Studies of direct thrombin inhibitors and low-molecular weight heparin (LMWH) are underway. A low-dose heparin to achieve an ACT of 250 to 300 seconds is used in the presence of GP IIb/IIIa inhibitors. However, if no GP IIb/IIIA agents are used, a higher heparin dose is given to achieve an ACT of 350 seconds. ACTs are repeated every 20 minutes given the hypercoagulable states of STEMI.

Use of Intra-Aortic Balloon Pump (IABP)

Routine use of IABP has shown not to be beneficial in managements of patients with AMI (PAMI-2) (45). However, continued ischemia, hypotension, congestive heart failure, severe ventricular dysfunction with multivessel disease, and mechanical complications such as ventricular septal defects or severe mitral regurgitation remain indications for adjunctive use of patients with IABP.

Use of Percutaneous Left Ventricular Assist Device (p-VAD)

A recent study comparing IABP support to p-VAD in 41 patients with revascularized AMI complicated by cardiogenic shock demonstrated that hemodynamic and metabolic parameters could be reversed more effectively with p-VAD. However, this was at the expense of a higher incidence of complications as severe bleeding and limb ischemia and no difference in 30-day mortality (IABP 45% vs. p-VAD 43%, $P = 0.86$) (46). At our institution, p-VAD remains a valuable tool in patients with continued shock despite IABP and inotropic support after revascularization or as a bridge to surgery.

MANAGEMENT OF NO REFLOW

Importance of TIMI III flow pre- and postprocedure. In an analysis of the PAMI trials, in-hospital events (reinfarction, TVR, and death) as well as 1-year events (reinfarction and death) were more common in patients with <TIMI III flow at the end of the primary PCI. On multivariate analysis, predictors of <TIMI III flow included age, diabetes, symptom onset to emergency room presentation, initial TIMI ≤1 flow, and left ventricular ejection fraction <50% (47). On the other hand, an analysis of the same studies in patients who presented with TIMI grade 3 flow on arrival at the catheterization laboratory (16%) demonstrated a greater left ventricular ejection fraction and a less likelihood of developing heart failure. The 6-month mortality was also reduced in these patients (48).

Intracoronary verapamil (100 to 200 micrograms), adenosine (600 to 2400 micrograms given as intracoronary boluses), nitroprusside (50 micrograms up to 200 micrograms), epinephrine (1 cc of 1/10,000 concentration), and abciximab (bolus dose given intracoronary) are all used in the presence of no or slow reflow. However, there are no randomized trials to support their use (Table 12-3).

MANAGEMENT OF NO REFLOW

May include one or more of the following:
–Repeated boluses of intracoronary adenosine (60 μg
  boluses until 1200 to 2400 μg have been given). This is
  the favored method of managing no reflow in the patient
  with AMI because it can have the additional benefit of
  limiting infarct size. Heart block is frequent but resolves in
  seconds.
  (6 mg adenosine in 100 cc NS = 60 μg/cc, incremental
  doses of 1 cc q 1 minute)
–Intracoronary nitroprusside (50 μg doses up to 200 μg
  total) (watch for hypotension)
  0.25 ml (6.25 mg-use TB syringe) in 250 cc D5W = 25
  μg/cc, incremental doses of 1 cc
–Intracoronary abciximab (bolus dose)
–Repeated boluses of intracoronary verapamil (100–200 μg)
  (watch for bradycardia)
  1 cc (2.5 mg) in 10 cc NS = 250 μg/cc
–Intracoronary epinephrine, if no reflow occurs with
  hypotension (watch for hypertension and ventricular
  arrhythmia)
  (1:10,000 dilution, 1 cc in 10 cc = 10 μg/cc, incremental
  doses of 1 cc)
–Placement of intra-aortic balloon pump if blood pressure is
  low or multivessel disease is present with severe
  ventricular dysfunction.

MANAGEMENT OF REPERFUSION INJURY

Efforts to decrease the size of myocardial damage and limit reperfusion injuries have focused on delivery of hypothermia, hyperbaric oxygen, or adenosine. Circulatory hypothermia is delivered through a cooling catheter into the inferior vena cava. In the cooling as an adjunctive therapy to PCI in patients with AMI (COOL-MI) (12) and intravascular cooling adjunctive to PCI (ICE-IT) (13) trials, patients undergoing conventional primary PCI were compared with others who underwent systemic hypothermia in addition to primary intervention. Adverse events were similar in the two groups, and no differences were found regarding the study's primary end point (infarct size), although in the anterior infarction subgroup the infarct size was smaller in those patients where it was possible to quickly achieve a deep level of hypothermia. Similarly, liquid hyperbaric oxygen ($PO_2 = 600$) in the infarction culprit artery immediately proximal to the obstruction, following angioplasty, continuously over 90 minutes has been studied. The results of a small observational study (49) were not confirmed by a randomized study (Acute myocardial infarction with hyperoxemic therapy; AMI-HOT) where hyperbaric oxygen did not reduce the infarct size, although the hyperbaric oxygen reduced the infarct size in patients with <6 hours' evolution of symptoms (14). In a study of intravenous adenosine in patients undergoing primary PCI, clinical outcomes were not significantly improved with adenosine, although infarct size was reduced with a 3-hour 70-microgram/kg/min adenosine infusion, a finding that correlated with fewer adverse clinical events (50). Further studies need to be conducted to evaluate that finding. Management of arrhythmias in the cardiac catheterization is outlined in Table 12-4.

EMERGENCY CORONARY BYPASS SURGERY

Left main disease, failed angioplasty, the presence of mechanical complications, and three-vessel proximal coronary artery disease (particularly with a low ejection fraction and diabetes) remain the gold standard for referral to bypass surgery as reported in the guidelines (15). Surgery is rarely immediately performed after restoration of coronary flow with only angioplasty (failed PCI, subtotal occlusion of left main). PAMI studies have demonstrated that most patients with three vessel coronary disease are treated with PCI. After treatment with stenting, the three-vessel disease is now converted to two-vessel disease, and CABG may be avoided. Only 5% of patients with STEMI are initially referred for CABG, and these patients have a patent infarct vessel with complex disease not amenable to PCI (Table 12-5).

TABLE 12-4

MANAGEMENT OF ARRHYTHMIAS IN THE CATHETERIZATION LABORATORY

Support head of table if CPR is performed (ineffective CPR can occur due to "diving board effect" of the pedestal table)

V-fibrillation and tachycardia: Prompt defibrillation/DC cardioversion and CPR, amiodarone bolus IV and then drip, lidocaine (prophylactic lidocaine should not be used)

Bradyarrhythmias, persistent bradycardia, and hypotension (Bezold–Jarisch reflex): atropine, temporary TV pacemaker

Atrial fibrillation: beta-blocker (if no hypotension)

Idioventricular rhythm: no treatment needed

TABLE 12-5

ANGIOGRAPHIC EXCLUSIONS PRECLUDING PERFORMANCE OF PCI

Unprotected left main >60%

Proximal multivessel disease in a patient who has TIMI-3 flow, if pain free and CABG is best

Infarct vessel stenosis <70% and TIMI-3 flow

Infarct vessel supplies small amount of myocardium

POSTPROCEDURAL PATHWAYS

Admission

Several risk scores determine outcome and thus in-hospital placement of patients following PCI for AMI. Patients with low-risk features as determined by the PAMI risk score (51) (age <70, EF > 45%, <3-vessel CAD, no SVG occlusion, and no persistent arrhythmias) or the CADILLAC risk score (52) (EF >40%, no renal insufficiency, Killip class I, final TIMI flow III, age <65, no anemia, <3-vessel disease) can be safely transferred to a step-down unit with a target discharge of 3 days (53). However, high-risk patients require CCU admission with a target discharge of 5 days.

Vascular Access Management

Early sheath removal is strongly recommended. Vascular sheaths should be removed when the ACT <190 seconds. Anticoagulation may be resumed after 4 to 6 hours from sheath removal for other indications (atrial fibrillation, prosthetic valves, large MI, poor left ventricle function, residual thrombus). If the GP IIb/IIIa inhibitors are being used, heparin should not be restarted after the procedure. Minidose heparin may be given subcutaneously while patients are in bed rest for prophylaxis against deep venous thrombosis.

Adjunctive Pharmacology

Aspirin, clopidogrel, beta-blockers, statins, angiotensin-converting enzyme inhibitors (ACEI), and aldosterone antagonists have all been shown to improve clinical outcomes, including mortality, following primary PCI. Their extremely important adjunctive role for short- and long-term outcomes is highlighted in the recent guidelines for management of patients with AMI (14).

Imaging

Two-dimensional (2D) echocardiogram and cardiac magnetic resonance imaging (MRI) provide baseline assessment of cardiac function and may be used as a reference for long-term follow-up. The latter technique has gained more support at our institution because it provides a one-stop assessment of function and viability with outstanding resolution. However, the role of echocardiogram in rapid assessment of a sudden hemodynamic instability, given its portable nature, is highlighted in the recent guidelines (14).

Long-Term Follow-up

Cardiac rehabilitation is of utmost importance in patients following AMI. Addressing the psychological concerns of patients (anxiety, depression, and financial impact) is as important as the clinical management. A recent study from our institution demonstrated that the most important predictor of short-term return to work is being a U.S. citizen, together with single-vessel disease and lack of smoking. Long-term return to work was also governed by country of employment, but also lack of angina (54). Various studies have also highlighted the importance of addressing the psychological sequel as well as the clinical sequel of AMI (55).

CONCLUSION

Recent advances in primary PCI for patients with STEMI have confirmed the validity of this technique for management of patients with AMI. Time to revascularization remains an important determinant of outcome. The benefit of adjunctive pharmacological (facilitated PCI) or mechanical therapies (cooling, hyperbaric oxygen, thrombectomy, distal protection) prior to or during the procedure has not been striking with only marginal accomplishments. Rapidly achieving TIMI-3 flow remains the major determinant of clinical outcome. In patients with cardiogenic shock, hemodynamic support using IABP and/or p-VAD may be required and improves outcomes. Continuation of clinically proven medical therapy, including antiplatelet therapy, beta-blockers, ACEI, and statins, as well addressing the psychological impact of this disease extends the benefits of primary PCI in the long run.

References

1. Keeley EC, Boura JA, Grines CL. Primary angioplasty versus intravenous thrombolytic therapy for acute myocardial infarction: a quantitative review of 23 randomized trials. Lancet 2003;361:13–20.
2. Andersen HR, Nielsen TT, Rasmussen K, et al, DANAMI-2 Investigators. A comparison of coronary angioplasty with fibrinolytic therapy in acute myocardial infarction. N Engl J Med 2003;349:733–742.
3. Widimsky P, Budesinsky T, Vorac D, et al, PRAGUE Study Group Investigators. Long distance transport for primary angioplasty vs immediate thrombolysis in acute myocardial infarction. Final results of the randomized national multicentre trial PRAGUE-2. Eur Heart J 2003;24:94–104.
4. Widimsky P, Groch L, Zelyzko M, et al. Multicentre randomized trial comparing transport to primary angioplasty vs immediate thrombolysis vs combined strategy for patients with acute myocardial infarction presenting to a community hospital without a catheterization laboratory. Eur Heart J 2000;21:823–883.
5. Grines CL, Cox DA, Stone GW, et al. Coronary angioplasty with or without stent implantation for acute myocardial infarction. Stent Primary Angioplasty in Myocardial Infarction Study Group. N Engl J Med 1999;341:1949–1956.
6. Stone GW, Grines CL, Cox DA, et al. (CADILLAC) trial comparison of angioplasty with stenting, with or without abciximab, in acute myocardial infarction. N Engl J Med 2002;346:957–966.
7. Montalescot G, Barragan P, Wittenberg O, et al. Admiral investigators. Abciximab before direct angioplasty and stenting in myocardial infarction regarding acute and long-term follow-up platelet glycoprotein IIb/IIIa inhibition with coronary stenting for acute myocardial infarction. N Engl J Med 2001;344(25):1895–1903.
8. Antoniucci D, Migliorini A, Parodi G, et al. Abciximab-supported infarct artery stent implantation for acute myocardial infarction and long-term survival: a prospective, multicenter, randomized trial comparing infarct artery stenting plus abciximab with stenting alone. Circulation 2004;109(14):1704–1706.
9. Stone GW. Primary angioplasty in acute myocardial infarction with distal protection of the microcirculation: principal results from the prospective, randomized EMERALD trial. Presented at the annual scientific session of the American College of Cardiology. New Orleans, LA, March 2004.
10. Orego et al. The Dethrombosis to Enhance Reperfusion in Myocardial Infarction (DEAR-MI). Presented at the Annual Scientific Session of the Transcatheter Therapeutics meeting. Washington DC, September 2004.
11. Ali A. Rheolytic thrombectomy vs conventional PCI in MI. J Am Coll Cardiol 2005;45:798–799.
12. Dixon SR, Rizik DG, Griffin JJ, et al, The COOL-MI Investigators. A prospective, randomized trial of mild hypothermia during primary percutaneous intervention for acute myocardial infarction (COOL-MI): one-year clinical outcome. J Am Coll Cardiol 2004;43 (Suppl 1):A251.
13. Grines CL. Intravascular cooling adjunctive to percutaneous coronary intervention for acute myocardial infarction (ICE-IT). Annual Scientific Session of the Transcatheter Therapeutics meeting. Washington DC, September 2004.
14. O'Neill WW. Acute myocardial infarction with hyperoxemic therapy (AMI-HOT): a prospective randomized, multicenter trial. Presented at the annual scientific session of the American College of Cardiology. New Orleans, LA, March 2004.
15. Antman EM, Anbe DT, Armstrong PW, et al. ACC/AHA guidelines for the management of patients with acute myocardial infarction-executive summary. Circulation 2004;110:588–636.
16. Nallamothu B, Bates E, Herrin J, et al. Times to treatment in transfer patients undergoing primary percutaneous coronary intervention in the United States: National registry of Myocardial Infarction (NRMI)-3/4 analysis. Circulation 2005;111:761–767.
17. Brodie BR, Stone GW, Morice MC, et al., Stent Primary Angioplasty in Myocardial Infarction Study Group. Importance of time to reperfusion on outcomes with primary coronary angioplasty for acute myocardial infarction (results from the Stent Primary Angioplasty in Myocardial Infarction Trial). Am J Cardiol 2001;88:1085–1090.
18. O'Neill WW. Does a 90-minute door-to-balloon time matter? Observations from four current reperfusion trials. Presented at the annual scientific session of the American College of Cardiology. Orlando, FL, March 2005.
19. Schomig A, Mehilli J, Antoniucci D, et al. Mechanical reperfusion in patients with acute myocardial infarction presenting more than 12 hours from symptom onset: a randomized controlled trial. JAMA 2005;293(23):2865–2872.
20. Becker RC. Antiplatelet therapy in coronary heart disease: emerging strategies for the treatment and prevention of acute myocardial infarction. Arch Pathol Lab Med 1993;117:89–96.
21. Liem A, Zijlstra F, Ottervanger JP, et al.. High dose heparin as pretreatment for primary angioplasty in acute myocardial infarction: the Heparin in Early Patency (HEAP) randomized trial. J Am Coll Cardiol 2000;35:600–604.
22. De Luca G, Suryapranata H, Stone GW, et al. Abciximab as adjunctive therapy to reperfusion in acute ST-segment elevation myocardial infarction: a meta-analysis of randomized trials. JAMA 2005;293(14):1759–1765.
23. Sutton AGC, Campbell PG, Graham R, et al. A randomized trial of rescue angioplasty versus a conservative approach for failed fibrinolysis in ST-segment elevation myocardial infarction (MERLIN). J Am Coll Cardiol 2004;44:287–296.
24. Gershlick A. Resuce angioplasty versus conservative treatment or repeat thrombolysis (REACT). Presented at the annual scientific session of the American Heart Association. New Orleans, LA, November 2004.
25. Schomig A, Ndrepepa G, Mehilli J, et al. A randomized trial of coronary stenting versus balloon angioplasty as a rescue intervention after failed thrombolysis in patients with acute myocardial infarction. J Am Coll Cardiol 2004;44:2073–2079.
26. Le May MR. Combined angioplasty and pharmacological intervention versus thrombolysis alone in myocardial infarction (CAPITAL AMI). Presented at the annual scientific session of the American College of Cardiology. New Orleans, LA, March 2004.
27. Kastrati A, Mehilli J, Schlotterbeck K, et al. Early administration of reteplase plus abciximab vs abciximab alone in patients with acute myocardial infarction referred for percutaneous coronary intervention. JAMA 2004;291:947–954.
28. van't Hof AWJ, Ernst N, de Boer MJ, et al. Facilitation of primary coronary angioplasty by early start of a glycoprotein IIb/IIIa inhibitor: results of the ongoing Tirofiban in myocardial infarction evaluation (ON-TIME) trial. Eur Heart J 2004;25;837–846.
29. Fernandez-Aviles F, Alonso JJ, Castro-Beiras A, et al. Routine invasive strategy within 24 hours of thrombolysis versus ischemia guided conservative approach for acute myocardial infarction with ST-segment (GRACIA-1): a randomized controlled trial. Lancet 2004;364:1045–1053.
30. Sabatine MS, Cannon CP, Gibson CM, et al. Addition of clopidogrel to aspirin and fibrinolytic therapy for myocardial infarction with ST-segment elevation. N Engl J Med 2005;352(12):1179–1189.
31. COMMIT collaborative group. Addition of clopidogrel to aspirin in 45 852 patients with acute myocardial infarction: randomized placebo-controlled trial. Lancet 2005;366:1607–1621.
32. Leong JY, Baker RA, Shah PJ, et al. Clopidogrel and bleeding after coronary artery bypass graft surgery. Ann Thorac Surg 2005;80(3):928–933.
33. Yusuf S, Zhao F, Mehta SR, et al. The Clopidogrel in Unstable Angina to Prevent Recurrent Events Trial Investigators: Effects of Clopidogrel in Addition to Aspirin in Patients With Acute Coronary Syndromes Without ST-Segment Elevation (CURE). N Engl J Med 2001;345:494–502.

34. Steinhubl SR, Berger PB, Mann JT 3rd, et al. Clopidogrel for the reduction of events during observation. *JAMA* 2002;288:2411–2420.
35. Fonarow GC, Wright RS, Spencer FA, et al. Effect of statin use within the first 24 hours of admission for acute myocardial infarction on early morbidity and mortality. *Am J Cardiol* 2005; 96:611–616.
36. Halkin A, Grines CL, Cox DA, et al. Impact of intravenous beta-blockade before primary angioplasty on survival in patients undergoing mechanical reperfusion therapy for acute myocardial infarction. *J Am Coll Cardiol* 2004;43(10):1780–1787.
37. Kernis SJ, Harjai KJ, Stone GW, et al. Does beta-blocker therapy improve clinical outcomes of acute myocardial infarction after successful primary angioplasty? *J Am Coll Cardiol* 2004;43(10):1773–1779.
38. Loubeyre C, Morice MC, Lefevre T, et al. A randomized comparison of direct stenting with conventional stent implantation in selected patients with acute myocardial infarction. *J Am Coll Cardiol* 2002;39:15–21.
39. Briguori C, Sheiban I, de Gregorio J, et al. Direct coronary stenting without predilation. *J Am Coll Cardiol* 1999;34:1910–1915.
40. Moschi G, Migliorini A, Trapani M, et al. Direct stenting without predilatation in acute myocardial infarction. *Eur Heart J* 2000;21 Suppl:P2847.
41. Spaulding C. Trial to assess the use of the cypher stent in acute myocardial infarction treated with balloon angioplasty (TYPHOON). Presented at the annual scientific session of the American College of Cardiology, March 2006.
42. Dirksen MT. Paclitaxel-eluting stent versus conventional stent for STEMI (PASSION). Presented at the annual scientific session of the American College of Cardiology, March 2006.
43. García E, for the Xamine ST Investigators. Final results of the Xamine ST study. *Am J Cardiol* 2004;94 Suppl 6A:E154.
44. Neumann FJ, Blasini R, Schmitt C, et al. Protection devices in PCI treatment of myocardial infarction for salvage of endangered myocardium (PROM-ISE). Presented at the annual scientific sessions of the American College of Cardiology. New Orleans, LA, March 2004.
45. Stone GW, Marsalese D, Brodie BR, et al. A prospective, randomized evaluation of prophylactic intraaortic balloon counterpulsation in high risk patients with acute myocardial infarction treated with primary angioplasty.
46. Thiele H, Sick P, Boudriot E, et al. Randomized trial of intra-aortic balloon support with a percutaneous left ventricular assist device in patients with revascularized acute myocardial infarction complicated by cardiogenic shock. *Eur Heart J* 2005;26(13):1276–1283.
47. Mehta RH, Harjai KJ, Cox D, et al. Clinical and angiographic correlates and outcomes of suboptimal coronary flow inpatients with acute myocardial infarction undergoing primary percutaneous coronary intervention. *J Am Coll Cardiol* 2003;42(10):1739–1746.
48. Stone GW, Cox D, García E, et al. Normal flow (TIMI-3) before mechanical reperfusion therapy is an independent determinant of survival in acute myocardial infarction: analysis from the primary angioplasty in myocardial infarction trials. *Circulation* 2001;104:636–641.
49. Bartorelli AL. Hyperbaric oxygen administration in AMI. *Am J Cardiovasc Drugs* 2004;4:253–263.
50. Ross AM, Gibbons RJ, Stone GW, et al. A randomized, double-blinded, placebo-controlled multicenter trial of adenosine as an adjunct to reperfusion in the treatment of acute myocardial infarction (AMISTAD-II). *J Am Coll Cardiol* 2005;45(11):1775–1780.
51. Addala S, Grines CL, Dixon SR, et al. Predicting mortality in patients with ST-elevation myocardial infarction treated with primary percutaneous coronary intervention (PAMI risk score). *Am J Cardiol* 2004;93:629–632.
52. Halkin A, Singh M, Nikolsky E, et al. Prediction of mortality after primary percutaneous coronary intervention for acute myocardial infarction: the CADILLAC risk score. *J Am Coll Cardiol* 2005;45:1397–1405.
53. Grines CL, Marsalese DL, Brodie B, et al. Safety and cost-effectiveness of early discharge after primary angioplasty in low risk patients with acute myocardial infarction. PAMI-II Investigators. Primary angioplasty in myocardial infarction. *J Am Coll Cardiol* 1998;31(5):967–972.
54. Abbas AE, Brodie B, Stone G, et al. Frequency of returning to work one and six months following percutaneous coronary intervention for acute myocardial infarction. *Am J Cardiol* 2004;94(11):1403–1405.
55. Hamilton GA, Seidman RN. A comparison of the recovery period for women and men after an acute myocardial infarction. *Heart Lung* 1993; 22:308–315.

Second Primary Angioplasty in Myocardial Infarction (PAMI-II) Trial Investigators. *J Am Coll Cardiol* 1997;29:1459–1467.

CHAPTER 13 ■ PRIMARY PCI AT COMMUNITY HOSPITALS WITHOUT ON-SITE CARDIAC SURGERY

NANCY SINCLAIR AND THOMAS P. WHARTON, JR.

RATIONALE FOR PRIMARY PERCUTANEOUS
    CORONARY INTERVENTION AT HOSPITALS
    WITHOUT CARDIAC SURGERY
BUILDING CRITICAL PATHWAYS FOR A SUCCESSFUL
    COMMUNITY HOSPITAL PRIMARY PCI PROGRAM
Establish an Acute Myocardial Infarction Protocol Team
Develop a Primary PCI Critical Pathway
Develop Operator and Institutional Criteria for Primary PCI
Establish Clinical and Angiographic Selection Criteria for Primary
    PCI and for Emergency Transfer for Coronary Artery Bypass
    Graft (CABG)
Establish Position Profiles, Expectations, and Training Programs
    for CCL Staff
Set Up a Fine-Tuned Emergency Triage System in the Emergency
    Department
Develop a Catheterization Laboratory Primary PCI Protocol
Establish an Ongoing Program to Improve Door-to-Balloon Times
Develop an Acuity-Based Procedure-Bumping Protocol
Create an Emergency Transfer Protocol and Establish Formal
    Agreements That Ensure Rapid Transfer to a Cardiac Surgery
    Center
Establish In-Hospital Management Pathways
Initiate Processes and Tracking Tools for Data Gathering and
    Analysis, Case Review, and Quality Assurance
CONCLUSIONS

RATIONALE FOR PRIMARY PERCUTANEOUS CORONARY INTERVENTION AT HOSPITALS WITHOUT CARDIAC SURGERY

Primary percutaneous coronary intervention (PCI) is now widely regarded as the reperfusion strategy of choice for patients with ST-segment elevation acute myocardial infarction (STEMI) when delivered rapidly and expertly (1). Primary PCI results in lower rates of death, stroke, recurrent ischemia, and reinfarction compared with fibrinolytic therapy. Yet data from the National Registries of Myocardial Infarction (NRMI) indicate that only 20% of patients with STEMI are treated with primary PCI in the United States (2,3). Over one-third of patients with STEMI still do not receive any type of reperfusion therapy. The emergence of primary PCI as lifesaving therapy without its effective dissemination into the community clearly represents an urgent public health problem.

Most patients with acute myocardial infarction (AMI) present to community hospitals without cardiac surgery programs (4). Primary PCI is seldom available at these hospitals, and many states still have regulations that restrict PCI to surgical centers. Thus patients that present to hospitals without on-site PCI have two reperfusion options: (a) fibrinolytic therapy, now widely regarded as suboptimal when immediate and expert PCI is available, or (b) rapid transfer or prehospital ambulance triage to a primary PCI center. For the appreciable number of patients that are not candidates for fibrinolytic therapy, the second option is the only one available.

Two recent randomized trials from Denmark (5) and Prague (6) compared rapid transfer to a PCI center versus local fibrinolytic therapy for patients with acute STEMI presenting to hospitals without PCI programs. (Interestingly, two of the seven PCI centers in the Prague study did not have cardiac surgery capability.) These trials, and a recent meta-analysis that included these and similar trials (7), demonstrated superior outcomes in patients with STEMI that were transferred rapidly for primary PCI compared to those randomized to fibrinolytic therapy.

Unfortunately, these strategies of early rapid transfer and prehospital ambulance triage to PCI centers have many limitations. Their use is generally confined to urban areas because the transport time must be short. Air transport, especially in the northern parts of the country, is not always a reliable option. Prehospital ambulance triage is also not an option in the 50% of AMI patients that do not arrive by ambulance (8). In addition, there could be considerable liability problems associated with interhospital transport or triage of unstable patients with AMI. Even when effective rapid transport is available, some AMI patients are too unstable to travel. In the transfer studies from Denmark and Prague, 4% and 1% of patients, respectively, were too unstable to travel, and some of these patients died; deaths during transfer also occurred (5,6). Patients too unstable to transfer, which are the highest-risk of all patients with AMI, are the very ones that should benefit the most from primary PCI if it were available at the point of first presentation. Patients with cardiogenic shock are at particular risk during interhospital transfer and often can be too unstable to transfer. Rapid primary PCI can be lifesaving in this group. The Should We Emergently Revascularize Occluded Coronaries for Cardiogenic Shock (SHOCK) study (9) demonstrated that the group randomized to mechanical revascularization within the first 6 hours of infarction had the greatest survival advantage of all subgroups.

In addition to the risk and sometimes the barrier of transfer, another problem with transfer for PCI is the delay in reperfusion. Recent data from NRMI unfortunately shows that door-to-balloon times in the United States are still 71 minutes longer for patients transferred for primary PCI than for those receiving PCI at the point of first presentation (10). Because the transfer delay in NRMI was approximately 1 hour greater than that seen in the Denmark and Prague studies, the data from these European randomized trials that showed superiority of transfer for PCI over local fibrinolytic therapy may not even be applicable to most hospitals in the United States (11).

Door-to-balloon times of 2.5 to 3 hours, as seen in patients transferred for PCI in the United States, are associated with a 60% increase in mortality compared to less than 2 hours (12). In fact, 85% of patients transferred for primary PCI in the NRMI registries did not receive it within 120 minutes (13). In striking contrast, nine published studies of primary PCI at hospitals with off-site backup, which include an aggregate of 5,750 patients, indicate that primary PCI at such centers can be performed within 56 to 110 minutes of first presentation (14–23). No study demonstrates median door-to-balloon times of longer than 110 minutes for nonsurgical hospitals.

As noted earlier, the risk, delay, and possibility of barrier of transfer are compounded, sometimes prohibitively, if the nearest PCI center is geographically remote.

For these reasons more and more hospitals in the United States that have cardiac catheterization laboratories but not cardiac surgery are starting to perform primary PCI on-site routinely as the treatment of choice for AMI. The American College of Cardiology/American Heart Association STEMI Guidelines (24) now designate primary PCI at hospitals without off-site cardiac surgical backup with a "class IIb" indication (usefulness/efficacy less well established by evidence/opinion), provided that at least 36 primary PCI procedures per year are performed at such hospitals, that the interventionalist performs at least 75 procedures per year, that procedures are performed within 90 minutes of presentation, and that there is a proven plan for rapid access to a cardiac surgical center. These guidelines also list further operator, institutional, and angiographic selection criteria for such hospitals, adapted from criteria that we have proposed (17). Our currently recommended criteria, including clinical criteria for emergent angiography, are listed in Tables 13-1 to 13-3.

There are at least 15 studies and registry reports of primary PCI at hospitals without cardiac surgery programs for off-site cardiac surgery, all of which indicate that community hospitals can deliver primary PCI safely, effectively, and rapidly, with outcomes that are similar to those reported from cardiac surgery centers (14–23,25–32). There are no reports that demonstrate the opposite. It is reasonable to expect that the benefits of increasing the speed of delivery and greater access to expert primary PCI should far outweigh any theoretical risk of having off-site rather than on-site cardiac surgery backup. The inherently lower interventional volumes of smaller hospitals may not detract from outcomes if primary PCI is performed as first-line therapy by high-volume interventionalists that regularly perform elective intervention. An institutional volume of primary PCI of more than 33 to 48 procedures per year, readily achievable at dedicated community hospital programs, correlates with improved mortality rates (12,33–36). In addition, community hospitals without on-site cardiac surgery may be able to perform primary PCI faster than larger centers both during regular working hours and during nights and weekends (37). Possible reasons for potentially greater efficiency of smaller hospitals may include more direct communication between the emergency physician and the cardiologist with less bureaucracy, decreased travel times if the catheterization team lives nearby, and greater flexibility in a catheterization laboratory schedule that may not be as congested.

There is a clear need to increase the availability of primary PCI. There is also a clear potential to accomplish this because well over 600 community hospitals in the United States have cardiac catheterization laboratories without cardiac surgery (38). Currently, PCI is being performed at certain hospitals with off-site cardiac surgery backup in 36 states, and programs are about to start in 3 others. Many of these programs are also offering nonemergent PCI, which will increase interventional volumes and thus should improve outcomes, in addition to improving access to PCI for patients with other high-risk acute coronary syndromes (39).

TABLE 13-1

OPERATOR AND INSTITUTIONAL CRITERIA FOR PRIMARY PCI PROGRAMS AT HOSPITALS WITH OFF-SITE CARDIAC SURGERY BACKUP

1. Experienced high-volume interventionalists.
2. Experienced nursing and technical CCL staff with training in interventional laboratories.
3. Well-equipped and well-stocked CCL, with IABP support on-site.
4. Experienced CCU nursing staff, comfortable with invasive hemodynamic monitoring and IABP management.
5. Formalized protocols and agreements for emergency transfer of patients to the nearest cardiac surgical facility (Tables 13-7 and 13-8).
6. Full support from hospital administration in fulfilling the preceding institutional requirements.
7. Rigorous clinical and angiographic selection criteria for PCI and for emergency transfer (Tables 13-2 and 13-3).
8. Performance of primary PCI as the treatment of first choice for STEMI to ensure streamlined care paths and increased case volumes.
9. Primary PCI coverage on a 24-hour, 7-day per week basis.
10. Performance of at least three to four primary PCI procedures per month.
11. Ongoing outcomes analysis and formalized periodic case review.
12. Participation in a national data registry such as the American College of Cardiology National Cardiovascular Data Registry.

CABG, coronary artery bypass graft; CCL, cardiac catheterization laboratory; CCU, cardiac care unit; IABP, intra-aortic balloon pump; PCI, percutaneous coronary intervention; STEMI, ST-segment acute myocardial infarction.
Adapted from Wharton et al (1999). Printed with permission from Wharton, Sinclair, copyright 2004.

The objective of this chapter is to propose standards, critical pathways, protocols, and care maps that will enable more of these hospitals to set up safe and effective primary PCI programs if they can meet the necessary standards. Hospitals that initiate interventional programs that rigorously follow the highest standards and protocols such as the ones that we outline here should be able to achieve outcomes that are comparable to PCI outcomes from the best high-volume surgical centers (30). Ensuring the highest quality in the delivery of PCI at all hours, which is well reflected in the achievement of rapid door-to-balloon times regardless of shift, is likely to save more lives than the theoretical advantage of having on-site cardiac surgery.

BUILDING CRITICAL PATHWAYS FOR A SUCCESSFUL COMMUNITY HOSPITAL PRIMARY PCI PROGRAM

Launching a successful program for primary PCI at a community hospital requires the commitment and collaboration of all

TABLE 13-2

CLINICAL SELECTION CRITERIA FOR EMERGENT CORONARY ANGIOGRAPHY WITH PCI WHEN INDICATED

Clinical Inclusion Criteria

- >30 min of ischemic pain not controlled by conventional medications (ASA, NTG, beta-blockers, and heparin)

and/or

- ECG with ≥2.0 mV of ischemic ST-segment deviation in two or more contiguous leads (there is no time limit on duration of pain if patient has ongoing chest pain, ST-segment deviation with preserved R waves in two or more infarct leads, or cardiogenic shock)

Clinical Exclusion Criteria

- Lack of vascular access
- Inability to obtain informed consent
- Severe dementia or coma (excepting patients with successful cardioversion of out-of-hospital ventricular fibrillation in the field, regardless of acute mental status)
- Any serious illness with life expectancy of only a few weeks

Developed by Wharton TP, Exeter Hospital, Exeter, NH. Printed with permission from Wharton TP. Copyright 2005.

TABLE 13-3

ANGIOGRAPHIC SELECTION FOR PRIMARY PCI AND EMERGENCY AORTOCORONARY BYPASS SURGERY AT HOSPITALS WITH OFF-SITE CARDIAC SURGERY BACKUP

Avoid intervention in:

- Patients with severe left main disease proximal to infarct-related lesion.
- Extremely long or angulated target lesions with TIMI grade 3 flow at high risk for PCI failure.
- Lesions in other than the infarct artery (unless they appeared to be flow-limiting in patients with hemodynamic instability or ongoing symptoms).
- Lesions with TIMI grade 3 flow that are not amenable to stenting in patients with left-main or three-vessel disease who will require coronary bypass surgery.

Transfer emergently for coronary bypass surgery patients with:

- High-grade residual left main or three-vessel coronary disease and clinical or hemodynamic instability after PCI of occluded vessels when appropriate and preferably with intra-aortic balloon pump support.
- Failed or unstable PCI result and ongoing ischemia, with intra-aortic balloon pump support during transfer.

PCI, percutaneous coronary intervention; TIMI, thrombolysis in myocardial infarction.
Adapted from Wharton et al (1999). Printed with permission from Wharton, Sinclair, copyright 2004.

members of the health care team. Before starting a PCI program, cardiologists, emergency department (ED) and paramedical staff, cardiac catheterization laboratory (CCL) staff, primary care physicians, cardiac nurses, cardiac rehabilitation staff, and hospital administrators need to develop a uniform standard of care for patients with AMI from the point of first patient contact through discharge planning and follow-up. Vigorous and ongoing quality improvement processes are also required to ensure a safe and effective program. The common goal is to extend all essential elements of the treatment of acute MI to patients throughout all areas of the hospital.

The essential elements that must be established and developed include

- *An AMI protocol team*
- *A primary PCI critical pathway*
- *Operator and institutional criteria for primary PCI*
- *Clinical and angiographic selection criteria for primary PCI and for emergency transfer for coronary bypass surgery*
- *Position profiles, defined expectations, and training programs for CCL staff*
- *A fine-tuned emergency triage system in the ED*
- *A catheterization laboratory primary PCI protocol*
- *An ongoing program to improve door-to-balloon times*
- *An acuity-based, procedure-bumping protocol*
- *An emergency transfer protocol and formal agreements that ensure rapid transfer to a cardiac surgery center*
- *In-hospital AMI management pathways, to include the development of patient care protocols, standing orders, and assessment tools from admission to discharge*
- *Processes and tracking tools for data gathering and analysis, case review, and quality assurance*

Let us examine each element of this process individually. Examples are given of critical pathways and care maps for the primary PCI program at Exeter Hospital, Exeter, New Hampshire, which is a 100-bed hospital with a 25-minute travel time to the nearest cardiac surgical facility.

Establish an Acute Myocardial Infarction Protocol Team

The first step in launching a primary PCI program is to set up a multidisciplinary AMI protocol team. The goal of this team is to develop the critical pathways and care plans needed to care for the patient with AMI from the first prehospital contact all the way through to hospital discharge. These critical pathways and care plans, such as the examples included in this chapter, will have to be individualized to fit the circumstances of the hospital and thus will require multidisciplinary input. The members of the AMI protocol team should include physicians, nurses, and technical staff from the cardiology and ED departments, the emergency medical services (EMS) paramedics and technicians, the CCL, the critical care unit (CCU), the telemetry unit, cardiac rehabilitation, the blood laboratory, pharmacy and case management, along with key members of the hospital administration. The initial commitment of resources to establish an on-call system (if not already in place), to recruit sufficient well-trained CCL personnel, and to fund the stocking of the CCL with interventional equipment and supplies requires the full support of an informed hospital administration, who may need to be educated regarding the clinical value of such a program.

Develop a Primary PCI Critical Pathway

The AMI protocol team should review the current literature and standards on the care of the patient with AMI and adapt these latest research results to their development of the central critical pathway for primary PCI. The team should incorporate newer modalities, techniques, and adjunctive medical therapies into this pathway as the current standard of care evolves. In addition, the team should review their institution's latest outcomes, which are available at the Centers for Medicare and Medicaid Studies (CMS) national Web-based database (40). This resource was designed to inform consumers about the performance of local hospitals in their care of patents with AMI. Special emphasis should be placed on examining and improving the hospital's compliance with currently established standards of care, including the percentage of patients offered reperfusion therapy, the times-to-reperfusion, rates of PCI success and complications, the percentage of AMI patients given medications such as aspirin, beta-blockers, angiotensin-converting enzyme inhibitors (ACEIs), angiotensin receptor blockers (ARBs), and lipid-lowering agents and the percentage

offered antismoking advice, cardiac teaching, and rehabilitation. Nursing and educational care plans should be revised to mirror these objectives. The team should provide educational sessions for hospital staff and referral services such as visiting nurses, skilled nursing facility staff, and cardiac rehabilitation staff to review these pathways and understand the new expectations, procedures, and equipment involved in the development of the PCI program and the follow-up utilization of evidenced-based therapies.

Exeter Hospital's critical pathway for primary PCI is shown in Figure 13-1. Key features of Exeter's pathways and care maps include protocols for the EMS paramedics in the field and the ED physicians that will optimize treatment and reduce time to reperfusion.

The cardiac catheterization procedure itself is streamlined to assess the coronary anatomy rapidly while attending to the medical treatment of the patient. With primary PCI chosen as

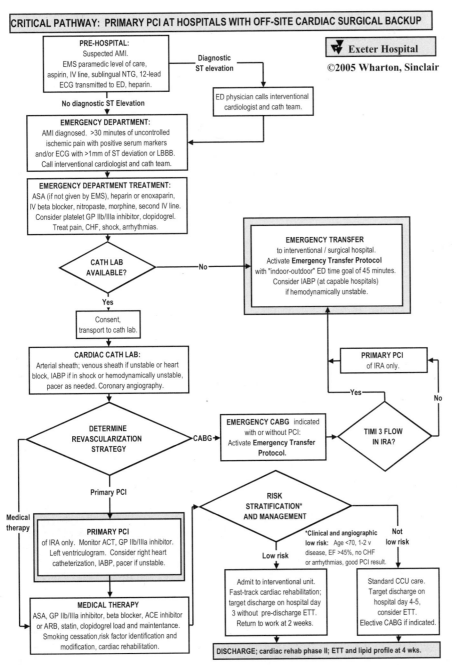

FIGURE 13-1. Critical pathway from prehospital contact through to hospital discharge for the primary PCI program at Exeter Hospital, Exeter, NH, which is a community hospital with off-site cardiac surgery backup. The use of fibrinolytic therapy has been excluded from this critical pathway. ACE, angiotensin-converting enzyme; ACT, activated clotting time; AMI, acute myocardial infarction; ASA, aspirin; BP, blood pressure; CABG, coronary artery bypass graft; CCU, cardiac care unit; CHF, congestive heart failure; ED, emergency department; EF, ejection fraction; ECG, electrocardiogram; EMS, emergency medical services; ETT, exercise tolerance test; GP, glycoprotein; IABP, intra-aortic balloon pump; IRA, infarct-related artery; IV, intravenous; LBBB, left bundle-branch block; NTG, nitroglycerin; PCI, percutaneous coronary intervention; TIMI, thrombolysis in myocardial infarction. (Printed with permission from Wharton TP and Sinclair N. Copyright 2005.)

the reperfusion strategy, the goal of intervention is the immediate establishment of stable and brisk (TIMI grade 3) flow.

After the procedure, the patient can be effectively risk-stratified and triaged to appropriate in-hospital management according to clinical and angiographic features as listed in Figure 13-1. Patients with low-risk clinical and angiographic features can avoid admission to the CCU, avoid predischarge exercise testing, be targeted for discharge on hospital day 3, and return to work within 2 weeks (41).

In the (hopefully infrequent) event that the CCL or interventionalist(s) is not available, the ED will be notified proactively. The ED physician will then discuss transfer. The decision regarding which patients with AMI should be transferred to an interventional center should be individualized and made in conjunction with the cardiologist.

Develop Operator and Institutional Criteria for Primary PCI

The AMI protocol team should develop operator, institutional, clinical, and angiographic criteria such as those listed in Tables 13-1 to 13-3 (17). The team should review local state regulations and national guidelines for primary PCI in the treatment of AMI (42). Invasive and noninvasive cardiologists, credentialing staff, and hospital administration should develop credentialing criteria based on national guidelines and regional standards. Fundamental to any interventional program is a state-of-the-art CCL, with optimal digital imaging systems, equipped with a broad array of interventional and supportive equipment (Table 13-4), and staffed by experienced and well-trained nursing and technical personnel (Table 13-5).

A commitment to provide primary PCI on a 24-hour, 7-day per week basis will avoid inconsistency in following the critical pathway for primary PCI and should reduce the potential for a lower standard of care. A single care plan for the treatment of AMI will eliminate the "door-to-decision" time; the resultant increase in procedural volumes will accelerate the learning curve for ED staff and CCL team members and operators. This will result in decreased times to reperfusion and improvement of procedural outcomes (12). A higher institutional volume of primary PCI (more than 33 to 48 procedures per year) correlates with faster door-to-balloon times and improved mortality rates (34,35).

Establish Clinical and Angiographic Selection Criteria for Primary PCI and for Emergency Transfer for Coronary Artery Bypass Graft (CABG)

Cardiologists should develop clinical and angiographic criteria for primary PCI and transfer for bypass surgery, such as those listed in Tables 13-2 and 13-3; these criteria should be documented in the patient care standards manual. We recommend immediate coronary angiography in all patients who present with a clinical picture of AMI, even if electrocardiogram (ECG) changes are not diagnostic, if they have ongoing ischemic pain for more than 30 minutes not controlled by conventional medications. Patients with AMI without ST-segment elevation on ECG represent a particularly high-risk group and are not appropriate for fibrinolytic therapy (43). These patients have greatly improved outcomes when admitted to hospitals with an early invasive rather than a conservative therapy (44). In addition, because the progression rate of necrosis in AMI varies considerably with the degree of baseline antegrade flow and collateral flow, and because the time of transition between un-

TABLE 13-4

ESSENTIAL AND SPECIAL EQUIPMENT REQUIREMENTS

Necessary for Performance of Primary Intervention	• Biphasic defibrillator/cardioverter with external pacing • Fully equipped code cart • Temporary pacemaker equipment • Intra-aortic balloon pump • Thrombectomy equipment and devices • Covered stents in the event of perforation • Femoral closure and compression devices • Intravascular catheter retrieval devices • Capability for photographic reproduction of cine frames for patients and staff.
Advisable for Performance of Nonemergent Intervention	• Pressure wire equipment for assessment of coronary fractional flow reserve • Intravascular ultrasound at the discretion of the operator • Distal protection devices
Unnecessary Outside Tertiary Center	• Rotational atherectomy • Directional atherectomy • Laser • Intracoronary radiation • Valvuloplasty equipment • Septal closure devices

stable angina and AMI is sometimes hard to identify, we suggest that there be no time cutoff for reperfusion therapy if symptoms or signs of ongoing myocardial necrosis or cardiogenic shock are present (45–47). The goal of these criteria is to maximize coronary reperfusion opportunities while minimizing the possibility of causing new myocardial jeopardy (a "surgical emergency") by procedures performed without on-site cardiac surgery.

Establish Position Profiles, Expectations, and Training Programs for CCL Staff

Nursing, technical, and paramedic CCL staff must be experienced in handling acutely ill patients and comfortable with interventional equipment. Training and performance requirements of the staff are summarized in Table 13-5. All members of the CCL team will have acquired or will be provided experience in dedicated interventional laboratories. Cardiac catheterization laboratory team members not already experienced in interventional procedures should be sent on rotation by formal arrangement to the referral surgical hospital for observation and "hands-on" experience in a busy interventional laboratory. For maximal flexibility with a small CCL staff, all personnel should be cross trained in all the CCL skills and responsibilities. Individuals will have their own areas of expertise and can serve as mentors to others with other skills.

TABLE 13-5

TRAINING AND PERFORMANCE REQUIREMENTS FOR CCL STAFFING (RN, RCIS, RADIOLOGY TECHNOLOGIST, AND PARAMEDIC) FOR PRIMARY PCI PROGRAMS AT HOSPITALS WITHOUT ON-SITE CARDIAC SURGERY

1. Each member will have acquired or will be provided experience in established interventional laboratories.[a]

2. Each member will have ACLS certification and complete IV certification and be competent in cardiac rhythm monitoring and the operation of temporary pacemakers and defibrillators.

3. Each member will be able to monitor the patient's medical condition and administer IV medications, including vasoactive drips and conscious sedation, under the direction of the physician.

4. Each member will be able to serve as scrub assistant to the physician, including performing coronary artery injections, panning the table, and handling of interventional equipment.

5. Each member will be competent with the operation of invasive hemodynamic monitoring equipment and the interpretation of data obtained from it.

6. Each member will be competent with the setting up, operation, timing, and troubleshooting of the IABP.

7. Each member will be familiar with the operation of the digital imaging system, including troubleshooting, acquiring and archiving digital images or images on cine film, and preparing angiograms on CD.

8. Each member will be competent with the operation of in-laboratory blood testing equipment including oximeters, ACT measurement devices, and other bedside blood testing as available.

9. Each member will reside within 30 minutes of the hospital. Pagers and cell phones will be provided.

10. Each member will participate in a 24-hour, 7-day per week call schedule.

11. Each member will be expected to communicate effectively with families, nursing units, and tertiary referral centers and to initiate the transfer protocol when needed.

12. Each member will be available to accompany patients requiring transfer to cardiac surgery when the CCTT team is incomplete or unavailable, including serving as the IABP operator.

13. Each member will be expected to continue education to maintain the skills needed in the laboratory. Each member will be given educational opportunities to learn the latest medical and technical modalities for the treatments of the cardiovascular patient.

14. Each member will be familiar with the institution's guidelines and credentialing criteria for invasive and interventional procedures.

15. Each member will be in-serviced and meet established competencies of new adjunctive devices, medications, and therapies as they are introduced to the CCL armamentarium.

16. Each member will participate in reporting of clinical indicators and in quality improvement projects.

ACLS, advanced cardiac life support; ACT, activated clotting time; CCTT, critical care transportation team; CCL, cardiac catheterization laboratory; CD, compact disc; IABP, intra-aortic balloon pump; IV, intravenous; PCI, percutaneous coronary intervention; RCIS, registered cardiac interventional specialist; RN, registered nurse.
[a]CCL team members not already experienced in interventional procedures could be sent on rotation and by formal arrangement to the referral surgical hospital for observation and "hands-on" experience in a busy interventional laboratory.
Developed by Wharton TP, (Sinclair-) McNamara N, Hiett D, CCL staff, and Human Resources Department, Exeter Hospital, Exeter, NH. Printed with permission from Exeter Hospital. Copyright 1993.

All members of the team should work toward this goal. Ideally, every team member should be able to operate diagnostic imaging equipment, hemodynamic monitoring and recording equipment, temporary pacemakers, defibrillators, the intra-aortic balloon pump (IABP), and other specialized equipment that the lab may have (Table 13-4); serve as scrub assistant to the physician performing the procedure; assist in medical monitoring and management of the patient, including administering medications; provide written documentation of the procedure; and interface with families, nursing units, and tertiary referral centers.

Hospital administration, interventional cardiologists, and the CCL staff must invest in and commit fully to providing the resources necessary to launch and maintain effective, state-of-the-art, 24-hour, 7-day per week primary PCI coverage. The delay and staffing limitations for off-hour procedures at community hospitals need not worsen PCI success rates, complications, or major in-hospital clinical outcomes (37,48,49).

Accomplishing Intensive Staffing on a Shoestring Budget

Community hospitals, with only two or three members of a smaller CCL staff on call, will find it critical to deploy ED and CCU nurses, nursing supervisors, and respiratory therapists to help at off hours with unstable patients. These highly skilled patient-care providers can contribute to the management of medications and drips, assist with documentation during the CCL procedure, assist with airways and ventilator management, and provide other general patient care. Enlisting the participation of these non-CCL personnel improves continuity of care and is cost-effective: these same nurses and therapists would likely have been involved with the care of these patients whether or not the patient was in the CCL. Hospital staff members interested in helping the CCL team in these off-hours cases should be encouraged to watch patients and be given the opportunity for CCL training.

In regions where it is difficult to recruit trained CCL personnel, other interested hospital staff members should be actively recruited and encouraged to join a 6-month CCL training program to ensure viability of the team.

Set Up a Fine-Tuned Emergency Triage System in the Emergency Department

The ED is the "command center" for the AMI (Fig. 13-1). Starting with a prehospital protocol for AMI (Table 13-6), paramedics in the field administer aspirin and heparin and transmit the ECG to the ED physician. This prehospital ECG can greatly reduce time-to-diagnosis and thus the time-to-reperfusion, which can be expected to improve survival (50–53). In addition, because some patients with initial ST-segment elevation arrive at the ED pain free with a normal ECG (10% to 15% of patients with AMI reperfuse with aspirin and other conservative measures), documenting ST-segment elevation at initial prehospital contact can confirm the diagnosis of such patients.

The ED is notified of the incoming patient with AMI, and the AMI critical pathway is initiated (Fig. 13-1). The ED physician contacts the predesignated interventional cardiologist on call immediately for patients with suspected AMI, and the unit coordinator pages the CCL team. These pages should go out simultaneously, even before the patient arrives, if diagnostic acute ST-segment elevation is present on ECG. One of the more correctable causes of delay in "door-to-balloon time" is the time that it takes to call the interventional cardiologist. The ED physician should call as soon as the clinical diagnosis is made and should not worry about "false alarms," which are rare.

The ED will be notified proactively whenever the interventional cardiologist or CCL will not be available to facilitate prompt consideration of transfer to an interventional center (see Fig. 13-1 and the earlier discussion, "Develop a Primary PCI Critical Pathway"). A suggested emergency transfer protocol is shown in Table 13-7, and elements of a transfer agreement and protocols for interhospital collaboration are shown in Table 13-8, as discussed in a separate section later.

Treatment protocols for paramedics and ED staff facilitate

TABLE 13-6

PREHOSPITAL PROTOCOL FOR AMI[a]

*911 is activated for suspected AMI: Local response to include activation of **paramedic** level of EMT care[b]*
- Administer oxygen
- Complete brief history and physical examination, record vital signs
- *–Administer four 81-mg ASA tablets (total 325 mg) chewed*
- Establish IV
- **NTG** SL if SBP >100 mm Hg and patient not in shock.
- Report history, physical examination findings, vital signs to ED physician
- *12-lead ECG immediately acquired and transmitted by cell phone to ED physician (50–53)[c]*
- If AMI is confirmed: administer heparin (5,000 U) IV bolus
- **ACLS** protocols per routine.
- **Fluids, atropine** for bradycardia with hypotension
- **Morphine** (2 to 4 mg) IV for uncontrolled chest pain
- Consider metoprolol 5 mg IV over 2 to 5 minutes unless heart rate <60 or SBP <100 mm Hg. Repeat every 5 minutes as tolerated for total of 15 mg
- Avoid intubation by nasal route: this greatly increases the risk of bleeding if GP IIb/IIIa platelet inhibitors or fibrinolytics are used
- *Document all clinical data including ST-segment elevation, time of pain onset, patient's physical appearance and vital signs on arrival, and interventions in the field*
- *While patient with ST-segment elevation is en route, paramedic verifies with ED physician that interventionalist and CCL team are available; ED physician calls cardiologist and CCL to plan for primary PCI on ED arrival[d]*

ACLS, advanced cardiac life support; AMI, acute myocardial infarction; ASA, aspirin; CCL, cardiac catheterization laboratory; ED, emergency department; ECG, electrocardiogram; EMT, emergency medical technician; GP, glycoprotein; IV, intravenous; NTG, nitroglycerin; PCI, percutaneous coronary intervention; SBP, systolic blood pressure; SL, sublingual.
[a]*Italics highlight measures that reduce time-to-reperfusion for primary PCI.*
[b]If no paramedic level of care is available in the community, consider establishing a hospital-based paramedic program.
[c]Ambulances should be equipped with ECG system capable of transmission to ED for all chest pain calls; this can greatly reduce time-to-diagnosis, time-to-reperfusion, and possibly mortality (50–53). Patient with initial ST-segment elevation may arrive to ED pain free with a normal ECG because 10% to 15% of patients with AMI may reperfuse with aspirin and other conservative measures. Documenting ST-segment elevation at initial prehospital contact can influence immediate triage.
[d]One of the more correctable causes of delay in "door-to-balloon time" is the time that it takes to call the interventional cardiologist. Do not worry about "false alarms," which are rare.
Developed by Wharton TP, Sinclair N, Mastromarino J, Luizzi P, and ED and EMT Committees, Exeter Hospital, Exeter, NH. Printed with permission from Exeter Hospital. Copyright 2005.

TABLE 13-7

EMERGENCY TRANSFER PROTOCOL TO CARDIAC SURGERY CENTER

CCL circulator initiates rapid transfer protocol on physician decision for immediate transfer and places the following calls on pages simultaneously:
- Call to cardiac surgeon at receiving cardiac surgery center
- Call to cardiac surgery clinical coordinator at receiving center
- Call ED to activate CCTT[a] and EMS ambulance provider[b]

Cardiologist provides clinical information to cardiac surgeon and obtains agreement to accept patient.

Cardiologist obtains consent from patient or family member for immediate transfer to cardiac surgery center.

In CCL
- Rapid mobilization is initiated (all hands on deck!). Help will be needed from unit coordinator, nursing supervisor, and social worker.
- Sheaths and balloon pumps are sewn in place; IVs, pressure lines, and infusion pumps are organized; patient is placed on stretcher.
- Report to CCTT to review patient status. Physician confirms the level of care required for the patient in collaboration with the CCTT: RN and/or paramedic level.
- CCL RN accompanies patient with multiple drips if CCTT RN is unavailable.
- CCL laboratory staff member or unit coordinator assembles necessary transfer information: copy of chart, cine films or CD of angiogram, copy of chest x-ray film, CCL log of procedure, and handwritten catheterization report. Transcriptionist faxes transfer summary to accepting surgical center.
- Nursing report is given to receiving cardiac center, including status of patient, lists of IV drips and doses, equipment, and treatments. Admission status is reconfirmed, ETA given, and destination unit in receiving hospital is provided.
- Cardiologist completes Patient Transfer Orders Out of Facility (Fig. 13-3) and Medicare Inter-Facility Patient Transfer form (CC. 272) if needed.
- Family is provided with directions to receiving facility and names of contact persons there.
- For medical problems during transfer, the interventionalist or ED physician at the sending institution should be contacted from the ambulance unless other formal arrangements are made.
- Five minutes before arrival at cardiac center, EMS notifies center of ETA, and center confirms in-hospital destination: ED, OR, CCU, or CCL.
- Patient is transferred to designated unit.
- Written documentation of all clinical data during transport recorded.

ACLS, advanced cardiac life support; CCL, cardiac catheterization laboratory; CCTT, cardiac care transport team: CCU, cardiac care unit; CD, compact disc; ECG, electrocardiogram; ED, emergency department; EMS, emergency medical services; ETA, estimated time of arrival; IABP, intra-aortic balloon pump; IV, intravenous; OR, operating room; RN, registered nurse.
[a]A hospital-based CCTT, consisting of critical care nurses, paramedics, and CCL personnel, all with IABP expertise.
[b]EMS ambulance provider must have available and/or be able to accommodate the following: portable cardiac ECG and pressure monitoring, sufficient oxygen supply, suction, multiple drips, ACLS drugs, resuscitation equipment, defibrillator, and IABP.
Developed by Wharton TP, Sinclair N, Sheridan S, and CCL staff, Luizzi P and ED staff, Exeter Hospital, Exeter, NH. Printed with permission from Exeter Hospital. Copyright 2005.

urgent triage and treatment (Tables 13-6 and 13-9). The use of transdermal rather than intravenous (IV) nitroglycerin and the avoidance of a heparin drip after initial bolus are two measures that can simplify nursing care in the ED. Creation of an emergency chest pain assessment record (Fig. 13-2) provides an efficient method of documentation for the permanent medical record, avoids duplication of documentation, and decreases questions asked by the CCL staff. This assessment record provides the ED staff and CCL with clinical information, a list of medications given in the ED, and test results, along with documentation of event times. All these data will be useful in outcomes analysis and ongoing cardiology registries and studies.

The ED nursing staff should create a list of all supplies that are likely to be needed in the initial ED treatment of patients with AMI and organize a portable "AMI box" to contain all these medications, IV equipment and tubing, and other essentials. This should include all documentation tools (Fig. 13-2) to prevent loss or duplication of information and to save valuable time. Use of this AMI box will prevent unnecessary distraction in searching for supplies while caring for the acutely ill AMI patient in the ED.

Members of the team should also conduct educational sessions with the EMS and ED staff, with explanation of the AMI critical pathway, protocols, standing orders, and emergency chest pain assessment record. Special emphasis should be placed on the goal of the critical pathway to improve time to reperfusion, which will enhance outcomes because coronary artery occlusion is causing progressive death of the heart muscle: "Time is myocardium."

TABLE 13-8

ELEMENTS OF A CARDIAC TRANSFER AGREEMENT AND INTERHOSPITAL COLLABORATION FOR PRIMARY PCI PROGRAMS AT HOSPITALS WITH OFF-SITE CARDIAC SURGERY BACKUP: A PROVEN PLAN FOR RAPID ACCESS TO CARDIAC SURGERY

1. Cardiologist will establish a good working relationship with cardiac surgeons at receiving facility.[a]
2. Cardiac surgeons from referral cardiac surgery hospital will formally agree to provide cardiac surgery backup for urgent and emergent cases at all hours.
3. Surgeon will ensure that the patient will be accepted for services based on factors such medical condition, capacity of surgeons to provide services at the time of request, and availability of facility and staff resources.
4. Cardiologist will review with surgeon the potential needs and risks of the patient being transferred for emergency care.
5. Referring facility will establish a rigorous medical protocol (Table 13-7) for the safe and rapid transfer of patients to receiving cardiac surgery hospital.
6. EMS ambulance supplier will be formally contracted to be available on-site within 15 to 20 minutes of a call on a 24-hour, 7-day per week basis.
7. The hospital's transport team will include critical care nurses, paramedics, and CCL personnel with

IABP expertise. All members of the team should be ACLS certified.
8. EMS ambulance provider will have available and/or be able to accommodate the following: portable cardiac ECG and pressure monitoring, sufficient oxygen supply, suction, multiple drips, ACLS drugs, resuscitation equipment, defibrillator, and IABP.
9. Transferring physician will obtain consent from patient or appropriate consenting party.
10. Review of transferred patients will be ongoing and include feedback from referring facility regarding problems in transfer process, teaching opportunities through catheterization conferences, and periodic review of the outcomes of the surgical program with special emphasis on outcomes of transferred patients.
11. Cardiac surgeon will be credentialed to visit patients and families at referring hospital to review medical options if time allows.
12. Hospital administrations from both referring and accepting facilities will endorse the transfer agreement.

[a]Cardiologists must collaborate with their cardiac surgeons to ensure a seamless transition of care from the primary hospital to the surgical center. Measures to foster a good working relationship include the surgeon's attendance at cardiac catheterization conferences and becoming credentialed at the referring hospital. This will enable bedside consultation on nonemergent in-patients with review of treatment options with cardiologists, patients, and families and encourage frequent personal interaction between the surgeon and the cardiologist. A very important element of this relationship will also include outcomes feedback from the surgeon to the referring cardiologist.
ACLS, advanced cardiac life support; CCL, cardiac catheterization laboratory; ECG, electrocardiogram; EMS, emergency medical services; IABP, intra-aortic balloon pump; PCI, percutaneous coronary intervention.
Developed by Wharton TP, Sinclair N, Hiett D, and Cresta D. Exeter Hospital, Exeter, NH. Printed with permission from Exeter Hospital. Copyright 1993.

Periodic ED meetings and CCL conferences should be scheduled to examine current topics in AMI care and evaluate cases. The team should welcome comments; allow time for problem solving and suggestions from ED staff, EMS staff, CCL staff, and ED physicians; and involve them in quality improvement processes.

Develop a Catheterization Laboratory Primary PCI Protocol

The protocol in the CCL, such as the one that we suggest in Table 13-10, should be directed toward rapid assessment of the coronary anatomy and rapid triage to the most appropriate therapy: primary PCI, medical therapy, or transfer for CABG surgery (Table 13-3). Simultaneous to this must be intensive attention to the medical treatment of the patient. When primary PCI is chosen as the reperfusion strategy, the goal of intervention is the immediate establishment of TIMI grade 3 flow while reducing to an absolute minimum the chance that new myocardial jeopardy could be created by the procedure itself.

Establish an Ongoing Program to Improve Door-to-Balloon Times

The time it takes from hospital arrival to the first balloon inflation, the "door-to-balloon time," can be regarded as the

best single indicator of the overall quality of a PCI program. Other monitored indicators that use the frequency of events that have a low incidence, such as PCI failures and major complications, may not provide a statistically meaningful basis for comparison of outcomes in small populations to national standards.

The efficiency of care delivery in every phase of the emergency care of the AMI patient, from prehospital care through early ED management—including speed of diagnosis and speed in notifying the CCL team—to the time for readying the CCL and team (including team travel time in off-hours cases) to the time from CCL arrival to first intervention, determines the overall door-to-balloon time. The AMI protocol team (described earlier) should ensure the tracking of the times of ED arrival, first ECG, call to cath team, and cath lab arrival for every patient and should periodically review these intervals to see where opportunities for improvement may exist. Table 13-11 includes the goals for these various time intervals and our suggestions as to how processes may be improved to shorten these intervals. Any interval more than 20% above the goal should be investigated to eliminate correctable systemic problems and introduce new efficiencies.

1. Time from First Patient Contact to Diagnosis

This first interval is the variable that is most difficult to control. ED staff must be trained and continually encouraged to perform ECGs within 5 minutes of ED arrival in patients with

TABLE 13-9

EMERGENCY DEPARTMENT PROTOCOL FOR AMI[a]

See **prehospital management protocol for AMI** (Table 13-6), which includes
- Paramedic level of care[b]
- Establish IV, administer oxygen
- NTG SBP >100 mm Hg and patient not in shock
- **ASA** (325 mg) chewed
- 12-lead ECG while en route; transmit to ED[c]

ED physician should page cardiologist and CCL team simultaneously—even before patient arrives—if diagnostic acute ST-segment elevation is present on ECG, even if transmitted from field(50–53)[d]

In ED
–*Rapid assessment, rapid call to CCL team/cardiologist for all patients with clinical impression of AMI who meet clinical selection criteria (Table 13-6)*
- **ASA** (325 mg) chewed if not given during prehospital management
Give ASA rectally if intubated
- **NTG** SL **nitropaste** for ongoing pain or hypertension
Omit IV NTG for simplification; avoid routine multiple doses of NTG
(Hypotension is all too common in this scenario)
- **Heparin** 70 U/kg bolus without continuous infusion.
Avoid heparin drip for simplification; ACT will be titrated with further heparin in CCL
- **Clopidogrel** (300 to 600 mg) at this time or after intervention, at operator discretion
- Establish second IV
- **Metoprolol** (5 mg) IV every 5 minutes × 3 doses unless pulse <55, BP <100, or wheezing
- **Morphine** or **fentanyl** PRN pain; may cause nausea (lower incidence of nausea with fentanyl)
- **Prochlorperazine** and **atropine** PRN
- **ACLS** protocols per routine
- **Fluids, atropine** for bradycardia with hypotension; phenylephrine (pure alpha agonist) for refractory hypotension
- GP IIb/IIIa platelet inhibitors may be started in ED in collaboration with cardiologist
- Consider **fibrinolytics** in cases of a delay of over 45 min in transferring the patient to the CCL
- Avoid intubation by nasal route: this greatly increases the risk of bleeding if GP IIb/IIIa agents or fibrinolytics are used
- Document all clinical data and therapy on Emergency Chest Pain Assessment Record (Fig. 13-2)

ACLS, advanced cardiac life support; ACT, activated clotting time; AMI, acute myocardial infarction; ASA, aspirin; CCL, cardiac catheterization laboratory; ECG, electrocardiogram; ED, emergency department; GP, glycoprotein; IV, intravenous; NTG, nitroglycerin; po, by mouth; PRN, as needed; PCI, percutaneous coronary intervention; SBP, systolic blood pressure; SL, sublingual.
[a]*Italics highlight measures that reduce time-to-reperfusion for primary PCI.*
[b]If no paramedic level of care is available in the community, consider establishing a hospital-based paramedic program.
[c]Ambulances should be equipped with ECG system capable of telephonic transmission to ED for all chest pain calls; this can greatly reduce time-to-diagnosis, time-to-reperfusion, and possibly mortality (50–53). Patient with initial ST-segment elevation may arrive to ED pain free with a normal ECG, because 10% to 15% of AMIs reperfuse with aspirin and other conservative measures. Documenting ST-segment elevation at initial contact can influence immediate triage.
[d]One of the more correctable causes of delay in "door-to-balloon time" is the time that it takes to call the interventional cardiologist. Do not worry about "false alarms," which are rare.
Developed by Wharton JP, Sinclair N, Vigdor C, ED physicians, and EMT and ED Committees. Exeter Hospital, Exeter, NH. Printed with permission from Exeter Hospital. Copyright 2005.

suspicious symptoms and to present the ECG to the ED physician as soon as it is performed. The one single factor that can most dramatically decrease the time to reperfusion is making the diagnosis in the ambulance and calling in the CCL team before the patient's arrival. The identification of patients with STEMI in the field can save a great deal of time. During regular working hours, the CCL can be prealerted to clear any elective cases quickly (see acuity-based bumping protocol section, following). During off-hours, the cardiac catheterization team can be called and be en route to the hospital, and sometimes arrive

there, even before the patient arrives. Transmitting ECGs in from the field has clearly shown, both in our hands and in the literature (50–52), to result in significantly faster door-to-balloon times. We endorse protocols such as those of the Cardiac Alert Program (52) of Aurora, Colorado, which can serve as a model for future EMS and hospital AMI critical care pathways. The time to diagnosis can be reduced by 30 to 40 minutes by prehospital diagnosis in patients brought in by ambulance from a distance. If the CCL team can be called prior to the patient's arrival, it is not unreasonable to expect a door-to-

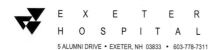

E X E T E R
H O S P I T A L

5 ALUMNI DRIVE • EXETER, NH 03833 • 603-778-7311

CHEST PAIN ASSESSMENT RECORD - PAGE 1 of 2

Room _____

Name							
Triage Acuity I II III IV V							

	TRIAGE TIME	ROOM TIME	ED/MD TIME	CALL TIME

Arrived Via   ☐ PRIVATE VEHICLE   ☐ AMBULANCE

Chief Complaint / Present Illness

SEEN BY MD

Childhood Immunizations   ☐ CURRENT   ☐ NA

TETANUS   ☐ < 5 Years ☐ > 5 Years   ☐ _____

Allergies/Reactions   ☐ **See ADR Sheet or EMR**

Current Prescription Meds / OTC / Herbals   ☐ None

Daily ASA ☐ No ☐ Yes   Taken today ☐ No ☐ Yes

☐ **Refer Medication Reconciliation List**

Objective Data

Medical History ☐ None

Self / EMS Treatment   ☐ None ☐ See EMS Run Sheet

Time 1st ECG: _____   ☐ Pre-Admission ECG

Temp ☐ TM ☐ PO ☐ PR	Pulse	Resp	BP R｜L	Weight

O2 Sat _____%   ☐ RA   ☐ O2 _____ L / M   ☐ NA   Height

Skin ☐ Warm & Dry   ☐ _____
Color ☐ WNL   ☐ _____
Integrity ☐ Intact   ☐ See Objective Data

☐ Recent GI Bleed	☐ CAD	☐ CHF
☐ MI	☐ DM	☐ Angina
☐ HTN	☐ Stroke	☐ CABG _____
☐ Pacemaker	☐ PCI	

Smoker ☐ No   ☐ Yes _____ Yrs _____ PPD

Respiratory   ☐ WNL   ☐ Smoker ☐ _____

Family History   ☐ None
☐ CAD   ☐ DM   ☐ Other _____

Mental Status ☐ Alert & Oriented   ☐ _____

Communicable Diseases   ☐ No Known Risk
☐ At Risk _____

Pain Severity   Time of Pain Onset _____ 0 - 10 _____
                  Pain on Arrival _____ 0 - 10 _____
☐ Numeric   ☐ Visual   Intensity (0 - 10) _____
☐ Behavioral ☐ Descriptive   (See Objective Data)

Symptoms: Anorexia, Fever, Persistent Cough,
       Bloody Sputum, Weight Loss or Night Sweats.

Stressors/Domestic Issues   ☐ No Known Risk
☐ At Risk _____

Radiation of Pain   ☐ No   ☐ Yes, to _____
Pain   ☐ Constant   ☐ Intermittent
Changes with ☐ Deep Breath   ☐ Movement ☐ None
Associated Symptoms _____

Support Available   ☐ Yes ☐ No
Learning Barriers/Needs _____

Triage Nurse Signature	**Time**

Cardiovascular Monitor Rhythm	**Abdominal Assessment** ☐ WNL ☐ See Objective Data	**Lung Assessment** ☐ WNL ☐ See Objective Data	**Pulses** Radial L ____ + R ____ + Femoral L ____ + R ____ +

_____

RN Signature	**Time**

ASM Form #168 (6/06)

FIGURE 13-2. Emergency chest pain assessment record developed at Exeter Hospital, Exeter, NH, in 1996. A form such as this provides a more efficient method of documentation for the permanent medical record, avoids duplication of documentation, and provides vital information to the emergency department (ED) staff and catheterization laboratory staff, including clinical information, medications given in the (*continues*)

Time	IV / PO Intake	Absorbed	Time	Output	Total
Total Intake			Total Output		

MEDICATION	DOSE	ROUTE	TIME	INITIALS	MEDICATION	DOSE	ROUTE	TIME	INITIALS
ASPIRIN	81 mg 4 tab	Chewed			MORPHINE		IVP		
NITRO	1/	SL			MORPHINE		IVP		
NITRO	1/	SL			MORPHINE		IVP		
NITRO	1/	SL			PLAVIX	300MG	Oral		
NITRO PASTE		DERMAL			IIb IIIa INHIBITOR:				
NITRO DRIP		IVPB			MED IV BOLUS		IV Drip Rate		
HEP BOLUS	Units	IVP			LYTIC BOLUS:				
HEP DRIP	Units/HR	IVPB					IVP		
LOPRESSOR		IVP			LYTIC INFUSION:				
LOPRESSOR		IVP					IVPB		
LOPRESSOR		IVP			LOVENOX	1 MG/KG	SC		

SIGNATURE _____ RN   SIGNATURE _____ MD   TIME _____

Pain Severity (P) 0 - 10   **Level of Sedation (LOS)**   1 - awake   2 - drowsy   3 - easy to arouse   4 - difficult to arouse   5 - unable to arouse

Time	Vital Signs	P / LOS	Continued Assessment

Discharge   ☐ Patient / Guardian Understands / Accepts Plan of Care   ☐ AMA   ☐ Other _____

Admission   To CCL Time_____   Room Number_____   Valuables_____   ☐ Home   ☐ c̄ Patient

Referrals   ☐ Social Work   ☐ VNA   ☐ Seacoast Mental Health   ☐ Safe Place   ☐ Victims Inc.

RN Signature   **Time**

FIGURE 13-2. (*continued*) ED, test results, and documentation of event times. Much of this data will be necessary for reporting outcomes to ongoing cardiology registries and studies. (Printed with permission from Exeter Hospital, Exeter, NH. Copyright 2005.)

TABLE 13-10

CATHETERIZATION LABORATORY PROTOCOL FOR PRIMARY PCI.

1. Abbreviated history and physical examination in ED. Complete chest pain assessment sheet to send to CCL with patient.
2. Cardiologist to obtain informed consent in the ED from patient or family, discussing risks, benefits, alternative therapies, and that transfer to a cardiac surgery institution would be required if emergency surgery were needed.
3. CCL team to alert ED as soon as they arrive; plan for patient transfer to CCL within 5 minutes of arrival. (CCL is always left in a state of readiness.)
4. Enforce acuity-based bumping protocol when an elective procedure is in progress in the CCL.
5. Rapid transfer to CCL after informed consent.
6. For off-hours cases with only two CCL team members on call, a CCU or ED nurse or paramedic is predesignated to be available to assist in managing medications, drips, and acute nursing care problems.
7. If patient is intubated or in danger of respiratory compromise, respiratory therapist must stay with patient during procedure.
8. ED nurse, nursing supervisor, or social worker to counsel family during procedure.
9. Uninterrupted ECG monitoring during changeover from portable transport monitor to CCL system.
10. Ensure patient has been pretreated with heparin, ASA, and 300 to 600 mg clopidogrel (unless operator prefers deferring clopidogrel loading dose until after intervention).
11. Rapid preparation of both groins for bilateral access if IABP is

necessary. Clipping can be done in ED while waiting for CCL to be readied.
12. Administer appropriate additional narcotics and sedation.
13. Administer IV beta-blockers if not given in ED and no contraindications.
14. Continue vigorous medical management, monitoring of oxygen saturation, blood pressure support with fluids and pressors, treatment of congestive heart failure, etc., as indicated.
15. Place arterial sheath.
16. IABP placement if in shock with introduction of second arterial sheath via opposite groin.
17. Femoral venous sheath placement if hemodynamically unstable or pacemaker likely to be needed.
18. Arterial blood for gasses if respiratory or acid-base status is unstable.
19. Give heparin boluses to assure ACT of 200 to 250 seconds. Repeat ACT every 30 minutes during the procedure to titrate subsequent heparin boluses.
20. Administer GP IIb/IIIa platelet inhibitors if not already given in the ED, or unless diagnosis is uncertain.
21. Immediate angiography of both coronary arteries with low-osmolar ionic contrast; limit injections to the minimal number required to define anatomy.
22. Rapid identification and assessment of the IRA.
23. Immediate decision on therapeutic action: PCI, emergent transfer for surgery (with antecedent PCI if IRA is occluded unless downstream from severe left main coronary lesion), or initial medical therapy.

24. Open the IRA before doing the LV gram, unless the IRA has initial TIMI grade 3 flow or the culprit lesion is unclear, in which case performing LV gram before intervention can influence interventional strategy.
25. Establish coronary flow with guide wire or low-pressure/undersized balloon inflations to define distal anatomy before final selection of balloon or stent stenting.
26. Use of thrombectomy device for large thrombus burden after establishing flow, at the discretion of the operator.
27. Use of drug-eluting stents is at the discretion of operator.
28. Flow-limiting lesions in tandem with the culprit lesion in the same arterial segment should also be addressed.
29. Avoid stenting if balloon angioplasty result is stable and patient will require CABG surgery in the near future.
30. If angiographic indications for emergent bypass surgery are present, activate emergency transfer protocol (Table 13-7) while performing any necessary intervention.
31. Avoid intervention in arteries other than the IRA unless lesions appear to be flow-limiting or patient has ongoing ischemia or hemodynamic instability.
32. Right heart catheterization with balloon-tipped catheter left indwelling if hemodynamically unstable.
33. LV gram in all cases except severe hemodynamic instability or severe renal insufficiency.
34. Initial loading dose (300 to 600 mg) of clopidogrel is given in CCL if not already given in ED.

ACT, activated clotting time; ASA, aspirin; CABG, coronary artery bypass graft; CCL, cardiac catheterization laboratory; CCU, cardiac care unit; ECG, electrocardiogram; ED, emergency department; GP, glycoprotein; IABP, intra-aortic balloon pump; IRA, infarct-related artery; IV, intravenous; LV gram, left ventriculogram; PCI, percutaneous coronary intervention; TIMI, thrombolysis in myocardial infarction.
Developed by Wharton TP, Sinclair N, Hiett D, Deboard D, Wason L, and the CCL staff. Exeter Hospital, Exeter, NH. Printed with permission from Wharton TP, Sinclair N. Copyright 2005.

balloon time of 50 to 60 minutes, even in off-hours, rather than 80 to 90 minutes if the patient arrives in the ED without prior diagnosis (53).

2. Time from Diagnosis to Calling the CCL Team

This should be 5 minutes or less if the ED physician is empowered to call the interventional cardiologist and the CCL team

directly as soon as the diagnosis of STEMI is made, even before the patient arrives if the diagnosis is made in the field. (The time from "diagnosis to decision" is reduced to zero if the decision is already made in advance to offer primary PCI as first-line treatment of choice to all patients with STEMI.)

3. Time from Calling the Team to CCL Arrival, and

TABLE 13-11

IMPROVING DOOR-TO-BALLOON TIMES

Interval/Time Goal	Steps to Streamline Process
1. First Contact to Diagnosis 5 minutes	• Regional educational programs on recognition of STEMI are established • EMS-developed chest-pain protocols are implemented (Table 13-6) • EMS classes in ECG interpretation are conducted • Rapid ECG assessment is performed in the field • ECG is transmitted from the ambulance to the ED • EMS communicates directly with ED physician • Bloods are drawn in the ambulance • ASA, IV beta-blockers, heparin bolus are administered in ambulance • If no ECG in field, this is obtained in ED within 5 minutes of arrival and is immediately shown to ED physician
2. Diagnosis to Calling Cath Team 5 minutes	• "Diagnosis-to-decision" time is eliminated: all patients with STEMI are treated with primary PCI • ED physician is empowered and expected to page directly the interventionalist and CCL team when diagnosis of acute STEMI is made, even prior to patient arrival • One page number is dialed to page all CCL personnel
3. Call To CCL Arrival 40 minutes	• CCL team lives ≤30 minutes from CCL • Team is paged with text-message of key information, i.e.: diagnosis, physician, location of patient, adjunctive services needed such as pacemaker, IABP, respiratory therapy • CCL team members confirm page received • ED physician begins to explain diagnosis, coronary angiography, and PCI to patient and family before arrival of interventionalist • Informed consent is obtained for the cardiac catheterization, possible PCI, IABP, and transfer to surgical center if needed • Omit IV NTG and heparin drip after bolus for simplification; avoid routine multiple doses of NTG. ACT will be titrated with further heparin in CCL • GP IIb/IIIa inhibitors are administered in ED • ED nurses clip both femoral areas if CCL not yet ready • ED secretary enters computer order for left heart catheterization to enable quick boot-up of CCL imaging equipment • CCL team calls ED to transport patient when nearly ready to accept patient • Completed Chest Pain Assessment Sheet (Fig. 13-2)
4. CCL Arrival to First Intervention 30 minutes	• CCL is left clean and "ready to go" • Basic angiographic and interventional supplies are set out on counter • Certain medication drips, such as phenylephrine, are premixed • Completed Chest Pain Assessment Sheet (Fig. 13-2) is available in CCL as a ready source of information about patient • Nursing supervisor or ED nurse provides extra pair of hands during setup, to aid in procurement of medications, equipment, communication with family members • CCL control desk has easy access to computerized lab results • Cordless hospital telephone is provided for circulating nurse • Physician scrubs while patient is being draped • Angiography of IRA is performed first to allow selection and preparation of interventional equipment while non-IRA is imaged • Left ventriculogram is deferred until after intervention unless needed for infarct localization

AMI, acute myocardial infarction; ASA, aspirin; CCL, cardiac catheterization laboratory; ECG, electrocardiogram; ED, emergency department; EMS, emergency medical services; GP, glycoprotein; IABP, intra-aortic balloon pump; IRA, infarct-related artery; IV, intravenous; NTG, nitroglycerin; PCI, percutaneous coronary intervention; STEMI, ST-segment elevation myocardial infarction.
Developed by Wharton TP, Sinclair N, Mechem D and CCL Staff, Luizzi P, Scalese C, Mastromarino J, Siegart W. Exeter Hospital, Exeter, NH. Printed with permission from Wharton TP, Sinclair N, Exeter Hospital. Copyright 2005.

4. Time from CCL Arrival to First Intervention

These two intervals are straightforward to address, standardize, and streamline: an experienced interventionalist and team that cover the CCL 24/7 should be able to obtain informed consent and move the patient into the CCL within 40 minutes of being called, even during off-hours, and should be able to perform the first intervention within 25 to 30 more minutes.

Develop an Acuity-Based Procedure-Bumping Protocol

Community hospitals with only one CCL are often busy with elective procedures scheduled throughout the day. When initiating a primary PCI program, all physicians performing procedures in the CCL should mutually develop and agree to follow

TABLE 13-12

CATHETERIZATION LABORATORY ACUITY-BASED PROCEDURE BUMPING PROTOCOL

Purpose: To permit rapid interventional treatment of the most critically ill patients while providing appropriately timed care to less-acute patients.

Policy: All physicians, CCL staff, and administration shall agree in advance to adhere to this acuity-based bumping protocol. This may mean the postponement of elective procedures or the interruption of elective procedures already in progress.

Classification of priority: Patients are classified as follows

Class A: Immediate priority
1. Acute high-risk AMI
   a. Hemodynamically compromised (shock or preshock, pulmonary edema)
   b. Heart block
   c. Anterior AMI
   d. Fibrinolytic ineligible
2. Suspected pulmonary embolus with hemodynamic instability
3. Cardiac tamponade
4. Acute aortic dissection requiring angiography

Class B: Emergent priority
1. Hemodynamically stable AMI other than anterior
2. Acute limb ischemia
3. Crescendo TIAs or stroke with abnormal carotid ultrasound

Class C: Urgent priority
1. Unstable angina within 24 hours
2. Inferior vena cava filters or venography for deep venous thrombosis

Protocol:

Class A: Immediate transfer to CCL with interruption of elective procedures in progress on stable patients. Interrupted patients with indwelling sheaths will be returned to the CCL after completion of the emergency procedure. Scheduled elective procedures not yet started will be postponed or rescheduled.

Class B: Transfer to CCL within a 30-minute window. Procedures in progress will be finished expeditiously.

Class C: Transfer to CCL on completion of the case in progress.

Transfers from other hospitals:

Patients being transferred in will be triaged according to the preceding classification system. Class A patients expected with an estimated time of arrival within 40 minutes will have the CCL room vacated and held open for direct admission. All others will be evaluated in the ED for transfer to the CCL according to the preceding system.

AMI, acute myocardial infarction; CCL, cardiac catheterization laboratory; CCU, cardiac care unit; ED, emergency department, TIA, transient ischemic attack.

Developed by Wharton TP, Thomas T, and Sullivan N. Exeter Hospital, Exeter, NH. Printed with permission from Exeter Hospital. Copyright 1993.

an acuity-based procedure bumping protocol such as the one we propose in Table 13-12. Having these agreements will avoid delays in treating immediate priority patients while lessening dissatisfaction caused by scheduling conflicts.

Create an Emergency Transfer Protocol and Establish Formal Agreements That Ensure Rapid Transfer to a Cardiac Surgery Center

About 3% to 5% of patients undergoing immediate coronary angiography will need to be transferred for emergency CABG surgery, almost always because of critical anatomy discovered by the angiogram rather than because of procedural mishap (14–17,23,26,27). Formal transfer agreements and protocols for interhospital collaboration must be in place for the expeditious transfer of these patients (Tables 13-7 and 13-8; Fig. 13-3), when the CCL is not available, or in the rare event of a CCL complication (e.g., abrupt vessel closure or coronary perforation). The goal of these emergency transfer protocols is to ensure the fastest possible response once the decision is made to transfer the patient, whether from the ED or the CCL.

The institution should consider establishing a hospital-based critical care transport team (CCTT), consisting of critical care nurses, paramedics, and CCL personnel, all with IABP expertise. The EMS ambulance service must be able to quickly (<15 minutes) provide to the site a vehicle that has available and/or is able to accommodate the following equipment: portable cardiac ECG and pressure monitoring, sufficient oxygen supply, suction, multiple drips, advanced cardiac life support (ACLS) drugs, resuscitation equipment, defibrillator, and IABP.

Cardiologists and the hospital administration must work with referral hospitals, especially their cardiac surgeons, to develop an atmosphere of collaboration and trust to ensure a seamless transition of care from the community hospital to the surgical center. The cardiac surgeon should be invited to attend cardiac catheterization conferences at the community hospital and hopefully will be credentialed there. This will enable the surgeon to consult on less-emergent in-patients and review treatment options with patients and families to help them make decisions on therapy before transfer. A very important element of this relationship will include feedback from the surgical center to the community hospital physicians on surgical outcomes

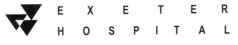

E X E T E R
H O S P I T A L

EXETER, NH 03833 • 603-778-7311

PHYSICIAN ORDERS
Patient Transfer Orders

Allergies (Allergen and Reaction)	Weight

Date / Time	ORDERS
	Transfer to _____ **Receiving unit** _____
	Staff required:
	☐ EMT-I (IV Only) ☐ Paramedic ☐ Paramedic and Nurse ☐ IABP Team
	☐ Cardiac Monitor
	☐ Pulse Oximetry Titrate 02 to keep saturation ≥ 92%
	☐ Vital Signs q 15 minutes unless indicated:
	Medications
	Pain:
	☐ NTG 1/150 gr sl q 5 min x3 prn chest pain
	☐ Start or Titrate NTG gtt to alleviate chest pain and maintain SBP > _____
	☐ Morphine _____ mg IV q _____ prn
	☐ Demerol _____ mg IV q _____ prn
	Nausea:
	☐ prochlorperazine _____ mg IV q _____ prn
	☐ promethazine _____ mg IV q _____ prn
	Other Meds: ☐ _____
	☐ _____
	☐ _____
	☐ IV Fluid _____ @ _____ cc/hr
	☐ Maintain all current IV drips.
	Blood Products:
	Vent Settings:
	Mode _____ FIO2 _____ TV _____ RR _____ PEEP _____ Other _____
	Full Code Unless Indicated:
	Physician/Practitioner Signature _____ Time _____ Date _____

EH 1/1999

FIGURE 13-3. Standing orders for patient transfer out of Exeter Hospital, Exeter, NH. (Printed with permission from Exeter Hospital, Exeter, NH. Copyright 1999.)

clinical follow-up, discussion of case studies, and newer cardiac surgical techniques and procedures.

Establish In-Hospital Management Pathways

Risk stratification and management protocols for the patient with AMI after intervention (Fig. 13-1; Table 13-13) should be developed to provide the team with a clear clinical pathway for each patient.

Interventionalists should institute standing orders that address the care to be provided after primary PCI (Fig. 13-4). The potential for groin bleeding will require the development of sheath protocols and standing orders (Fig. 13-5) for quick detection and control. Accompany this with education programs in the use of in-lab closure devices, femoral compression devices, hemodynamic monitoring, medication in-services, and IABP modules and training.

High-risk patients with AMI admitted to the CCU require intensive care and monitoring. Critical care nurses must learn new skills, because patients will often come to the CCU with femoral sheaths, pulmonary lines, temporary pacemakers, and/or IABPs. Cardiac shock patients that might have died without primary PCI may remain on multiple drips and support technology for several days. Nurses will be continually challenged to maintain their skills at the highest level.

Low-risk patients with AMI (for example, patients <70 years of age with 1- to 2-vessel coronary artery disease that have an ejection fraction >45% and no congestive heart failure or arrhythmias, a good PCI result with TIMI grade 3 flow, and no major dissection or residual thrombus) can be admitted to an interventional unit, then to telemetry (41). This group, perhaps one-half of all patients with AMI treated with primary PCI, has a low mortality rate of only 0.3%. These patients at low risk can safely avoid CCU care and predischarge exercise testing, and be discharged on hospital day 3 with return to work in 2 weeks. These measures will save an average of $2,000 per patient in total hospital costs, while decreasing the loss of wages and disability payments (41).

Telemetry and cardiac rehabilitation staff must originate fast-track educational programs for patients at low risk, who are often discharged after only 2 or 3 days in the hospital, and thus may tend to minimize the importance of their MI. Standing orders for cardiac rehabilitation phases I and II should be in-

---

TABLE 13-13

IN-HOSPITAL MANAGEMENT AND RISK-STRATIFICATION PROTOCOL AFTER PRIMARY PCI

1. Communicate with family, primary physician, and ED staff immediately after procedure. Providing photographs of IRA before and after intervention is especially helpful.
2. Stratify patients into **low risk** (those with age <70 year, 1–2 vessel CAD, EF >45%, no CHF or arrhythmias, good PCI result, TIMI grade 3 flow, and no major dissection or residual thrombus) and **high risk** (all others).
3. Patients at low-risk can be transferred to step-down or interventional unit if they have received a femoral closure device or if the nurses are able to care for sheaths. Patients at high risk go to CCU.
4. Early sheath removal in 3 hours or when ACT is <180 sec.
5. No heparin infusion immediately after procedure if sheaths are to be removed early or if GP IIb/IIIa platelet inhibitors are used. Low-dose weight-adjusted heparin protocol may be started 3 hours after sheath removal for lesions at high risk of rethrombosis, at operator discretion.
6. Start maintenance aspirin, clopidogrel, beta-blockers, ACE inhibitors, and statins if no contraindications. Loading dose of clopidogrel is given in ED or CCL.
7. Consider weight-adjusted heparin or enoxaparin after completion of GP IIb/IIIa infusion for patients who have suboptimal interventional result, residual intracoronary thrombus burden, apical left ventricular dyskinesis, CHF, or bedridden status.
8. Follow platelet counts beginning 4 to 6 hours after procedure to ensure thrombocytopenia has not been induced by heparin or GP IIb/IIIa platelet inhibitors.
9. Cardiac rehabilitation consultation for all patients.
10. A "fast-track" cardiac rehabilitation program should be established to meet the special needs of patients with low-risk AMI, who are often discharged on day 3 after AMI. If discharged without a consult to cardiac rehabilitation, provide a follow-up phone to the patient for education and encouragement to enroll in cardiac rehabilitation.
11. Target patients at low risk for discharge on hospital day 3.
12. Predischarge exercise testing only for high-risk patients.

Positive reinforcement after the procedure is particularly important for ED physicians, nurses, and paramedics (e.g., providing photographs, report of "door-to-balloon" time, praise of rapid and efficient care, if warranted; constructive troubleshooting if problems occurred).

ACE, angiotensin-converting enzyme; ACT, activated clotting time; AMI, acute myocardial infarction; CAD, coronary artery disease; CCU, coronary care unit; CHF, congestive heart failure; ED, emergency department; EF, ejection fraction; GP, glycoprotein; IRA, infarct-related artery; IV, intravenous; PCI, percutaneous coronary intervention; TIMI, thrombolysis in myocardial infarction.
Developed by Wharton TP and Sinclair N, Exeter Hospital, Exeter, NH. Printed with permission from Wharton TP, Sinclair N. Copyright 2005.

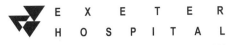

Cardiac
Unstable Angina, AMI, PCI Orders
Confirm/document allergies on the Allergy Documentation Sheet

PATIENT ORDERS

Status: ☐ Inpatient ☐ Outpatient Observation (pt anticipated to meet d/c requirements w/in 24hrs) ☐ SCU ☐ PCU ☐ Telemetry

Diagnosis/Procedure:_____

Physician/Practitioners: Admitting:_____ Attending: _____ Primary MD/DO:_____

Enact all numbered orders. If order is not to be enacted draw a line through. Check box to activate optional orders.

1. Consult ☒ Cardiac Rehab ☐ Dietitian ☐ Case Manager; ☐ Cardiologist (physician must call); ☐ other:_____

2. Precautions: ☒ Standard ☐ Other_____ (refer to isolation manual)

3. Diet: ☐ Advance to cardiac diet as tolerated ☐ Intake and Output ☐ Monitor I & O Hourly

4. Activity: ☐ as tolerated ☐ see post-cath/PCI section below ☐ Other_____

5. Vital Signs: Q4h, except do not awaken unless indicated.

6. ☐ O$_2$ @ 2L/m nasal cannula or non-re-breather mask 8-10L/m; titrate to keep 02 sat >93%. Pulse oximetry PRN.

7. Continuous Cardiac Monitoring, rhythm strip Q6 hours and as indicated.

8. Chest Pain Guidelines (TX.212) and Critical Clinical Practice Guidelines (TX.274)

Labs and Diagnostic Testing (IF not performed in ER)

1. CBC w/ Diff; CPK Total and MB, Basic Metabolic Profile (BMP) on admission and in a.m.

☐ Troponin at 0h, 6-8h, and 24h; coordinate with PTTA draws

2. Baseline PTTA and PT.

3. Lipid Profile, Liver profile, U/A in a.m. if not yet sent ☐ HbA1C ☐ Magnesium level

4. Test all stools for occult blood and record in progress notes

5. EKG for hospital admission, on arrival to unit post cath (if done), and Q AM x 2 days.

☐ Portable CXR now ☐ Portable CXR in AM

☐ Cardiac Echo

☐ Exercise Test (type_____) at (time_____) if no further pain and EKG and enzymes negative.

 Call physician/practitioner when exercise test completed or if it must be cancelled.

Medications:

1. IV Fluid: ☐ Med Lock ☐ See Post Cath Orders below ☐ IV:_____ @ _____cc's/hr x_____ cc's, then med lock

☒ ASA 325 mg po q AM.

☐ Heparin protocol ☐ low dose protocol

☐ enoxaparin 1mg/kg sc q12hrs

☐ IV NTG: titrate to keep BP:_____

Beta blocker: _____

ACE inhibitor: _____

Lipid Rx: _____

Potassium: _____

Magnesium: _____

☐ Morphine 5-10 mg IV q 15 min PRN pain, anxiety.

GP IIb/IIIa inhibitor: _____

☐ Resume all previously ordered medications

☐ clopidogrel 300 mg po stat. OR ☐ Plavix 600 mg po stat

☐ clopidogrel 75 mg po daily

☐ esomeprazole 40 mg po now and daily.

☐ famotidine 20 mg IV now and bid.

☐ temazepam 30 mg po qhs PRN, MR x1 PRN for sleep

☐ lorazepam 0.5mg - 1 mg IV or po q 4 hrs PRN for anxiety.

☐ prochlorperazine 5-10 mg IV q 4 hrs PRN nausea/vomiting

☐ sublimaze 50 mcg - 100 mcg IV q 15 min PRN pain, anxiety.

If Post-Cath or Post-PCI: (See Vascular Sheath/IABP order sheets as appropriate.)

1. Femostop for any bleeding. ☐ Vascular sheath protocol; draw all bloods from sheath.

2. Bed rest x ____ hours after sheaths removed.

3. IV normal saline at 150 cc/hr x 1,000 cc's, or:_____

4. Foley catheter PRN if patient has not voided by 3 h post cath.

☐ Start heparin 3 hrs after sheaths out, no bolus: ☐ standard protocol ☐ low dose protocol

☐ See Additional Order Sheet

Physician/Practitioner Signature_____ Time_____ Date_____

Read all telephone/verbal orders back to the physician/practitioner in their entirety

EH (12/2004)

FIGURE 13-4. Standing orders for patients admitted with myocardial infarction, other acute coronary syndromes, and/or after coronary intervention at Exeter Hospital, Exeter, NH. (Printed with permission from Exeter Hospital, Exeter, NH. Copyright 2004.)

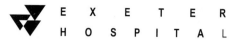

E X E T E R

H O S P I T A L

EXETER, NH 03833 • 603-778-7311

PHYSICIAN ORDERS
Vascular Sheath / IABP

Allergies (Allergen and Reaction)	Weight

Date / Time	**ORDERS** (carry out all orders except those with blank checkbox)
	1. VS q 15 min x 4, q 30 min x 2, then q 1 hr if stable.
	2. Monitor q 1 hr.: VS, pulse, temp, color mobility of extremity distal to sheath.
	3. Monitor mean arterial pressure, systolic, diastolic & mean PA pressure q 1 hr; mean PC wedge q ___ hrs. CO/CI q shift. (as applicable)

	4. Lab Work: Draw all bloods from sheaths, except IABP. ☐ Nurses draw all ABG's from IABP.
	   a. Complete CBC with platelets q AM.
	   b. ☐ H/ H q 6 PM (Draw with PTT's whenever possible).
	   c. U/A qod.

	5. Heparin protocol ☐ Standard dose ☐ Low dose ☐ No bolus
	6. Change sheath dressing every day. Clean with Betadine and apply transparent dressing. Only 1 piece of gauze between puncture site and transparent dressing, unless active oozing.

	7. Bleeding:
	   a. Inspect site q 30 min x 4 hrs, then q 1 hr if no signs of bleeding.
	   b. Watch for concealed trickle of blood down crease in groin. Place 4 x 4 in groin. Inspect sheet under patient q 1 hr.
	   c. For oozing not controlled in 30 minutes (i.e., rate of one-soaked 4x4 per hour); remove dressing; apply balloon compression device.
	   d. Outline hematomas q 2 hrs; call physician if enlarging.

	8. Notify Physician Immediately for:
	   a. Prolonged CP or any flank pain.
	   b. Unstable VS.
	   c. Bleeding.
	   d. Altered color, temp, pulses or sensation in the extremities.
	   e. Severe pain in or around the puncture site.
	   f. U/O < 30cc/hr or if pt. Has not voided 3hrs post -cath.
	   g. Hives, dyspnea, itching.
	   h. If most recent Hct. Is above 35 and falls 5 pts.
	   i. If most recent Hct. Is below 35 and falls 3 pts.
	   j. Any signs of blood in IABP tubing.
	   k. If nonfunctioning IABP can not be corrected within 15 minutes.

	After sheath removal: 9. Patient to remain in bed for 6 hours (2 hr if groin closure device used). Head of bed may be flexed 30°.
	10. The extremity distal to the puncture site will remain extended straight for 6 hours.
	11. ☐ Patient may shower on the evening following sheath removal.

Physician/Practitioner Signature_____   Time_____   Date_____

EH 3/2001

FIGURE 13-5. Standing orders for patients with vascular sheaths or intra-aortic balloon pump (IABP) at Exeter Hospital, Exeter, NH. (Printed with permission from Exeter Hospital, Exeter, NH. Copyright 2001.)

cluded on the post-MI/postintervention order sheet (Fig. 13-4). All patients should be encouraged on discharge to enroll in the phase II cardiac rehabilitation program for risk factor modification and supervised exercise.

Discharge teaching handouts should be created that document and emphasize established standards of care for patients with AMI such as smoking cessation counseling; medications including aspirin, beta-blockers, ACE inhibitors/ARBs, statins, and antiplatelet agents; signs and symptoms that require a call to the doctor; diet; activity; daily weights (if appropriate); and follow-up appointments.

Initiate Processes and Tracking Tools for Data Gathering and Analysis, Case Review, and Quality Assurance

The institution should enroll in a national or regional data registry such as the American College of Cardiology National Cardiovascular Data Registry (NCDR) or The Northern New England Cardiovascular Disease Study Group. Maintaining ongoing data collection and outcomes analysis is particularly important for institutions that are performing unconventional or controversial procedures (e.g., primary PCI without on-site cardiac surgery). An appropriate data collection tool should include the following information on each patient: demographic information, clinical presentation, initial treatment, time intervals (ED arrival, angiography, first intervention), coronary anatomy, medications, therapies chosen and reasons, results of PCI, CCL complications, in-hospital complications, in-hospital mortality, and further procedures or cardiac surgery.

In addition to retrospective data review, positive reinforcement and feedback immediately after each procedure is particularly important to provide to ED physicians, nurses, and paramedics (e.g., providing photographs, report of "door-to-balloon" time, praise of rapid and efficient care, if warranted; constructive troubleshooting if problems occurred).

The use of data tracking tools allows identification of areas for improvement, such as suboptimal times to reperfusion and groin bleeding complications. When identified, constructive steps can be taken. For example, at Exeter Hospital we decreased bleeding complications more than fourfold despite aggressive use of glycoprotein IIb/IIIa platelet inhibitors with the initiation of weight-based heparin protocols, fluoroscopy for femoral puncture, postprocedural standing orders (Figs. 13-4 and 13-5), femoral compression devices, and most importantly, in-lab sheath removal using femoral closure devices. We also continually strive to improve our times-to-reperfusion using more streamlined prehospital and ED protocols (Tables 13-6 and 13-9 to 13-11). These have resulted in a 17% improvement in our median "door-to-balloon" time. This process of outcomes analysis can also be used to gauge the effects of new policies and procedures, new equipment and medical therapies, and new educational programs.

Key members of the AMI protocol team must take responsibility for spearheading these quality improvement efforts and for communicating the outcomes of the program to the medical community on an ongoing basis. Continuous quality improvement processes will prevent complacency and continue to stimulate the development of new goals in the care of the patient with AMI.

CONCLUSIONS

Because of its broader applicability, safety, and efficacy, primary PCI can and should be offered as the standard-of-care

for patients with AMI at well-qualified hospitals that do not have cardiac surgery. Primary PCI can be provided safely and effectively at such hospitals, with outstanding outcomes that are similar to those reported from high-volume surgical centers.

A uniform commitment to immediate and routine triage of patients with AMI from the ED to the CCL as first-line therapy around the clock will improve times-to-reperfusion, increase institutional primary PCI volumes, streamline acute critical care pathways, and ensure optimal emergency management of the AMI patient. These beneficial effects should improve outcomes and mortality in patients with AMI (12,33–35).

Achieving a successful primary PCI program in a community hospital requires the intensive collaboration and commitment of all members of the health care team. Critical pathways and care plans covering every aspect of management of the AMI patient, from first contact through discharge, coupled with ongoing assessment of evolving protocols to improve patient care, continuous educational programs, and ongoing data gathering and analysis are required to provide safe and effective interventional treatment of AMI. These elements are especially imperative for interventional programs at centers without on-site cardiac surgery.

Offering this potentially lifesaving therapy to more patients with AMI in more hospitals throughout the country can provide a substantial health care benefit to society.

References

1. Keeley EC, Boura JA, Grines CL. Primary angioplasty versus intravenous thrombolytic therapy for acute myocardial infarction: a quantitative review of 23 randomised trials. *Lancet* 2003;361:13–20.
2. Rogers WJ, Canto JG, Lambrew CT, et al. Temporal trends in the treatment of over 1.5 million patients with myocardial infarctions in the U.S. from 1990–1999. *J Am Coll Cardiol* 2000;36:2056–2063.
3. Brodie BR. Primary percutaneous intervention at hospitals without onsite cardiac surgery. *J Am Coll Card* 2004;43:1951–1953.
4. Mehta RH, Stalhandske EJ, McCargar PA, et al. Elderly patients at highest risk with acute myocardial infarction are more frequently transferred from community hospitals to tertiary centers: reality or myth? *Am Heart J* 1999;138:688–695.
5. Andersen HR, Nielsen TT, Rasmussen K, et al. A comparison of coronary angioplasty with fibrinolytic therapy in acute myocardial infarction. *N Engl J Med* 2003;349:733–742.
6. Widimsky P, Budesinsky T, Vorac D, et al. Long distance transport for primary angioplasty vs immediate thrombolysis in acute myocardial infarction. *Eur Heart J* 2003;24:94–104.
7. Dalby M, Bouzamondo A, Lechat P, et al. Transfer for primary angioplasty versus immediate thrombolysis in acute myocardial infarction: a meta-analysis. *Circulation* 2003;108:1809–1814.
8. Canto JG, Zalenski RJ, Ornato JP, et al. Use of emergency medical services in acute myocardial infarction and subsequent quality of care. Observations from the National Registry of Myocardial Infarction 2. *Circulation* 2002;106:3018–3023.
9. Hochman JS, Sleeper LA, Webb JG, et al. Early revascularization in acute myocardial infarction complicated by cardiogenic shock. SHOCK Investigators. Should we emergently revascularize occluded coronaries for cardiogenic shock? *N Engl J Med* 1999;341:625–634.
10. Gibson CM. NRMI and current treatment patterns for ST-elevation myocardial infarction. *Am Heart J* 2004;148:S29–S33.
11. Hermann HC. Transfer for primary angioplasty: the importance of time. *Circulation* 2005;111:718–720.
12. Cannon CP, Gibson CM, Lambrew CT, et al. Relationship of symptom-onset-to-balloon time and door-to-balloon time with mortality in patients undergoing angioplasty for acute myocardial infarction. *JAMA* 2000;283:2941–2947.
13. Nallamothu BK, Bates ER, Herrin J, et al. Times to treatment in transfer patients undergoing primary percutaneous coronary intervention in the United States. National Registry of Myocardial Infarction (NRMI)-3/4 analysis. *Circulation* 2005;111:761–767.
14. Weaver WD, Litwin PE, Martin JS, et al. Use of direct angioplasty for treatment of patients with acute myocardial infarction in hospitals with and without on-site cardiac surgery. *Circulation* 1993;88:2067–2075.
15. Weaver WD, Parsons L, Every N, et al. Primary coronary angioplasty in hospitals with and without surgery backup. *J Invasive Cardiol* 1995;7:34F–39F.
16. Smyth DW, Richards AM, Elliott JM. Direct angioplasty for myocardial

infarction: one-year experience in a center with surgical back-up 220 miles away. *J Invasive Cardiol* 1997;9:324–332.

17. Wharton TP, McNamara NS, Fedele FA, et al. Primary angioplasty for the treatment of acute myocardial infarction: experience at two community hospitals without cardiac surgery. *J Am Coll Cardiol* 1999;33:1257–1265.

18. Ribichini F. Experiences with primary angioplasty without on site-cardiac surgery. *Semin Interv Cardiol* 1999;4:47–53.

19. Ribichini F, Steffenino G, Dellavalle A. Primary angioplasty without surgical back-up at all. Results of a five years experience in a community hospital in Europe (abstract). *J Am Coll Cardiol* 2000;35:364A.

20. Aversano T, Aversano LT, Passamani E, et al. Thrombolytic therapy vs primary percutaneous coronary intervention for myocardial infarction in patients presenting to hospitals without on-site cardiac surgery: a randomized controlled trial. *JAMA* 2002;287:1943–1951.

21. Aversano T. Primary angioplasty at hospitals without cardiac surgery: C-PORT Registry outcomes (abstract). *Circulation* 2003;108:IV–613.

22. Sanborn TA, Jacobs AK, Frederick PD, et al. Comparability of quality-of-care indicators for emergency coronary angioplasty in patients with acute myocardial infarction regardless of on-site cardiac surgery (Report from the National Registry of Myocardial Infarction). *Am J Cardiol* 2004;93:1335–1339.

23. Wharton TP Jr, Grines LL, Turco MA, et al. Primary Angioplasty in Acute Myocardial Infarction at Hospitals With No Surgery On-Site (the PAMI-No SOS study) versus transfer to surgical centers for primary angioplasty. *J Am Coll Cardiol* 2004;43:1943–1950.

24. Antman EM, Anbe DT, Armstrong PW, et al. ACC/AHA guidelines for the management of patients with ST-elevation myocardial infarction—Executive Summary. A report of the American College of Cardiology/American Heart Association Task Force on Practice Guidelines (Committee to Revise the 1999 Guidelines for the Management of Patients With Acute Myocardial Infarction). *JACC* 2004;44:671–719.

25. Iannone LA, Anderson SM, Phillips SJ. Coronary angioplasty for acute myocardial infarction in a hospital without cardiac surgery. *Tex Heart Inst J* 1993;20:99–104.

26. Weaver WE, for the MITI project investigators. PTCA in centers without surgical backup—outcome, logistics and technical aspects. *J Invasive Cardiol* 1997;9:20B–23B.

27. Brush JE, Thompson S, Ciuffo AA, et al. Retrospective comparison of a strategy of primary coronary angioplasty versus intravenous thrombolytic therapy for acute myocardial infarction in a community hospital without cardiac surgical backup. *J Invasive Cardiol* 1996;8:91–98.

28. Moquet B, Huguet RG, Cami G, et al. Primary angioplasty in acute myocardial infarction: a one-year experience in a small urban community. *Arch Mal Coeur Vaiss* 1997;90:11–15.

29. Politi A, Zerboni S, Galli M, et al. Primary angioplasty in acute myocardial infarction: experience and results in the first 1,000 consecutive patients. *Ital Heart J Suppl* 2003;4:755–763.

30. Kutcher MA, Klein LW, Wharton TP, et al. Clinical outcomes in coronary angioplasty centers with off-site versus on-site cardiac surgery capabilities: a preliminary report from the American College of Cardiology-National Cardiovascular Data Registry (abstract). *J Am Coll Cardiol* 2004;43:96a.

31. Singh M, Ting HH, Berger PB, et al. Rationale for on-site cardiac surgery for primary angioplasty: a time for reappraisal. *J Am Coll Cardiol* 2002;39:1881–1889.

32. Wennberg DE, Lucas FL, Siewers AE, et al. Outcomes of percutaneous coronary interventions performed at centers without and with onsite coronary artery bypass graft surgery. *JAMA* 2004;292:1961–1968.

33. Every NR, Maynard C, Schulman K, et al. The association between institutional primary angioplasty procedure volume and outcome in elderly Americans. *J Invasive Cardiol* 2000;12:303–308.

34. Canto JG, Every NR, Magid DJ, et al. The volume of primary angioplasty procedures and survival after acute myocardial infarction. *N Engl J Med* 2000;342:1573–1580.

35. Magid DJ, Calonge BN, Rumsfeld JS, et al. Relation between hospital primary angioplasty volume and mortality for patients with acute MI treated with primary angioplasty vs thrombolytic therapy. *JAMA* 2000;284:3131–3138.

36. Vakili BA, Kaplan R, Brown DL. Volume-outcome relation for physicians and hospitals performing angioplasty for acute myocardial infarction in New York State. *Circulation* 2001;104:2171–2176.

37. Magid DJ, Wang Y, Herrin J, et al. Relationship between time of day, day of week, timeliness of reperfusion, and in-hospital mortality for patients with acute ST-segment elevation myocardial infarction. *JAMA* 2005;294:803–812.

38. Sheldon WC. Trends in cardiac catheterization laboratories in the United States. *Catheter Cardiovasc Interv* 2001;53:40–45.

39. Wharton TP Jr. Nonemergent percutaneous coronary intervention with off-site surgery backup: an emerging new path to access. *Crit Pathways in Cardiol* 2005;4:98–106.

40. Hospital Compare; a quality tool for adults including people with Medicare. United States Department of Health & Human Services; 2005. Available at http:www.hospitalcompare.hhs.gov/. Accessed May 19, 2006.

41. Grines CL, Marsalese DL, Brodie B, et al. Safety and cost-effectiveness of early discharge after primary angioplasty in low risk patients with acute myocardial infarction. PAMI-II investigators. Primary angioplasty in myocardial infarction. *J Am Coll Cardiol* 1998;31:967–972.

42. Smith SC Jr, Dove JT, Jacobs AK, et al. ACC/AHA guidelines for percutaneous coronary intervention: executive summary and recommendations: a report of the American College of Cardiology/American Heart Association Task Force on Practice Guidelines (Committee to Revise the 1993 Guidelines for Percutaneous Transluminal Coronary Angioplasty). *J Am Coll Cardiol* 2001;37:2215–2238.

43. The TIMI Study Group. Effects of tissue plasminogen activator and a comparison of early invasive and conservative strategies in unstable angina and non–Q-wave myocardial infarction: results of the TIMI IIIB trial. Thrombolysis in myocardial ischemia. *Circulation* 1994;89:1545–1556.

44. Scull GS, Martin JS, Weaver WD, et al, for the MITI Investigators. Early angiography versus conservative treatment in patients with non-ST elevation acute myocardial infarction. *J Am Coll Cardiol* 2000;35:895–902.

45. Antman EM, Anbe DT, Armstrong PW, et al. ACC/AHA guidelines for the management of patients with ST-elevation myocardial infarction—Executive Summary: a report of the American College of Cardiology/American Heart Association Task Force on Practice Guidelines (Committee to Revise the 1999 Guidelines for the Management of Patients With Acute Myocardial Infarction). *JACC* 2004;44:684.

46. Schomig A, Mehilli J, Antoniucci, D, et al. Mechanical reperfusion in patients with acute myocardial infarction presenting more than 12 hours from symptom onset. A randomized controlled trial. *JAMA* 2005;293:2965–2972.

47. Gibbons RJ, Grines CL. Acute PCI for ST-segment elevation myocardial infarction. Is later better than never? *JAMA* 2005;293:2930–2932.

48. McNamara NS, Hiett D, Allen B, et al. Can community hospitals provide effective primary PTCA coverage at all hours? *J Am Coll Cardiol* 1997;29:91A(abst).

49. McNamara NS, Wharton TP Jr, Johnston J, et al. Can hospitals with no surgery on site provide effective infarct intervention at all hours? The PAMI-No SOS experience. *Circulation* 1998;98:I-306–I-307(abst).

50. Kereiakes DJ, Gibler WB, Martin LH, et al. Relative importance of emergency medical system transport and the prehospital electrocardiogram on reducing hospital time delay to therapy for acute myocardial infarction: a preliminary report from the Cincinnati Heart Project. *Am Heart J* 1992;123:835–840.

51. Canto JG, Rogers WJ, Bowlby LJ, et al. The prehospital electrocardiogram in acute myocardial infarction: is its full potential being realized? *J Am Coll Cardiol* 1997;29:498–505.

52. Bull GW, Wilcox D. Cardiac alert. *JEMS* 2002;27:2–7,31.

53. Bradley EH, Roumanis SA, Radford MJ, et al. Achieving door-to-balloon times that meet quality guidelines. *J Am Coll Cardiol* 2005;46:1236–1241.

CHAPTER 14 ■ APPROACH TO THE PATIENT WITH COMPLICATED MYOCARDIAL INFARCTION

RICHARD C. BECKER

SETTING THE STAGE FOR COMPLICATIONS
Fundamental Concepts
Cellular Characteristics of Wound Healing
EARLY RISK CHARACTERIZATION
Identification of Patients at High Risk
Non–ST-Segment Elevation MI
RECURRENT ISCHEMIA AND INFARCTION
Recurrent Ischemia
Management
MYOCARDIAL REINFARCTION
Management
CORONARY ANGIOGRAPHY AND PERCUTANEOUS
    CORONARY INTERVENTIONS
Surgical Revascularization
MYOCARDIAL AND MECHANICAL COMPLICATIONS
Right Ventricular Infarction
Management
Left Ventricular Dysfunction
Diastolic Dysfunction
MECHANICAL COMPLICATIONS
Ventricular Septal Rupture
Left Ventricular Free-Wall Rupture
Mitral Regurgitation
Left Ventricular Dilation and Aneurysm Formation
Pseudoaneurysm
PERICARDIAL COMPLICATIONS
Pericarditis
Early Postinfarction Pericarditis
Postmyocardial Infarction Syndrome (Dressler's Syndrome)
Thromboembolic Complications
Pulmonary Embolism
Systemic Embolism
ELECTRICAL COMPLICATIONS
Rhythm and Conduction Disturbances
TREATMENT COMPLICATIONS
Hemorrhage
Antiplatelet Therapy
Heparin Compounds
Hirudin and Other Direct Thrombin Antagonists
Warfarin
Fibrinolytic Therapy
Recombinant Activated Factor VII for Uncontrolled Bleeding

Acute coronary syndromes (ACS) are best defined as atherothrombotic disorders of the coronary arterial system. Although the underlying pathoanatomic substrate exhibits features of chronicity developing slowly over decades, the defining events of plaque disruption, intraluminal thrombosis, and distal embolization are acute and occur suddenly, often without warning. For this reason, clinicians involved directly in the management of patients with ACS must be well versed in a broad range of diagnostic and treatment strategies to rapidly provide the highest possible level of care.

Acute myocardia infarction (MI) is not infrequently complicated by potentially lethal events that can be categorized as vascular (recurrent coronary thrombosis, cardioembolism, or venous thromboembolism), myocardial or mechanical (ventricular dilation, aneurysm formation, pump failure, ventricular septal rupture, papillary muscle rupture, free-wall rupture), pericardial (pericarditis), electrical (heart block, bradyarrhythmias, tachyarrhythmias) and metabolic (Table 14-1 and Fig. 14-1). Most complications occur within the initial 72 hours of infarction; however, the early risk period extends to include the first 4 to 6 weeks. Pharmacologic treatments, including antithrombotic agents and fibrinolytics, can also cause complications that require prompt management. Critical pathways, which represent a readily available and implementable means to facilitate consistently high levels of care among patients with complicated MI, are highlighted in this chapter.

SETTING THE STAGE FOR COMPLICATIONS

Fundamental Concepts

Acute MI, caused most often by coronary arterial thrombosis that impairs myocardial blood flow and tissue perfusion and less commonly as a result of excessive myocardial oxygen demand, is defined pathologically as an irreversible change or death of an individual cell (myocyte) or, in most cases, group of cells. The necrotic process can be identified approximately 6 hours from the onset of myocardial hypoperfusion and is characterized initially by a heavy infiltration of neutrophils that persists for approximately 48 hours. Within 7 days of infarction, the myocardium thins as necrotic tissue is steadily removed by mononuclear cells and phagocytes. Granulation tissue infiltrates the involved region 1 week later and, in essence, covers the entire area by 3 to 4 weeks. Over time (typically within 12 to 16 weeks), the zone of infarction contracts to become a thin, white, firm scar (1–4).

Cellular Characteristics of Wound Healing

The infiltration of inflammatory cells, an immediate response to tissue injury in acute MI, includes neutrophils, lymphocytes, macrophages, and fibroblasts. Collagen degradation, also an early response to myocardial necrosis, involves matrix metalloproteases (MMP) that reside within the myocardium in latent forms (5–8). The abrupt release of inflammatory mediators and MMP contribute to coronary arterial thrombosis and plaque instability, respectively, providing, at least in part, one

TABLE 14-1

COMPLICATIONS OF ACUTE MYOCARDIAL INFARCTION

Vascular complications

Recurrent ischemia
Recurrent infarction

Myocardial complications

Diastolic dysfunction
Systolic dysfunction
Congestive heart failure
Cardiogenic shock
Right ventricular infarction
Ventricular cavity dilation
Aneurysm formation (true, false)

Mechanical complications

Left ventricular free-wall rupture
Ventricular septal rupture
Papillary muscle rupture with acute mitral
regurgitation

Pericardial complications

Pericarditis
Dressler's syndrome
Pericardial effusion

Thromboembolic complications

Mural thrombosis
Systemic thromboembolism
Deep vein thrombosis
Pulmonary embolism

Electrical complications

Ventricular tachycardia
Ventricular fibrillation
Supraventricular tachyarrhythmias
Bradyarrhythmias
Atrioventricular block (1, 2, or 3 degree)

Metabolic Complications

Hyperglycemia
Diabetic ketoacidosis

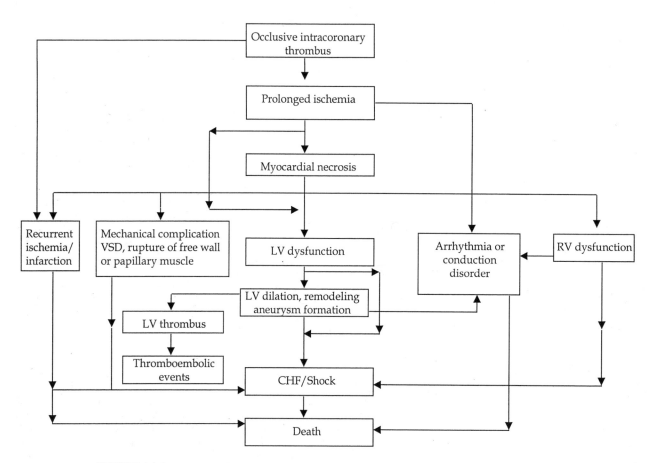

FIGURE 14-1. Pathobiologic and clinical sequence of events in myocardial infarction. CHF, congestive heart failure; LV, left ventricular; RV, right ventricular; VSD, ventricular septal defect.

explanation for the heightened propensity for thromboembolic events that persists following an initial event. These same mediators may also play a role in cellular apoptosis (programmed myocyte death). The inflammatory infiltrate, coupled with a significant degree of surrounding edema, creates a profound effect on electrical conduction and refractory periods. Beyond the "irritability" of necrotic myocardium that can cause *automatic* ventricular arrhythmias, the differing characteristics of injured and healthy myocardium existing "side-by-side" create "dispersion of refractoriness"—the substrate for *re-entrant* ventricular arrhythmias, including ventricular tachycardia and ventricular fibrillation. Lastly, collagenase activity within the myocardium, although designed to permit "rebuilding" of the damaged area, may initially weaken the infarct zone, increasing the risk of cardiac rupture.

The fibrous stage of wound healing follows an initial inflammatory stage. Increased synthesis of fibrillar type III collagen and, over the subsequent days to weeks, type I collagen, provides an organized "scaffold" for scar development that follows. It is during this stage that most myocardial remodeling takes place, including expansion of both the infarct- and noninfarct-related zones, leading to aneurysm formation and ventricular dilation.

In the final stage, fibrillar fibronectin and collagen are deposited and by 4 to 6 weeks most of the necrotic myocardium has been removed and replaced by fibrous scar tissue. As with the initial or inflammatory stage, the late scarring stage is characterized by marked heterogeneity of repolarization and refractory periods, creating a permissive environment for malignant arrhythmias.

EARLY RISK CHARACTERIZATION

A vital component of clinical practice and critical care medicine is an ability to anticipate complications either of the MI itself or of its treatment. The development and utilization of risk-assessment scales facilitates a response to potentially life-threatening events and represents the logical "first" step in patient-specific management pathways.

Identification of Patients at High Risk

Early Clinical Phase

Risk stratification schemes for patients with ST-segment elevation MI (STEMI) have been developed by several experienced clinical trial groups, highlighting the importance of patient demographics, medical history, clinical features, and the presenting electrocardiogram (ECG). The Thrombolysis in Myocardial Infarction (TIMI) study investigators (9) established a risk score that predicted, with considerable accuracy, the occurrence of early morbidity and mortality.

Predictors of early (30-day) mortality were also established by the GUSTO (Global Utilization of Streptokinase and tPA for Occluded Coronary Arteries) investigators (10). In a trial including more than 40,000 patients with acute MI, age was identified as the most significant factor, with death rates of 1.1% in the youngest decile (<45 years) and 20.5% in patients more than 75 years of age. Overall, five characteristics contained 90% of the prognostic information in the baseline clinical data—they included age, lower systolic blood pressure, higher Killip class, elevated heart rate, and anterior site of infarction (Figs. 14-2 and 14-3).

The National Registry of Myocardial Infarction (NRMI) risk assessment assignment was developed as a readily available, bedside clinical "scorecard" for rapid triage and management. Predictors of adverse in-hospital clinical outcomes were identified from more than 100,000 patients with MI (11).

Presenting Surface Electrocardiogram

Clinicians have recognized for some time that the sum of ST-segment "shifts" on the presenting ECG is a reliable marker of infarction size and, as a result, can provide important diagnostic (and prognostic) information. The initial ECG may also contain evidence of a prior MI, identifying patients at increased risk for an early adverse outcome (Fig. 14-4) (12). ST-segment area also provides prognostic information.

Cardiac Enzyme Analysis

Biochemical markers of myocardial necrosis approximate infarction size and, in general, provide an estimate of clinical

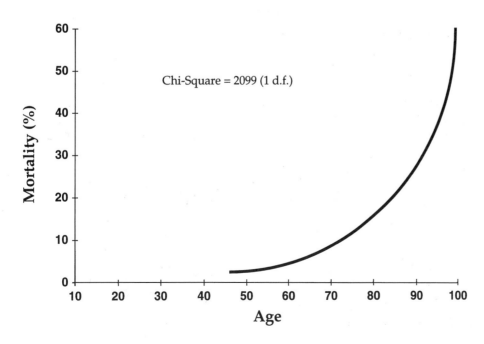

FIGURE 14-2. Relationship between age and mortality (30-day) in the Global Utilization of Streptokinase and tPA for Occluded Coronary Arteries (GUSTO)-1 study. (From Anderson RD, Ohman EM. Successful identification and management of high-risk patients with acute myocardial infarction. *J Thromb Thrombolysis* 1996;3:271–278, with permission.)

Chi-Square = 2099 (1 d.f.)

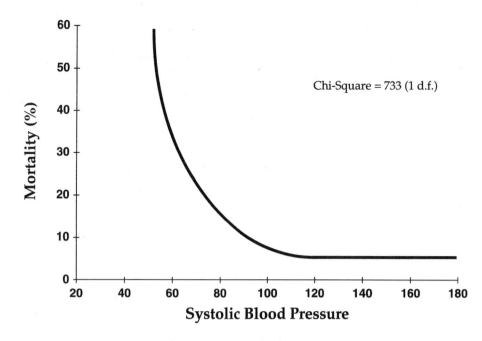

FIGURE 14-3. Relationship between presenting systolic blood pressure and mortality (30-day) in the Global Utilization of Streptokinase and tPA for Occluded Coronary Arteries (GUSTO)-1 study. (From Anderson RD, Ohman EM. Successful identification and management of high-risk patients with acute myocardial infarction. *J Thromb Thrombolysis* 1996;3:271–278, with permission.)

outcome. The alteration of pharmacokinetics, particularly for creatine kinase (CK), following coronary reperfusion has complicated the picture somewhat. In essence, when calculated correctly, the "area under the curve" does provide prognostic information, but this measurement requires time (serial CK determinations) and effort.

The prognostic value of cardiac-specific troponin T and I among patients with unstable angina and non–ST-segment elevation MI is recognized; however, data from the Global Use of Strategies To open Occluded Arteries (GUSTO) IIA trial (13) also suggest that an elevated troponin T (>0.1 ng/mL) on hospital presentation correlates strongly and independently with hospital mortality among patients with STEMI.

Inflammatory Markers

The measurement of inflammatory markers represents an important tool that links the triad of atherosclerosis, inflammation, and thrombosis. Recent observations with the acute phase reactant amyloid A protein in all likelihood will open the door to a vast array of markers that ultimately can be used to determine the "activity" of disease and direct response to treatment (14).

Risk for Stroke

Stroke is the most feared and devastating complication of fibrinolytic therapy (15). Overall, 60% of patients with hemor-

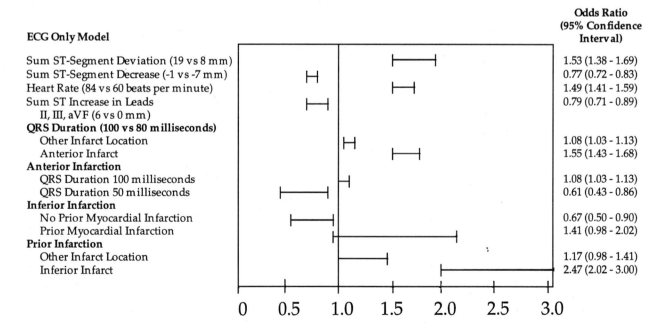

FIGURE 14-4. Electrocardiographic model to determine risk for 30-day mortality after acute myocardial infarction. The sum of ST-segment deviation was the most powerful predictor of a poor outcome. (From Hathaway WR, Peterson ED, Wagner GS, et al. Prognostic significance of the initial electrocardiogram in patients with acute myocardial infarction. *JAMA* 1998;279:387–391, with permission.)

TABLE 14-2

RISK FACTORS AND PREDICTORS OF HEMORRHAGIC STROKE FOLLOWING THROMBOLYSIS: GUSTO-1 TRIAL

Age

Low body weight

Prior cerebrovascular disease

Diastolic blood pressure

History of hypertension (particularly with increased age)

Combination fibrinolytic therapy

Systolic blood pressure

Tissue plasminogen activator (compared with streptokinase)

GUSTO, Global Utilization of Streptokinase and tPA for Occluded Coronary Arteries: Phase 1 Trial.

From Gore JM, Granger CB, Simoons ML, et al. Stroke after thrombolysis. Mortality and functional outcomes in the GUSTO-1 trial. *Circulation* 1995;92:2811–2818, with permission.

rhagic stroke die, whereas 25% are left with at least a moderate degree of disability (Table 14-2).

Non–ST-Segment Elevation MI

The medical community has placed considerable emphasis on the early management of patients with STEMI or bundle branch block MI because of the profound impact of early reperfusion on patient outcome. It has become clear that patients with non–ST-segment elevation MI also require careful consideration, not solely because of their recognized risk for cardiac events over the subsequent 6 to 12 months, but also because a substantial number of patients are at risk for in-hospital death.

A total of 183,113 patients with non–ST-segment elevation MI were identified in NRMI-2 (16). Risk factors for in-hospital death included advanced age (odds ratio [OR] 1.51), female sex (OR 1.20), history of diabetes (OR 1.22), prior congestive heart failure (OR 1.30), and Killip class II, III, and IV (OR 1.61, 1.94, and 21.4, respectively) (Table 14-3).

TABLE 14-3

PREDICTORS OF IN-HOSPITAL DEATH (AFTER 24 H)[a]

Variable	Odds ratio	95th CI
Aspirin (<24 h)	0.46	0.43–0.48
Oral beta-blocker (<24 h)	0.59	0.55–0.63
ACE inhibitor (<24 h)	0.66	0.62–0.71
Normal ECG	0.78	0.70–0.85
ST-segment depression	1.13	1.06–1.20
Prior stroke	1.39	1.29–1.49
Killip class III or IV	8.72	8.56–8.80

ACE, angiotensin-converting enzyme; CI, confidence interval; ECG, electrocardiogram.
[a]Multivariate logistic regression analysis.

RECURRENT ISCHEMIA AND INFARCTION

Recurrent Ischemia

The two most common cardiac causes of recurrent chest pain among hospitalized patients with acute MI are acute pericarditis and myocardial ischemia; the latter occurs more often and is a marker of poor outcome. Recurrent myocardial ischemia occurs in 15% to 20% of patients and is typically transient (17). It does, however, identify patients with a persistently unstable atherosclerotic plaque and heightened thrombotic potential, as well as those with multivessel coronary artery disease or compromised collateral circulation (18).

Patients with recurrent ischemia can be further stratified according to ECG changes, hemodynamic stability, and overall clinical status. Three distinct categories of patients have been identified as being at increased risk for postinfarction angina and reinfarction: (a) patients with non–ST-segment elevation MI, (b) patients receiving fibrinolytic therapy, and (c) patients with multiple cardiac risk factors (19). The incidence of postinfarction angina is nearly twice as high after non–ST-segment elevation MI (25% to 35%) than after ST-segment elevation or bundle branch block MI (15% to 20%). Patients treated with fibrinolytics have a 20% to 30% incidence of recurrent ischemia and a 4% to 5% incidence of reinfarction, even with the concomitant use of aspirin and adjunctive anticoagulant strategies (20).

Management

Recurrent ischemia must be recognized promptly and managed aggressively. Pain relief is best approached in the context of myocardial oxygen supply and demand. Based on this fundamental construct, myocardial oxygen demand can be lowered by decreasing heart rate, inotropic state (using intravenous or oral beta-blockers), and preload (most commonly with nitrate preparations). Morphine sulfate, in low doses, is also useful in early management. A calcium channel blocker can be added, if needed, to control heart rate, to prevent episodic coronary vasospasm, or as an alternative to beta-blocker therapy when absolute contraindications exist. Antiplatelet (aspirin ± clopidogrel) therapy should be continued and anticoagulation with intravenous unfractionated heparin or low-molecular-weight heparin (LMWH) instituted (or continued) for patients with ischemic chest pain at rest. In addition, consideration should be given to the addition of a GP IIb/IIIa antagonist. Anxiolytics such as benzodiazepines can also be used, as needed, to reduce anxiety and provide mild sedation. The goals of therapy are to reduce mean arterial blood pressure and heart rate by approximately 10% to 20%, but not to a level where coronary arterial perfusion pressure is compromised. In clinically unstable patients with evidence of congestive heart failure, volume status must be assessed carefully and treated appropriately.

When aggressive pharmacologic therapy does not alleviate the myocardial ischemia or if concomitant hemodynamic instability exists, early diagnostic coronary angiography is recommended. Consideration should also be given to inserting an intra-aortic balloon pump to improve myocardial perfusion and serve as a "bridge" to definitive therapy (revascularization, correction of mechanical defects) in hemodynamically unstable patients and those with angina refractory to medical therapy

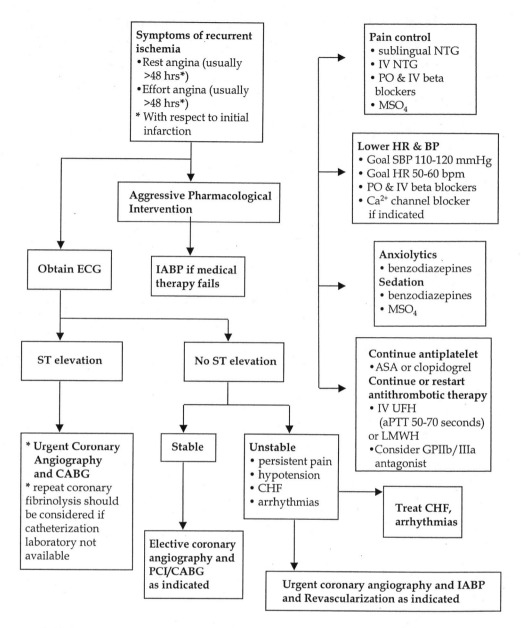

FIGURE 14-5. The management of recurrent ischemia is determined by clinical signs and symptoms, electrocardiographic features, hemodynamic status, and angiographic findings. ASA, aspirin; CABG, coronary artery bypass grafting; CHF, congestive heart failure; HR, heart rate; MSO_4, morphine sulfate; NTG, nitroglycerin; PCI, percutaneous coronary intervention; SBP, systolic blood pressure.

Serial ECGs and clinical assessment are recommended to guide optimal management (Fig. 14-5).

MYOCARDIAL REINFARCTION

Reinfarction represents a recurrent atherothrombotic event with subsequent myocardial necrosis. The diagnosis can be difficult to confirm within the initial 24 hours of the index event because serum cardiac markers have not yet returned to a normal range. Thus, confirmation must be established in the context of an existing elevation with further (usually twofold) elevation of cardiac enzymes above a prior level (determined within the previous 6 hours). Beta-adrenergic blockers have been shown to reduce the risk of reinfarction, whereas fibrino-lytic therapy is associated with a slightly increased risk

(21,22). Heart-rate-slowing calcium channel blockers may reduce the rate of reinfarction among patients with preserved left ventricular (LV) function after acute MI, whereas the role of unfractionated heparin is controversial (23). In contrast, the available data strongly support the ability of LMWH and GP IIb/IIIa receptor antagonists to reduce the likelihood of recurrent MI in patients with non–ST-segment elevation MI and possibly in STEMI or bundle branch block MI as well (24,25).

Management

The clinical approach to recurrent MI, as with recurrent myocardial ischemia, is determined by the patient's overall clinical status and early indicators of injury (Fig. 14-6).

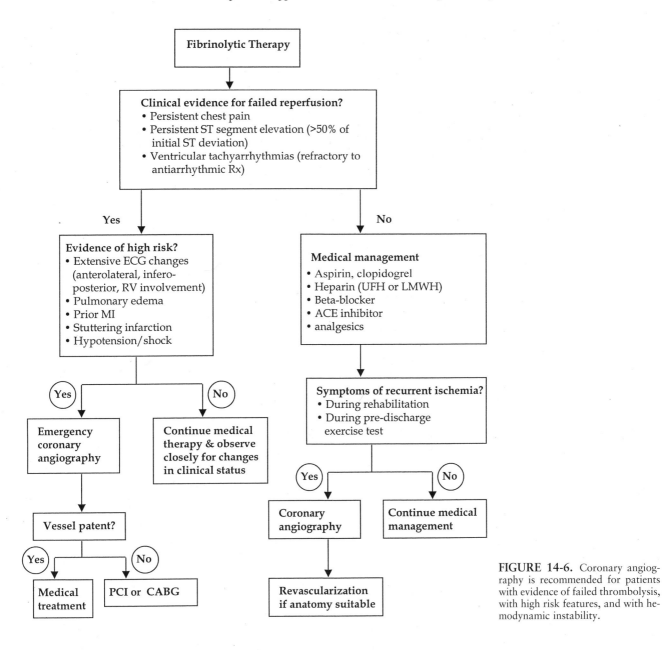

FIGURE 14-6. Coronary angiography is recommended for patients with evidence of failed thrombolysis, with high risk features, and with hemodynamic instability.

CORONARY ANGIOGRAPHY AND PERCUTANEOUS CORONARY INTERVENTIONS

Early recurrent myocardial ischemia, persistent ST-segment elevation (>50% of maximal ST-segment deviation), hemodynamic instability, and ventricular tachyarrhythmias refractory to antiarrhythmic therapy are indications for early coronary angiography (26). The American College of Cardiology/American Heart Association Guidelines for Coronary Angiography and Percutaneous Coronary Intervention are outlined in Table 14-4.

Surgical Revascularization

Although the procedure is typically reserved for a carefully selected patient, outcomes following emergent surgical revascularization have improved over time as a result of increasing experience; the application of mechanical, hemodynamic, or circulatory support measures; and advanced methods of myocardial protection and anesthetic management (Table 14-5).

Surgical intervention for mechanical complications of MI and cardiac transplantation will be discussed in a subsequent section.

MYOCARDIAL AND MECHANICAL COMPLICATIONS

Right Ventricular Infarction

Right ventricular (RV) infarction encompasses a complex spectrum of pathologic and clinical presentations, ranging from asymptomatic mild RV dysfunction to overt cardiogenic shock. RV infarction complicates 35% to 50% of inferior MIs, which in turn make up 40% to 50% of all acute MIs. The diagnosis of RV extension is important because of its association with a higher mortality rate (25% to 30%) (27). Only a small percentage (~5%) of patients with acute MI present with isolated RV infarction.

TABLE 14-4

EARLY INVASIVE EVALUATION IN PATIENTS WITH STEMI

Class I

1. Coronary arteriography should be performed in patients with spontaneous episodes of myocardial ischemia or episodes of myocardial ischemia provoked by minimal exertion during recovery from STEMI (Level of Evidence: A).

2. Coronary arteriography should be performed for intermediate- or high-risk findings on noninvasive testing after STEMI (Level of Evidence: B).

3. Coronary arteriography should be performed if patients are sufficiently stable before definitive therapy of a mechanical complication of STEMI, such as acute MR, VSD, pseudoaneurysm, or LV aneurysm (Level of Evidence: B).

4. Coronary arteriography should be performed in patients with persistent hemodynamic instability (Level of Evidence: B).

5. Coronary arteriography should be performed in survivors of STEMI who had clinical heart failure during the acute episode but subsequently demonstrated well-preserved LV function (Level of Evidence: C).

Class IIa

1. It is reasonable to perform coronary arteriography when STEMI is suspected to have occurred by a mechanism other than thrombotic occlusion of an atherosclerotic plaque. This would include coronary embolism, certain metabolic or hematological diseases, or coronary artery spasm (Level of Evidence: C).

2. Coronary arteriography is reasonable in STEMI patients with any of the following: diabetes mellitus, LVEF less than 0.40, CHF, prior revascularization, or life-threatening ventricular arrhythmias (Level of Evidence: C).

Class IIb

1. Catheterization and revascularization may be considered part of a strategy of routine coronary arteriography for risk assessment after fibrinolytic therapy (Level of Evidence: C).

From Antman EM, Anbe DT, Armstrong PW, et al. ACC/AHA guidelines for the management of patients with ST-elevation myocardial infarction—executive summary: a report of the American College of Cardiology/American Heart Association Task Force on Practice Guidelines (Writing Committee to Revise the 1999 Guidelines for the Management of Patients With Acute Myocardial Infarction). *J Am Coll Cardiol* 2004;44:671–719, with permission.

The clinical triad of hypotension, clear lung fields, and increased jugular venous pressure in a patient experiencing an inferior MI strongly supports the diagnosis of RV extension. A right-sided S_3 gallop or Kussmaul's sign (distention of the jugular veins during inspiration) may also be present on physical examination. Other potential clinical features of RV infarction include tricuspid regurgitation, sinoatrial (SA) or atrioventricular (AV) nodal conduction disturbances, and AV dissociation. The ECG reveals ST-segment elevation of more than 0.5 mm in V_4R. A Q wave in this lead is considered a nonspecific finding. Other available modalities that can be used to diagnose RV infarction include thallium or sestamibi perfusion imaging, echocardiography, cardiac magnetic resonance imaging (MRI), and through hemodynamic measurements obtained using a pulmonary artery catheter.

Complications of acute RV infarction, in most instances, are a manifestation of both LV and RV dysfunction, as well as increased parasympathetic tone (Table 14-6). Overt cardiogenic shock, although occurring rarely, is the most serious complication. High-degree AV block is not uncommon and identifies a patient at particularly high risk. Atrial fibrillation occurs in one-third of patients with RV infarction as a result of concomitant right atrial infarction or dilation caused by volume and pressure overload. Other potential complications of RV infarction include ventricular septal rupture (particularly in patients with concomitant transmural posterior septal infarction), RV thrombus formation with subsequent pulmonary embolism, tricuspid regurgitation, and a high incidence of pericarditis, most likely because of the frequent transmural injury pattern of the thin-walled RV. The development of a right-to-left shunt through a patent foramen ovale is a complication unique to RV infarction and should be suspected when severe hypoxia is not responsive to supplemental oxygen therapy (28).

Management

As with all ST-segment elevation MI, the initial approach to patients with RV infarction must address the need for early reperfusion therapy directed at limiting infarct size (Fig. 14-7). Fibrinolytic therapy and primary angioplasty, when successful, improve RV ejection fraction and reduce the incidence of complete heart block. If hemodynamic compromise is present, measures should be implemented to maintain RV preload, reduce RV afterload, and support the dysfunctional RV with pharmacologic inotropic agents. The requirement for volume (preload-dependent state) differentiates the treatment of RV infarction

TABLE 14-5

1. Timing of Surgery

Class IIa

1. In patients who have had a STEMI, CABG mortality is elevated for the first 3 to 7 days after infarction, and the benefit of revascularization must be balanced against this increased risk. Patients who have been stabilized (no ongoing ischemia, hemodynamic compromise, or life-threatening arrhythmia) after STEMI and who have incurred a significant fall in LV function should have their surgery delayed to allow myocardial recovery to occur. If critical anatomy exists, revascularization should be undertaken during the index hospitalization (Level of Evidence: B).

The Writing Committee believes that if stable STEMI patients with preserved LV function require surgical revascularization, then CABG can be undertaken within several days of the infarction without an increased risk.

2. Arterial Grafting

Class I

1. An internal mammary artery graft to a significantly stenosed left anterior descending coronary artery should be used whenever possible in patients undergoing CABG after STEMI (Level of Evidence: B).

3. CABG for Recurrent Ischemia After STEMI

Class I

1. Urgent CABG is indicated if the coronary angiogram reveals anatomy that is unsuitable for PCI (Level of Evidence: B).

4. Elective CABG Surgery after STEMI in Patients with Angina

Class I

1. CABG is recommended for patients with stable angina who have significant left main coronary artery stenosis (Level of Evidence: A).

2. CABG is recommended for patients with stable angina who have left main equivalent disease: significant (at least 70%) stenosis of the proximal left anterior descending coronary artery and proximal left circumflex artery (Level of Evidence: A).

3. CABG is recommended for patients with stable angina who have three-vessel disease (survival benefit is greater when LVEF is less than 0.50) (Level of Evidence: A).

4. CABG is beneficial for patients with stable angina who have one- or two-vessel coronary disease without significant proximal left anterior descending coronary artery stenosis but with a large area of viable myocardium and high-risk criteria on noninvasive testing (Level of Evidence: B).

5. CABG is recommended in patients with stable angina who have two-vessel disease with significant proximal left anterior descending coronary artery stenosis and either ejection fraction less than 0.50 or demonstrable ischemia on noninvasive testing (Level of Evidence: A).

From Antman EM, Anbe DT, Armstrong PW, et al. ACC/AHA guidelines for the management of patients with ST-elevation myocardial infarction—executive summary: a report of the American College of Cardiology/American Heart Association Task Force on Practice Guidelines (Writing Committee to Revise the 1999 Guidelines for the Management of Patients With Acute Myocardial Infarction). *J Am Coll Cardiol* 2004;44: 671–719, with permission.

TABLE 14-6

POTENTIAL COMPLICATIONS OF RIGHT VENTRICULAR INFARCTION

Cardiogenic shock

High-degree atrioventricular block

Atrial fibrillation or atrial flutter

Ventricular tachycardia or fibrillation

Ventricular septal rupture

Right ventricular thrombus with or without pulmonary embolism

Tricuspid regurgitation

Pericarditis

Right-to-left shunt via patent foramen ovale

from that of "pure" LV infarction. Volume expansion is the mainstay of therapy, with the goal of maintaining a right atrial or central venous pressure between 12 and 15 mm Hg. Normal saline (250 to 500 mL) given as a bolus should be used acutely, with an appreciation that a large volume of fluid may be required to sufficiently increase RV filling pressure, LV preload, and cardiac output. If volume support does not produce hemodynamic improvement, a pulmonary artery catheter may be required to guide further management.

Patients with persistent hypotension (despite volume resuscitation) may benefit from inotropic support with either dobutamine or dopamine. Because of their potential to reduce preload, vasodilators, including nitroglycerin and morphine sulfate, routinely used in the management of LV infarctions, should be used with great caution in patients with RV infarction. Another crucial factor in sustaining adequate preload is the maintenance of AV synchrony. In patients with high-degree AV block, dual-chamber pacing may be required, particularly if ventricular pacing does not cause an improvement in the patient's overall clinical status (29). Atrial fibrillation can cause profound hemodynamic deterioration, necessitating prompt cardioversion. In patients with biventricular failure, circulatory support using intra-aortic balloon counterpulsation may be required followed by coronary angiography and either percuta-

+ If hemodynamically unstable, refer to Figure 14-9, 14-10, and 14-12
+ Refer to Figure 6
++ Refer to Figure 5
+++ Non-complicated MI

	Day 0 Emergency Department	Day 0 CCU	Day 1 CCU	Day 2+++ Step Down Unit	Day 3+++ Step Down Unit	Pre-Discharge +++
Assessment	• Vitals • Continuous ECG monitoring • Secure venous access	• Vitals q2-4° • Continuous ECG monitoring	• Vitals q4° • Continuous ECG monitoring	• Vitals q8°	• Vitals q8°	• Vitals AM
Benchmark	• Reperfusion Rx* • Salvage myocardium • Treat arrhythmias • Maintain hemodynamic stability	• Pain relief* • Hemodynamically stable • Oxygenating	• Afebrile* • Hemodynamically stable • Oxygenating	• No recurrent chest pain++ • No sign of CHF • No arrhythmias	• Ambulating without difficulty	• Discuss EMS options • Discuss recommendation for seeking medical care
Medication	• ± fibrinolytic + • ß-blocker • Aspirin • Unfractionated Heparin	• Heparin • Aspirin, clopidogrel • ß-blocker • ACE-inhibitor • Statin	• Heparin (SC) • Aspirin, clopidogrel • ß-blocker • ACE-inhibitor • Statin	• Aspirin, clopidogrel • ß-blocker • ACE-inhibitor • Statin	• Aspirin, clopidogrel • ß-blocker • ACE-inhibitor • Statin	• Medication education • Prescriptions (including sublingual nitroglycerin)
Laboratory Tests	• CBC • Chem-20 • CK, CK-MB • ± Troponin • Lipid profile • INR, aPTT	• CBC • Chem-6 • CK, CK-MB q8° X 3 • APTT	• CBC • Chem-7	• Chem-7	• Chem-7	• Fasting lipid profile • CRP 4 weeks post-discharge
Diagnostic/ Interventional Procedures	• 12-lead ECG • ± echocardiogram • ± coronary angiography • ± IABP (for shock)	• 12-lead ECG • ± echocardiogram • ± coronary angiography • ± IABP (for shock)	• 12-lead ECG	• 12-lead ECG	• Modified ETT • ± coronary angiography	• Standard ETT 2 weeks post-discharge • ± echocardiograpm
Nutrition	• NPO	• NPO	• AHA Step II	• AHA Step II	• AHA Step II	• AHA Step II
Activity	• Bed rest	• Bed rest	• Bed to chair	• Ambulate.	• Routine activity	• Routine activity
Case Management	• Notify primary care physician • Notify case manager	• Notify social services	• Cardiac rehabilitation consult	• Lipid management • Family education • Smoking cessation	• Nutrition consult	• Discuss medication/ insurance coverage • Notify primary care physician • Schedule return visit

FIGURE 14-7. Acute cardiac care-interdisciplinary management pathway for STEMI.

neous or surgical intervention as the findings and clinical status dictate (Fig. 14-8).

Left Ventricular Dysfunction

The extent of LV compromise, which correlates directly with the extent of myocardial damage, is a major determinant of clinical outcome (Fig. 14-9). Anterior site of infarction is commonly associated with extensive LV damage, reduced ventricular performance, and reduced survival. The Killip classification separates patients into four distinct groups based on existing clinical signs and symptoms of LV failure. Increasing Killip class, which represents progressively severe LV compromise, is associated strongly with a poor prognosis (Table 14-7).

The immediate functional consequences of acute myocardial ischemia and infarction include both systolic and diastolic ventricular dysfunction; either can compromise ventricular performance and lead to congestive heart failure. Diastolic dysfunction (impaired ventricular relaxation) occurs uniformly in patients with acute MI, but is clinically evident in only 20% to 30% of patients. When it does occur, diastolic dysfunction often precedes systolic dysfunction and is the most common cause of early congestive heart failure. Systolic dysfunction, also known as pump failure (typically forward and backward failure), is a serious complication of acute MI. The sudden loss

of contractile function decreases stroke volume and increases end-systolic volume, end-diastolic volume, and diastolic filling pressure. The clinical manifestations of systolic dysfunction include decreased forward flow (perfusion) and increased backward flow (pulmonary congestion and edema).

The loss of contractile function in the initial minutes to hours of MI is potentially reversible, particularly with successful coronary reperfusion. Myocardial "stunning" as a cause for systolic dysfunction is also a reversible component of myocardial dysfunction (30). Stunned myocardium, in some instances, responds to pharmacologic inotropic stimulation (31).

Hemodynamic instability associated with LV systolic dysfunction is an indication for placement of a pulmonary artery catheter to determine intracardiac pressures, cardiac output, and systemic vascular resistance and to guide patient management. A diagnosis of LV failure is supported by increased pulmonary artery (particularly diastolic) and pulmonary capillary wedge pressures (PCWP), decreased cardiac index, and an elevated systemic vascular resistance.

Cardiogenic shock complicates 5% to 15% of all infarctions (32) and typically occurs when myocardial necrosis involves more than 40% of the LV (33). It is the most common cause of in-hospital death among patients with MI, with a mortality rate exceeding 50%. Clinically, cardiogenic shock is characterized by hypotension and hypoperfusion of vital organs. Hemo-

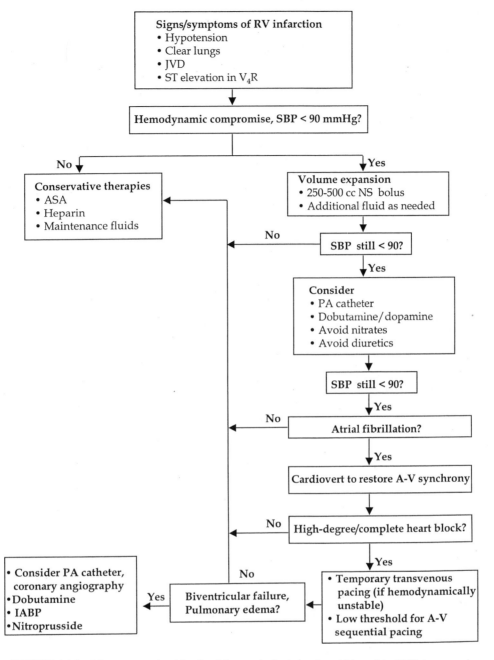

FIGURE 14-8. Management algorithm for right ventricular infarction. ASA, aspirin; IABP, intra-aortic balloon pump; JVD, jugular venous distention; NS, normal saline; PA, pulmonary artery; SBP, systolic blood pressure.

dynamic disturbances as measured by a pulmonary artery catheter include elevated PCWP and a markedly reduced cardiac output (Tables 14-8 and 14-9). Complications of acute MI other than severe LV dysfunction can also cause cardiogenic shock, including extensive RV infarction, ventricular septal rupture, papillary muscle rupture or ischemic papillary muscle dysfunction with severe mitral regurgitation, and ventricular free-wall rupture with cardiac tamponade.

Diastolic Dysfunction

The comprehensive management of LV diastolic dysfunction must concomitantly address ongoing myocardial ischemia and pulmonary congestion. Intravenous furosemide is considered the diuretic of choice for patients not previously receiving diuretics. Larger doses may be required among patients previously on diuretic therapy and for those with compromised renal function. Excessive diuresis should be avoided to prevent a decline in coronary arterial perfusion pressure.

Beta-blockade is an important treatment consideration in patients with isolated ischemic diastolic dysfunction. Beta-blockers not only reduce myocardial oxygen demand, but also improve LV compliance (lusitropy) and reduce LV filling pressures and, as a result, pulmonary congestion. Caution is recommended when systolic and diastolic dysfunction coexist. In this setting, diuresis should be achieved before initiating beta-blocker therapy.

Preload- and afterload-reducing agents can be used to reduce pulmonary venous pressures. Nitroprusside is an arterio-

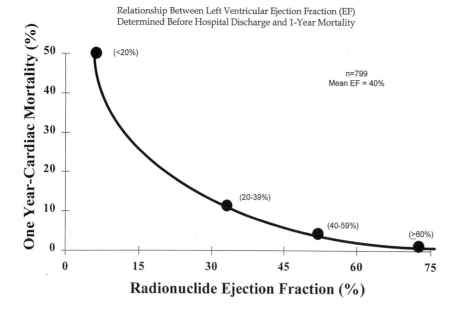

Relationship Between Left Ventricular Ejection Fraction (EF)
Determined Before Hospital Discharge and 1-Year Mortality

FIGURE 14-9. Left ventricular performance is the strongest independent predictor of long-term mortality following acute myocardial infarction. (From Multicenter Postinfarction Research Group. Risk stratification and survival after myocardial infarction. *N Engl J Med* 1983; 309:331, with permission.)

lar and venodilator that lessens both afterload and preload. This agent is particularly useful in situations where ischemic diastolic dysfunction complicates existing systolic dysfunction. Nitroglycerin reduces preload and improves both coronary arterial blood flow and myocardial perfusion. For this reason, it is an important therapeutic adjunct in patients with ischemia-mediated congestive heart failure. Because of rapid titratability, intravenous administration is preferred in the coronary care unit setting.

The management of LV systolic dysfunction, when severe, is dictated by specific hemodynamic disturbances as reflected in PCWP, cardiac output (CO), systemic vascular resistance, and systemic blood pressure (BP) (Table 14-10). However, in most patients with uncomplicated MI and mild LV failure, invasive hemodynamic monitoring is not required. Frequent assessment is needed of the patient's cardiopulmonary status, mental status, skin and mucous membranes, cardiac rhythm and heart rate, oxygenation, and urine output. In most patients with systolic dysfunction that is mild in severity, conventional therapy with morphine; nasal oxygen; intravenous, oral, or transdermal nitrates; and gentle diuresis will yield clinical improvement.

The initial management of patients with severe congestive heart failure must include a careful evaluation of oxygenation and acid–base balance; occasionally, endotracheal intubation with ventilatory support is necessary. In the setting of severe LV dysfunction associated with hypotension, intravenous inotropic agents (e.g., dopamine and dobutamine) should be administered. In addition to inotropic support, preload and afterload reduction may be required to augment forward flow and reduce pulmonary congestion. Diuretics and nitrates will diminish pulmonary congestion; however, overall improve-

TABLE 14-7

KILLIP CLASSIFICATION OF PATIENTS WITH ACUTE MYOCARDIAL INFARCTION

Class	Clinical definition	Patients at hospital admission (%)	Mortality[a] (%)
I	No clinical signs of heart failure	30–40	8
II	Rales over ≤50% of lungs, S₃ gallop	30–50	30
III	Rales over >50% of lungs, pulmonary edema	5–10	44
IV	Cardiogenic shock	10	80–100

[a]Prereperfusion or interventional era.
From Killip T, Kimball JT. Treatment of myocardial infarction in a coronary care unit. A two year experience with 250 patients. *Am J Cardiol* 1967;20:457–464.

TABLE 14-8

SIGNS, SYMPTOMS, AND COMMON CHARACTERISTICS OF CARDIOGENIC SHOCK

Clinical
Evidence of hypoperfusion
Cold, clammy, or mottled skin (livedo reticularis)
Impaired mentation (agitation, obtundation, confusion)
Oliguria (<30 mL/h)
Evidence of primary cardiac abnormality

Hemodynamic
Systolic blood pressure <90 mm Hg (mean arterial pressure <65 mm Hg or >20% decrease from baseline)
PCWP ≥20 mm Hg
CI <2.0 L /min/m²[a]

[a] While receiving inotropic support.

CI, cardiac index; PCWP, pulmonary capillary wedge pressure.

TABLE 14-9

HEMODYNAMIC PARAMETERS IN COMMONLY ENCOUNTERED CLINICAL SITUATIONS (IDEALIZED)[a]

CI	SVR	RA	PVR	RV	PA	PAWP	AO
Normal							
≥2.5	1,500	0–6	≤250	25/0–6	25/6–12	6–12	130/80
Hypovolemic shock							
<2.0	>1,500	0–2	≤250	15–20/0–2	15–20/2–6	2–6	≤90/60
Cardiogenic shock							
<2.0	>1,500	8	≤20	50/8	50/35	35	≤90/60
Septic shock							
Early							
≥2.5	<1,500	0–2	<250	20–25/0–2	20–25/0–2	0–6	≤90/60
Late							
<2.0	>1,500	0–4	>250	25/4–10	25/4–10	4–10	≤90/60
Acute massive pulmonary embolism							
<2.0	>1,500	8–12	>450	50/12	50/12–15	≤12	≤90/60
Cardiac tamponade							
<2.0	>1,500	12–18	≤250	25/12–18	25/12–18	12–18	≤90/60
AMI without LVF							
≤2.5	1,500	0–6	≤250	25/0–6	25/12–18	≤18	140/90
AMI with LVF							
>2.0	>1,500	0–6	>250	30–40/0–6	30–40/18–25	>18	140/90
Biventricular failure secondary to LVF							
~2.0	>1,500	>6	>250	50–60/>6	50–60/25	18–25	120/80
RVF secondary to RVI							
<2.0	>1,500	12–20	>250	30/12–20	30/12	<12	≤90/60
Cor pulmonale							
<2.0	>1,500	>6	>500	80/>6	80/35	<12	100/60
Idiopathic pulmonary hypertension							
<2.0	>1,500	0–6	>500	80–100/0–6	80–100/40	<12	100/60
Acute VSR[b]							
<2.0	>1,500	6	>250	60/6–8	60/35	30	≤90/60

AMI, acute myocardial infarction; AO, aortic; CI, cardiac index; LVF, left ventricular failure; PA, pulmonary artery; PAWP, pulmonary artery wedge pressure; PVR, pulmonary vascular resistance; RA, right atrium; RV, right ventricle; RVI, right ventricular infarction; RVF, right ventricular failure; SVR, systemic vascular resistance; VSR, ventricular septal rupture.
[a]Hemodynamic profile seen in approximately one-third of patients in late septic shock.
[b]Confirmed by appropriate RA–PA oxygen saturation step-up.
From Voyce S. *Intensive care medicine.* Philadelphia: Lippincott-Raven Publishers; 2004, with permission.

ment in CO may not occur, and in fact, systemic BP may decrease. Nitroprusside, through a reduction of both preload and afterload, will commonly increase CO, reduce LV end-diastolic pressure, and alleviate pulmonary congestion. In the early hours of acute MI, when ischemia often contributes substantially to LV dysfunction, nitroglycerin is a preferred agent as it causes a greater degree of venodilation than does nitroprusside. The phosphodiesterase inhibitors amrinone and milrinone exhibit inotropic and vasodilating properties and, for this reason,

should be considered, particularly in patients with reduced LV systolic function who have been treated previously with beta-blockers. Inotropic and vasodilator therapies must be carefully titrated to maintain a systolic BP of at least 90 mm Hg (mean arterial pressure ≥65 mm Hg). Once BP has remained stable for 60 to 90 minutes, diuresis can usually be initiated safely.

Patients with severe LV dysfunction, depressed CO, elevated LV diastolic pressure, a mean systemic BP less than 65 mm Hg (or reduced by ≥30% of baseline), and evidence of vital

TABLE 14-10

INDICATIONS FOR HEMODYNAMIC MONITORING ASSESSMENT FOLLOWING ACUTE MYOCARDIAL INFARCTION

Class I

1. Pulmonary artery catheter monitoring should be performed for the following:

   a. Progressive hypotension, when unresponsive to fluid administration or when fluid administration may be contraindicated (Level of Evidence: C).

   b. Suspected mechanical complications of STEMI, (i.e., VSD, papillary muscle rupture, or free wall rupture with pericardial tamponade) if an echocardiogram has not been performed (Level of Evidence: C).

2. Intra-arterial pressure monitoring should be performed for the following:

   a. Patients with severe hypotension (systolic arterial pressure less than 80 mm Hg) (Level of Evidence: C).

   b. Patients receiving vasopressor/inotropic agents (Level of Evidence: C).

   c. Cardiogenic shock (Level of Evidence: C).

Class IIa

1. Pulmonary artery catheter monitoring can be useful for the following:

   a. Hypotension in a patient without pulmonary congestion who has not responded to an initial trial of fluid administration (Level of Evidence: C).

   b. Cardiogenic shock (Level of Evidence: C).

   c. Severe or progressive CHF or pulmonary edema that does not respond rapidly to therapy (Level of Evidence: C).

   d. Persistent signs of hypoperfusion without hypotension or pulmonary congestion (Level of Evidence: C).

   e. Patients receiving vasopressor/inotropic agents (Level of Evidence: C).

2. Intra-arterial pressure monitoring can be useful for patients receiving intravenous sodium nitroprusside or other potent vasodilators (Level of Evidence: C).

Class IIb

1. Intra-arterial pressure monitoring might be considered in patients receiving intravenous inotropic agents (Level of Evidence: C).

Class III

1. Pulmonary artery catheter monitoring is not recommended in patients with STEMI without evidence of hemodynamic instability or respiratory compromise (Level of Evidence: C).

2. Intra-arterial pressure monitoring is not recommended for patients with STEMI who have no pulmonary congestion and have adequate tissue perfusion without use of circulatory support measures (Level of Evidence: C).

From Antman EM, Anbe DT, Armstrong PW, et al. ACC/AHA Guidelines for the management of patients with ST-elevation myocardial infarction—executive summary: a report of the American College of Cardiology/American Heart Association Task Force on Practice Guidelines (Writing Committee to Revise the 1999 Guidelines for the Management of Patients With Acute Myocardial Infarction). *J Am Coll Cardiol* 2004;44:671–719, with permission.

organ hypoperfusion, by definition, have cardiogenic shock. Hypoxemia is common in this setting and should be corrected using supplemental oxygen with a low threshold for endotracheal intubation in the setting of progressive hemodynamic deterioration and severe acidemia. Although intravenous vasopressors including norepinephrine may be required to achieve a mean systemic BP of 70 mm Hg or greater, mechanical circulatory support is a preferred management adjunct in patients with cardiogenic shock and features of active myocardial ischemia (intra-aortic balloon counterpulsation is a Class I indication). Early angiography followed by revascularization (percutaneous coronary intervention [PCI] or coronary artery bypass grafting [CABG]) is a particularly attractive management strategy in patients less than 75 years of age (34) if it can be performed within 36 hours of MI onset and 18 hours of shock onset (Fig. 14-10).

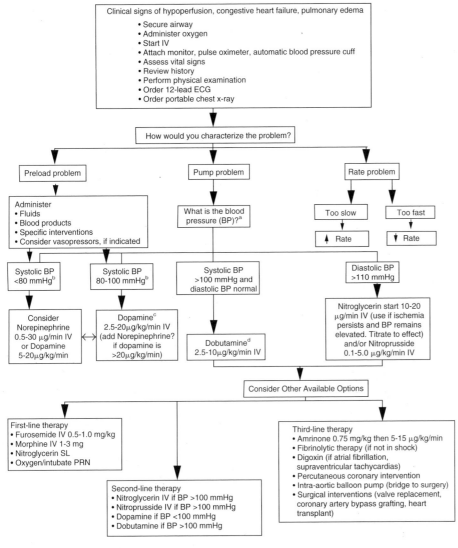

FIGURE 14-10. Stepwise approach to cardiogenic shock.

MECHANICAL COMPLICATIONS

The most commonly encountered mechanical complications of acute MI include ventricular septal rupture (VSR), LV free-wall rupture, mitral regurgitation (MR), and LV aneurysm formation. Papillary muscle and chordal rupture (causing acute MR), VSR, and free-wall rupture, when they occur, commonly do so suddenly within the first week of infarction, whereas aneurysm formation is slow and progressive in nature. In general, patients with acute mechanical complications have smaller infarctions than patients who develop pump failure or malignant ventricular arrhythmias (1). Sudden or rapidly progressive hemodynamic deterioration with systemic hypotension, congestive heart failure, and hypoperfusion should raise suspicion of an acute mechanical defect. The echocardiogram (transthoracic, transesophageal) is an important diagnostic tool that should be used early in the evaluation of patients suspected of having mechanical defects (Fig. 14-11).

Ventricular Septal Rupture

Rupture of the ventricular septum occurs in 2% to 4% of patients with MI and is responsible for 5% of all in-hospital deaths. Although VSR usually occurs between 3 and 5 days postinfarction, the greatest risk is actually within the first 24 hours. Early occurrence is particularly common among patients who have received fibrinolytic therapy. Risk factors for VSR include first infarction, advanced age, history of hypertension, and female sex. Inferior wall infarction is most often associated with posterior septal rupture, whereas distal septal and apical ruptures are more likely to occur following an anterior site of infarction.

Clinically, acute VSR is characterized by new-onset congestive heart failure in the presence of a new, harsh holosystolic murmur; however, patients may exhibit a relatively small degree of pulmonary congestion because of left-to-right shunting. The extent of hemodynamic compromise is determined by the combined defect size and reduced ventricular performance. A diagnosis of VSR can be made using Doppler echocardiography

Potential Sites of Cardiac Rupture After Acute Myocardial Infarction

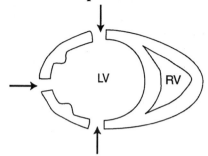

A. Left Ventricular Free Wall Rupture

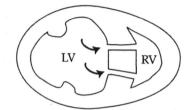

B. Ventricular Septal Rupture

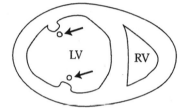

C. Papillary Muscle Rupture

FIGURE 14-11. Cardiac rupture, a potentially lethal complication of myocardial infarction, can involve the (**A**) left ventricular free wall, (**B**) ventricular septum, or (**C**) papillary muscle.

or detection of an oxygen saturation "step-up" between the right atrium and the RV or pulmonary artery during RV catheterization. An oxygen step-up of greater than 10% indicates a significant left-to-right shunt at the ventricular level.

Management

The immediate supportive treatment of VSR includes intravenous fluid administration and inotropic therapy (dopamine or dobutamine) in combination with afterload reduction using nitroprusside or, more commonly, intra-aortic balloon counterpulsation. Although surgical repair represents the definitive treatment, operative mortality is high, ranging from 20% to 70%. Preoperative shock and inferoposterior infarction, particularly with RV dysfunction, are risk factors for a poor surgical outcome following surgery. Emergency repair should be considered when either pulmonary edema or cardiogenic shock is present, but deferred repair is preferable among hemodynamically stable patients. Although aggressive and early surgery leads to the highest survival rates, many patients have a complicated postoperative course and prolonged hospitalization (35). Percutaneous VSR closure is under investigation.

When VSR is suspected, echocardiography with color flow Doppler imaging should be performed as soon as possible to confirm the diagnosis, establish the coexistence of other cardiac abnormalities (mitral regurgitation, pericardial effusion), and provide estimates of both RV and LV systolic function. If a decision is made to proceed with surgical repair, coronary angiography should be performed in anticipation of concomitant revascularization. Left ventriculography may not be necessary if echocardiography provides adequate information on LV performance and the existence of concomitant valvular abnormalities.

Left Ventricular Free-Wall Rupture

Rupture of the LV free wall occurs in 1% to 2% of patients, but is responsible for 10% to 15% of in-hospital deaths. After cardiogenic shock from LV pump failure and ventricular arrhythmias, it is the most common cause of death. In addition, rupture of the LV free wall occurs eight to ten times more frequently than rupture of either a papillary muscle or the ventricular septum. Autopsy series have shown that the lateral wall is the most common site of rupture. Similar to acute VSR, risk factors for free-wall rupture include age more than 70 years, female sex, hypertension, first MI, and transmural infarction in the absence of collateral vessels (36,37).

The clinical presentation among patients with ventricular free-wall rupture ranges from sudden hypotension with pulseless electrical activity and death from cardiac tamponade to transient chest discomfort and bradyarrhythmias. The patient frequently develops signs of systemic hypoperfusion, jugular venous distention, pulsus paradoxus, and distant heart sounds. Episodes of chest pain with diaphoresis and nausea can herald subacute or impending free-wall rupture. The diagnosis is most often suggested clinically and confirmed by echocardiography, pericardiocentesis (revealing hemopericardium), or at the time of emergent surgery.

Management

Patients suspected of having LV free-wall rupture and systemic hypotension should receive intravenous fluid. A large volume is commonly required to increase ventricular preload and maintain CO. Vasopressor support must follow without delay if the hemodynamic status does not improve. Emergent pericardiocentesis can be a lifesaving maneuver in patients with abrupt pulseless electrical activity; however, surgical intervention remains the definitive treatment (38).

Mitral Regurgitation

Acute MR is associated with a poor prognosis (39). With moderate to severe MR, the 1-year survival rate is approximately 50%. Although the diagnosis is typically suggested by the presence of a new holosystolic murmur, up to 50% of the patients with severe MR do not have an audible murmur. Because of the frequency of "silent" MR, the clinician must maintain a high index of suspicion in patients with unexplained hypotension or pulmonary edema.

The papillary muscle is the cardiac structure that ruptures least frequently; however, this event is associated with rapid hemodynamic deterioration because the compromised LV is unable to compensate for the excessive volume load imposed by the incompetent mitral valve. Because the posteromedial papillary muscle receives its blood supply solely from the posterior descending artery (usually as a branch of the right coronary artery), it is susceptible to ischemia, necrosis, and rupture. The anterolateral papillary muscle has a dual blood supply provided by the left anterior descending and left circumflex coronary arteries and, therefore, is less susceptible to ischemic dysfunction and injury.

Management

Patients with acute MR causing congestive heart failure or overt cardiogenic shock require hemodynamic monitoring and pharmacologic inotropic or vasopressor therapy. Intra-aortic balloon counterpulsation should be considered for hemodynamic support and to serve as a bridge to coronary angiography and surgical intervention. Serial echocardiography can be used to determine progression and to assess overall LV compensation in relatively stable patients. Moderate to severe MR, particularly when unresponsive to pharmacologic and supportive measures, should be addressed surgically (40); however, concomitant mitral valve replacement (or repair, if feasible) and bypass grafting, even in experienced hands, are associated with a high surgical mortality rate. The potential role of percutaneous repair requires further consideration.

The management of patients with mechanical complications of acute MI is summarized in Figure 14-12.

Left Ventricular Dilation and Aneurysm Formation

Infarct "expansion" occurs acutely (in the first few days following MI) and results in dilation and thinning of the infarcted segment (41). This event must be distinguished from infarct "extension" (or reinfarction). Clinically, these two complications of MI may present similarly (electrocardiographic ST-segment changes and hemodynamic disturbances); however, infarct expansion is not accompanied by re-elevation of cardiac enzymes as is the case with infarct extension. Infarct expansion usually occurs in the setting of transmural, anterior infarction; it is proportional to the size of the MI and portends a greater likelihood of death.

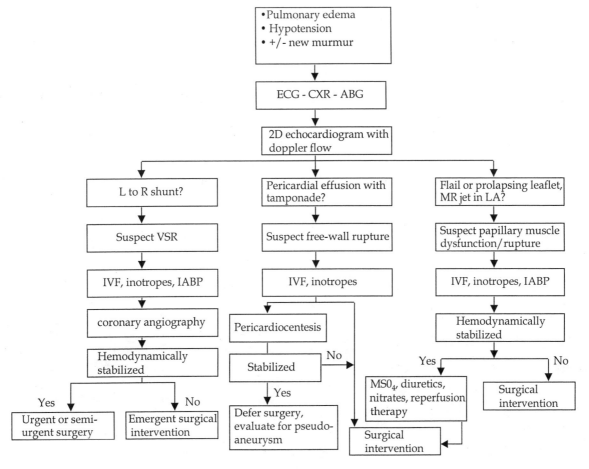

FIGURE 14-12. The management of patients with postinfarction mechanical complications is determined by the site of the involvement and the degree of hemodynamic compromise.

LV dilation and remodeling, which occurs more insidiously, is a progressive process that begins shortly after the acute event and continues over the subsequent weeks to months. Following acute injury, the ventricle dilates in an effort to maintain CO. Unfortunately, progressive dilation causes increased wall stress, which in turn leads to further cavity enlargement, decompensation, and impaired performance.

Management

Efforts to reduce wall stress through reductions in preload and afterload are important. Early treatment with intravenous nitroglycerin and angiotensin-converting enzyme (ACE) inhibitors is effective, particularly the latter (42,43), which exert most of their effects at the tissue level. Aldosterone receptor antagonists also exhibit beneficial effects.

At an extreme end of a spectrum that characterizes LV remodeling is aneurysm formation. The prevalence of LV aneurysms following MI, as estimated from postmortem studies, is between 3% and 15%. The location is typically anterior, anteroapical, or apical. Aneurysms can be asymptomatic or associated with angina pectoris, arrhythmias (including malignant ventricular dysrhythmias), cardioembolism, or congestive heart failure. A diagnosis is most often confirmed by two-dimensional echocardiography or contrast ventriculography. Cardiac MRI is also a useful tool.

Patients developing ventricular aneurysms should be treated in a manner similar to others with MI (beta-blocker, ACE inhibitor, aspirin). Pharmacologic therapies should not be based solely on the presence of an aneurysm, but according to the presence of congestive heart failure, mural thrombi, or life-threatening ventricular arrhythmias. Occasionally, surgical resection and myoplasty are indicated to correct refractory heart failure, recurrent life-threatening arrhythmias, and recurrent systemic emboli, despite anticoagulant therapy. Aneurysmectomy is usually combined with coronary arterial bypass grafting, and in patients with concomitant ventricular arrhythmias, the line of resection should be guided by electrophysiologic mapping. The role of left ventricular partition devices, either in early prevention or late progression, is under investigation.

Pseudoaneurysm

Pseudoaneurysms, also referred to as "false" aneurysms, are a rare complication of acute MI and, in essence, represent a "contained rupture" of the ventricular free wall. Clot forms in the pericardial space, and an aneurysmal wall consisting of organized thrombus and pericardium prevents hemorrhage within the mediastinum. Unlike a true ventricular aneurysm, a pseudoaneurysm has a narrow base (neck) and the risk of rupture (recurrent rupture) is high. The pseudoaneurysm, which has the potential to progressively expand, is clinically silent in most instances, but can cause congestive heart failure, an abnormal bulge on the cardiac silhouette, persistent ST-segment elevation within the region of infarction, or systolic murmurs (44).

The diagnosis of LV pseudoaneurysm can be established by two-dimensional echocardiography, ventriculographic radionuclide studies, cardiac MRI, or contrast left ventriculography.

Management

In addition to the pharmacologic management of congestive heart failure and life-threatening arrhythmias, anticoagulation should be discontinued because of the risk of rupture. Surgical resection with or without bypass grafting is recommended. The potential for percutaneous closure will require further consideration.

PERICARDIAL COMPLICATIONS

Pericarditis

Pericardial inflammation, which is common following acute MI, typically manifests in either an acute or subacute form. Although pericarditis is less common with the advent of reperfusion therapy, it nevertheless must be recognized and diagnosed promptly.

Early Postinfarction Pericarditis

The most common manifestation of pericarditis is chest pain that characteristically is aggravated by inspiration, swallowing, coughing, and lying flat and is lessened when the patient sits up and leans forward. Fever, generally less than 38.6°C, can accompany postinfarction pericarditis and typically lasts for several days (45). A scratchy one-, two-, or three-component pericardial friction rub is often appreciated along the left sternal border. Concave upward ST-segment elevation in five or more ECG leads supports the diagnosis. Although sinus tachycardia is the most common accompanying rhythm abnormality, a wide variety of dysrhythmias, including atrial fibrillation, have been described (46). A small pericardial effusion, identified by transthoracic echocardiography, is not uncommon following MI, and its presence or absence neither confirms nor excludes the diagnosis of pericarditis.

Management

The pain of pericarditis usually responds promptly to aspirin or a nonsteroidal anti inflammatory agent, which should be administered for approximately 5 to 7 days. Aspirin represents the treatment of choice and is given at a dose of 650 mg every 4 to 6 hours. Indomethacin also provides effective symptom relief; however, it can cause increased coronary vascular resistance, competes with aspirin for an important COX-1 acetylation site, and in experimental animal models, causes thinning of the infarct zone. Corticosteroids should be avoided whenever possible because of their association with myocardial rupture and recurrent symptoms after discontinuation. Colchicine is a potential alternative when aspirin is not tolerated or, in rare instances, contraindicated because of true allergy. Although anticoagulant therapy is not an absolute contraindication, it must be used cautiously to minimize the risk of hemorrhagic transformation (47) (Table 14-11). If a pericardial effusion develops or progresses, anticoagulant therapy should be discontinued immediately.

TABLE 14-11

MANAGEMENT OF EARLY POSTINFARCTION PERICARDITIS AND DRESSLER'S SYNDROME*

Distinguish postinfarction pericarditis from recurrent myocardial ischemia or infarction

Aspirin: 160–325 mg daily, as high as 650 mg every 4 to 6 h if required, with decreasing doses as symptoms permit

Indomethacin 25–50 mg three times daily, to be used in severe cases

Morphine sulfate or other oral analgesia for severe pain

Avoid corticosteroids whenever possible

*See text.

Postmyocardial Infarction Syndrome (Dressler's Syndrome)

Dressler's syndrome typically occurs between 2 and 12 weeks after the initial event and may follow either ST-segment elevation or non–ST-segment elevation MI (although it is rare following the latter). The overall frequency of Dressler's syndrome has diminished substantially with the advent of reperfusion therapy.

The clinical features of Dressler's syndrome are fever, pleuritic chest pain, and polyserositis. Pleural and pericardial friction rubs, lasting from several days to weeks, can be appreciated. Pericardial and pleural effusions are present in most patients, and although they are typically small, large hemorrhagic effusions have been described. Dressler's syndrome is an immune-mediated phenomenon.

Management

The pharmacologic approach to Dressler's syndrome is similar to that of early postinfarction pericarditis; however, a course of oral corticosteroid therapy more often is needed for complete symptom relief. Nevertheless, treatment should begin with aspirin or nonsteroidal anti-inflammatory agents, and if steroids are used, they should be gradually tapered off over 1 to 4 weeks. Unfortunately, recurrences are common, often requiring reinstitution of corticosteroids with a more gradual tapering. Drainage procedures may be necessary for large pleural effusions that compromise overall pulmonary performance.

Thromboembolic Complications

Thromboembolism, a recognized complication of acute MI, occurs in 5% to 10% of patients. Both arterial and venous events can occur, with LV mural thrombi accounting for most systemic emboli, and RV or deep vein thrombi serving as a nidus for pulmonary embolism.

Pulmonary Embolism

The prevalence of deep venous thrombosis (DVT) among patients with acute MI is reported to be between 18% and 38% (48). Risk factors in this setting include large infarctions in any location, anterior infarctions, congestive heart failure, and complicated infarctions—each associated with a systemic inflammatory response, prolonged immobilization, and venous stasis. In addition to traditional risk factors, reduced CO also predisposes to DVT. The diagnosis is particularly challenging in critically ill patients, who typically suffer from a variety of active medical problems. Early reports suggested that 10% to 15% of all patients with DVT experienced a pulmonary embolism, and 3% to 6% had fatal events. More recent estimates are less impressive but still concerning, with rates of 3% to 5% and 1%, respectively.

Early mobilization, as clinical status permits, and prophylactic anticoagulation are recommended for all patients experiencing acute MI, particularly those with prior events or known thrombophilias. The management of venous thromboembolism is outlined in Chapter 22.

Systemic Embolism

The prevalence of systemic embolism in patients with MI is approximately 5% (49). Emboli to the cerebral, renal, mesenteric, iliofemoral, or other arterial beds can occur, typically originating from mural thrombi within the LV (50). Left atrial appendage thrombi are a potential source of emboli in patients

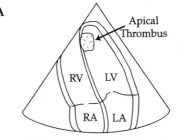

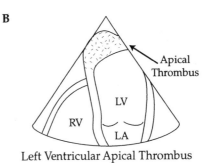

FIGURE 14-13. Thrombi developing within the left ventricular apex can be (A) well-defined and partially mobile, or (B) laminated along the endocardial surface. LA, left atrium; LV, left ventricle; RA, right atrium; RV, right ventricle.

with atrial fibrillation. The predilection of the ventricular apex for thrombus development is caused by localized inflammation (from the infarction) and stagnant blood flow. Although depressed LV function and chamber dilation are not absolute prerequisites for thrombus formation, both contribute substantially to the process (51).

LV thrombi typically develop within the first three postinfarction days, but can form later. Systemic embolization occurs, on average, 14 days after infarction and is relatively rare after 6 weeks in the absence of clinical heart failure and LV chamber dilation. The diagnosis of mural thrombus is most often made by two dimensional echocardiography (Fig. 14-13). Atheroembolism, presenting as intestinal ischemia, acute renal failure, and/or painful digits (in the presence of patent peripheral vessels), can complicate fibrinolytic therapy or angiography.

Management

Patients with systemic embolism, particularly those with a documented cardiac source or in whom a high index of suspicion for cardioembolism is seen, should be systemically anticoagulated with unfractionated or LMWH heparin, followed by warfarin (target INR 2 to 3) for 6 to 12 months. A longer treatment duration may be indicated for patients with persistently depressed ejection fractions (<30%). Long-term anticoagulation is recommended for patients with chronic atrial fibrillation and those with prior cardioembolism. Neuroimaging and vascular imaging may be particularly useful when the cause of stroke is not evident (Table 14-12).

ELECTRICAL COMPLICATIONS

Rhythm and Conduction Disturbances

Abnormalities of cardiac rhythm and conduction, which are common following MI, can be life-threatening. Before hospital

TABLE 14-12

MANAGEMENT OF VENTRICULAR TACHYARRHYTHMIAS

Class I

1. Ventricular fibrillation (VF) or pulseless VT should be treated with an unsynchronized electric shock with an initial monophasic shock energy of 200 J; if unsuccessful, a second shock of 200 to 300 J should be given, and then, if necessary, a third shock of 360 J (Level of Evidence: B).

Class IIa

1. It is reasonable that VF or pulseless VT that is refractory to electrical shock be treated with amiodarone (300 mg or 5 mg/kg, IV bolus) followed by a repeat unsynchronized electric shock (Level of Evidence: B).
2. It is reasonable to correct electrolyte and acid-base disturbances (potassium greater than 4.0 mEq/L and magnesium greater than 2.0 mg/dL) to prevent recurrent episodes of VF once an initial episode of VF has been treated (Level of Evidence: C).

Class IIb

1. It may be reasonable to treat VT or shock-refractory VF with boluses of intravenous procainamide. However, this has limited value due to the length of time required for administration (Level of Evidence: C).

Class III

1. Prophylactic administration of antiarrhythmic therapy is not recommended when using fibrinolytic agents (Level of Evidence: B).

There is no convincing evidence that the prophylactic use of lidocaine reduces mortality, and the prior practice of routine (prophylactic) administration of lidocaine to all patients with known or suspected STEMI has been largely abandoned. VF should be treated with an unsynchronized electric shock using an initial monophasic shock energy of 200 J. If this is unsuccessful, a second shock using 200 to 300 J and, if necessary, a third shock using 360 J are indicated (160).

b. Ventricular Tachycardia

Class I

1. Sustained (more than 30 seconds or causing hemodynamic collapse) polymorphic VT should be treated with an unsynchronized electric shock with an initial monophasic shock energy of 200 J; if unsuccessful, a second shock of 200 to 300 J should be given, and if necessary, a third shock of 360 J (Level of Evidence: B).
2. Episodes of sustained monomorphic VT associated with angina, pulmonary edema, or hypotension (blood pressure less than 90 mm Hg) should be treated with a synchronized electric shock of 100 J initial monophasic shock energy. Increasing energies may be used if not initially successful. Brief anesthesia is desirable if hemodynamically tolerable (Level of Evidence: B).

b. Aggressive normalization of serum potassium to greater than 4.0 mEq/L and of magnesium to greater than 2.0 mg/dL (Level of Evidence: C).
c. If the patient has bradycardia to a rate less than 60 beats per minute or long QTc, temporary pacing at a higher rate may be instituted (Level of Evidence: C).

Class IIb

1. It is may be useful to treat sustained monomorphic VT not associated with angina, pulmonary edema, or hypotension (blood pressure less than 90 mm Hg) with a procainamide bolus and infusion (Level of Evidence: C).

Class III

1. The routine use of prophylactic antiarrhythmic drugs (i.e., lidocaine) is not indicated for suppression of isolated ventricular premature beats, couplets, runs of accelerated idioventricular rhythm, or nonsustained VT (Level of Evidence: B).
2. The routine use of prophylactic antiarrhythmic therapy is not indicated when fibrinolytic agents are administered (Level of Evidence: B).

Management Strategies for VT. Cardioversion is always indicated for episodes of sustained hemodynamically compromising VT (161). Episodes of sustained VT that are somewhat better tolerated hemodynamically may initially be treated with drug regimens, including amiodarone or procainamide.

d. Implantable Cardioverter Defibrillator Implantation in Patients after STEMI

Class I

1. An implantable cardioverter-defibrillator (ICD) is indicated for patients with VF or hemodynamically significant sustained VT more than 2 days after STEMI, provided the arrhythmia is not judged to be due to transient or reversible ischemia or reinfarction (Level of Evidence: A).
2. An ICD is indicated for patients without spontaneous VF or sustained VT more than 48 hours after STEMI whose STEMI occurred at least 1 month previously, who have an LVEF between 0.31 and 0.40, demonstrate additional evidence of electrical instability (e.g., nonsustained VT), and have inducible VF or sustained VT on electrophysiological testing (Level of Evidence: B).

Class IIa

1. If there is reduced LVEF (0.30 or less), at least 1 month after STEMI and 3 months after coronary artery revascularization, it is reasonable to implant an ICD in post-STEMI patients without spontaneous VF or sustained VT more than 48 hours after STEMI (Level of Evidence: B).

(continues)

TABLE 14-12

CONTINUED

3. Sustained monomorphic VT not associated with angina, pulmonary edema, or hypotension (blood pressure less than 90 mm Hg) should be treated with:

   a. Amiodarone: 150 mg infused over 10 minutes (alternative dose 5 mg/kg); repeat 150 mg every 10 to 15 minutes as needed. Alternative infusion: 360 mg over 6 hours (1 mg/min), then 540 mg over the next 18 hours (0.5 mg/min). The total cumulative dose, including additional doses given during cardiac arrest, must not exceed 2.2 g over 24 hours (Level of Evidence: B).

   b. Synchronized electrical cardioversion starting at monophasic energies of 50 J (brief anesthesia is necessary) (Level of Evidence: B).

Class IIa

1. It is reasonable to manage refractory polymorphic VT by:

   a. Aggressive attempts to reduce myocardial ischemia and adrenergic stimulation, including therapies such as beta-adrenoceptor blockade, IABP use, and consideration of emergency PCI/CABG surgery (Level of Evidence: B).

Class IIb

1. The usefulness of an ICD is not well established in STEMI patients without spontaneous VF or sustained VT more than 48 hours after STEMI who have a reduced LVEF (0.31 to 0.40) at least 1 month after STEMI but who have no additional evidence of electrical instability (e.g., nonsustained VT) (Level of Evidence: B).

2. The usefulness of an ICD is not well established in STEMI patients without spontaneous VF or sustained VT more than 48 hours after STEMI who have a reduced LVEF (0.31 to 0.40) at least 1 month after STEMI and additional evidence of electrical instability (e.g., nonsustained VT) but who do not have inducible VF or sustained VT on electrophysiological testing (Level of Evidence: B).

Class III

1. An ICD is not indicated in STEMI patients who do not experience spontaneous VF or sustained VT more than 48 hours after STEMI and in whom the LVEF is greater than 0.40 at least 1 month after STEMI (Level of Evidence: C).

From Antman EM, Anbe DT, Armstrong PW, et al. ACC/AHA Guidelines for the management of patients with ST-elevation myocardial infarction—executive summary: a report of the American College of Cardiology/American Heart Association Task Force on Practice Guidelines (Writing Committee to Revise the 1999 Guidelines for the Management of Patients With Acute Myocardial Infarction). *J Am Coll Cardiol* 2004;44:671–719, with permission.

arrival, ventricular tachycardia and fibrillation account for most sudden cardiac deaths. Both tachyarrhythmias and bradyarrhythmias are encountered in the hospital phase of acute MI, and most patients experience one or more conduction abnormalities (25%) or rhythm disturbances (90%) in the first 24 hours. The cause of electrical complications is multifactorial, including myocardial ischemia, necrosis, altered autonomic tone, hypoxia, electrolyte and acid–base disturbances, and adverse drug effects.

Management

The general goal of therapy in the setting of rhythm and conduction disturbances is to return heart rate and AV synchrony to their normal state (Tables 14-13 and 14-14).

The use of temporary transvenous pacing in the setting of acute MI is determined by the specific bradyarrhythmia or conduction disturbance, the presence of hemodynamic compromise, and the site of infarction. Transcutaneous pacing systems are suitable for stable patients judged to be at low to moderate risk for progressive AV block. Transcutaneous modalities are also attractive among patients who have received fibrinolytic therapy, given their added risk for vascular and hemorrhagic complications. Temporary pacing in the early stages of MI does not automatically translate to a requirement for permanent pacemaker placement.

TREATMENT COMPLICATIONS

Hemorrhage

Antithrombotic and fibrinolytic therapy, by design but not by intention, impair both thrombotic potential (a goal of treatment) and hemostatic capacity (an unwanted effect).

Antiplatelet Therapy

Bleeding events associated with disorders of primary hemostasis most often involve the skin, joint spaces, and mucous membranes; however, the gastrointestinal and genitourinary tracts and central nervous system are occasionally involved. Bleeding severity is directly related to the cumulative degree of platelet dysfunction, integrity of the vasculature, and status of thrombin-generating coagulation pathways. In general, an isolated acquired platelet defect is not commonly the sole cause of life-threatening hemorrhage.

The template bleeding time has been employed as a general estimate of platelet function; however, it is nonspecific and vulnerable to technical errors. Laboratory-based platelet aggregation studies can also be performed if time allows. The evolution of bedside assays and point-of-care platelet aggregometers, particularly the PFA-100, provide a readily available means to rapidly diagnose platelet abnormalities, particularly those related to pharmacologic inhibition.

Preconditions for rFVIIa Administration

Hematological parameters. As rFVIIa acts on the patient's own clotting mechanism, its administration should be considered after blood component therapy has achieved the following:

1. Fibrinogen levels of ≥ 50 mg dL^{-1} (preferably 100 mg dL^{-1})
2. Platelet levels of $\geq 50,000 \times 10^9$ L^{-1} (preferably $100,000 \times 10^9$ L^{-1}) (Table 14-15)

pH. Clinical and laboratory evidence suggests that the efficacy of rFVIIa decreases at a pH of ≤ 7.1. Hence, correction of the pH to ≥ 7.2 is recommended prior to its administration.

TABLE 14-13

MANAGEMENT OF SUPRAVENTRICULAR ARRHYTHMIAS

Class I

1. Sustained atrial fibrillation and atrial flutter in patients with hemodynamic compromise or ongoing ischemia should be treated with one or more of the following:

   a. Synchronized cardioversion with an initial monophasic shock of 200 J for atrial fibrillation and 50 J for flutter, preceded by brief general anesthesia or conscious sedation whenever possible (Level of Evidence: C).

   b. For episodes of atrial fibrillation that do not respond to electrical cardioversion or recur after a brief period of sinus rhythm, the use of antiarrhythmic therapy aimed at slowing the ventricular response is indicated. One or more of these pharmacological agents may be used:

      i. Intravenous amiodarone (Level of Evidence: C).

      ii. Intravenous digoxin for rate control principally for patients with severe LV dysfunction and heart failure (Level of Evidence: C).

Sustained atrial fibrillation and atrial flutter in patients with ongoing ischemia but without hemodynamic compromise should be treated with one or more of the following:

   a. Beta-adrenergic blockade is preferred, unless contraindicated (Level of Evidence: C).

   b. Intravenous diltiazem or verapamil (Level of Evidence: C).

   c. Synchronized cardioversion with an initial monophasic shock of 200 J for atrial fibrillation and 50 J for flutter, preceded by brief general anesthesia or conscious sedation whenever possible (Level of Evidence: C).

For episodes of sustained atrial fibrillation or flutter without hemodynamic compromise or ischemia, rate control is indicated. In addition, patients with sustained atrial fibrillation or flutter should be given anticoagulant therapy. Consideration should be given to cardioversion to sinus rhythm in patients with a history of atrial fibrillation or flutter prior to STEMI (Level of Evidence: C).

Re-entrant paroxysmal supraventricular tachycardia, because of its rapid rate, should be treated with the following in the sequence shown:

   a. Carotid sinus massage (Level of Evidence: C).

   b. Intravenous adenosine (6 mg given over 1 to 2 seconds; if no response, 12 mg IV after 1 to 2 minutes may be given; repeat 12 mg dose if needed (Level of Evidence: C).

   c. Intravenous beta-adrenergic blockade with metoprolol (2.5 to 5.0 mg every 2 to 5 minutes to a total of 15 mg over 10 to 15 minutes) or atenolol (2.5 to 5.0 mg over 2 minutes to a total of 10 mg in 10 to 15 minutes) (Level of Evidence: C).

   d. Intravenous diltiazem (20 mg [0.25 mg/kg]) over 2 minutes followed by an infusion of 10 mg/h) (Level of Evidence: C).

   e. Intravenous digoxin, recognizing that there may be a delay of at least 1 hour before pharmacological effects appear (8 to 15 mcg/kg [0.6 to 1.0 mg in a person weighing 70 kg]) (Level of Evidence: C).

Class III

1. Treatment of atrial premature beats is not indicated (Level of Evidence: C).

From Antman EM, Anbe DT, Armstrong PW, et al. ACC/AHA Guidelines for the management of patients with ST-elevation myocardial infarction—executive summary: a report of the American College of Cardiology/American Heart Association Task Force on Practice Guidelines (Writing Committee to Revise the 1999 Guidelines for the Management of Patients With Acute Myocardial Infarction). *J Am Coll Cardiol* 2004;44: 671–719, with permission.

Body Temperature

rFVIIa retains its activity in the presence of hypothermia; hence, the latter does not limit is use. Nonetheless, body temperature should be restored to physiological values whenever possible.

rFVIIA and Surgical Hemostasis

1. It is recommended that rFVIIa be administered as an adjunctive therapy to concomitant surgical measures, as the agent arrests coagulopathic, rather than surgical, bleeding.
2. If packing was performed, unpacking should be considered before administration of rFVIIa. This is recommended because the cessation of diffuse coagulopathic bleeding induced by rFVIIa and the hemodynamic improvement that follows may serve to expose surgical bleeding sites that could not be previously identified.
3. For the same reason, if hemorrhage is encountered outside the operating room, angiography or a "second look" should be considered (depending on the clinical circumstances) to rule out surgical bleeding. There are cases where administration of rFVIIa alone, prior to, or even without surgical intervention led to cessation or marked decline in the rate of bleeding.

Dosage

The recommended dose of rFVIIa for treatment of massive bleeding is approximately 120 (100 to 140) $\mu g\ kg^{-1}$ administered intravenously over 2 to 5 minutes.

Repeat Dosage

If hemorrhage persists beyond 15 to 20 minutes following the first administration of rFVIIa, an additional dose of approximately 100 $\mu g\ kg^{-1}$ should be considered.

If the response remains inadequate following a total dose of >200 $\mu g\ kg^{-1}$, the preconditions for rFVIIa administration should be rechecked, if possible, and corrected as necessary before a third dose is considered. If this is not feasible, the empirical administration of fresh frozen plasma (10 to 15 mL kg^{-1} or 4 to 6 U for 70 kg), cryoprecipitate (1 to 2 U for 10 kg^{-1} or 10 to 15 U for 70 kg), and platelets (1 to 2 U for 10 kg^{-1} or 10 to 15 U for 70 kg) should be considered, and the pH and calcium should be checked and corrected. Only after these measures have been applied should a third dose of rFVIIa 100 $\mu g\ kg^{-1}$ be administered.

TABLE 14-14

MANAGEMENT OF CONDUCTION DISTURBANCES AND BRADYARRHYTHMIAS

Class I

1. Prompt resuscitative measures, including chest compressions, atropine, vasopressin, epinephrine, and temporary pacing, should be administered to treat ventricular asystole. (Level of Evidence: B)
2. Use of permanent pacemakers

PERMANENT PACING FOR BRADYCARDIA OR CONDUCTION BLOCKS ASSOCIATED WITH STEMI

Class IIa

1. Permanent ventricular pacing is indicated for persistent second-degree AV block in the His-Purkinje system with bilateral bundle-branch block or third-degree AV block within or below the His-Purkinje system after STEMI (Level of Evidence: B).
2. Permanent ventricular pacing is indicated for transient advanced second- or third-degree infranodal AV block and associated bundle-branch block. If the site of block is uncertain, an electrophysiological study may be necessary (Level of Evidence: B).
3. Permanent ventricular pacing is indicated for persistent and symptomatic second- or third-degree AV block (Level of Evidence: C).

Class IIb

1. Permanent ventricular pacing may be considered for persistent second- or third-degree AV block at the AV node level (Level of Evidence: B).

Class III

1. Permanent ventricular pacing is not recommended for transient AV block in the absence of intraventricular conduction defects (Level of Evidence: B).
2. Permanent ventricular pacing is not recommended for transient AV block in the presence of isolated left anterior fascicular block (Level of Evidence: B).
3. Permanent ventricular pacing is not recommended for acquired left anterior fascicular block in the absence of AV block (Level of Evidence: B).
4. Permanent ventricular pacing is not recommended for persistent first-degree AV block in the presence of bundle-branch block that is old or of indeterminate age (Level of Evidence: B).

SINUS NODE DYSFUNCTION AFTER STEMI

Class I

1. Symptomatic sinus bradycardia, sinus pauses greater than 3 seconds, or sinus bradycardia with a heart rate less than 40 bpm and associated hypotension or signs of systemic hemodynamic compromise should be treated with an intravenous bolus of atropine 0.6 to 1.0 mg. If bradycardia is persistent and maximal (2-mg) doses of atropine have been used, transcutaneous or transvenous (preferably atrial) temporary pacing should be instituted (Level of Evidence: C).

From Antman EM, Anbe DT, Armstrong PW, et al. ACC/AHA Guidelines for the management of patients with ST-elevation myocardial infarction—executive summary: a report of the American College of Cardiology/American Heart Association Task Force on Practice Guidelines (Writing Committee to Revise the 1999 Guidelines for the Management of Patients With Acute Myocardial Infarction). *J Am Coll Cardiol* 2004;44:671–719, with permission.

TABLE 14-15

ADMINISTRATION GUIDELINES FOR RECOMBINANT FVIIA

1. The blood bank should be immediately alerted to incidents of massive bleeding to facilitate timely preparation of the various blood components required.

2. rFVIIa should be administered as early as possible (after conventional treatments have failed to arrest bleeding) and should be given in conjunction with transfusion of packed red blood cells to avoid further loss of clotting factors, exacerbation of acidosis, and further lowering of body temperature (all of which adversely affect hemostasis and prognosis).

TABLE 14-16

SUGGESTED DOSE OF PROTAMINE TO NEUTRALIZE ANTICOAGULANT EFFECTS OF ENOXAPARIN[a]

Last dose of enoxaparin (1.0 mg/kg)

| ≤8 h | >8 h and ≤12 h | >12 h |

Protamine dose[b] 1 mg protamine/1 mg enoxaparin, 0.5 mg protamine/1 mg enoxaparin may not be required

Fresh frozen plasma may be required in patients with life-threatening hemorrhage.

[a]The potential risk of rapid neutralization must be weighed against the perceived benefit.
[b]Protamine neutralizes the anti-IIa effects of enoxaparin (and other low-molecular-weight heparins).

Monitoring

Currently, there is no laboratory method for monitoring the effect of rFVIIa. The best available indicator of rFVIIa efficacy is the arrest of hemorrhage judged by visual evidence, hemodynamic stabilization, and a reduced demand for blood components. The PT is expected to shorten, frequently below the normal expected range (as there is TF in the test tube), but this does not reflect efficacy. Thromboelastography and thrombin generation are future candidate tests for evaluation of efficacy of rFVIIa.

The initial approach to bleeding complications should center on the site, extent, and clinical impact. As with any hemorrhage, the source should be identified, the offending agent discontinued (when feasible), and local measures (manual pressure, suturing) explored first. Thereafter, treatment is dictated by the severity of the event. Platelet transfusions, either with or without DDAVP, to increase VWF multimers, should be given for serious or life-threatening hemorrhage.

Profound thrombocytopenia (platelet counts <2,000/mm^3) has been observed with the GP IIb/IIIa antagonists. The largest clinical experience is with abciximab. Most patients have responded to discontinuation of the medication and platelet transfusions. Intravenous immunoglobulin (Ig) and corticosteroid therapy do not affect the natural history of the acute disorder; however, delayed thrombocytopenia (>2 weeks after exposure) has been described (after abciximab administration) and is immune mediated. Accordingly, intravenous Ig and/or prednisone therapy should be considered. Fibrinogen supplementation with cryoprecipitate or fresh frozen plasma represents an important first-line treatment when major hemorrhage occurs during administration of the small-molecule GP IIb/IIIa inhibitors, eptifibatide, and tirofiban.

Heparin Compounds

Mild to moderate bleeding should initially prompt a reduction in the unfractionated heparin dose (particularly if the activated partial thromboplastin time is excessively prolonged) or an interruption of the infusion for a brief period of time (30 to 60 minutes). More severe hemorrhage may require complete discontinuation or, with life-threatening hemorrhage, neutralization with protamine sulfate (1 mg/100 U heparin administered in the preceding 4 hours). However, in patients with active coronary heart disease, a careful risk-to-benefit assessment must be undertaken, considering the risks of coronary thrombosis versus those of bleeding. It may be in the patient's best interest to continue systemic anticoagulation, particularly if the bleeding is not serious or life threatening and can be controlled

adequately with local measures (e.g., manual pressure over a site of vascular trauma).

Protamine sulfate (1 mg/100 U anti-Xa) can also be administered to neutralize partially the anticoagulant effects of LMWH. It is important to recognize that the neutralization is incomplete (~60%). Fresh frozen plasma should be administered in the setting of life-threatening bleeding to correct any residual hemostatic impairment (Table 14-16).

The neutralization of heparinoids (e.g., danaparoid sodium) and the very LMWH, fondaparinux, are even more challenging, given their long circulating half-lives and poor (or absent in the case of fondaparinux) response to protamine. As with LMWH preparations, fresh frozen plasma (10 to 15 mL/kg) should be administered for serious or life-threatening bleeding complications. Plasmapheresis has been used successfully to remove danaparoid sodium in several patients following bypass surgery complicated by uncontrolled hemorrhage.

Hirudin and Other Direct Thrombin Antagonists

There are no known antidotes for lepirudin, bivalirudin, or argatroban, creating potentially serious life-threatening challenges when bleeding occurs. Beyond immediate discontinuation of the drug, fresh frozen plasma should be considered as a source of clotting factors. Plasmapheresis should be considered for life-threatening hemorrhage.

Warfarin

The anticoagulant effect of warfarin can be reduced or entirely reversed by lowering the dose, discontinuing treatment, administering vitamin K, or replacing the defective coagulation factors with fresh frozen plasma or prothrombin concentrate. The severity of bleeding and inherent risks of reduced anticoagulation should dictate the course of action (Table 14-17).

Fibrinolytic Therapy

Even with careful patient selection and close monitoring, hemorrhagic events do occur. Routine management includes volume and BP support as well as a prompt and thorough search for the site of bleeding. Abdominopelvic or head computed tomography scans may be useful in the diagnosis and management of major hemorrhagic events. Life-threatening hemor-

TABLE 14-17

MANAGEMENT OF PROLONGED INR ASSOCIATED WITH WARFARIN THERAPY[a]

INR	<6.0	6.0–10.0	>10.0	>20.0
Clinical profile[a]	No bleeding	No bleeding	No bleeding	No bleeding
Recommended approach	Omit next 1–2 doses of warfarin	Vitamin K 1–2 mg s.c.	Vitamin K 3–5 mg s.c.	Vitamin K 5–10 mg s.c.
	↓	↓↓		
	Repeat INR in 8 h	Repeat INR in 6 h	Repeat INR in 6 h	
	Consider additional vitamin K	Consider additional vitamin K	Consider additional vitamin K	

INR, international normalized ratio; IV, intravenous; s.c., subcutaneous.
[a]For rapid reversal of anticoagulant effect because of life-threatening hemorrhage, fresh frozen plasma or prothrombin concentrates should be administered. Concomitant administration of vitamin K (3–5 mg IV given over 60 to 90 minutes) is also recommended.

rhage warrants prompt intervention. Heparin should be discontinued and neutralized with protamine sulfate. Fresh frozen plasma is an excellent source of factors V and VIII, α_2-antiplasmin, and plasminogen-activator inhibitor. Cryoprecipitate (8 to 10 U) is the preferred source of fibrinogen (200 to 250 mg/10 to 15 mL) and factor VIII (80 U/10 to 15 mL). If the platelet count is low (<80,000/mm^3), platelets (6 U random donor) should be given. If indicated, DDAVP (0.3 μg/kg IV over 20 minutes) can be used to correct qualitative platelet abnormalities. Persistent and potentially life-threatening hemorrhage unresponsive to standard measures (outlined previously) may require antifibrinolytic therapy. This intervention should be used with caution because serious thrombotic complications can be precipitated. Alpha-aminocaproic acid (Amicar) and tranexamic acid are the most frequently used agents (Fig. 14-14).

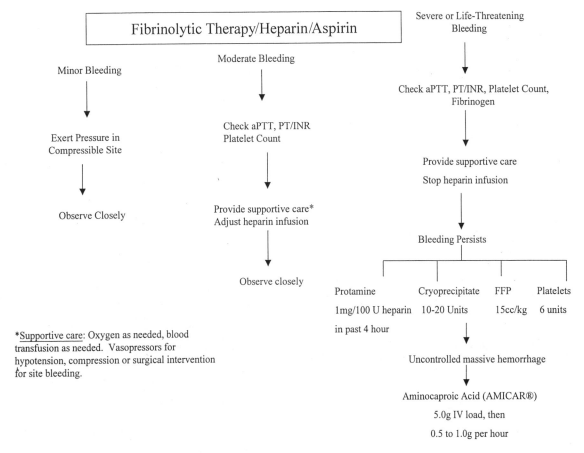

FIGURE 14-14. A recommended approach to the management of patients with hemorrhagic complications following fibrinolytic (and adjunctive antithrombotic) therapy.

Recombinant Activated Factor VII for Uncontrolled Bleeding

Recombinant activated factor VII is approved by the U.S. Food and Drug Administration for hemophilic patients with existing inhibitors (to factor VIII). Its off-label use as a hemostatic agent for massive/life-threatening hemorrhage developing in a wide variety of clinical settings continues to expand. General guidelines for the administration of rFVIIa have been proposed (Table 14-15) (52).

References

1. Braunwald E. *Heart disease: a textbook of cardiovascular medicine*, Vol. 2. Philadelphia: WB Saunders; 1984:1262–1300.
2. Buja LM, Willerson JT. Clinicopathological correlates of acute ischemic heart disease syndromes. *Am J Cardiol* 1981;47:343–356.
3. Fishbein MC, Maclean D, Maroko PR. The histopathological evolution of myocardial infarction. *Chest* 1978;73:843–849.
4. Henson DE, Najafi H, Callaghan R, et al. Myocardial lesions following open heart surgery. *Arch Pathol* 1969;88:423–430.
5. Tyagi SC, Ratajska A, Weber KT. Myocardial matrix metalloproteinase(s): localization and activation. *Mol Cell Biochem* 1993;126:49–59.
6. Cleutjens JPM, Kandala JC, Guarda E, et al. Regulation of collagen degradation in the rat myocardium after infarction. *J Mol Cell Cardiol* 1995;27:1281–1292.
7. McCormick RJ, Musch TI, Bergman BC, et al. Regional differences in LV collagen accumulation and mature cross-linking after myocardial infarction in rats. *Am J Physiol* 1994;266:H354–H359.
8. Finesmith TH, Broadley KN, Davidson JM. Fibroblasts from wounds of different stages of repair vary in their ability to contract a collagen gel in response to growth factors. *J Cell Physiol* 1990;144:97–107.
9. Mueller HS, Cohen LS, Braunwald E, et al. Predictors of early morbidity and mortality after thrombolytic therapy of acute myocardial infarction. Analyses of patient subgroups in the Thrombolysis in Myocardial Infarction (TIMI) Trial, Phase II. *Circulation* 1992;85:1254–1264.
10. Lee KL, Woodlief LH, Topol EJ, et al. Predictors of 30-day mortality in the era of reperfusion for acute myocardial infarction. Results from an international trial of 41,021 patients. *Circulation* 1995;91:1659–1668.
11. Becker RC, Burns M, Gore JM, for the NRMI-2 Investigators. Early assessment and in-hospital management of patients with acute myocardial infarction at increased risk for adverse outcomes: a nationwide perspective of current clinical practice. *Am Heart J* 1998;135:786–796.
12. Hathaway WR, Peterson ED, Wagner GS, et al. Prognostic significance of the initial electrocardiography in patients with acute myocardial infarction. *JAMA* 1998;279:387–391.
13. Ohman EM, Armstrong PW, Christenson RH, et al. Cardiac troponin T levels for risk stratification in acute myocardial ischemia. *N Engl J Med* 1996;335:1333–1341.
14. Morrow DA, Rifan N, Antman EM, et al. Serum amyloid A protein predicts early mortality in acute coronary syndromes: a TIMI 11A substudy. *J Am Coll Cardiol* 2000;35:358–362.
15. Gore JM, Granger CB, Simoons ML, et al. Stroke after thrombolysis. Mortality and functional outcomes in the GUSTO-1 trial. *Circulation* 1995;92:2811–2818.
16. Becker RC, Burns M, Every N, et al. Early clinical outcomes and routine management of patients with non–ST-segment elevation myocardial infarction: a nationwide perspective. *Arch Intern Med* 2001;161:601–607.
17. TIMI Study Group. Comparison of invasive and conservative strategies after treatment with intravenous tissue plasminogen activator in acute myocardial infarction. Results of the Thrombolysis in Myocardial Infarction (TIMI) Phase II Trial. *N Engl J Med* 1989;320:618.
18. Bosch X, Theroux P, Waters DD, et al. Early postinfarction ischemia: clinical, angiographic, and prognostic significance. *Circulation* 1987;5:988–995.
19. Gibson RS, Boden WE, Theroux P, et al. Diltiazem and reinfarction in patients with non–Q-wave myocardial infarction. Results of a double-blind, randomized, multicenter trial. *N Engl J Med* 1986;315:423–429.
20. Schaer DH, Ross AM, Wasserman AG. Reinfarction, recurrent angina and reocclusion after thrombolytic therapy. *Circulation* 1987;76:II–57.
21. ISIS-2 (Second International Study of Infarct Survival) Collaborative Group. Randomized trial of intravenous streptokinase, oral aspirin, both, or neither among 17,187 cases of suspected acute myocardial infarction: ISIS-2. *Lancet* 1988;2:349.
22. Gruppo Italiano per lo Studio della Streptochinasi nell'Infarto Miocardico (GISSI). Effectiveness of intravenous thrombolytic treatment in acute myocardial infarction. *Lancet* 1986;1:397.
23. Granger CB, Miller JM, Bovill EG, et al. Rebound increase in thrombin generation and activity after cessation of intravenous heparin in patients with acute coronary syndromes. *Circulation* 1995;91:1929–1935.
24. Antman EM, for the TIMI 14 investigators. Abciximab facilitates the rate and extent of thrombolysis: results of the TIMI 14 Trial. *Circulation* 1999;99:2720–2732.
25. Ross AM, Molhoek GP, Knudtson ML, et al. A randomized comparison of low molecular weight heparin and unfractionated heparin adjunctive to tPA thrombolysis and aspirin (HART-II). *Circulation* 2000;102:II–600.
26. Antman EM, Anbe DT, Armstrong PW, et al. ACC/AHA guidelines for the management of patients with ST-elevation myocardial infarction—executive summary: a report of the American College of Cardiology/American Heart Association Task Force on Practice Guidelines (Writing Committee to Revise the 1999 Guidelines for the Management of Patients With Acute Myocardial Infarction). *J Am Coll Cardiol* 2004;44:671–719.
27. Zehender M, Kasper W, Kauder E, et al. Right ventricular infarction as an independent predictor of prognosis after acute inferior myocardial infarction. *N Engl J Med* 1993;328:981–988.
28. Manno BV, Bemis CE, Carver J, et al. Right ventricular infarction complicated by right to left shunt. *J Am Coll Cardiol* 1983;1:554–557.
29. Love JC, Haffajee CI, Gore JM, et al. Reversibility of hypotension and shock by atrial or atrioventricular sequential pacing in patients with right ventricular infarction. *Am Heart J* 1984;108:5–13.
30. Braunwald E, Kloner RA. The stunned myocardium: prolonged postischemic ventricular dysfunction. *Circulation* 1982;66:1146.
31. Scott BD, Kerber RE. Clinical and experimental aspects of myocardial stunning. *Prog Cardiovasc Dis* 1992;35:61.
32. Goldberg RJ, Gore JM, Alpert JS, et al. Cardiogenic shock resulting form acute myocardial infarction: a fourteen-year community-wide perspective. *N Engl J Med* 1991;325:1117–1122.
33. Alonso DR, Scheidt S, Post M, et al. Pathophysiology of cardiogenic shock: quantification of myocardial necrosis, clinical, pathologic and electrocardiographic correlations. *Circulation* 1973;48:588–596.
34. Hochman JS, Sleeper LA, Webb JG, et al. Early revascularization in acute myocardial infarction complicated by cardiogenic shock. *N Engl J Med* 1999;341:625–634.
35. Skillington PD, Davies RH, Luf AJ, et al. Surgical treatment for infarct-related ventricular septal defects: improved early results combined with analysis of late functional status. *J Thorac Cardiovasc Surg* 1990;99:798–808.
36. Becker RC, Charlesworth A, Wilcox RG, et al. Cardiac rupture associated with thrombolytic therapy: impact of time to treatment in the late assessment of thrombolytic efficacy (LATE) study. *J Am Coll Cardiol* 1995;25:1063–1068.
37. Becker RC, Gore JM, Lambrew C, et al. A composite view of cardiac rupture in the United States: National Registry of Myocardial Infarction. *J Am Coll Cardiol* 1996;27:1321–1326.
38. Becker RC, Hochman JS, Cannon CP, et al. Fatal cardiac rupture among patients treated with thrombolytic agents and adjunctive thrombin antagonists. *J Am Coll Cardiol* 1999;33:479–487.
39. Tcheng JE, Jackman JD Jr, Nelson CL, et al. Outcome of patients sustaining acute ischemic mitral regurgitation during myocardial infarction. *Ann Intern Med* 1992;117:18–24.
40. Hendren WG, Nemec JJ, Lytle BW, et al. Mitral valve repair for ischemic mitral insufficiency. *Ann Thorac Surg* 1991;52:1246–1251.
41. Hutchins GM, Bulkley BH. Infarct expansion versus extension: two different complications of acute myocardial infarction. *Am J Cardiol* 1978;41:1127.
42. Pfeffer MA, Braunwald E, Moye LA, et al. Effect of captopril on mortality and morbidity in patients with left ventricular dysfunction after acute infarction. *N Engl J Med* 1992;327:669.
43. The Acute Infarction Ramipril Efficacy (AIRE) Study Investigators. Effect of ramipril on mortality and morbidity of survivors of acute myocardial infarction with clinical evidence of heart failure. *Lancet* 1993;342:821.
44. Martin RH, Almond CH, Saab S, et al. True and false aneurysms of the left ventricle following myocardial infarction. *Am J Med* 1977;62:418–424.
45. Krainin FM, Flessas AP, Spodick DH. Infarction-associated pericarditis: rarity of diagnostic electrocardiogram. *N Engl J Med* 1984;311:1211–1214.
46. Guillevin L, Valere PE. Pericarditis in acute myocardial infarction. *Lancet* 1976;1:429.
47. Guberman BA, Fowler NO, Engel PJ, et al. Cardiac tamponade in medical patients. *Circulation* 1981;64:633.
48. Miller RR, Lies JE, Carretta RF, et al. Prevention of lower extremity venous thrombus by early mobilization. *Ann Intern Med* 1976;84:700–703.
49. Gueret P, Bubourg O, Ferrier A, et al. Effects of full-dose heparin anticoagulation on the development of left ventricular thrombosis in acute myocardial infarction. *J Am Coll Cardiol* 1986;8:419.
50. Weinreich DJ, Burke JF, Pauletto FJ. Left ventricular mural thrombi complicating acute myocardial infarction: long-term follow-up with serial echocardiography. *Ann Intern Med* 1984;100:789.
51. Keating EC, Gross SA, Schlamowitz RA, et al. Mural thrombi in myocardial infarctions: prospective evaluation by two dimensional echocardiography. *Am J Med* 1983;74:989–995.
52. Martinowitz U, Michaelson M. Guidelines for the use of recombinant activated factor VII(rFVIIa) in uncontrolled bleeding: a report by the Israeli Multidisciplinary rFVIIa Task Force. *J Thromb Haemost* 2005;3:640–648.

CHAPTER 15 ■ CARDIAC CATHETERIZATION AND PERCUTANEOUS CORONARY INTERVENTION

CHRISTOPHER P. CANNON AND PATRICK T. O'GARA

INDICATIONS FOR CORONARY ANGIOGRAPHY
INDICATIONS FOR PERCUTANEOUS CORONARY INTERVENTION
PREOPERATIVE EVALUATION
INFORMED CONSENT
PREPARATION OF THE PATIENT
MANAGEMENT OF PATIENTS DURING THE PROCEDURE
MANAGEMENT OF THE PATIENT AFTER CARDIAC CATHETERIZATION AND PERCUTANEOUS CORONARY INTERVENTION
Cardiac Catheterization
Percutaneous Coronary Intervention

Coronary arteriography, the "gold standard" for identifying the presence or absence of stenoses caused by coronary artery disease (CAD), provides the most reliable anatomic information needed to determine the appropriateness of medical therapy, percutaneous coronary intervention (PCI), or coronary artery bypass graft (CABG) surgery. Coronary arteriography is performed by directly injecting radiopaque contrast material into the coronary arteries and imaging the coronary anatomy on 35-mm cinefilm or, more recently, digital recordings (1). It is estimated that more than two million patients will have coronary arteriography in the United States this year; of these, nearly 1 million will have PCI, using a variety of devices including conventional balloon angioplasty, atherectomy, or coronary stents.

The methods used to perform coronary arteriography have evolved substantially over the past few years. A number of factors have contributed to reduced complications and shorter hospitalization periods in patients having cardiac catheterization and PCI. More efficient preprocedural evaluation systems have been established, and many diagnostic tests are now performed in the preadmission testing centers, allowing patients "same-day" cardiac catheterization within 60 minutes after arrival to the cardiac catheterization laboratory. Smaller (5 to 6 Fr), high-flow injection catheters used during the procedure have replaced larger (8 Fr) thick-walled catheters. The reduced sheath size has allowed coronary arteriography, ambulation, and discharge within 6 to 8 hours following the procedure. The rapid sequence of events that occurs today in patients having cardiac catheterization and PCI lends itself to the establishment of "critical pathways" to coordinate the safe and efficient delivery of care in patients with symptomatic CAD. This chapter outlines the indications for cardiac catheterization and PCI and discusses the perioperative management in patients having these procedures.

INDICATIONS FOR CORONARY ANGIOGRAPHY

It is important to make certain that the patient has been referred to the cardiac catheterization suite with a clinical history and physical examination that warrant cardiac catheterization. Although the hemodynamic indications for cardiac catheterization are fairly clear (e.g., valvular heart disease, congestive heart failure [CHF]), indications for coronary arteriography are somewhat more vague. Appropriate guidelines for coronary arteriography have been outlined by a recent consensus statement of the American College of Cardiology (ACC) and American Heart Association (AHA) (1).

The following patients are candidates for coronary angiography.

1. Patients with suspected CAD who have stable angina or asymptomatic ischemia should undergo coronary arteriography if their angina is severe (Canadian Cardiovascular Society [CCS] class III–IV) or if they have "high-risk" criteria for adverse outcome on noninvasive testing.

    High-risk features include severe resting left ventricular (LV) dysfunction (LV ejection fraction [LVEF] <35%), or a standard exercise treadmill test demonstrating hypotension or ≥1- to 2-mm ST-segment depression associated with decreased exercise capacity (2) or an exercise-induced LVEF <35% (1). Stress imaging that demonstrates a large perfusion defect (particularly in the anterior wall), multiple defects, a large fixed perfusion defect with LV dilatation or increased thallium-201 lung uptake, or extensive stress or dobutamine-induced wall motion abnormalities also indicate high risk for an adverse outcome (1,3).

2. Patients resuscitated from sudden cardiac death, particularly those with residual ventricular arrhythmias, are also candidates for coronary arteriography, given the favorable outcomes associated with revascularization in these patients (1).

3. Patients with unstable angina who develop recurrent symptoms despite medical therapy or who are at "intermediate" or "high" risk of subsequent death or myocardial infarction (MI) are also candidates for coronary arteriography (1,4,5). High-risk features include prolonged, ongoing (>20 minutes) chest pain, pulmonary edema or worsening mitral regurgitation, dynamic ST-segment depression >1 mm, or hypotension (1). Intermediate-risk features include angina at rest (>20 minutes) relieved with rest or sublingual nitroglycerin, angina associated with dynamic electrocardiographic

changes, recent-onset angina with a high likelihood of CAD, pathologic Q waves or ST-segment depression <1 mm in multiple leads, or age >65 years (1).

4. Patients with Q-wave or non–Q-wave MI who develop spontaneous ischemia or with ischemia at a minimal workload or when the MI is complicated by CHF, hemodynamic instability, cardiac arrest, mitral regurgitation, or ventricular septal rupture should undergo coronary arteriography. Patients with angina or provocable ischemia after MI should also undergo coronary arteriography (6).

5. Patients presenting with chest pain of unclear cause, particularly those who have high-risk criteria on noninvasive testing, may benefit from coronary arteriography to diagnose or exclude the presence of significant CAD (1). Patients who have undergone prior revascularization should undergo coronary arteriography if suspicion exists of abrupt vessel closure or when recurrent angina develops with high-risk noninvasive criteria in patients who have undergone PCI within the past 9 months.

6. Coronary arteriography should be performed in patients scheduled to undergo noncardiac surgery who develop high-risk criteria on noninvasive testing, have angina unresponsive to medical therapy, develop unstable angina, or have equivocal noninvasive test results and are scheduled to undergo high-risk surgery. Coronary arteriography is also recommended for patients scheduled to undergo surgery for valvular heart disease or congenital heart disease, particularly those with multiple cardiac risk factors and those with infective endocarditis and evidence of coronary embolization (1).

7. Coronary arteriography should be performed annually in patients after cardiac transplantation in the absence of clinical symptoms because of the diffuse and asymptomatic nature of graft atherosclerosis (7). Coronary arteriography is useful in potential donors for cardiac transplantation whose age or cardiac risk profile increases the likelihood of CAD. Coronary arteriography often provides important diagnostic information about the presence of CAD in patients with intractable arrhythmias who are planned to undergo electrophysiologic testing or in patients who present with a dilated cardiomyopathy of unknown cause.

No absolute contraindications are seen for coronary arteriography (1), although cardiac catheterization should be performed with extreme caution in patients with unexplained fever, untreated infection, severe anemia with hemoglobin less than 8 g/dL, severe electrolyte imbalance, severe active bleeding, uncontrolled systemic hypertension, digitalis toxicity, previous contrast allergy but no pretreatment with corticosteroids, or ongoing stroke. Other relative contraindications include acute renal failure, decompensated CHF, severe coagulopathy, and active endocarditis (1).

Risk factors for significant complications after catheterization include advanced age, as well as several general medical, vascular, and cardiac characteristics. Patients with these risk factors should be monitored closely for a minimum of 18 to 24 hours after coronary arteriography, and admission is indicated in patients with severe renal insufficiency (creatinine >2.0 mg/dL) for fluid hydration, uncompensated CHF for diuresis, or advanced age. Coronary arteriography performed under emergency conditions is associated with a higher risk of procedural complications. Careful discussion of the risks and benefits of the procedure and its alternatives should be reviewed with the patient and family in all circumstances before coronary arteriography is performed.

INDICATIONS FOR PERCUTANEOUS CORONARY INTERVENTION

The major value of coronary revascularization, whether performed by surgical or percutaneous methods, is the relief of symptoms and signs of ischemic CAD caused by obstructive epicardial disease. A careful assessment of the risks and benefits of coronary revascularization must be reviewed with the patient and family members, if appropriate, before these procedures are performed. The following guidelines for the performance of PCI and CABG have been published by the ACC/AHA (8,9).

1. Patients who are asymptomatic or have only mild symptoms are generally best treated with medical therapy, unless one or more significant lesions subtend a large area of viable myocardium that is shown using objective noninvasive testing, the patient prefers to maintain an aggressive lifestyle or has a high-risk occupation, and the procedure can be performed with a high chance of success and low likelihood of complications (8).

2. Patients with classes II to IV angina, particularly those who are refractory to medical therapy, are suitable candidates for coronary revascularization, provided that the lesion subtends a moderate to large area of viable myocardium by noninvasive testing (8).

3. In selected patients with unstable angina or non–ST-elevation MI, PCI may improve prognosis, although it is not clear whether routine PCI is indicated in all patients with acute coronary syndromes (10–12).

4. Cardiac catheterization and selective coronary revascularization in patients who have received thrombolytic therapy is indicated for those with recurrent ischemia, those who present with or develop cardiogenic shock, or those who failed to develop signs of reperfusion after thrombolytic administration (6,13).

PREOPERATIVE EVALUATION

Once the appropriate indications have been established and the risk factors have been determined by the clinician, the patient should be prepared for the catheterization procedure. With the availability of high-resolution playback systems now available with digital angiographic systems, immediate interpretation of the coronary anatomy is available, and PCI is often performed in appropriate patients at the same sitting. As result, patients should be prepared for both coronary angiography and PCI.

INFORMED CONSENT

It is incumbent on the physician to fully explain the risks and benefits of the cardiac catheterization and PCI to the patient before the procedure. It is often useful to include family members in this discussion. Major complications (e.g., death, MI) are exceedingly uncommon (<0.3%) after routine coronary arteriography (Table 15-1). In two large registries of patients having femoral artery catheterization, death occurred in 0.10% to 0.14%, MI in 0.06% to 0.07%, cerebral ischemia or neurologic complications in 0.07% to 0.14%, contrast reactions in 0.23%, and local vascular complications in 0.24% to 0.46% (14,15). The incidence of death during coronary arteriography is higher in the presence of left main coronary artery (LMCA) disease (0.55%), in the presence of LVEF <30% (0.30%), and in patients with New York Heart Association functional class IV (0.29%). More recent registries have identified equivalent

TABLE 15-1

RISKS OF CARDIAC CATHETERIZATION

Risk factor	SCAI registry (%)
Mortality	0.11
Myocardial infarction	0.05
Cerebrovascular accident	0.07
Arrhythmias	0.38
Vascular complications	0.43
Contrast reaction	0.37
Hemodynamic complications	0.26
Perforation of heart chamber	0.03
Other complications	0.28
Total of major complications	1.70

SCAI, Society for Cardiac Angiography and Intervention.

complication rates despite increasing age and acuity of illness (16). The risk of clinically significant coronary air embolus during diagnostic coronary arteriography is low, occurring in less than 0.1% of cases. If the syndrome of coronary air embolus and air lock does occur, 100% oxygen by nonrebreathing face mask should be administered, which allows resorption of smaller amounts of air within 2 to 4 minutes. Morphine sulfate can be given for pain relief. Ventricular arrhythmias associated with air embolus can be treated with lidocaine and direct current cardioversion.

The risk factors for PCI are slightly higher than for coronary arteriography alone. Death occurs in less than 0.5% of elective procedures, and the frequency of periprocedural Q-wave MI is approximately 1% to 2%. The need for emergency CABG has been reduced substantially in recent years and is now less than 1% in most centers. Other complications (e.g., groin site bleeding, contrast-induced nephropathy, and lesser degrees of myocardial necrosis) occur in an additional 5% of patients after PCI.

PREPARATION OF THE PATIENT

Before coronary angiography, comorbid conditions (e.g., CHF, diabetes mellitus, or renal insufficiency) should be stable. A baseline electrocardiogram (ECG), electrolyte and renal function tests, complete blood count, and coagulation parameters should be reviewed before coronary arteriography and PCI. We recommend the following procedural preparations by the patient and clinician.

1. Patients should refrain from eating or drinking after midnight on the evening before the procedure. The patient may take the usual antihypertensive medications and antianginal medication on the morning of the procedure with a small sip of water. A period of fasting (>6 hours) is generally required for conscious sedation in patients having elective coronary arteriography and PCI.
2. Adequate preprocedural fluid hydration is needed in patients at high risk for contrast-induced nephrotoxicity (18), particularly in those patients with prior renal insufficiency, diabetes mellitus, dehydration before the procedure, CHF, larger volumes of contrast, and those with recent (<48 hour) contrast administration (19,20). In patients with baseline renal insufficiency (creatinine >1.5 mg/dL), use of nonionic contrast agents is associated with a lower incidence of contrast nephropathy (21).
3. Patients with a prior history of radiocontrast allergy should also be treated with two doses of prednisone

(60 mg, or its equivalent) on the night before and 2 hours before the procedure, based on a randomized study showing that patients given methylprednisolone (32 mg) 12 hours and 2 hours before contrast exposure had a lower (6.4%) incidence of allergic reactions than patients treated with a single dose of methylprednisolone 2 hours before contrast exposure (9.4%) or placebo (9%) (P <0.001) (22). Diphenhydramine (50 mg) and cimetidine (300 mg) should also be given before the procedure (23).
4. Patients who may have PCI immediately following coronary angiography should receive aspirin (100 to 325 mg) at least 2 hours before the procedure. A few good substitutes for aspirin are available, although pretreatment with ticlopidine or clopidogrel may be used as an alternative in aspirin-sensitive patients. It should be noted that aspirin desensitization can be performed in patients with a history of an allergic reaction to aspirin.
5. Clopidogrel pre-treatment is recommended in the ACC/AHA/SCAI Guidelines. 300 mg loading dose 6–12 hours prior to PCI has been used extensively, but 600 mg at least two hours pre-PCI has also been but tested (8).
6. Warfarin sodium should be discontinued at least 3 days before elective coronary arteriography, and the international normalized ratio should be less than 2.0 before arterial puncture. Patients at increased risk for systemic thromboembolism on withdrawal of warfarin (e.g., those with atrial fibrillation, mitral valve disease, or a history of systemic thromboembolism) can be treated with intravenous unfractionated heparin or subcutaneous low-molecular-weight heparin (LMWH) in the periprocedural period.
7. After informed consent has been obtained, we recommend that the patients receive diazepam (2.5 to 10 mg) orally, and diphenhydramine, 25 to 50 mg orally 1 hour before the procedure. Conscious sedation in the catheterization laboratory can also be performed using intravenous midazolam (0.5 to 2 mg) and fentanyl (25 to 50 µg), which are useful agents to provide sedation during the procedure if oral premedications are not given.
8. Those patients who are receiving intravenous unfractionated heparin should have their infusion discontinued just before the procedure. Patients who are receiving LMWH can safely have coronary angiography, but additional anticoagulation during PCI should be tailored to the timing of the most recent LMWH dose. Although intravenous heparin is no longer required during routine coronary arteriography (17), patients at increased risk for thromboembolic complications, including those with severe aortic stenosis, critical peripheral arterial disease, or arterial atheroembolic disease or those undergoing procedures requiring prolonged (>1 to 2 minutes) use of guidewires in the central circulation, can be given intravenous heparin (3,000 to 5,000 U). Patients having brachial or radial artery catheterization may also be given intra-arterial unfractionated heparin (2,000 to 5,000 U). Frequent (every 30 to 60 seconds) flushing of catheters with contrast medium or heparinized saline will avoid the formation of microthrombi within the catheter tip.
9. In the event that anticoagulation needs to be reversed, the anticoagulant effect of unfractionated heparin can be reversed with protamine (1 mg for every 100 U of heparin). Protamine can cause anaphylaxis or serious hypotensive episodes in approximately 2% of patients. Protamine should not be administered to patients with prior exposure to NPH insulin, because of an increased

risk of adverse effects, or in patients with a history of unstable angina, with a high-risk coronary anatomy, or have undergone coronary arteriography via the brachial or radial arteries.

10. After the procedure, femoral sheaths can be removed once the anticoagulant effect of heparin has dissipated (activated clotting time [ACT] <150 to 180 seconds).

MANAGEMENT OF PATIENTS DURING THE PROCEDURE

Patients should be kept modestly sedated during the procedure to reduce their anxiety. When complications do occur, the response should be coordinated with all the catheterization laboratory staff. A few of these complications are discussed next.

Allergic reactions to radiocontrast agents can be classified as mild (grade I: single episode of emesis, nausea, sneezing, or vertigo); moderate (grade II: hives, multiple episodes of emesis, fevers, or chills); or severe (grade III: clinical shock, bronchospasm, laryngospasm or edema, loss of consciousness, hypotension, hypertension, cardiac arrhythmias, angioedema, or pulmonary edema) (22). Although mild or moderate reactions occur in approximately 9% of patients, severe reactions are uncommon (0.15% to 0.7%) (19,20). Contrast reactions can be more difficult to manage in patients receiving beta-blocker therapy. Hives and urticaria can be managed with diphenhydramine (25 to 50 mg) intravenously, and hypotension can be managed with subcutaneous epinephrine (0.3 mL of a 1:1,000 dilution). Shock can be treated with intravenous epinephrine (3 mL of a 1:10,000 solution).

Patients can develop angina during coronary arteriography because of ischemia induced by tachycardia, hypertension, contrast agents, microembolization, coronary spasm or enhanced vasomotor tone, or dynamic platelet aggregation. Sublingual (0.3 mg), intracoronary (50 to 200 µg), or intravenous (25 µg/minute) nitroglycerin can be given to patients with a systolic blood pressure higher than 100 mm Hg. Patients without contraindications to beta-blockers (e.g., bradycardia, bronchospasm, or LV dysfunction) can be given intravenous metoprolol (2.5 to 5.0 mg) or propranolol (1 to 4 mg). Intra-aortic balloon counterpulsation is also a useful adjunct in patients with coronary ischemia and left main coronary artery disease, cardiogenic shock, or refractory pulmonary edema.

In patients undergoing PCI who are not given adjunct glycoprotein (GP) IIb/IIIa inhibitors, sufficient intravenous unfractionated heparin should be given to maintain the ACT between 250 and 300 seconds using the Hemochron device (International Technidyne) and 300 and 350 seconds using the Hemochron device. If GP IIb/IIIa inhibitors are given, ACT of more than 200 seconds generally suffices. Based on these studies, GP IIb/IIIa inhibitors should be considered in all patients having coronary intervention, including those having stent implantation. They are particularly beneficial in diabetics; patients with unstable angina with elevated troponins, dynamic ECG changes, or ongoing rest pain; and in those patients with acute MI undergoing primary angioplasty.

MANAGEMENT OF THE PATIENT AFTER CARDIAC CATHETERIZATION AND PERCUTANEOUS CORONARY INTERVENTION

Reduced arterial sheath sizes, reduced anticoagulation, and arterial closure devices have allowed more rapid ambulation in patients undergoing cardiac catheterization and PCI.

Cardiac Catheterization

Most patients can be discharged the same day after diagnostic cardiac catheterization. Following femoral artery catheterization, the 5 to 6 Fr catheter can be removed manually immediately, and following a period of 6 hours of bedrest with the leg extended, ambulation can be undertaken. Shorter (1 to 3 hours) periods of bedrest are indicated after the procedure if arterial closure devices (e.g., Angio-Seal [Kensey-Nash Corp., Exton, PA], VasoSeal [Datascope Corp., Montvale, NJ], or Perclose [Abbott Laboratories Co., Redwood City, CA]) are used, but the cost of these devices ($100 to $250) has prevented their widespread clinical use at our institution. No studies have shown a decreased complication rate with new closure devices compared with manual compression.

Because of the administration of radiocontrast agents during coronary angiography, 1 to 2 L of one-half normal saline should be administered intravenously after the procedure. The patient should also be encouraged to drink fluids. In patients with renal insufficiency or CHF, intravenous furosemide (20 to 80 mg) can be given to initiate a force diuresis and clearance of the radiocontrast agents.

With no signs of bleeding from the arterial puncture site, the patient can be discharged home. Patients undergoing femoral artery catheterization should be counseled to avoid lifting objects weighing more than 10 pounds for the ensuing 48 hours and driving a car for 72 hours. The patient should also be counseled about signs of rebleeding from the access site and to watch for signs of redness, tenderness, expanding ecchymosis, or extreme tenderness. On occasion, pseudoaneurysms develop after hospital discharge, and a low threshold for vascular ultrasound should be undertaken in patients who present with symptoms.

Percutaneous Coronary Intervention

Patients undergoing PCI are generally kept in the hospital overnight, although outpatient PCI has been successfully undertaken at some institutions with extensive follow-up networks. In patients undergoing balloon angioplasty or atherectomy alone, aspirin (80 to 325 mg daily) is recommended for secondary prevention of coronary events. In those patients receiving a coronary stent, clopidogrel 300–600 mg loading dose preprocedure, followed by 75 mg daily for 1 year ideally to prevent subacute stent thrombosis. An absolute minimum duration 1, 3, or 6 months for bare metal, sirolimus coated, or paclitaxel-coated stents is needed (8).

Similar to patients undergoing cardiac catheterization, patients undergoing PCI should also receive 1 to 2 L of one-half normal saline, and patients with renal insufficiency and CHF may also need intravenous furosemide. In the absence of angiographic complications, patients do not require anticoagulation after PCI, and the sheaths should be removed when the ACT is less than 150 seconds. Vascular closure devices, which are used more often after PCI, allow ambulation 4 to 6 hours after the procedure. In addition, some clinicians routinely use the radial artery for access, which allows ambulation immediately after the procedure. With no signs of bleeding from the arterial puncture site, the patient can be discharged home the following morning, with the same precautions given those patients undergoing cardiac catheterization.

It is important to emphasize to patients with CAD that atherosclerosis is a ubiquitous disease that manifests clinical symptoms only late in its pathogenic development. Ischemia management in patients with symptomatic CAD should have two major objectives: (a) to relieve the flow-limiting stenosis causing ischemia using stents, balloon catheter, atherectomy devices, or radiation therapy to provide an effective long-term outcome at the site of arterial narrowing, and (b) to prevent further episodes of death and MI, which requires aggressive, systemic lipid reduction therapy. Patients, specialists, and primary care physicians each need to take accountability for risk factor modification after coronary revascularization. It should be emphasized to the patient that atherosclerosis is a lifelong disease, and the measures to improve coronary flow by percutaneous or surgical methods are just palliative—definitive therapy may be too late once symptoms have developed. The objective should be to lower the low-density lipoprotein-cholesterol (LDL-C) to less than 70 mg/dL in all patients. Once lipid-lowering therapy is begun, regular surveillance according to the National Cholesterol Education Program (NCEP) guidelines should be undertaken to make certain that the treatment goal of LDL-C less than 70 mg/dL is achieved. At the very least, patients with CAD should have a keen awareness of the prognostic implications for maintaining aggressive dietary and pharmacologic approach to lipid-lowering therapy after cardiac catheterization and PCI.

Acknowledgment

The authors wish to acknowledge Jeffrey J. Popma as the author of this chapter in the previous edition, which was the basis for this chapter.

References

1. Scanlon P, Faxon DP, Audet A-M, et al. ACC/AHA guidelines for coronary angiography. *J Am Coll Cardiol* 1999;33:1756–1824.
2. Fletcher GF, Balady G, Froelicher VF, et al. Exercise standards: a statement for healthcare professionals from the American Heart Association. *Circulation* 1995;91:580–615.
3. Travin MI, Boucher CA, Newell JB, et al. Variables associated with a poor prognosis in patients with an ischemic thallium-201 exercise test. *Am Heart J* 1993;125:335–344.
4. Braunwald E. Unstable angina. A classification. *Circulation* 1989;80(2):410–414.
5. Braunwald E, Jones RH, Mark DB, et al. Diagnosing and managing unstable angina. *Circulation* 1994;90:613–622.
6. Madsen JK, Grande P, Saunamäki K, et al. Danish multicenter randomized study of invasive versus conservative treatment in patients with inducible ischemia after thrombolysis in acute myocardial infarction (DANAMI). *Circulation* 1997;96(3):748–755.
7. Fish RD, Nabel EG, Selwyn AP, et al. Responses of coronary arteries of cardiac transplant patients to acetylcholine. *J Clin Invest* 1988;81:21–31.
8. Smith SC, Jr., Feldman TE, Hirshfeld JW, Jr., et al. ACC/AHA/SCAI 2005 Guideline Update for Percutaneous Coronary Intervention-Summary Article: A Report of the American College of Cardiology/American Heart Association Task Force on Practice Guidelines (ACC/AHA/SCAI Writing Committee to Update the 2001 Guidelines for Percutaneous Coronary Intervention). *J Am Coll Cardiol* 2006;47(1):216–235.
9. Eagle KA, Guyton RA, Davidoff R, et al. ACC/AHA 2004 guideline update for coronary artery bypass graft surgery: summary article: a report of the American College of Cardiology/American Heart Association Task Force on Practice Guidelines (Committee to Update the 1999 Guidelines for Coronary Artery Bypass Graft Surgery.) *Circulation* 2004;110(9):1168–1176.
10. Anderson HV, Cannon CP, Stone PH, et al. One year results of the thrombolysis in myocardial infarction (TIMI) IIIB clinical trial. *J Am Coll Cardiol* 1995;26:1643–1650.
11. Boden WE, O'Rourke RA, Crawford MH, et al. Outcomes in patients with acute non–Q-wave myocardial infarction randomly assigned to an invasive as compared with a conservative management strategy. *N Engl J Med* 1998;338(25):1785–1792.
12. Invasive compared with non-invasive treatment in unstable coronary artery disease: FRISC II prospective randomised multicentre study. *Lancet* 1999;354:708–715.
13. Ryan T, Faxon DP, Gunnar RM, et al. Guidelines for percutaneous transluminal coronary angioplasty: a report of the American College of Cardiology/American Heart Association Task Force on Assessment of Diagnostic and Therapeutic Cardiovascular Procedures. *J Am Coll Cardiol* 1988;12:529–545.
14. Coronary Artery Surgery Study (CASS). A randomized trial of coronary artery bypass surgery: survival data. *Circulation* 1983;68:939–950.
15. Klinke WP, Kubac G, Talibi T, et al. Safety of outpatient catheterizations. *Am J Cardiol* 1985;56:639–641.
16. Johnson LW. Cardiac catheterization 1991. *Cathet Cardiovasc Diagn* 1993;28:219–220.
17. Davis K, Kennedy JW, Kemp HG Jr, et al. Complications of coronary arteriography. *Circulation* 1979;59:1105–1112.
18. Solomon R, Werner C, Mann D, et al. Effects of saline, mannitol, and furosemide to prevent acute decreases in renal function induced by radiocontrast agents. *N Engl J Med* 1994;331:1416–1420.
19. Taliercio CP, McCallister SH, Holmes DR, et al. Nephrotoxicity of nonionic contrast media after cardiac angiography. *Am J Cardiol* 1989;64:815–816.
20. Brogan WC III, Hillis LD, Lange RA. Contrast agents for cardiac catheterization: conceptions and misconceptions. *Am Heart J* 1991;122:1129–1135.
21. Hill JA, Winniford M, Cohen MB, et al. Multicenter trial of ionic versus nonionic contrast media for cardiac angiography. *Am J Cardiol* 1993;72(11):770–775.
22. Lasser ED, Berry CC, Talner LB, et al. Pretreatment with corticosteroids to alleviate reactions to intravenous contrast material. *N Engl J Med* 1987;317:845–849.
23. Hill JA, Lambert CR, Pepine CJ. Radiographic contrast agents. In: Pepine CJ, Hill JA, Lambert CR, eds. *Diagnostic and therapeutic cardiac catheterization.* Baltimore: Williams & Wilkins; 1994:182–194.

CHAPTER 16 ■ PATHWAYS FOR CORONARY ARTERY BYPASS SURGERY

RASHID M. AHMAD, FRANCES WADLINGTON, TIFFANY STREET, JAMES P. GREELISH, JORGE M. BALAGUER, AND JOHN G. BYRNE

BACKGROUND
PREOPERATIVE PATHWAY
History
Physical Examination
Studies and Laboratory Evaluation
POSTOPERATIVE PATHWAY
Day of Surgery
Initial Postoperative Assessment
EXTUBATION GUIDELINES
Postoperative Day 1
Postoperative Days 2 to 4
Postoperative Day 4
MANAGEMENT GUIDELINES FOR ATRIAL
    FIBRILLATION
Prophylaxis
Treatment

BACKGROUND

The development of "critical pathways" in coronary artery bypass graft (CABG) surgery was initiated primarily in response to cost pressures created by managed care and changes in health care reimbursement. It was felt that the implementation of pathways or clearly defined and reproducible care goals would improve efficiency, decrease costs, and maintain or improve quality. The use of these pathways supplemented existing guidelines and practice standards that had evolved over time. CABG was an early opportunity for application of critical pathways because this operation is frequently performed, is resource intensive, and care processes do not differ significantly from patient to patient. Specific goals are shown in Table 16-1 (1).

A multidisciplinary team consisting of cardiac surgeons, cardiologists, nurses, physical therapists, midlevel providers, and case managers provided input for developing the critical pathway at Vanderbilt University Medical Center. Measurable goals and outcomes included time to extubation following surgery, length of stay, utilization of laboratory tests, chest x-rays, electrocardiograms, and diagnostic studies including pulmonary function tests and carotid duplex studies. Particular emphasis was placed on four key outcomes (Table 16-2).

The critical pathway is a collection of task categories that include assessment, consults, tests, activity, medications, treatments, diet, education, and discharge. Currently at our institution, clinical documentation is computerized and notes are written electronically with discrete capture of the events and stored in a database as well as in the hospital's electronic record. This system allows statistical assessment of a patient's postoperative course. Analysis of variance provides the clinician with insight into critical steps in the care process and provides a platform for continuous improvement.

Implementation of the critical pathway is one element in a multifactorial approach to improving efficiency and quality and reducing length of stay (2). Although there are no controlled trials demonstrating the benefits of critical pathway implementation in cardiac surgery, rapid recovery and early discharge is increasingly becoming the standard of care, and most evidence suggests that outcomes are improved (3).

The basic elements of a given critical pathway can be incorporated into order sets or into practice guidelines. Our current pathways and guidelines have evolved to reflect our experience as well as nationally accepted standards of care (4). It should be emphasized that pathways, protocols, and guidelines represent commonly agreed-on standards of care at a particular institution. Therefore, minor differences may exist in critical pathways at differing institutions depending on the infrastructure of the ancillary services and personnel.

Practice standards in pathways may not have the support of prospective randomized trials and consequently remain open to modification. Patients with significant complications or pre-existing medical problems may not always be candidates for pathways or guidelines. Recognizing that certain comorbidities may significantly affect and require alteration from a critical pathway to generate a "subpathway" is essential for individualizing care for patients. The clinical judgment of the physi-

TABLE 16-1

SPECIFIC GOALS FOR CRITICAL PATHWAYS

1. Selecting a "best practice" when practice styles vary unnecessarily.
2. Defining standards for the expected duration of hospital stay and for the use of tests and treatments.
3. Examining the inter-relations among the different steps in the care process to find ways to coordinate or decrease the time spent in the rate-limiting steps.
4. Giving all hospital staff a common "game plan" from which to view and understand their various roles in the overall care process.
5. Providing a framework for collecting data on the care process so that providers can learn how often and why patients do not follow an expected course during their hospitalization.
6. Decreasing nursing and physician documentation burdens.
7. Improving patient satisfaction with care by educating patients and their families about the plan of care and involving them more fully in its implementation.

TABLE 16-2

CABG CRITICAL PATHWAY—KEY OUTCOMES

Postoperative Day	Outcome
Day of Surgery	Extubation
Postoperative day 1	Transfer to intermediate care telemetry unit
Postoperative day 2	Removal of pacing wires
Postoperative day 3	Ambulate 300 feet TID
Postoperative day 4	Discharge from hospital

cian and associated health care providers should rarely be substituted by a "recipe" pathway. This chapter will summarize current pathways and guidelines for uncomplicated CABG surgery at Vanderbilt University Medical Center. Guidelines for new-onset atrial fibrillation have been also included because it occurs so frequently.

PREOPERATIVE PATHWAY

Patients are now typically admitted for elective CABG surgery on the day of surgery. For patients undergoing more urgent surgery, the basic elements of the pathway are incorporated in the preoperative order set (Table 16-3A). As noted previously,

TABLE 16-3A

PREOPERATIVE ORDER SET

Pre-op for: Tomorrow
Diet: House, NPO after midnight
VS q4h please obtain height and weight.
Activity: As tolerated
Allergies: NKDA
IV: Saline lock
Anesthesia consult
12-Lead EKG
Radiology: Chest PA & Lateral
Laboratory Tests:
 CBC with platelet count
 PT, PTT if pt on heparin or Coumadin
 Electrolytes: BUN, creatine, glucose, calcium, SGOT, SGPT, bilirubin
 Hemoglobin A1C
 Urine analysis
 Urine drug screen
 Type and cross match four bags PRBC
Cardiac chipping & prep chin to toes. Hibiclens shower night before surgery and morning of surgery
Keep HOB at 30 degrees.
NTG 1/150 1 TAB SL × 1 PRN chest pain
Medications:
 Continue beta-blockers, heparin, NTG
 Bactroban ointment to each nare on night before and morning of surgery
 Ambien 5 to 10 mg PO qhs prn insomnia
 Ancef 2 grams IV to the OR this patient
Call HO for T >101, SBP >160, SBP <90, HR >100, RR >30, Chest pain

there may be slight institutional differences for critical pathways, and Table 16-3B shows the preoperative CABG order set at the Nashville Veterans Administration Hospital, an affiliate of Vanderbilt University Medical Center.

Patients undergoing CABG should undergo a preoperative history and physical examination. In addition, standard hematologic and chemistry profiles, urinalysis, an electrocardiogram (ECG), and a chest x-ray should be obtained (a lateral film is mandatory for all reoperations to assess proximity of the heart to the sternum). In addition to coronary angiography, an assessment of left ventricular (LV) function (left ventriculography or echocardiography) is typically made. Other studies (e.g., carotid Doppler studies or pulmonary function tests for patients with history of smoking or asthma) may be performed if dictated by the preoperative evaluation. It has become extremely important to capture and document a patient's comorbidities for accurate assessment of risk as well as for financial reimbursement.

There are several key elements of the preoperative assessment that influence perioperative management and determine morbidity and mortality risk. They include the following.

TABLE 16-3B

NASHVILLE VETERANS ADMINISTRATION PREOPERATIVE ORDERS

1. Initiate the Cardiac Surgery Protocols Pre-op for: _____ (date)
   a. BMP, magnesium, CBC, coagulation panel (PT, PTT, INR), hepatic panel, UA with sediment, ABG, and 12-lead ECG
   Type and cross for 4 units PRBCs, 3 units Platelets, 2 units FFP
   Chest x-Ray: AP and lateral and pre-op op swabs for MRSA (nasal) and VRE (rectal)
   Obtain pulmonary function tests, echocardiogram, carotid duplex if patient history warrants need.
2. Head to toe Hibiclen's shower/wash (not scrub) night before surgery; no powder or deodorant
3. Bactroban nasal ointment both nares BID until pre-op nasal cultures return negative
4. Restoril 15 mg PO at bedtime × 1 dose as needed for sleep
5. Obtain patient's pre-op (stated) height and (measured) weight and document in patient's chart.
6. Please notify house officer if: T >100°F orally and occurs within 12 hours of planned surgery.
7. Replace potassium and magnesium according to cardiac surgery pre-op protocol.
8. NPO after midnight night before surgery, except for the following medications _____ .
9. If in-patient, please transport patient to OR on 2 L/min O_2 via nasal cannula
10. Immediate pre-op orders

A. Pre-op shave prep:
   All in-patients: On unit, electric shave prep: umbilicus, anterior chest wall, bilateral inner thighs to ankle night before surgery.

B. Pre-op antibiotics:
   Cefazolin 1 gm IV pre-op dose on call to the OR –or– Vancomycin 1 gm if patient has Beta Lactam/PCN allergy or if patient has positive MRSA cultures.

History

- Age
- Sex
- Obesity
- History of stroke or transient ischemic attack
- Peripheral vascular disease
- Diabetes mellitus
- Renal failure or insufficiency
- Liver disease
- Chronic obstructive pulmonary disease (COPD)
- Smoking and alcohol history
- Anginal symptoms
- Symptoms of congestive heart failure
- Previous thoracic surgery
- History of recent infection
- History of bleeding or thrombocytopenia
- Medications, particularly
  - Anticoagulants
  - Antiplatelet agents
  - Beta-blockers
  - Angiotensin-converting enzyme (ACE) inhibitors
  - Diuretics
  - Antiarrhythmics
  - Thyroid medication
  - Insulin and oral hypoglycemics
- Allergies

Physical Examination

- Neurologic deficits
- Evidence of pulmonary disease
- Bruits
- Murmurs
- Discrepancies in upper extremity blood pressure
- Signs of peripheral vascular disease
- Adequacy of peripheral arteries and veins for bypass conduit
- Presence of abdominal aortic aneurysm

Studies and Laboratory Evaluation

- Evidence of renal or hepatic dysfunction
- Electrolyte abnormalities
- Coagulation abnormalities, presence of anemia
- Evidence of infection
- Presence of left main coronary artery disease
- Left ventricular ejection fraction
- Valvular abnormalities
- Evidence of aortic calcification
- Evidence of heart failure, pulmonary infiltrates, or congestion

Four units of packed red blood cells are typically reserved for patients undergoing first-time coronary artery surgery, and additional units are reserved for reoperations. Patients are instructed not to eat or drink after midnight prior to undergoing surgery. In general, preoperative antihypertensive, antianginal, and antiarrhythmic medications are continued up until surgery, particularly heparin, nitroglycerin, and beta-blockers. A cephalosporin (e.g., cefazolin) should be given within 30 to 60 minutes of incision to maximize its efficacy. Intraoperatively, the prophylactic antibiotic should also be repeated at a dosing interval of two times the half-life of the drug (5).

Patient and family education is initiated as early as possible and continued throughout the patient's stay. Setting expectations early for the patient and family is critical for safely minimizing length of stay and ensuring successful outcomes.

POSTOPERATIVE PATHWAY

Day of Surgery

Upon arrival in the intensive care unit (ICU), surgeons and anesthesiologists communicate the details of the procedure to the nurses and physicians assuming the care of the patient. Hemodynamic, ECG, temperature, and pulse oximetry monitoring are established. Most of the basic elements of the critical pathway are incorporated into the postoperative order set (Table 16-4).

Initial Postoperative Assessment

Initial evaluation of the patient following surgery includes the following elements.

- ECG
- Chest x-ray
- Cardiac output (for depressed LV function, pulmonary hypertension)
  - Thermodilution or Fick method (if PA catheter in place)
  - Extremity perfusion, urine output, blood pressure
- Assessment of bleeding

TABLE 16-4

CORONARY ARTERY BYPASS GRAFTING POSTOPERATIVE ORDER SET

Admit to cardiac surgery intensive care unit
Diagnosis: s/p CABG
Initiate collaborative path
Allergies: NKDA
Condition: Stable
Continuous cardiac monitor
Continuous pulse oximetry
Continuous hemodynamic monitoring
Pacemaker wires attached to pacemaker; pacemaker on standby
Vital Signs q 15 min × 4 then q 1 hr
Neurovascular checks q 2 hrs
Temperature q 1h
CO/CI/SVR q 2h
NG tube pH, irrigate q 4h
Surgical Bra on all patients with breasts that strain the midline incision
I + O q 1h
Daily weight 0500
Activity: Soft restraints when intubated
    Elevate the HOB to 30 degrees when hemodynamically stable.
    Turn side to side, reposition q 2h
    Elevate vein harvest extremity on pillow
    Dangle within 2 hrs postextubation, if hemodynamically stable OOB to chair
    OOB to chair by 0900 POD 1 and thereafter
Respiratory
    Ventilator settings Mode: SIMV; FiO$_2$: 60%; TV: 10 cc/kg; Rate: 14; PEEP: 5 cm H$_2$O

- Laboratory studies
  - Arterial blood gas
  - Mixed venous blood gas (if PA catheter in place)
  - Complete blood count; electrolytes blood urea nitrogen (BUN), creatinine, glucose

Hypothermic (temp <36°C) patients are actively warmed (6). Arterial blood gases are obtained every 4 hours until the patient is extubated, unless clinical circumstances dictate more frequent assessment. Hemoglobin and potassium levels are obtained with each blood gas. Coagulation tests do not need to be repeated if there is no significant bleeding. Aspirin is given within 1 hour postoperatively if there is no evidence of active bleeding (7). Vasoactive medications are weaned as tolerated. In the absence of complications, early extubation is attempted.

EXTUBATION GUIDELINES

Early extubation can shorten ICU stays, reduce respiratory complications, and lower costs (8). In the absence of complications, patients can be safely extubated within 4 to 6 hours. This is facilitated by the use of short-acting anesthetic agents (e.g., propofol). Nonsteroidal anti-inflammatory drugs (NSAIDs) (indomethacin and ketorolac) can provide significant analgesia without sedation and can reduce narcotic requirements (9). NSAIDs should be avoided in patients with renal insufficiency, recent peptic ulcer disease, or significant postoperative bleeding. Patients may be extubated when adequate oxygenation and ventilation are maintained, secretions are manageable, and nonpulmonary contraindications to extubation are absent (Table 16-5).

Postoperative Day 1

Evaluation of the patient on postoperative day (POD) 1 includes the following elements:

1. Vital signs, weight, fluid balance
2. ECG
3. Chest x-ray
4. Cardiac output
   Thermodilution or Fick method (if PA catheter in place)
   Extremity perfusion, urine output, blood pressure
5. Chest tube output
6. Laboratory studies
   Arterial blood gas
   Mixed venous blood gas (if PA catheter in place and thermodilution output is marginal)
   Complete blood count; electrolytes BUN, creatinine, glucose

Beta-blockers are started on all patients unless there are contraindications (see management guidelines for atrial fibrillation, following). Aspirin is continued. ACE inhibitors are started for patients with low ejection fraction (<40%). Caution is exercised in patients with a history of renal insufficiency. Most patients are started on a diuretic with potassium replacement. Pain control is assessed.

Pulmonary artery catheters are removed if cardiac output is adequate and the patient is not requiring inotropic medications. Patients are mobilized from bed to chair. Diet is initiated with clear fluids and advanced as tolerated.

In the absence of complications, Foley catheter and central line are removed, and patients are transferred to a step-down

---

TABLE 16-5

EXTUBATION PATHWAY FOR CABG PATIENTS

1. **Arrival to ICU**
   a. When patient temperature is ≥35, discontinue Propofol and raise HOB 30 degrees as BP allows
   b. ABG 15 minutes after arrival. If the ABG meets the following criteria:
      - pH >7.35
      - PaO_2 ≥65
      - PCO_2 <45
   c. Decrease IMV to 8 and wean FiO_2 to 40% keeping SaO_2 ≥92%
2. **Weaning criteria**
   a. Does the patient meet the following weaning criteria?
      - No evidence of ischemia by 12-lead ECG
      - Normothermic (≥36°C)
      - Chest tube output <100 cc/hr
      - SaO_2 ≥92% on FiO_2 <50%
      - Awake and following commands
      - Conscious and able to raise head
      - Bilateral hand grasps, leg lifts
      - Gag reflex present
      - Secretions are absent to minimal and easily cleared
      - Stable hemodynamics: MAP >60 and <100; HR >70 and <110; CI ≥2.0
      - No hemodynamically significant dysrhythmias
      - Without significant pain
      - UOP ≥0.5 ml/kg/hr
      - Manageable airway secretions
      - Total respiratory rate ≥12
   b. If patient meets the preceding criteria, decrease IMV to 4 and monitor minute ventilation. Patient must maintain minute ventilation ≥6.5 liters. If patient unable to maintain minute ventilation, return to IMV = 8
3. **CPAP**
   a. After 30 minutes on IMV = 4, if patient continues to meet all criteria in Step Two, then place patient on CPAP for 30 minutes and obtain ABG
4. **Extubation**
   a. Notify house officer with ABG results and for extubation order
   b. Criteria for extubation:
      - Awake and following commands; able to lift head off pillow
      - pH >7.35
      - PaO_2 ≥65
      - $PaCO_2$ ≤48
      - SaO_2 ≥92% on FiO_2 ≤50%

unit (SDU), which has telemetry monitoring. Table 16-6 is the order set for transfer to the SDU.

Postoperative Days 2 to 4

Evaluation of the patient on postoperative days 2 to 4 includes the following elements:

1. Vital signs, weight, fluid balance
2. Chest x-ray and ECG is obtained the day before discharge
3. Laboratory studies
   Complete blood count; electrolytes BUN, creatinine, glucose

TABLE 16-6

CORONARY ARTERY BYPASS GRAFTING TRANSFER TO STEP-DOWN ORDER SET

Transfer to step-down unit, Cardiac Surgery Service
Diagnosis: s/p CABG
NKDA
Condition: Stable
Vital signs: q 4 hours
Cardiac telemetry
    O2 sats q 4 hours
    Blood glucose as directed
    Titrate FIO$_2$ to keep O$_2$ sat >92%, notify attending for increase oxygen needs
I + O q 4 hours to include chest tube drainage
Daily weight

Activity:
    Ambulate in halls TID goal at least 300 ft
    Cardiac rehab to begin seeing pt on POD 1
    OOB by 0900 and with all meals
    Ambulate independently QID on POD 2–4
    Limit sitting (with legs down) to meals and bathroom only
Cough and deep breathe q 2 hours while awake
Remove dressing morning of POD 2
Chest tube site care qd POD 1 to POD 4.
Pacing wire care: Cleanse with soap and water q 24hrs

Tubes and drains:
    Chest tube to suction measure output q 4 hrs
    Foley to gravity. Remove on POD 1

Diet: Advance as tolerated cardiac diet
IV: Saline lock

Medications:
Metoprolol 12.5 mg
Aspirin enteric coated 325 mg
Furosemide
Initiate statin
ACE inhibitor
Percocet prn pain
Colace (docusate sodium) 100 mg PO TID prn constipation
MOM (magnesium hydroxide) 30 mL PO QD prn constipation

Tests
EKG POD 1
CXR after chest tube removal

Beta-blockers, diuretics, ACE inhibitors, and electrolyte replacements are adjusted each morning and as indicated. Statin medications are begun once the patients are tolerating a cardiac diet. Patients are mobilized and ambulated at least 300 feet TID. Pacing wires and chest tubes are removed on POD 2. Chest tubes are removed if the patient has been mobilized and if the chest tube output has been less than 150 cc for the previous 8 hours. Need for rehabilitation facility or home resources are identified on POD 1 to 2, and arrangements are facilitated throughout the remainder of the hospital stay.

Postoperative Day 4

Discharge from hospital to home or other inpatient facility.

MANAGEMENT GUIDELINES FOR ATRIAL FIBRILLATION

Atrial fibrillation is a common complication of surgery in the chest; it occurs in approximately one-third of patients following CABG surgery. Prophylaxis and treatment are controversial, although the use of beta-blockers for prophylaxis is generally accepted (10–12). The guidelines outlined following are based on the recognition that postoperative atrial fibrillation is generally well tolerated and self-limited and represents one attempt to standardize therapy.

Prophylaxis

A beta-blocker (metoprolol) should be started or resumed in all patients on POD 1 following cardiac surgery unless specific contraindications exist (13). Patients receiving beta-blockers preoperatively are two times more likely to develop atrial fibrillation postoperatively if the medication is not restarted (14).
    Contraindications include:

    Hemodynamic compromise
    Inotropic support
    AV block (PR interval >0.24, second- or third-degree block)
    Known history of beta-blocker-induced bronchospasm

Metoprolol 12.5 mg PO (orally) BID or QID is a suggested starting dose. Patients should be assessed daily and the dosage adjusted to ensure effective beta-blockade. If patients do not experience significant atrial arrhythmias, they should be transitioned to BID dosing or their preoperative beta-blocker by POD 3 or 4.

Treatment

Initial Assessment

The management of atrial fibrillation should be guided by the answers to the following three questions.
    1. Is the patient symptomatic? Atrial fibrillation is generally well tolerated, and overaggressive management can cause significant morbidity. Nonetheless, the first step in the management of atrial fibrillation is an assessment of its hemodynamic significance. Significant symptoms may respond to rate control alone or may require chemical or electrical cardioversion. Monitor for:

- Hypotension
- Changes in mental status
- Decreased urine output
- Decreased peripheral perfusion
- Anginal symptoms
- Decreased cardiac output or increased filling pressures

    2. What are the precipitating factors? Appropriate management of atrial fibrillation requires identification and treatment of potential risk factors. Atrial fibrillation can result from:

- Beta-blocker withdrawal
- Ischemia
- Atrial distension
- Increased sympathetic tone
- Electrolyte imbalances, particularly hypokalemia and hypomagnesemia (frequently precipitated by diuresis)
- Acid–base disturbances
- Sympathomimetic medications (inotropes, bronchodilators)

- Pneumonia, atelectasis
- Pulmonary embolism

3. What are the goals of therapy? Hemodynamic stability is the primary goal. For most patients, rate control is sufficient because 90% of patients with new-onset atrial fibrillation following cardiac surgery will be in normal sinus rhythm (NSR) in 6 weeks (15). Evidence of hemodynamic compromise or interference with recovery should prompt chemical or electrical cardioversion.

Drug Therapy

Although there are several options, one should remember that single drug therapy is generally better than multidrug therapy.

1. **Beta-blockers:** Metoprolol should be first-line therapy in most patients and can be given either PO or intravenously (IV). Metoprolol should be titrated to effect with a heart rate goal of less than 100 beats/minute at rest. The suggested treatment for new-onset rapid atrial fibrillation is 5 to 10 mg IV or 50 mg PO, followed by 25 mg PO every 6 hours and titrated upward, until NSR or adequate rate control is achieved. Additional doses of intravenous metoprolol may be needed. Some patients may require up to 200 mg/day PO.

2. **Calcium channel blockers:** For patients who cannot tolerate beta-blockers, diltiazem is the agent of choice. It should be initiated as a bolus at 0.25 mg/kg IV, followed by a continuous infusion 5 to 15 mg/hr as tolerated. A second bolus of 0.35 mg/kg may be needed. The combination of metoprolol and diltiazem is occasionally necessary to achieve adequate rate control, but should be used cautiously given concerns for hypotension or bradycardia.

3. **Antiarrhythmic:** Amiodarone can cause hypotension, especially in patients with LV systolic dysfunction, when given rapidly by intravenous infusion. Therefore, an amiodarone bolus of 150 mg should be administered over 30 minutes, followed by an infusion of 1 mg/kg for 6 hours, then 0.5 mg/hr. Intravenous amiodarone should be administered only by a central route and not via a peripheral line. Oral amiodarone should be substituted as soon as possible. An ECG should be obtained to monitor for QTc prolongation. Amiodarone can be weaned over a 6-week period and stopped to maximize its benefits and minimize the toxicity associated with its administration (16–19). Recent studies suggest reduction in the incidence of postoperative atrial fibrillation for patients who receive amiodarone prophylactically. It can be given orally several days before elective surgery or as an intravenous bolus at the time of induction (20).

Direct Current Cardioversion

Direct current cardioversion should be used emergently for the treatment of hemodynamically unstable atrial fibrillation, starting at 200 J (synchronous). Sedation (e.g., propofol) should be used. In patients with atrial wires who are in atrial flutter, overdrive pacing can be attempted. Biphasic cardioversion has a higher success rate for cardioversion.

Anticoagulation

Patients who remain in atrial fibrillation for more than 48 hours or who have paroxysmal atrial fibrillation should be started on warfarin in the absence of contraindications. Patients who require a permanent pacemaker should be transitioned to warfarin with intravenous heparin.

References

1. Pearson SD, Goulart-Fisher D, Lee TH. Critical pathways as a strategy for improving care: problems and potential. *Ann Intern Med* 1995;123(12): 941–948.
2. Cohn LH, Rosborough D, Fernandez J. Reducing costs and length of stay and improving efficiency and quality of care in cardiac surgery. *Ann Thorac Surg* 1997;64(6 Suppl):S58–60; discussion S80–82.
3. Cowper PA, Peterson ED, DeLong ER, et al. Impact of early discharge after coronary artery bypass graft surgery on rates of hospital readmision and death. The Ischemic Heart Disease (IHD) patient Outcomes Research Team (PORT) Investigators. *J Am Coll Cardiol* 1997;30(4):908–913.
4. Eagle KA, Guyton RA, Davidoff R, et al. ACC/AHA guidelines for coronary artery bypass graft surgery: a report of the American College of Cardiology/American Heart Association Task Force on Practice Guidelines (Committee to Revise the 1991 Guidelines for Coronary Artery Bypass Graft Surgery). *J Am Coll Cardiol* 1999;34:1262–1346.
5. Kreter B, Woods M. Antibiotic prophylaxis for cardiothoracic operations: meta-analysis of thirty years of clinical trials. *J Thorac Cardiovasc Surg* 1992;104:590–599.
6. Frank SM, Fleischer LA, Breslow MJ, et al. Perioperative maintenance of normothermia reduces the incidence of morbid cardiac events. *JAMA* 1997; 277:1127–1134.
7. Lorenz RL, Schacky CV, Weber M, et al. Improved aortocoronary bypass patency by low-dose aspirin (100 mg daily): effects on platelet aggregation and thromboxane formation. *Lancet* 1984;1:1261–1264.
8. Lee JH, Kim KH, vanHeeckeren DW, et al. Cost analysis of early extubation after coronary bypass surgery. *Surgery* 1996;120(4):611–617.
9. Ready LB, Brown CR, Stahlgren LH, et al. Evaluation of intravenous ketorolac administered by bolus or infusion for treatment of postoperative pain. A double-blind, placebo-controlled, multicenter study. *Anesthesiology* 1994;80:1277–86.
10. Hogue CW, Hyder ML. Atrial fibrillation after cardiac operation: risks, mechanisms, and treatment. *Ann Thorac Surg* 2000;69:300–306.
11. Eagle KA, Guyton RA, Davidoff R, et al. ACC/AHA 2004 guideline update for coronary artery bypass graft surgery: summary article: a report of the American College of Cardiology/American Heart Association Task Force on Practice Guidelines (Committee to Update the 1999 Guidelines for Coronary Artery Bypass Graft Surgery). *Circulation* 2004;110:1168–1176.
12. Lucio EA, Flores A, Blacher C, et al. Effectiveness of metoprolol in preventing atrial fibrillation and flutter in the postoperative period of coronary artery bypass graft surgery. *Arq Bras Cardiol* 2004;82:42–46,37–41.
13. Kowey PR, Taylor JE, Rials SJ, et al. Meta-analysis of the effectiveness of prophylactic drug therapy in preventing supraventricular arrhythmia early after coronary artery bypass grafting. *Am J Cardiol* 1992;69:963–965.
14. Ali IM, Sanalla AA, Clark V. Beta-blocker effects on postoperative atrial fibrillation. *Eur J Cardiothorac Surg* 1997;11:1154–1157.
15. Andres TC, Reimold SC, Berlin JA, et al. Prevention of supraventricular arrhythmias after coronary artery bypass surgery: a meta-analysis of randomized control trials. *Circulation* 1991;84:236–244.
16. Eagle KA, Guyton RA, Davidoff R, et al. ACC/AHA 2004 guideline update for coronary artery bypass graft surgery: summary article: a report of the American College of Cardiology/American Heart Association Task Force on Practice Guidelines (Committee to Update the 1999 Guidelines for Coronary Artery Bypass Graft Surgery). *Circulation* 2004;110:1168–1176.
17. Kerstein J, Soodan A, Qamar M, et al. Giving IV and oral amiodarone perioperatively for the prevention of postoperative atrial fibrillation in patients undergoing coronary artery bypass surgery: the GAP study. *Chest* 2004;126:716–724.
18. Auer J, Weber T, Berent R, et al. A comparison between oral antiarrhythmic drugs in the prevention of atrial fibrillation after cardiac surgery: the pilot study of prevention of postoperative atrial fibrillation (SPPAF), a randomized, placebo-controlled trial. *Am Heart J* 2004;147:636–643.
19. Giri S, White CM, Dunn AB, et al. Oral amiodarone for prevention of atrial fibrillation after open heart surgery, the Atrial Fibrillation Suppression Trial (AFIST): a randomised placebo-controlled trial. *Lancet* 2001;357:830–836.
20. Mitchell LB, Exner DV, Wyse DG, et al. Prophylactic oral amiodarone for the prevention of arrhythmias that begin early after revascularization, valve replacement, or repair: PAPABEAR: a randomized controlled trial. *JAMA* 2005;294(24):3093–3100.

CHAPTER 17 ■ ACUTE AORTIC SYNDROMES

PIOTR SOBIESZCZYK AND PATRICK T. O'GARA

EPIDEMIOLOGY AND PATHOPHYSIOLOGY
NATURAL HISTORY
CLINICAL PRESENTATION
DIAGNOSIS
TREATMENT
CLINICAL PATHWAY FOR MANAGEMENT OF
    SUSPECTED ACUTE AORTIC SYNDROMES

Nontraumatic acute aortic syndromes (AAS) comprise a group of diagnostically elusive and highly lethal, albeit relatively uncommon, disorders. Aortic dissection (AD), aortic intramural hematoma (IMH), and aortic penetrating ulcer constitute this group. They are difficult to diagnose by clinical criteria alone and require a high index of suspicion and a low threshold for utilization of imaging tests to avoid the high price of erroneous diagnosis. Traumatic aortic injuries, such as deceleration injury and penetrating or blunt trauma, are usually recognized during the standard trauma evaluation pathways and are not the subject of this chapter.

EPIDEMIOLOGY AND PATHOPHYSIOLOGY

Aortic dissection is the most common of the three acute aortic syndromes with an estimated U.S. annual incidence of 3.5/100,000 (1). The exact incidence is likely much higher because sudden death is often the only manifestation. Aortic dissection was described as early as 1761 during the autopsy of King George II of England (2), but the actual term is credited to Laennec's description in 1826 (3). The dissection of the aortic wall is caused by a disruption or tear of the intimal layer through which the underlying weakened media is exposed to pulsatile systemic pressure and propagation of the tear. The resultant intimal flap divides the aorta into true and false lumens. The location of the tear usually occurs at the site of highest stress, the right lateral wall of the proximal aorta in type A dissection and the ligamentum arteriosum in type B dissection. Any process weakening the integrity of the medial layer will predispose to AD (Table 17-1). Hereditary connective tissue disorders such as Marfan syndrome or Ehlers-Danlos syndrome weaken the aortic media by inducing cystic medial degeneration. Chronic hypertension, smoking, dyslipidemia, and cocaine use degrade the elastic components of the media, leaving the stiffer wall vulnerable to the pulsatile forces of the cardiac cycle. Inflammatory vasculitides and iatrogenic aortic injury (4) also weaken the wall and increase the risk of AD. Aortic dissection can also complicate the course of patients with coarctation or bicuspid aortic valve disease. It has also been reported in pregnancy.

More recently, IMH and penetrating aortic ulcer (PAU) have received increasing recognition. These syndromes frequently coexist, raising the question whether IMH and PAU are indeed independent lesions. The preponderance of data supports an independent etiology for these syndromes (5). Aortic IMH was first described in 1920 (6), but its prevalence has been under-recognized due to the limitations of traditional contrast angiography. The recognition of IMH has been advanced by the newer, more precise tomographic imaging techniques. In the largest registry of acute AD, IMH was

TABLE 17-1

CONDITIONS ASSOCIATED WITH INCREASED RISK OF NONTRAUMATIC ACUTE AORTIC SYNDROMES

Degeneration of the aortic wall
Age
Tobacco use
Chronic hypertension
Cocaine
Connective tissue disorders
Marfan syndrome
Ehlers-Danlos syndrome
Familial aortic aneurysm disease
Familial annuloaortic ectasia
Inflammatory disorders
Giant cell arteritis
Takayasu's arteritis
Behçet's disease
Iatrogenic aortic injury
Catheter-mediated injury
Aortic cross-clamping
Congenital disorders of the aorta
Bicuspid aortic valve
Aortic coarctation
Other causes
Pregnancy
Turner's syndrome
Noonan's syndrome

diagnosed in about 6% of the patients (7), but other, more inclusive, series suggest that IMH may represent as many as 20% to 30% of the acute aortic syndromes (8–11). Aortic IMH is caused by rupture of the vasovasorum in the aortic wall or by extension of a PAU into the media. A hematoma within an intact aortic wall has no communication with the lumen and no outlet for decompression. Hypertension and older age are the most common risk factors for IMH (7).

Penetrating aortic ulcer was first recognized in 1934 (12). It accounts, in some series, for 8% of acute aortic syndromes (13). PAU results from erosion of an atherosclerotic lesion through the intima and beyond the elastic lamina of the arterial wall. It is a disease of older patients with established systemic arteriosclerosis and arterial calcification (14,15). It is often associated with abdominal aortic aneurysms, which are present in up to 40% of PAU patients (5).

NATURAL HISTORY

The natural history and prognosis of AAS are directly related to the segment of aorta involved. The Stanford classification categorizes the AAS into those involving the ascending aorta and arch (type A) and those involving exclusively the descending aorta distal to the ligamentum arteriosum (type B). Aortic syndromes identified within 2 weeks of onset of symptoms are defined as acute, whereas those identified later are considered chronic.

When untreated, AD carries a high mortality rate, which increases by 1% per hour in the first 24 hours, rises to 50% at 1 week, and reaches 90% after 3 months (16). Aggressive surgical and medical treatment of AD can reduce the early mortality rates to 15% to 25% (17–19) and increase 5-year survival rates to between 50% to 70% (18,20,21). Type A dissection accounts for 65% of ADs. It remains a particularly lethal disorder with a 35% in-hospital mortality rate, particularly in patients presenting with shock, tamponade, renal failure, abnormal electrocardiogram (ECG), peripheral pulse deficits, or advanced age (22,23). Patients with type B AD fare better, with a 13% in-hospital mortality rate, which increases in patients presenting with the triad of hypotension, branch vessel involvement, and absence of pain (24). The risk of early rupture is relatively low, but in the chronic phase the injured aorta undergoes remodeling and aneurysmal transformation and rupture accounts for 30% of late deaths (25). Persistent patency of the false lumen and pressurization of this compartment is associated with progressive aortic dilatation and worse long-term survival (26). Patients with Marfan syndrome constitute 5% of AD patients, are more likely to suffer from type A dissection (27), and have a higher rate of subsequent complications and late death (28).

Data on the natural history of IMH and PAU come from observational studies with heterogeneous patient populations and variable stages of presentation. IMH primarily affects the descending aorta in older patients (7). The natural history of the aortic IMH is variable and characterized by dynamic changes leading to regression and healing, extension of the hematoma, progression to classic dissection, frank rupture, or aneurysmal remodeling. The site of injury in IMH is closer to the adventitial layer and may explain the observed higher risk of rupture for IMH compared with AD (29). In general, type A IMH is associated with worse outcomes compared to type B IMH (9,30). The hospital mortality associated with type A IMH exceeds that of type B, reported to be 34% versus 14%, with most deaths occurring within the first 72 hours (7,10,31). Type A IMH is associated with higher rates of rupture and progression to frank dissection than type B IMH (32) and carries a prog-

nosis similar to type A AD (31,33–35). Type A IMH may progress to AD in 25% of patients and to aortic rupture in 28% (14,15). Several series suggest a more benign outcome for some type A IMH patients, with mortality rates below 10% with medical therapy alone (8,32,36–38). However early surgical intervention remains the recommended treatment for type A IMH. Medical therapy may be an alternative in elderly patients with multiple comorbidities and high perioperative risk.

Type B IMH follows a more benign course (14,15,39). Evangelista et al followed 68 patients with predominantly type B IMH over a mean period of 45 months (40). A third of the lesions regressed completely, 54% developed various aneurysmal changes, and only 12% progressed to classic AD. Most of the regression occurred in the first 6 months after presentation. In another cohort, 57% of patients showed regression, 40% showed progressive aortic dilatation, 13% progressed to frank dissection, and 7% developed rupture (41). Other series suggest progression to dissection in up to 33% of patients (20,11,31,33). The prognosis of medically treated type B IMH appears to be no different from that for type B dissection (7). The actuarial 10-year survival rate for type B IMH can reach 85% (42).

The morphological characteristic most predictive of IMH evolution is the initial aortic diameter. A smaller aortic caliber, specifically less than 40 to 50 mm, and aortic wall thickness below 10 mm predict regression and healing (40,41,43–45). Progression of IMH into aneurysmal disease may be predicted by signs of intrinsic weakness in the wall, such as larger diameter on presentation, absence of intramural echolucency, and the presence of an ulcerated atherosclerotic plaque (40). The coexistence of IMH with an aortic ulceration, a finding more common in the descending aorta, carries a worse prognosis (46).

Although some aortic ulcerations are asymptomatic and incidentally found on computed tomography (CT) angiograms (47), PAU often presents as an aggressive lesion. As an AAS, this dynamic lesion may remain stable or rapidly progress and evolve into other lesions (15,48–50). Exposure of the media and elastic lamina to pulsatile flow may transform the ulcer into dissection or IMH, whereas penetration of the ulcer to the adventitia can lead to the formation of a pseudoaneurysm or rupture. A PAU can progress to an aortic aneurysm with an average annual aortic growth rate ranging from 0.2 to 0.33 cm (47,51). Clinical outcomes are also related to the anatomic location of the ulcer. PAU is predominantly found in the descending thoracic aorta. In the ascending aorta, PAU has been associated with a 57% rate of progression to dissection or rupture, whereas that rate is 12% for type B lesions (14,15). The risk of aortic rupture exceeds that typical for AD (13) and may be particularly high in ulcers >2 cm wide and >1 cm deep (30,46). In some series, up to 38% of patients with either type A or B PAU rapidly progressed to rupture (51).

CLINICAL PRESENTATION

Acute aortic syndromes present with myriad nonspecific symptoms confounding even experienced physicians. Symptoms range from chest and back pain to those caused by end-organ ischemia as anatomical consequences of aortic injury and occlusion of aortic branch vessels. Lesions of the descending aorta are less likely to present with cardiac complications and are more likely to cause renal and mesenteric ischemia. Although ischemic complications are less common in patients with PAU and IMH (51), it is virtually impossible to differentiate between

TABLE 17-2

PRESENTING SYMPTOMS AND CLINICAL FINDINGS IN PATIENTS WITH AAS

| | Aortic Dissection | | Intramural Hematoma | | Penetrating Aortic Ulcer |
	Type A	Type B	Type A	Type B	
Symptoms					
Chest pain	79%	63%	79%	50%	80%
Back pain	47%	64%	26%–64%	68%	80%
Abdominal pain	22%	43%	5%	7%–30%	uncommon
Syncope	13%	4%	4%	6%	uncommon
Cerebral ischemia	6%–10%	2%	uncommon	uncommon	uncommon
Clinical Findings					
Hypertension	36%	70%	53%	53%	common
Hypotension	12%	2%–3.5%	27%	13%	uncommon
Pulse deficits	19%	9%–21%	17%		uncommon
Aortic regurgitation	44%	12%	12%–26%	4%	uncommon
Tamponade	13%	1.5%	22%–50%	0	uncommon
Pericardial effusion	22%–48%	uncommon	50%–88%	3%–11%	uncommon
Congestive heart failure	9%	3%	9%	3%	uncommon
Myocardial infarction	9%	3%	0%	0%	0%

the three syndromes on the basis of symptoms alone (Table 17-2).

Chest and back pain predominate as the presenting symptoms and are present in over 70% of all patients with AAS. As many as 10% of patients with dissection present with syncope. Pulse deficits correlate with increased mortality rate and can be found in 20% and 30% of patients with type A and type

B dissection, respectively (52). Malperfusion syndromes occur in up to 22% of patients and can involve coronary, mesenteric, cerebral, and peripheral arteries, depending on the location and extent of aortic injury (24). Compression of the true lumen can compromise perfusion of the lower body, inducing renal ischemia and difficult to control hypertension (Fig. 17-1). Spinal cord ischemia causing paraplegia can occur in 3% of

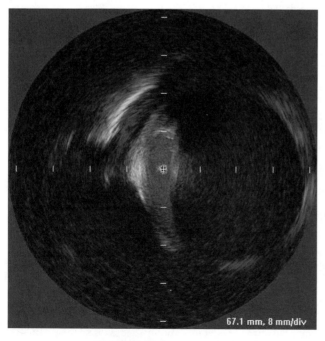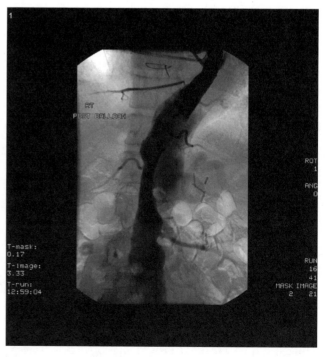

FIGURE 17-1. Compression of the true lumen can compromise perfusion of the lower body, inducing renal ischemia and difficult to control hypertension.

type B dissections patients. Several clinical features are more specific for type A lesions and include pericardial effusion, tamponade, and aortic regurgitation.

DIAGNOSIS

There are currently no clinically useful serologic markers indicative of aortic injury. The diagnosis of the AAS relies, therefore, on a high index of clinical suspicion and appropriate use of imaging tests. Nevertheless, three potential biochemical markers have shown some diagnostic promise in early clinical experience.

D-dimer reflects the activation of the endogenous fibrinolytic pathways and can be released as a consequence of liberation of tissue factor from the dissected aortic wall and thrombosis of the false lumen. In two small series combining 26 patients with AD, D-dimer had a 100% sensitivity, 68% specificity, and a negative predictive value of 100% (53,54). However, its short half-life jeopardizes recognition of subacute or delayed presentation. Moreover, the test did not distinguish dissection from pulmonary embolism. The low specificity and poorly defined diagnostic thresholds as well as lack of prospective data

limit its clinical utility at present. The combination of elevated D-dimer and the chest x-ray derived ratio of mediastinal to thoracic diameter has been suggested as a reliable tool to differentiate patients with acute coronary syndromes and AD (55).

Elastin is an integral structural component of the aortic wall and has been investigated as a potential marker of compromised aortic wall integrity. In a retrospective study, the specificity of this marker has been demonstrated to reach 99%, positive predictive value of 94% and negative predictive value of 98% (56). A time-consuming assay and lack of prospective evaluation hinder clinical use of this test. Elastin would also not be expected to be elevated in IMH where the elastin rich media is not exposed to the circulation.

Smooth muscle myosin heavy-chain protein rises rapidly and falls within 24 hours of AD. This time-sensitive assay can reach a sensitivity of 90% and specificity of 98% when compared with healthy controls, but the specificity falls in comparison to patients with acute coronary syndromes (57,58). Interestingly, levels of this protein are only elevated in type A dissection and are not useful in type B dissection (57).

A clinical prediction model for AD using immediate onset of pain, aortic widening on chest x-ray, and pulse deficits or

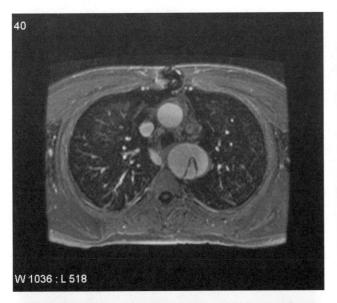

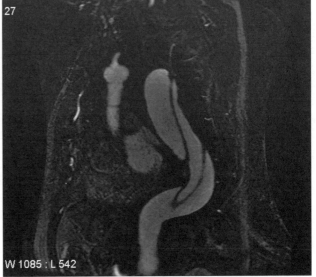

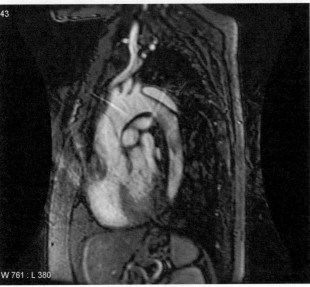

FIGURE 17-2. The diagnosis of AD rests on identification of a dissection flap with a clear entry point.

blood pressure differential can help in identification of AD (59). Imaging, however, remains the diagnostic gold standard. Chest radiography is not a reliable diagnostic modality, having low sensitivity and specificity for AD and hematoma (60). Contrast x-ray angiography has been replaced by transesophageal echocardiography, CT-angiography, and magnetic resonance angiography (MRA). The selection of one of these imaging modalities must depend on local expertise and availability as well as applicability in a given clinical scenario.

The diagnosis of AD rests on identification of a dissection flap with a clear entry point (Fig. 17-2). By virtue of its availability in the emergency room, CT is the first imaging study obtained in 63% of patients, followed by transesophageal echocardiography (TEE) in 32%, aortography in 4%, and magnetic resonance imaging (MRI) in 1%. Most patients, however, have a second imaging modality, with TEE in 58%, CT in 17%, and MRI in 10% (61). The sensitivity and specificity of TEE in the diagnosis of ascending AD are 96% to 98% and 100%, respectively (10,62–64). The sensitivity and specificity of CT for AD ranges from 93% to 100% and 87% to 100% respectively (65,66). Magnetic resonance angiography is of limited use in the emergency room setting, but is an excellent tool for long-term follow-up, with specificity and sensitivity ranging from 98% to 100% (66,67) (Table 17-3).

Diagnosis of IMH is made by identifying the intramural accumulation of blood, aortic wall thickening exceeding 7 mm in a circular or crescentic shape, and the absence of intimal flap (Fig. 17-3). Central displacement of the intimal calcification is often seen (31,33,68). On CT, IMH appears as a crescentic or circumferential high attenuation lesion in the aortic wall, which does not enhance after contrast administration. Diagnostic sensitivity and specificity of the three imaging modalities in identifying IMH approach 100% (31,69–71). CT may be slightly less accurate in identifying an intimal flap and thus may overestimate the incidence IMH (66). MRI uses T1 and T2 sequences to identify methemoglobin and provide information regarding the age of the IMH. TEE for IMH is remarkably accurate for detection of intimal flaps and is accurate in distinguishing IMH from dissection (8,10,11).

TREATMENT

Any patient suspected of an AAS requires immediate stabilization, reduction of aortic wall stress, and identification of the location and extent of the aortic injury. Type A dissection is a surgical emergency, and timely operative repair results in a 30-day mortality of 25% to 30%, a superior outcome compared to the 50% mortality rate observed with medical therapy alone. In type B dissection, on the other hand, medical therapy is associated with a 1-month mortality rate of 10% to 13%, whereas surgery carries a 25% to 30% mortality rate. These results also hold true for PAU and IMH, and the majority of reports recommend surgical intervention for type A lesions (30,31,34,72,73). A meta-analysis of 143 reported cases of IMH supported the findings that surgical treatment of type A IMH is associated with lower mortality than medical treatment (9). Treatment of type B IMH, on the other hand, carries a mortality rate of 13% with medical management versus 15% with surgical management (73).

Beta-blockers constitute the mainstay of medical therapy. In AD, beta-blockers reduce systolic pressure, wall stress, and the rate of pressure change (dP/dT), thus reducing the driving force of expansion and propagation of the hematoma. These benefits extend to IMH patients who experience reduced rates of progression and improved long-term outcomes (30,74). With appropriate use of medical and surgical therapy, 5-year survival in type A and B IMH reaches 80% and 90%, respectively (75).

High afterload increases wall stress, and blood pressure must be lowered aggressively. Additional antihypertensive agents, such as sodium nitroprusside, should be instituted only after achieving adequate beta-blockade to avoid rebound tachycardia and an increase in wall stress.

Surgical or endovascular treatment of acute and chronic type B aortic syndromes have been traditionally reserved for patients with malperfusion syndromes, recurrent pain, contained rupture, or rapid aneurysmal dilatation of the pressurized false lumen. Emergent surgical intervention for these indi-

---

TABLE 17-3

CHARACTERISTICS OF NONINVASIVE IMAGING MODALITIES COMMONLY USED IN DIAGNOSIS OF ACUTE AORTIC SYNDROMES

	Sensitivity (%)	Specificity (%)	Advantages	Disadvantages
TEE	96–98	100	Rapidly available. Additional information about aortic regurgitation, left ventricular function, pericardial effusion.	Operator dependent and invasive. Air in the trachea may interfere with arch imaging, unable to visualize distal aorta.
MRA	95–100	95–100	Accurate, 3D images, branch vessel visualization.	Relatively time consuming and not widely available; not suitable for unstable patients; requires breath hold and susceptible to motion artifact.
CTA	93–100	87–100	Widely available, rapid, and accurate. 3D images, branch vessel visualization.	Exposure to nephrotoxic contrast and radiation.

Adapted from Moore AG, et al. Choice of computed tomography, transesophageal echocardiography, magnetic resonance imaging, and aortography in acute aortic dissection: International Registry of Acute Aortic Dissection (IRAD). *Am J Cardiol* 2002;89(10):1235–1238; Nienaber CA, et al. The diagnosis of thoracic aortic dissection by noninvasive imaging procedures. *N Engl J Med* 1993;328(1):1–9; Nienaber CA, et al. Diagnosis of thoracic aortic dissection. Magnetic resonance imaging versus transesophageal echocardiography. *Circulation* 1992;85(2):434–447; Erbel R, et al. Echocardiography in diagnosis of aortic dissection. *Lancet* 1989;1(8636):457–461.

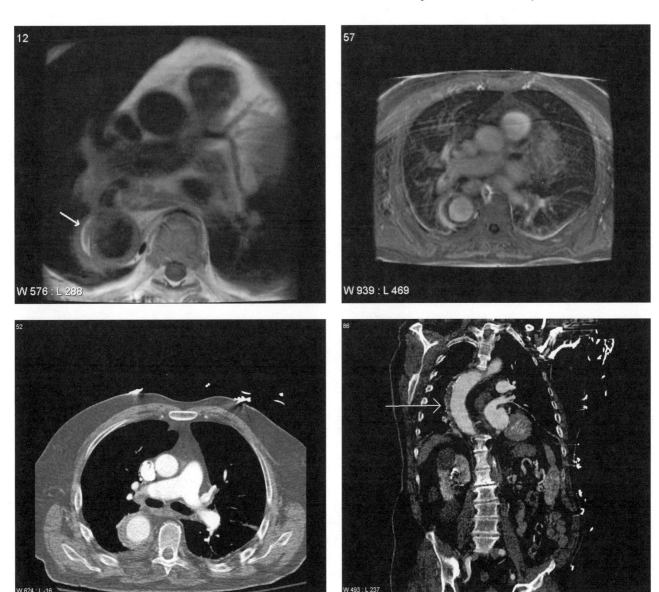

FIGURE 17-3. Diagnosis of IMH is made by identifying the intramural accumulation of blood, aortic wall thickening exceeding 7 mm in a circular or crescentic shape, and the absence of intimal flap.

cations can double the mortality rates (76,77), and less-invasive endovascular approaches have become increasingly popular. These include balloon fenestration of the false lumen for decompression and augmentation of flow in the true lumen or placement of a stent graft to seal the site of intimal tear and promote thrombosis of the false lumen. Clinical experience with endovascular stent graft implantation has been steadily growing since it was first described in 1999 (78). In general, stent grafting is associated with high technical success and low complication rates (79). Patient selection plays a crucial role in determining outcomes of stent grafting, and whether this approach should be used more widely awaits the results of randomized studies comparing medical and endovascular therapy (80).

Long-term follow-up of patients with aortic disease is critical to their long-term survival. Most of the late mortality results from remodeling and progression of aortic disease. Serial imaging of surgically repaired and medically managed aortas should

be performed with CT or MR at discharge, 3 months, 6 months, 12 months, and annually thereafter.

CLINICAL PATHWAY FOR MANAGEMENT OF SUSPECTED ACUTE AORTIC SYNDROMES

Successful management of patients presenting with AAS rests on high index of suspicion, timely evaluation, and rapid institution of the appropriate therapy. Any delay in diagnosis and treatment translates into higher mortality. Clinical history and physical exam alone are insufficient to establish the diagnosis. Furthermore, they will raise the suspicion of AAS in only 65% of patients (81). Clinicians must be vigilant for the possibility of aortic disease in patients presenting with chest and back pain and focal ischemic syndromes and use the imaging tests at their disposal. Despite advances in imaging modalities and

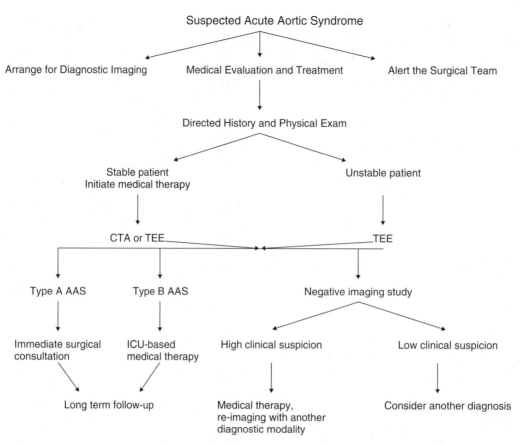

FIGURE 17-4. A critical pathway algorithm can help streamline the triage and management of AAS patients.

surgical and endovascular techniques, aortic syndromes continue to confound physicians and claim lives. Implementation of a critical pathway algorithm can help streamline the triage and management of this complex group of patients (Fig. 17-4).

References

1. Clouse WD, Hallett JW Jr, Schaff HV, et al. Acute aortic dissection: population-based incidence compared with degenerative aortic aneurysm rupture. *Mayo Clin Proc* 2004;79(2):176–180.
2. Nicholls F. Observations concerning body of the late majesty. *Philos Trans* 1762;52:265.
3. Gore I. Pathogenesis of dissecting aneurysm of the aorta. *AMA Arch Pathol* 1952;53(2):142–153.
4. Januzzi JL, Sabantine MS, Eagle KA, et al. Iatrogenic aortic dissection. *Am J Cardiol* 2002;89(5):623–626.
5. Coady MA, Rizzo JA, Elefteriades JA. Pathologic variants of thoracic aortic dissections. Penetrating atherosclerotic ulcers and intramural hematomas. *Cardiol Clin* 1999;17(4):637–657.
6. Krukenberg E. Beitrage zur Frage des Aneurysma dissecans. *Beitr Patholog Anat Allg Pathol* 1920;67:329–351.
7. Evangelista A, Mukherjee D, Mehta RH, et al. Acute intramural hematoma of the aorta: a mystery in evolution. *Circulation* 2005;111(8):1063–1070.
8. Kang DH, Song JK, Song MG, et al. Clinical and echocardiographic outcomes of aortic intramural hemorrhage compared with acute aortic dissection. *Am J Cardiol* 1998;81(2):202–206.
9. Maraj R, Rerkpattanapipat P, Jacobs LE, et al. Meta-analysis of 143 reported cases of aortic intramural hematoma. *Am J Cardiol* 2000;86(6):664–668.
10. Keren A, Kim CB, Hu BS, et al. Accuracy of biplane and multiplane transesophageal echocardiography in diagnosis of typical acute aortic dissection and intramural hematoma. *J Am Coll Cardiol* 1996;28(3):627–636.
11. Vilacosta I, San Roman JA, Ferrieros J, et al. Natural history and serial morphology of aortic intramural hematoma: a novel variant of aortic dissection. *Am Heart J* 1997;134(3):495–507.
12. Shennan T. Dissecting aneurysms. Medical Research Council, special report series, 1934:193.
13. Coady MA, Rizzo JA, Hammond GL, et al. Penetrating ulcer of the thoracic aorta: what is it? How do we recognize it? How do we manage it? *J Vasc Surg* 1998;27(6):1006–1015; discussion 1015–1016.
14. von Kodolitsch Y, Nienaber CA. [Intramural hemorrhage of the thoracic aorta: diagnosis, therapy and prognosis of 209 in vivo diagnosed cases]. *Z Kardiol* 1998;87(10):797–807.
15. von Kodolitsch Y, Nienaber CA. [Ulcer of the thoracic aorta: diagnosis, therapy and prognosis]. *Z Kardiol* 1998;87(12):917–927.
16. Hirst AE Jr, Johns VJ Jr, Kime SW Jr. Dissecting aneurysm of the aorta: a review of 505 cases. *Medicine* (Baltimore) 1958;37(3):217–279.
17. Chirillo F, Marchiori MC, Andriolo L, et al. Outcome of 290 patients with aortic dissection. A 12-year multicentre experience. *Eur Heart J* 1990;11(4):311–319.
18. Svensson LG, Crawford ES, Hess KR, et al. Dissection of the aorta and dissecting aortic aneurysms. Improving early and long-term surgical results. *Circulation* 1990;82(5 Suppl):IV24–IV38.
19. Rizzo RJ, Aranki SF, Aklog L, et al. Rapid noninvasive diagnosis and surgical repair of acute ascending aortic dissection. Improved survival with less angiography. *J Thorac Cardiovasc Surg* 1994;108(3):567–574; discussion 574–575.
20. Doroghazi RM, Slater EE, DeSanctis RW, et al. Long-term survival of patients with treated aortic dissection. *J Am Coll Cardiol* 1984;3(4):1026–1034.
21. Glower DD, Fann JL, Speier RH, et al. Comparison of medical and surgical therapy for uncomplicated descending aortic dissection. *Circulation* 1990;82(5 Suppl):IV39–IV46.
22. Mehta RH, Suzuki T, Hagan PG, et al. Predicting death in patients with acute type A aortic dissection. *Circulation* 2002;105(2):200–206.
23. Mehta RH, O'Gara PT, Bossone E, et al. Acute type A aortic dissection in the elderly: clinical characteristics, management, and outcomes in the current era. *J Am Coll Cardiol* 2002;40(4):685–692.
24. Suzuki T, Mehta RH, Ince H, et al. Clinical profiles and outcomes of acute type B aortic dissection in the current era: lessons from the International Registry of Aortic Dissection (IRAD). *Circulation* 2003;108 (Suppl 1):II312–II317.

25. DeBakey ME, McCollum CH, Crawford ES, et al. Dissection and dissecting aneurysms of the aorta: twenty-year follow-up of five hundred twenty-seven patients treated surgically. *Surgery* 1982;92(6):1118–1134.

26. Bernard Y, Zimmermann H, Chocron S, et al. False lumen patency as a predictor of late outcome in aortic dissection. *Am J Cardiol* 2001;87(12):1378–1382.

27. Januzzi JL, Marayati F, Mehta RH, et al. Comparison of aortic dissection in patients with and without Marfan's syndrome (results from the International Registry of Aortic Dissection). *Am J Cardiol* 2004;94(3):400–402.

28. Yu HY, Chen YS, Huang SC, et al. Late outcome of patients with aortic dissection: study of a national database. *Eur J Cardiothorac Surg* 2004;25(5):683–690.

29. Uchida K, Imoto K, Takahashi M, et al. Pathologic characteristics and surgical indications of superacute type A intramural hematoma. *Ann Thorac Surg* 2005;79(5):1518–1521.

30. von Kodolitsch Y, Csosz SK, Koschyk DH, et al. Intramural hematoma of the aorta: predictors of progression to dissection and rupture. *Circulation* 2003;107(8):1158–1163.

31. Nienaber CA, von Kodolitsch Y, Petersen B, et al. Intramural hemorrhage of the thoracic aorta. Diagnostic and therapeutic implications. *Circulation* 1995;92(6):1465–1472.

32. Shimizu H, Yoshino H, Udagawa H, et al. Prognosis of aortic intramural hemorrhage compared with classic aortic dissection. *Am J Cardiol* 2000;85(6):792–795, A10.

33. Mohr-Kahaly S, Erbel R, Kearney P, et al. Aortic intramural hemorrhage visualized by transesophageal echocardiography: findings and prognostic implications. *J Am Coll Cardiol* 1994;23(3):658–664.

34. Muluk SC, Kaufman JA, Torchiana DF, et al. Diagnosis and treatment of thoracic aortic intramural hematoma. *J Vasc Surg* 1996;24(6):1022–1029.

35. Murray JG, Manisali M, Flamm SD, et al. Intramural hematoma of the thoracic aorta: MR image findings and their prognostic implications. *Radiology* 1997;204(2):349–355.

36. Song JK, Kim HS, Kang DH, et al. Different clinical features of aortic intramural hematoma versus dissection involving the ascending aorta. *J Am Coll Cardiol* 2001;37(6):1604–1610.

37. Song JK, Kim JS, Song JM, et al. Outcomes of medically treated patients with aortic intramural hematoma. *Am J Med* 2002;113(3):181–187.

38. Kaji S, Akasaka T, Horibata Y, et al. Long-term prognosis of patients with type A aortic intramural hematoma. *Circulation* 2002;106(12 Suppl 1):I248–I252.

39. Kaji S, Akasaka T, Katayama M, et al. Long-term prognosis of patients with type B aortic intramural hematoma. *Circulation* 2003;108 (Suppl 1):II307–II311.

40. Evangelista A, Dominguez R, Sebastia C, et al. Long-term follow-up of aortic intramural hematoma: predictors of outcome. *Circulation* 2003;108(5):583–589.

41. Sueyoshi E, Imada T, Sakamoto I, et al. Analysis of predictive factors for progression of type B aortic intramural hematoma with computed tomography. *J Vasc Surg* 2002;35(6):1179–1183.

42. Sueyoshi E, Sakamoto I, Fukuda M, et al. Long-term outcome of type B aortic intramural hematoma: comparison with classic aortic dissection treated by the same therapeutic strategy. *Ann Thorac Surg* 2004;78(6):2112–2117.

43. Nishigami K, Tsuchiya T, Shono H, et al. Disappearance of aortic intramural hematoma and its significance to the prognosis. *Circulation* 2000;102(19 Suppl 3):III243–III247.

44. Kaji S, Nishigami K, Akasaka T, et al. Prediction of progression or regression of type A aortic intramural hematoma by computed tomography. *Circulation* 1999;100(19 Suppl):II281–II286.

45. Evangelista A, Dominguez R, Sebastia C, et al. Prognostic value of clinical and morphologic findings in short-term evolution of aortic intramural hematoma. Therapeutic implications. *Eur Heart J* 2004;25(1):81–87.

46. Ganaha F, et al. Prognosis of aortic intramural hematoma with and without penetrating atherosclerotic ulcer: a clinical and radiological analysis. *Circulation* 2002;106(3):342–348.

47. Quint LE, Williams DM, Francis IR, et al. Ulcerlike lesions of the aorta: imaging features and natural history. *Radiology* 2001;218(3):719–723.

48. Harris JA, Bis KG, Glover JL, et al. Penetrating atherosclerotic ulcers of the aorta. *J Vasc Surg* 1994;19(1):90–98; discussion 98–99.

49. Braverman AC. Penetrating atherosclerotic ulcers of the aorta. *Curr Opin Cardiol* 1994;9(5):591–597.

50. Stanson AW, Kazmier J, Hollier LH, et al. Penetrating atherosclerotic ulcers of the thoracic aorta: natural history and clinicopathologic correlations. *Ann Vasc Surg* 1986;1(1):15–23.

51. Tittle SL, Lynch RJ, Cole PE, et al. Midterm follow-up of penetrating ulcer and intramural hematoma of the aorta. *J Thorac Cardiovasc Surg* 2002;123(6):1051–1059.

52. Bossone E, Rampoldi V, Nienaber CA, et al. Usefulness of pulse deficit to predict in-hospital complications and mortality in patients with acute type A aortic dissection. *Am J Cardiol* 2002;89(7):851–855.

53. Weber T, Rammer M, Auer J, et al. D-dimer in acute aortic dissection. *Chest* 2003;123(5):1375–1378.

54. Eggebrecht H, Naber CK, Bruch C, et al. Value of plasma fibrin D-dimers for detection of acute aortic dissection. *J Am Coll Cardiol* 2004;44(4):804–809.

55. Hazui H, Fukumoto H, Negoro N, et al. Simple and useful tests for discrimi-nating between acute aortic dissection of the ascending aorta and acute myocardial infarction in the emergency setting. *Circ J* 2005;69(6):677–682.

56. Shinohara T, Suzuki K, Okada M, et al. Soluble elastin fragments in serum are elevated in acute aortic dissection. *Arterioscler Thromb Vasc Biol* 2003;23(10):1839–1844.

57. Suzuki T, Katoh H, Tsuchio Y, et al. Diagnostic implications of elevated levels of smooth-muscle myosin heavy-chain protein in acute aortic dissection. The smooth muscle myosin heavy chain study. *Ann Intern Med* 2000;133(7):537–541.

58. Suzuki T, Katoh H, Watanabe M, et al. Novel biochemical diagnostic method for aortic dissection. Results of a prospective study using an immu-noassay of smooth muscle myosin heavy chain. *Circulation* 1996;93(6):1244–1249.

59. von Kodolitsch Y, Schwartz AG, Nienaber CA. Clinical prediction of acute aortic dissection. *Arch Intern Med* 2000;160(19):2977–2982.

60. von Kodolitsch Y, Nienaber CA, Dieckmann C, et al. Chest radiography for the diagnosis of acute aortic syndrome. *Am J Med* 2004;116(2):73–77.

61. Moore AG, Eagle KA, Bruckman D, et al. Choice of computed tomography, transesophageal echocardiography, magnetic resonance imaging, and aor-tography in acute aortic dissection: International Registry of Acute Aortic Dissection (IRAD). *Am J Cardiol* 2002;89(10):1235–1238.

62. Evangelista A, Garcia-del-Castillo H, Gonzalez-Alujas T, et al. Diagnosis of ascending aortic dissection by transesophageal echocardiography: utility of M-mode in recognizing artifacts. *J Am Coll Cardiol* 1996;27(1):102–107.

63. Ballal RS, Nanda NC, Gatewood R, et al. Usefulness of transesophageal echocardiography in assessment of aortic dissection. *Circulation* 1991;84(5):1903–1914.

64. Hashimoto S, Kumada T, Osakada G, et al. Assessment of transesophageal Doppler echography in dissecting aortic aneurysm. *J Am Coll Cardiol* 1989;14(5):1253–1262.

65. Cigarroa JE, Isselbacher EM, DeSanctis RW, et al. Diagnostic imaging in the evaluation of suspected aortic dissection. Old standards and new direc-tions. *N Engl J Med* 1993;328(1):35–43.

66. Nienaber CA, von Kodolitsch Y, Nicolas V, et al. The diagnosis of thoracic aortic dissection by noninvasive imaging procedures. *N Engl J Med* 1993;328(1):1–9.

67. Nienaber CA, Spielmann RP, von Kodolitsch Y, et al. Diagnosis of thoracic aortic dissection. Magnetic resonance imaging versus transesophageal echo-cardiography. *Circulation* 1992;85(2):434–447.

68. Harris KM, Braverman AC, Gutierrez FR, et al. Transesophageal echocar-diographic and clinical features of aortic intramural hematoma. *J Thorac Cardiovasc Surg* 1997;114(4):619–626.

69. Song JK. Diagnosis of aortic intramural haematoma. *Heart* 2004;90(4):368–371.

70. Alfonso F, Goicolea J, Aragoncillo P, et al. Diagnosis of aortic intramural hematoma by intravascular ultrasound imaging. *Am J Cardiol* 1995;76(10):735–738.

71. Sueyoshi E, Matsuoka Y, Sakamoto I, et al. Fate of intramural hematoma of the aorta: CT evaluation. *J Comput Assist Tomogr* 1997;21(6):931–938.

72. Robbins RC, McManus RP, Mitchell RS, et al. Management of patients with intramural hematoma of the thoracic aorta. *Circulation* 1993;88(5 Pt 2):II1–II10.

73. Sawhney NS, DeMaria AN, Blanchard DG. Aortic intramural hematoma: an increasingly recognized and potentially fatal entity. *Chest* 2001;120(4):1340–1346.

74. Nienaber CA, Richartz BM, Rehders T, et al. Aortic intramural haematoma: natural history and predictive factors for complications. *Heart* 2004;90(4):372–374.

75. Moizumi Y, Komatsu T, Motoyoshi N, et al. Clinical features and long-term outcome of type A and type B intramural hematoma of the aorta. *J Thorac Cardiovasc Surg* 2004;127(2):421–427.

76. Umana JP, Lai DT, Mitchell RS, et al. Is medical therapy still the optimal treatment strategy for patients with acute type B aortic dissections? *J Thorac Cardiovasc Surg* 2002;124(5):896–910.

77. Brandt M, Hussel K, Walluascheck KP, et al. Stent-graft repair versus open surgery for the descending aorta: a case-control study. *J Endovasc Ther* 2004;11(5):535–538.

78. Dake MD, Kato N, Mitchell RS, et al. Endovascular stent-graft placement for the treatment of acute aortic dissection. *N Engl J Med* 1999;340(20):1546–1552.

79. Eggebrecht H, Nienaber CE, Neuhauser M, et al. Endovascular stent-graft placement in aortic dissection: a meta-analysis. *Eur Heart J* 2006;27:489–498.

80. Eggebrecht H, Herold U, Kuhnt O, et al. Endovascular stent-graft treatment of aortic dissection: determinants of post-interventional outcome. *Eur Heart J* 2005;26(5):489–497.

81. Rosman HS, Patel S, Borzak S, et al. Quality of history taking in patients with aortic dissection. *Chest* 1998;114(3):793–795.

82. Hagan PG, Nienaber CE, Isselbacher EM, et al. The International Registry of Acute Aortic Dissection (IRAD): new insights into an old disease. *JAMA* 2000;283(7):897–903.

83. Armstrong WF, Bach DS, Carey L, et al. Spectrum of acute dissection of the ascending aorta: a transesophageal echocardiographic study. *J Am Soc Echocardiogr* 1996;9(5):646–656.

84. Erbel R, Engberding R, Daniel W, et al. Echocardiography in diagnosis of aortic dissection. *Lancet* 1989;1(8636):457–461.

CHAPTER 18 ■ INTENSIVE MANAGEMENT OF HYPERGLYCEMIA IN ACUTE CORONARY SYNDROME

VERA T. FAJTOVA

EPIDEMIOLOGY
Diabetes and Myocardial Infarction
Hyperglycemia First Noted in the Setting of ACS
Metabolic Implications of Newly Noted Hyperglycemia in the
    Setting of ACS
MECHANISM OF GLUCOSE TOXICITY
Myocardial Energy Balance: Effect of Hyperglycemia and Hypoxia
Vascular Function and Inflammation in Hyperglycemia
Electrophysiological Abnormalities Associated with Hyperglycemia
CLINICAL EVIDENCE OF GLUCOSE CONTROL IN
    CRITICAL ILLNESS AND ACS
Hyperglycemia and Critical Illness
Glucose Insulin Potassium (GIK) Infusions in ACS
Diabetes Mellitus and Acute Myocardial Infarction (DIGAMI)
    Studies
SUMMARY AND RECOMMENDATIONS

The connection between diabetes and macrovascular disease is well established. In 1931 Cruikshank noted an unusually high incidence of glycosuria in patients presenting with coronary thrombosis (1). Today over 20% of patients over the age of 35 with diabetes are known to suffer from coronary artery disease, and between 10% and 30% of patients presenting with acute coronary syndrome (ACS) have diabetes. Additional patients who present with ACS are found to be hyperglycemic. Both pre-existing diabetes and newly noted hyperglycemia in the setting of ACS is associated with a poor outcome. Evidence is accumulating that hyperglycemia is causative in the poor prognosis, and not merely an epiphenomenon that is associated with more severe underlying disease. Trials have assessed the potential benefit of controlling hyperglycemia in this setting with insulin or insulin and glucose infusions.

EPIDEMIOLOGY

Diabetes and Myocardial Infarction

Diabetes is associated with a considerable risk of coronary events and with a resultant poor outcome. The presence of diabetes is equivalent to the presence of pre-existing coronary artery disease (CAD) as a risk factor for future myocardial infarction (MI). Patients who have both diabetes and CAD are at the highest risk of coronary events. A 7-year follow-up study of Finnish men and women in late 1950s revealed an overall incidence of MI of 12.9%. Patients with no pre-existing CAD had an incidence of MI of 3.5%, whereas similar patients with diabetes had an incidence of MI of 20.2%, comparable to patients without diabetes but with pre-existing CAD who had an incidence of 18.8%. Patients with both CAD and diabetes had a 45% chance of having an MI during the observation period. The presence of diabetes was also associated with a poorer prognosis post-MI (2). Reviews of large cohorts of patients presenting with acute MI reveal that patients with diabetes have a higher 30-day (3) and 1-year (4) mortality. The prognosis is worse with the severity and duration of their diabetes (3,4). Patients with diabetes who survive an acute MI with left ventricular function compromise (ejection fraction less than 40%) have more cardiovascular events and deaths on long-term follow-up (3.5 years) than patients who do not have diabetes (5). The increased cardiovascular risk in patients with diabetes is well established.

Pre-existing diabetes is associated with worse prognosis after an MI, and acute hyperglycemia in the setting of an acute MI compounds this. Over 700 patients with diabetes admitted with non-Q-wave MI over a 10-year period were followed for 2 years. This comprised 16% of all patients admitted with a non-Q-wave MI. Patients in the highest blood glucose (BG) quartile (BG over 275 mg/dL, 15.3 mmol) were more likely to be women, had longer duration of diabetes (more than 10 years), had congestive heart failure on admission, were on treatment for hyperlipidemia, had a non-Q-wave MI, and had an elevated creatinine on admission (6). These patients had a higher hospital mortality, 30-day mortality, and 2-year mortality, with a hazard ratio of 2.46, 2.41, and 1.69, respectively, compared with the lowest quartile BG on admission (less than 153 mg/dL, 8.5 mmol) (6). However, hypoglycemia (BG less than 55, 3 mmol) was also associated with a higher 2-year mortality. The prognosis after an MI is worse with more severe hyperglycemia, prolonged duration of diabetes, and renal compromise.

Hyperglycemia First Noted in the Setting of ACS

Hyperglycemia is a complicating factor in many patients who present with ACS but are not known to have diabetes. Hyperglycemia in patients with established diabetes who present with ACS is anticipated and requires treatment. Hyperglycemia newly noted in the setting of ACS is also significant. In 1,664 consecutive patients presenting with acute MI hyperglycemia, defined as BG over 200 mg/dL (11.1 mmol), was noted in 11.1% of patients without diabetes and 62.5% patients with diabetes. Although diabetes was an independent predictor of in-hospital mortality, newly noted hyperglycemia was an even stronger predictor. In the whole population, predictors of mortality were the presence of peripheral vascular disease, use of insulin on admission, age, previous heart failure or MI, being female, and having renal compromise. Use of aspirin, beta-blockade, statin, and angiotensin-converting enzyme inhibition were protective. All patients presenting with an acute MI were included, regardless of whether they received percutaneous coronary intervention (7). Acute hyperglycemia in patients with and without diabetes was noted to be associated with higher risk of the "no-reflow" phenomenon, as measured by intracoronary myocardial contrast echocardiography after reperfusion. In that study blood glucose (BG) of 160 mg/dL (8.9 mmol) was a dividing point between patients with and without reflow. Lack of reflow was not related to glycosylated hemoglobin or the incidence of pre-existing diabetes mellitus. Patients with acute hyperglycemia also had significantly greater infarct size measured as a rise in creatine kinase and a decline in wall motion score, as determined by echocardiography (8). Similarly, acute hyperglycemia (over 180 mg/dL or 10 mmol) was associated with lower left ventricular ejection fraction (LVEF) on presentation and on discharge in patients with first anterior wall MI. The improvement in LVEF from admission to discharge was smaller in patients with hyperglycemia. However, a pre-existing diagnosis of diabetes mellitus did not predict acute or discharge LVEF. The 30-day mortality correlated with acute hyperglycemia, rising at levels over 144 mg/dL (8 mmol) at presentation, with the plasma glucose being an independent predictor of mortality (9). The same group also found that acute hyperglycemia abolished the benefits of ischemic preconditioning in patients presenting with the first anterior wall MI (10).

Meta-analysis of 15 studies revealed increased risk of death and pump failure following MI in patients with "stress hyperglycemia," but no diagnosis of diabetes prior to presentation. The risk of death was 3.9-fold higher in patients with BG 110 to 144 mg/dL (6.1 to 8 mmol) than in patients presenting with BG levels in the normal range, or under 110 mg/dL (6.1 mmol). Further increases of BG were also associated with increased risk of congestive heart failure and cardiogenic shock. The prognostic implications of hyperglycemia in patients with pre-existing diabetes were not as significant as in patients with hyperglycemia and not known to have diabetes (11).

Acute hyperglycemia can have implications on short- and long-term prognosis. An analysis of nearly 1,000 patients presenting with acute MI revealed a correlation between admission BG and postdischarge mortality (up to 50 months) but not in hospital death. Mortality increased by 4% for each 18 mg/dL (1 mmol) increase in BG for patients without known diabetes and 5% for patients with established diabetes (12). Glucose levels at presentation are more predictive of adverse cardiac outcome than a diagnosis of pre-existing diabetes. Hyperglycemia at presentation was noted to be a more important prognosticator than the presence of microvascular disease.

Metabolic Implications of Newly Noted Hyperglycemia in the Setting of ACS

It is estimated that about 30% of people with diabetes do not know that they have this disease. Hence, patients presenting with hyperglycemia may have diabetes that has yet to be diagnosed. Analysis of 146 patients presenting with acute MI and hyperglycemia revealed that 18.5% of patients had known diabetes, 9.2% of patients not previously diagnosed with diabetes were noted to have an elevated glycosylated hemoglobin on admission suggesting pre-existing hyperglycemia, and the rest had no evidence of pre-existing hyperglycemia. In this cohort acute hyperglycemia, along with reduced renal function, was

an independent predictor of 5- and 28-day mortality. Admission hyperglycemia was associated with higher mortality, whereas the glycosylated hemoglobin was not (13).

The risk of developing diabetes is increased after an MI. In patients without diabetes presenting with acute MI and BG less than 200 mg/dL (11.1 mmol), mild hyperglycemia at the time of hospitalization was predictive of persistent glucose intolerance on follow-up. Only 34% of these patients had normal glucose tolerance on follow-up, 25% had diabetes, and the remainder had impaired glucose tolerance. Glucose tolerance at the time of discharge was similar to glucose tolerance at 3-month follow-up (14). On 34-month follow-up, cardiovascular morbidity and mortality were associated with abnormal glucose tolerance, all eight deaths occurred in patients with abnormal glucose tolerance (15). In Finland, where a national health registry is used to track outcomes, 16% of men and 20% of women presenting with their first MI had diabetes. Those who did not have diabetes at the time of their MI had an increased risk of developing diabetes subsequently, a 2.3-fold increase for men and 4.3-fold increase for women (16). Abnormal glucose tolerance after MI predicted glucose intolerance on follow-up. Newly noted glucose intolerance was associated with high risk of future cardiovascular events.

MECHANISM OF GLUCOSE TOXICITY

Diabetes, with established chronic hyperglycemia, and new onset acute hyperglycemia are associated with more severe compromise in myocardial function and increased mortality after an MI. There are several possible mechanisms for this phenomenon. Stress, such as is noted with ACS, is associated with increased insulin resistance and tendency toward hyperglycemia. The counter-regulatory hormones, catecholamines, and glucocorticoids associated with stress inhibit insulin secretion and increase insulin resistance. This results in higher BG levels and high free fatty acid (FFA) levels. Any hyperglycemic state is a state of relative insulin deficiency. Insulin has various metabolic effects, including facilitating glucose uptake by tissues and suppression of FFA levels.

Myocardial Energy Balance: Effect of Hyperglycemia and Hypoxia

The beating heart has a large energy requirement: a 300-gram heart synthesizes and utilizes about 5 kg of adenosine triphosphate (ATP) each day. At any time the heart contains only about 750 mg of ATP, thus the turnover of ATP is rapid, and the heart requires a constant production of ATP. Normally FFAs are the substrate for 60% to 70% of myocardial oxygen consumption; however, in the diabetic heart this is up to 90%. Because there is no anaerobic pathway for the consumption of FFA, there is increased dependence on glucose oxidation in the setting of ischemia, leading to increased lactate production (17). Insulin deficiency, hyperglycemia, and high FFA levels result in impaired glucose uptake, glycolysis, impaired pyruvate oxidation, impaired lactate uptake, and greater dependency on fatty acid as a source of Krebs cycle substrates. Reducing dependence on fatty acid oxidation and increasing pyruvate oxidation would benefit the diabetic heart during and following ischemia (18). Improved glucose uptake is protective in the setting of myocardial stress. Transgenic mice that overexpressed the GLUT-1 glucose transporter had better survival in the setting of left ventricular stress and hypertrophy than wild-type mice (19). Insulin may act as an antiapoptotic mediator by activating protein kinase B, which has dual effects of increasing glucose uptake via increased translocation of the glucose transporter GLUT-4 to the plasma membrane and inhibition of the activation of proapoptotic peptide (20). Any compromise in the delivery and uptake of substrates for energy production, increase in reliance on oxidation, or slowing in the washout of toxic by-products will result in myocardial injury.

Vascular Function and Inflammation in Hyperglycemia

Acute hyperglycemia results in impaired vascular function. Peripheral vascular function has been studied under various conditions of experimental hyperglycemia. Flow-mediated vasodilation in the brachial artery was inhibited during an oral glucose tolerance test in human subjects with normal glucose tolerance, impaired glucose tolerance, or diabetes. The degree of flow-mediated vasodilation was inversely proportional to plasma glucose level (21). Hyperglycemia is associated with increased production of free radicals (superoxide anion), which results in the inactivation of nitric oxide (NO), an endothelium-derived vasodilator (22). Beckman and his colleagues noted impaired endothelium-dependent vasodilation in human volunteers in the presence of acute hyperglycemia. They studied methacholine chloride-stimulated forearm blood flow under euglycemic and hyperglycemic conditions and in the presence and absence of a protein kinase C-β inhibitor. Protein kinase C-β inhibits endothelium-dependent vasodilation by decreasing endothelium-derived NO synthesis. Because the inhibition of vasodilation in the presence of hyperglycemia was corrected with inhibition of protein kinase C-β, these authors concluded that acute hyperglycemia is associated with activation of protein kinase C-β and impaired NO synthesis (23). A possible mediator of increased oxidative stress may be the enzyme heme oxygenase, which catalyzes the oxidation of heme into biliverdin, carbon monoxide, and free iron. The presence of acute hyperglycemia is associated with lower levels of this cell-protective enzyme (24). While hyperglycemia is noted to reduce vascular relaxation in some sites, such as the forearm (25), this was not observed in the coronary microcirculation (26). This results in greater oxidative stress, decreased NO, and decreased endothelium-dependent vasodilatation.

Acute and chronic hyperglycemia is associated with higher inflammatory tone, a process that may accelerate plaque rupture and stimulate coagulation pathways (27,28). Inflammation is a precursor to ACS, is sustained long after the event, and is associated with poorer outcome (29). Patients with hyperglycemia in the setting of an acute MI had higher inflammatory markers and more evidence of cytotoxic T-cell activation than patients with BG levels under 126 mg/dL (7 mmol) (30). Hyperglycemia results in increased platelet adhesion and increased adhesiveness of the endothelium through the activation of endothelial adhesion molecules such as VCAM-1 (31). Hyperglycemic patients who received insulin had a smaller rise in C-reactive protein levels over 24 hours after MI (32). Treatment with glucose and insulin in patients presenting with acute MI and receiving reperfusion therapy resulted in an attenuated rise in inflammatory markers and plasminogen activator inhibitor-1 (33). Because acute insulin administration reduces inflammation in MI and reperfusion, insulin administration may be therapeutic in this setting.

Electrophysiological Abnormalities Associated with Hyperglycemia

Hyperglycemia predisposes the myocardium to rhythm abnormalities. Increased ST-segment elevation was noted in patients presenting with hyperglycemia and normal glycosylated hemoglobin levels (34). In experimental models hyperglycemia is associated with prolongation of the QT interval in vivo and in vitro (35,36).

Acute and chronic hyperglycemia are proinflammatory and prothrombogenic, attenuate endothelium-dependent vasodilation, and may be proarrhythmogenic. Treatment of hyperglycemia and treatment with insulin in the setting of acute MI corrects some of these abnormalities (Table 18-1).

CLINICAL EVIDENCE OF GLUCOSE CONTROL IN CRITICAL ILLNESS AND ACS

Hyperglycemia is common in critically ill patients. Until recently this was thought to be an adaptive response to illness. However, in vitro and in vivo observations suggest that hyperglycemia, even when transient, is deleterious. It is associated with increased inflammatory tone, decreased ability to ward off infections, nutritional deficits, and fluid and electrolyte derangements, as well as hypercoagulability and compromised vascular function.

Hyperglycemia and Critical Illness

The most aggressive treatment of hyperglycemia has been possible in intensive care units (ICUs), where insulin can be safely delivered intravenously with close monitoring. Patients treated aggressively with intravenous insulin have benefited from reduced infections and improved cardiovascular outcomes. Patients with newly discovered hyperglycemia in hospital, who do not have a history of diabetes, have a worse prognosis than patients who were normoglycemic or those who had established diabetes. The outcome measures include death, intensive unit stay, length of stay in hospital, and discharge to an institution rather than home. Over one-third of patients admitted to the hospital were noted to be hyperglycemic (fasting glucose over 125, 7 mmol; or random BG over 200 mg/dL; 11.1 mmol on two occasions), and one-third of these patients do not have a history of pre-existing diabetes (37). Patients with newly noted hyperglycemia had greater hospital mortality than patients with known diabetes or normal glucose levels (16%, 3%, and 1.7%, respectively). This effect held true in ICU and non-ICU patients (37).

The impact of hyperglycemia on infections was first demonstrated in postoperative patients. Patients who had at least one BG over 200 mg/dL had nearly triple the infection rate of those whose BG levels remained under 200 mg/dL (11.1 mmol) (38). Zerr, Furnary, and colleagues observed a higher rate of wound infections in patients undergoing heart surgery who had diabetes than those who did not. This difference was corrected with the use of intravenous insulin to control hyperglycemia (39,40). Subsequent reports also noted a reduced all-cause mortality rate with insulin infusion and glucose control, some of which may be attributed directly to improved cardiac function, such as reduction of congestive heart failure and arrhythmias (41). These studies were nonrandomized and focused on patients with diabetes, not on patients selected solely on glycemic levels. However, insulin treatment was targeted to achieve improved glucose levels, initially under 200 mg/dL (11.1 mmol) and subsequently under 150 mg/dL (8.3 mmol). Controlling hyperglycemia after cardiac surgery is associated with fewer infections and improved myocardial function.

Hyperglycemia is deleterious in a general intensive care population, and these patients benefit from aggressive glycemic control. Acute hyperglycemia, not the diagnosis of diabetes, was noted to be associated with greater mortality in a community hospital ICU (42). Treatment with intravenous insulin to a target BG of less than 140 resulted in a 29.3% decrease in mortality. Patients with sepsis, neurologic causes for admis-

TABLE 18-1

EFFECTS OF HYPERGLYCEMIA ON VASCULAR AND MYOCARDIAL FUNCTION

Direct effect of hyperglycemia	How noted	Ref.
Metabolic		
Increased lactate production	Swine—surgical model	17
Overexpression of GLUT 1 is protective in hypertrophied hearts	Myocardial hypertrophy induced with ascending aortic constriction in normal and transgenic mice, which overexpress GLUT1	19
Vascular function		
Impaired endothelium-dependent vasodilation, reversed with inhibition of protein kinase C-β, which decreases endothelium-derived NO synthesis	Human volunteers, methacholine chloride-stimulated forearm blood flow in the presence of euglycemia and 6 hrs of hyperglycemia	23
Increased production of the adhesion protein VCAM-1, blocked by inhibition of PKC beta activation	Human aortic endothelium in vitro	29
Flow-mediated vasodilation inhibited with OGTT, inversely proportional to plasma glucose level	Human subjects with NGT, IGT, and DM, brachial artery	21
No compromise in coronary vasodilation as measured by LAD peak flow	Normal men, hyperglycemic clamp with glucose infusion and octreotide, color Doppler echocardiography at rest and after dipyridamole stimulation	26
Lower levels of the cell-protective enzyme heme oxygenase, which catalyzes the oxidation of heme to biliverdin, carbon monoxide, and free iron	Normal and streptozotocin-treated hyperglycemic rats	24
Inflammation		
Pts with and without DM with BG >126 had higher troponin, CRP, IL-18, and evidence of cytotoxic T-cell activation than pts with ACS but no hyperglycemia; more abnormal in new hyperglycemia than in DM	108 pts presenting with ACS—hyperglycemia also associated with poorer myocardial function on echocardiogram	30
DM and high A1c is prothrombogenic	Patients with DM	27
CRP and A1c independently and additively predict major coronary event—MI, PCI, CABG, DEA, CVA, or death	Prospectively studied patients	28
Insulin (GIK) reduced CRP, serum amyloid A and plasminogen activator inhibitor-1 (PAI-1), creatine kinase and CK-MB rise in AMI	Patients presenting with ACS and receiving systemic fibrinolytics	33
CRP level lower in patients who received insulin/ glucose infusion to maintain BG <180 for 24 hrs	Patients presenting with ACS and either DM or BG = 7.8 (140).	32
Arrhythmia		
Increased ST elevation	10 patients with nl A1c, hyperglycemia with MI	34
Prolonged QT interval	Streptozotocin-induced DM in rats and normal hearts perfused with high-glucose solution	35
Prolonged QT interval, increased coronary perfusion pressure, lipid peroxidation, decreased mitochondrial superoxide dismutase activity	Isolated hearts perfused with glucose solution	36

sion, and sur-gical patients benefited significantly. Patients admitted to the ICU for cardiac reasons did not have a reduction in mortality; however, other cardiac indices and postdischarge prognosis was not evaluated (43). The most definitive trial of glycemic control in the ICU was a large randomized, controlled trial of predominantly surgical patients in Belgium. Patients were randomized to standard control, given insulin only if BG was sustained over 215 mg/dL (12 mmol), or to tight control, and treated with intravenous insulin to a target BG of 80 to 110 mg/dL (4.4 to 5.6 mmol). Nearly all (98.7%) of the patients randomized to the tight control group required insulin to maintain blood sugar levels below 110 mg/dL (5.6 mmol), highlighting the common occurrence of hyperglycemia in the critically ill patient. This study revealed survival and length-of-stay benefit for the patients in the tight control group, with very little hypoglycemia and no severe adverse events from tight glycemic

control. The patients who benefited the most from tight glycemic control were those who had the highest APACHE score and required a longer ICU length of stay (44). Subsequent analyses of this study attributed much of the benefit to removing the toxic effect of hyperglycemia rather than to the administration of insulin per se (45). An analysis of insulin dosages in ICU patients, mostly after cardiac surgery, revealed increased mortality and longer length of stay in patients who required more insulin; however, there was a benefit to maintaining BG under a derived cutoff near 145 mg/dL (8 mmol), regardless of the insulin required to do so. This suggested that the benefit was derived from glycemic control rather than insulin administration (46). Analysis of the effects of aggressive insulin administration reveals that the predominant effect of insulin in vivo is to suppress endogenous hepatic glucose production and to preserve endothelial function. This results in preservation of hepatocellular structure, better regulation of blood flow, and transendothelial trafficking of nutrients and biologically active molecules (47–50).

Glucose Insulin Potassium (GIK) Infusions in ACS

GIK infusions were proposed over 40 years ago to protect the ischemic myocardium by shifting metabolism from the most abundant fatty acids to the more easily metabolized glucose under anaerobic conditions (51). GIK infusions have been studied in patients recovering from cardiac arrest, cardiac surgery, and acute MI, both before and after the advent of thrombolysis and reperfusion therapy. The results of GIK trials in acute MI are inconsistent.

Although some studies have shown benefit in terms of immediate and long-term mortality or myocardial function, the results are not consistent, and more recent analysis of randomized trials do not support a benefit (52). GIK was evaluated as adjunctive therapy to percutaneous coronary intervention in patients with acute MI. This population included patients with diabetes, comprising 10% of the cohort. A solution of 20% glucose with 80 mmol potassium was infused at a rate of 3 mL/kg body weight/hr over 8 to 12 hours, with a separate insulin infusion titrated to BG of 126 to 198 mg/dL (7 to 11 mmol). Patients were taken to the catheterization laboratory after the initiation of infusion. There was no overall benefit to GIK infusion in terms of mortality; however, the subset of patients with no heart failure (Killip Class 1) had a survival benefit at 30 days (adjusted RR death 28%; 95% CI 10% to 77%) (53). The glycemic values in this patient population were not reported. The CREATE-ECLA study randomized over 20,000 patients to standard therapy versus high-dose GIK (25% glucose, 50 units regular insulin/L, 80 mEq potassium/L at 1.5 mL/kg) administered over 24 hours followed by 7 days of heparin. This was a multicenter study conducted in Latin America, China, India, and Pakistan. Again, there was no benefit on survival in this large study (54). The noted limitations of this study were the initiation of the GIK infusion after reperfusion therapy in nearly two-thirds of the patients, the relative hyperglycemia in the GIK group compared to the control group at 6 and 24 hours after randomization, and the relatively high overall mortality rate in the trial. However, separate analysis of the patients who received GIK early did not reveal a benefit. A meta-analysis of trials using GIK or glucose and insulin revealed that the greatest benefit was demonstrated when the investigators used insulin with the aim of controlling hyperglycemia rather than to give glucose and insulin as a substrate for myocardial metabolism. Trials that aimed to achieve glycemic control demonstrated a benefit in mortality, whereas those who used insulin in the form of GIK did not. In this meta-analysis, controlling hyperglycemia with intravenous insulin was beneficial in acute MI (52).

Although smaller studies demonstrate a benefit from administering GIK at high doses to patients in the setting of acute MI, large, controlled studies and meta-analysis of multiple studies do not reveal a benefit of this treatment beyond that of achieving glycemic control. This finding suggests that an appropriate balance of glucose and insulin is necessary for the recovering myocardium, rather than an oversupply of glucose along with insulin.

Diabetes Mellitus and Acute Myocardial Infarction (DIGAMI) Studies

Given the high prevalence of CAD in patients with diabetes, the poor prognosis after an MI in this population, and the presence of hyperglycemia on presentation with an acute MI, the DIGAMI investigators undertook a large, randomized trial to assess the benefits of glycemic control in patients with diabetes. The first study (DIGAMI-1) was designed to evaluate the benefit of glycemic control at the time of the MI, followed by long-term intensive insulin therapy. Patients with diabetes were randomized to standard management ($n = 314$) or tight control ($n = 306$). Those in the experimental arm received an infusion of 5% dextrose with insulin 160 units/L at a rate of 30 mL/hr, equivalent to about 4.8 units of insulin per hour. The infusion rate was titrated to a BG 126 to 180 mg/dL (7 to 10 mmol). The tight control group achieved BG levels of 173 (9.6 mmol), whereas those in the control group had mean glucose levels of 211 mg/dL (11.7 mmol). Those in the experimental group were discharged on multiple daily insulin injections with premeal regular insulin and bedtime delayed-action insulin, whereas those in the control arm remained on their usual therapy. All patients received state-of-the-art care, with thrombolysis and beta-blockers when possible (55). Follow-up revealed that intensive insulin therapy was associated with a 30% reduction in mortality, with benefit persisting for the entire 3.4-year period. Other predictors of increased risk of mortality in this study included age, diabetes duration, admission glucose, and admission glycosylated hemoglobin; however, previous MI, hypertension, smoking, or sex did not add independent predictive value (56,57).

To investigate if it was the acute control or the prolonged postdischarge management that resulted in improved survival, a second study, DIGAMI-2, was carried out. Patients with diabetes were randomized to three groups: intravenous insulin followed by long-term subcutaneous insulin therapy ($n = 474$), intravenous insulin followed by standard management ($n = 473$), and standard management ($n = 306$). Patients in all three groups had equivalent mortality at 30 days and 1, 2, and 3 years. However, patients in DIGAMI 2 were admitted with better metabolic control than those in DIGAMI 1, with an admission BG near 230 mg/dL (12.8 mmol) compared with 280 mg/dL (15.6 mmol), and glycosylated hemoglobin of 7.3 versus 8.1. The differential in glycemic control on intravenous insulin was maintained, but not on long-term follow-up after discharge. The difference in postdischarge metabolic control between those being aggressively treated and those on conventional therapy may not have been big enough to demonstrate a benefit (58). This study was aborted before the target enrollment could be achieved due to slow recruitment; however, it is unlikely that the final result would have been significantly different.

The key difference between the DIGAMI studies is the pre-MI and postdischarge glycemic control. The patients in DIGAMI-2 had lower BG levels and lower glycosylated hemoglobin levels on admission, and after discharge the control groups were treated more aggressively than in DIGAMI-1. It is likely that this improvement in glycemic control is responsible for diminishing differences between the experimental and control arms. With that in mind, we cannot discount the results of DIGAMI-1, but rather interpret the cumulative evidence in favor of tighter glycemic control.

SUMMARY AND RECOMMENDATIONS

Hyperglycemia in the setting of an acute MI is deleterious to recovery, resulting in greater cardiac compromise, and increased short- and long-term mortality. This is the case regardless of pre-existing diabetes and glycemic control. Achieving glycemic control with intravenous insulin has been shown to be beneficial in critical illness and possibly in acute MI. There

INSULIN INFUSION PROTOCOLS

Protocol Name	Date	Characteristics	Clinical setting	Glucose target	Outcome measures	Ref.
Watts	1987		ICU patients	120–180	Glycemic control	61
Portland	1997, 2001, 2003	Nurse managed	After cardiac surgery	150–200; 100–150 now 80–120	Deep wound infection, Mortality	39,40
Leuvlen	2001	Nurse managed with physician backup, some judgment allowed	ICU patients—predominantly surgical	80–110	Mortality	44
Glucommander	2003	Multiplier with computer-based algorithm, insulin dose multiplied according to patient's insulin resistance	ICU patients, perioperative, labor and delivery	100–150	Glycemic control	62
Yale IIP	2004	Nurse managed, change columns according to an estimation of insulin resistance	Medical/Surgical ICU patients	100–140	Glycemic control	63
Hartford	2004	Nurse managed	SICU	180–220	Glycemic control, nosocomial infections	64
Detroit	2004	Nurse managed	Cardiothoracic ICU	80–150	Glycemic control	65

is good clinical and experimental evidence that hyperglycemia is toxic and that controlling it with intravenous insulin is beneficial. Insulin itself has anti-inflammatory properties, and inflammation has a pathogenic role in ACS. Hyperglycemia is proinflammatory, is prothrombogenic, compromises vascular relaxation, and is arrhythmogenic. Treating hyperglycemia with an aggressive insulin regimen has been shown to be beneficial in the general ICU and after MI. Several different target levels for insulin therapy have been used, ranging from under 110 mg/dL (6 mmol) to under 200 mg/dL (11.1 mmol). The finding that hypoglycemia, even mild, may be associated with worse prognosis after an acute MI will limit how aggressive we can be in this setting. The consensus to target BG levels 80 to 110 mg/dL (4.4 to 6 mmol) in the ICU is not based on patients with ACS (59,60). Further studies to define an appropriate target for patients with ACS are necessary. For now, it is reasonable to achieve a target that can be inferred to be therapeutic from studies in other populations, as well as experimental and clinical observations in myocardial ischemia. This evidence supports a glycemic tagged of less than 145 mg/dL (8 mmol). It is essential that treatment be instituted immediately on presentation to improve vascular function, limit myocardial cell apoptosis, and increase the success of reperfusion therapy.

There are numerous published insulin infusion protocols, with a range of target BG levels and measured outcomes (Table 18-2) (39,40,44,61–65). Continuous insulin infusion therapy should be initiated if BG is noted to be over 145 or 150 mg/dL (8 to 8.3 mmol), regardless of the diagnosis of pre-existing diabetes. It is important to select a protocol that can be implemented immediately on presentation, used as a matter of routine, and managed throughout the hospital where a patient may travel, including the emergency department, catheterization laboratory, and telemetry floors. The protocol needs to be nurse-managed, and in most cases, bedside glucose monitoring

will ensure the safety and success of glycemic management. Careful monitoring for hypoglycemia and hypokalemia is required while administering intravenous insulin, especially if insulin bolus is needed for severe hyperglycemia. It is safe to transition to an effective subcutaneous or oral antihyperglycemic regimen when the patient is hemodynamically stable and able to take oral medication and nutrients. Although insulin administration itself is beneficial, glycemic control is the determining factor in improving prognosis.

References

1. Cruikshank N. Coronary thrombosis and myocardial infarction with glycosuria. *BMJ* 1931;1:618–619.
2. Haffner S, Lehto S, Ronnemaa T, et al. Mortality from coronary heart disease in subjects with type 2 diabetes and in nondiabetic subjects with and without prior myocardial infarction. *N Engl J Med* 1998;339:229–234.
3. Mak K, Moliterno DJ, Granger CB, et al. Influence of diabetes mellitus on clinical outcome in the thrombolytic era of acute myocardial infarction. *J Am Coll Cardiol* 1997;30:171–179.
4. Berger AK, Breall JA, Gersh BJ, et al. Effect of diabetes mellitus and insulin use on survival after acute myocardial infarction in the elderly (The Cooperative Cardiovascular Project). *Am J Cardiol* 2001;87:272–277.
5. Murcia AM, Hennekens CH, Lamas GA, et al. Impact of diabetes on mortality in patients with myocardial infarction and left ventricular dysfunction. *Arch Int Med* 2004;164:2273–2279.
6. Svensson A, McGuire D, Abrahamson P, et al. Association between hyper- and hypoglycaemia and 2 year all-cause mortality risk in diabetic patients with acute coronary events. *Eur Heart J* 2005;26:1255–1261.
7. Wahab N, Cowden EA, Pearce NJ, et al. Is blood glucose an independent predictor of mortality in acute myocardial infarction of the thrombolytic era? *J Am Coll of Cardiol* 2002;40:1748–1754.
8. Iwakura K, Ito H, Ikushima M, et al. Association between hyperglycemia and the no-reflow phenomenon in patients with acute myocardial infarction. *J Am Coll Cardiol* 2003;41:1–7.
9. Ishihara M, Inoue I, Kawagoe T, et al. Impact of acute hyperglycemia on left ventricular function after reperfusion therapy in patients with a first anterior wall acute myocardial infarction. *Am Heart J* 2003;146:674–678.

10. Ishihara M, Inoue I, Kawagoe T, et al. Effects of acute hyperglycemia on the ischemic preconditioning effect of prodromal angina pectoris in patients with a first anterior wall myocardial infarction. *Am J Cardiol* 2003;92:288–291.
11. Capes SE, Hunt D, Malmberg K, et al. Stress hyperglycemia and increased risk of death after myocardial infarction in patients with and without diabetes: a systematic overview. *Lancet* 2000;355:773–778.
12. Stranders I, Diamant M, van Gelder RE, et al. Admission blood glucose level as risk indicator of death after myocardial infarction in patients with and without diabetes mellitus. *Arch Int Med* 2004;164:982–988.
13. Hadjaj S, Coisne D, Muco G, et al. Prognostic value of admission plasma glucose and HbA1c in acute myocardial infarction. *Diabet Med* 2004;21:305–310.
14. Tenerz A, Norhammar A, Silveira A, et al. Diabetes, insulin resistance, and the metabolic syndrome in patients with acute myocardial infarction without previously known diabetes. *Diabetes Care* 2003;26:2770–2776.
15. Bartnik M, Malmberg K, Norhammar A, et al. Newly detected abnormal glucose tolerance: an important predictor of long-term outcome after myocardial infarction. *Eur Heart J* 2004;25:1990–1997.
16. Pajunen P, Koukkunen H, Ketonen M, et al. Five-year risk of developing clinical diabetes after first myocardial infarction; the FINAMI study. *Diabet Med* 2005;22:1334–1337.
17. Chavez PN, Stanley WC, McElfresh TA, et al. Effect of hyperglycemia and fatty acid oxidation inhibition during aerobic conditions and demand-induced ischemia. *AJP—Heart* 2003;284:1521–1527.
18. Stanley WC, Lopaschuk GD, McCormack JG. Review: regulation of energy substrate metabolism in the diabetic heart. *Cardiovasc Res* 1997;34:25–33.
19. Liao R, Jain M, Cui L, et al. Cardiac-specific overexpression of GLUT1 prevents the development of heart failure attributable to pressure overload in mice. *Circulation* 2002;106:2125–2131.
20. Sack MN, Yellon DM. Insulin therapy as an adjunct to reperfusion after acute coronary ischemia. A proposed direct myocardial cell survival effect independent of metabolic modulation. *J Am Coll Cardiol* 2003;41:1404–1407.
21. Kawano H, Mooyama T, Hirashima O, et al. Hyperglycemia rapidly suppresses flow-mediated vasodilation of brachial artery. *J Am Coll Cardiol* 1999;34:146–154.
22. Gutterman, DD. Vascular dysfunction in hyperglycemia. *Circ Res* 2002;90:5–11.
23. Beckman JA, Goldfine AB, Gordon MB, et al. Inhibition of protein kinase C beta prevents impaired endothelium-derived vasodilatation causes by hyperglycemia in humans. *Circ Res* 2001;90:107–111.
24. Di Filippo C, Marfells R, Cuzzocrea S, et al. Hyperglycemia in streptozotocin-induced diabetic rat increases infarct size associated with low levels of myocardial HO-1 during ischemia/reperfusion. *Diabetes* 2005;54:803–810.
25. Beckman JA, Goldfine AB, Gordon MB, et al. Ascorbate restores endothelium-dependent vasodilation impaired by acute hyperglycemia in humans. *Circulation* 2001;103:1618–1623.
26. Capaldo B, Galderisi M, Turco AA, et al. Acute hyperglycemia does not affect the reactivity of coronary microcirculation in humans. *J Clin Endocrinol Metab* 2005;90(7):3871–3876.
27. Seriello A, Taboga C, Giacomello R, et al. Fibrinogen plasma levels as a marker for thrombin activation in diabetes. *Diabetes* 1994;43:430–432.
29. Schillinger M, Exner M, Amighi J, et al. Joint effect of C-reactive protein and glycated hemoglobin in predicting future cardiovascular events of patients with advanced atherosclerosis. *Circulation* 2003;108:2323–2328.
29. Mulvihill NT, Foley JB. Inflammation in acute coronary syndromes. *Heart* 2002;87:201–204.
30. Marfella R, Siniscalchi M, Esposito K, et al. Effects of stress hyperglycemia on acute myocardial infarction. *Diabetes Care* 2003;26:3129–3135.
31. Kouroedov A, Eto M, Joch H, et al. Selective inhibition of protein kinase Cbeta2 prevents acute effects of high glucose on vascular cell adhesion molecule-1 expression in Human endothelial cells. *Circulation* 2004;110:91–96.
32. Wong VW, McLean M, Boyages SC, et al. C-reactive protein levels following acute myocardial infarction. *Diabetes Care* 2004;27:2971–2973.
33. Chaudhuri A, Janicke D, Wilson MF, et al. Anti-inflammatory and profibrinolytic effect of insulin in acute ST-segment-elevation myocardial infarction. *Circulation* 2004;109:849–854.
34. Gokhroo R, Mittal SR. Electrocardiographic correlates of hyperglycemia in acute myocardial infarction. *Int J Cardiol* 1989;22(2) 267–269.
35. D'Amico M, Marfella R, Nappo F, et al. High glucose induces ventricular instability and increases vasomotor tone in rats. *Diabetologia* 2001;44:464–470.
36. Di Filippo C, Cuzzocrea S, Marfella R, et al. M40403 prevents myocardial injury induced by acute hyperglycaemia in perfused rat heart. *Eur J Pharmacol* 2004;497(1):65–74.
37. Umpierrez GE, Isaacs SD, Bazargan N, et al. Hyperglycemia: an independent marker of in-hospital mortality in patients with undiagnosed diabetes. *J Clin Endocrinol and Metab* 2002;87(3):978–982.
38. Pomposelli JJ, Baxter JK 3rd, Babineau TJ, et al. Early postoperative glucose control predicts nosocomial infection rate in diabetic patients. *J of Parenter Enteral Nutr* 1998;22:77–81.
39. Zerr KJ, Furnary AP, Grunkemeier GL, et al. Glucose control lowers the risk of wound infection in diabetics after open heart operations. *Ann Thorac Surg* 1997;63(2):356–61.
40. Furnary AP, Zerr KJ, Grunkemeier GL, et al. Continuous intravenous insulin infusion reduces the incidence of deep sternal wound infection in diabetic patients after cardiac surgical procedures. *Ann Thorac Surg* 1999;67(2):352–360.
41. Furnay AP, Gao G, Grunkemeier GL, et al. Continuous insulin infusion reduces mortality in patients with diabetes undergoing coronary artery bypass grafting. *J Thorac Cardiovasc Surg* 2003;125(5):1007–1021.
42. Krinsley JS. Association between hyperglycemia and increased hospital mortality in a heterogeneous population of critically ill patients. *Mayo Clin Proc* 2003;78:1471–1478.
43. Krinsley JS. Effect of intensive glucose management protocol on the mortality of critically ill adult patients. *Mayo Clin Proc* 2004;79:992–1000.
44. Van den Berghe G, Wouters P, Weekers F, et al. Intensive insulin therapy in critically ill patients. *N Engl J Med* 2001;345:1359–1367.
45. Van den Berghe G, Wouters P, Bouillon R, et al. Outcome benefit of intensive insulin therapy in the critically ill: insulin dose versus glycemic control. *Crit Care Med* 2003;31(2):359–366.
46. Finney SJ, Zekveld C, Elia A, et al. Glucose control and mortality in critically ill patients. *JAMA* 2003;290:2041–2047.
47. Van den Berghe G. How does blood glucose control with insulin save lives in intensive care? *J Clin Investig* 2004;114:1187–1195.
48. Vanhorebeek I, De Vos R, Medotten D, et al. Protection of hepatocyte mitochondrial ultrastructure and function by strict blood glucose control with insulin in critically ill patients. *Lancet* 2005;365(9453):53–59.
49. Thorell A, Rooyackers O, Myrenfors P, et al. Intensive insulin treatment in critically ill trauma patients normalizes glucose by reducing endogenous glucose production. *J Clin Endocrinol and Metab* 2004;89:5382–5386.
50. Langouche L, Vanhorebeek I, Vlasselaers D, et al. Intensive insulin therapy protects the endothelium of critically ill patients. *J Clin Invest* 2005;115:2277–2286.
51. Sodi-Pallares D, Testelli MR, Fishleder BL, et al. Effects of an intravenous infusion of a potassium-glucose-insulin solution on the electrocardiographic signs of myocardial infarction. A preliminary clinical report. *Am J Cardiol* 1962;9:166–181.
52. Pittas AG, Siegel RD, Laue J. Insulin therapy for critically ill hospitalized patients. *Arch Int Med* 2003;164:2005–2011.
53. Van der Horst ICC, Zijlstra F, van't Hof AWJ, et al. Glucose-insulin-potassium infusion in patients treated with primary angioplasty for acute myocardial infarction. *J Am Coll Cardiol* 2003;42:784–791.
54. The CTEATE-ECLA Trial Group Investigators. Effect of glucose-insulin-potassium infusion on mortality in patients with acute ST-segment elevation myocardial infarction. *JAMA* 2005;293:437–446.
55. Malmberg K, Ryden L, Efendic S, et al. Randomized trial of insulin-glucose infusion followed by subcutaneous insulin treatment in diabetic patients with acute myocardial infarction (DIGAMI Study): effects on mortality at 1 year. *J Am Coll Cardiol* 1995;26:57–65.
56. Malmberg K. Prospective randomized study of intensive insulin treatment on long term survival after acute myocardial infarction patients with diabetes mellitus. *Brit Med J* 1997;314:1512–1515.
57. Malmberg K, Norhammar A, Wedel H, et al. Glycometabolic state at admission: important risk marker of mortality in conventionally treated patients with diabetes mellitus and acute myocardial infarction. Long-term results from the diabetes and insulin-glucose infusion in acute myocardial infarction (DIGAMI) study. *Circulation* 1999;99:2626–2632.
58. Malmberg K, Ryden L, Wedel H, et al. Intense metabolic control by means of insulin in patients with diabetes mellitus and acute myocardial infarction (DIGAMI 2): effects on mortality and morbidity. *Eur Heart J* 2005;26:650–661.
59. Clement S, Braithwaite SS, Magee MF, et al. Management of diabetes and hyperglycemia in hospitals. *Diabetes Care* 2004;27:553–591.
60. American College of Endocrinology Task Force on Inpatient Diabetes and Metabolic Control. American College of Endocrinology position statement on inpatient diabetes and metabolic control. *Endocr Pract* 2004;10:77–82.
61. Watts NB, Gebbard SS, Clark RV, et al. Postoperative management of diabetes mellitus: steady-state glucose control with bedside algorithm for insulin adjustment. *Diabetes Care* 1987;10:722–728.
62. The Glucommander. Presented at Diabetes Technology, San Francisco, CA; 2003. Available online at www.glucommander.com. Accessed May 23, 2006.
63. Goldberg PA, Siegel MD, Sherwin RS, et al. Implementation of a safe and effective insulin infusion protocol in a medical intensive care unit. *Diabetes Care* 2004;27:461–467.
64. Grey NJ, Perdrized GA. Reduction of nosocomial infections in the surgical intensive-care unit by strict glycemic control. *Endocr Pract* 2004;10:46–52.
65. Zimmerman CR, Mlynarek ME, Jordan JA, et al. An insulin infusion protocol in critically ill cardiothoracic surgery patients. *Ann Pharmacother* 2004;38:1123–1129.

CHAPTER 19 ■ MANAGEMENT OF ATRIAL FIBRILLATION AND ATRIAL FLUTTER

EYAL HERZOG AND JONATHAN S. STEINBERG

GOALS AND STRATEGIES IN MANAGING PATIENTS
WITH ATRIAL FIBRILLATION AND ATRIAL FLUTTER
BASED ON THE RACE PATHWAY
Initial Assessment
Assessment of Patient Hemodynamic Stability
Defining the Etiology and Pathophysiology of Atrial Fibrillation
and Atrial Flutter
Assessment of Duration of Atrial Fibrillation and Atrial Flutter
Restoring Sinus Rhythm-Cardioversion, Electrical or
Pharmacologic
Management of Patients with Atrial Fibrillation and Atrial Flutter
of More Than 48 Hours or of an Unknown Duration
Management of Permanent Atrial Fibrillation
Management of Atrial Flutter
Cardiac Imaging for Patients with Atrial Fibrillation and Atrial
Flutter
Prevention of Embolic Stroke with Anticoagulation Therapy Based
on Thromboembolic Risk Assessment
Rate Control Medication
Rhythm Control and Antiarrhythmic Drug Therapy
CONCLUSION

Atrial fibrillation (AF) is the most common cardiac rhythm disturbance encountered in clinical practice, and its prevalence is increasing as the population ages (1,2). Electrocardiographically, AF is characterized by an irregularly irregular ventricular rhythm, with an absence of discrete P-wave activity. Rather, undulating fibrillatory activity (f waves) are seen on the electrocardiogram between QRS complexes and T waves. Sometimes very small "f" waves are difficult to see unless a 12-lead electrocardiogram (ECG) is done (3). The American College of Cardiology (ACC), the American Heart Association (AHA), and the European Society of Cardiology (ESC) established guidelines in 2001 for the management of patients with AF (4).

Atrial flutter (Afl) is less common and is often associated with AF or occurs in an isolated pattern. Guidelines for its management were included in the ACC/AHA/ESC Guidelines for the Management of Patients with Supraventricular Arrhythmias (5). The electrocardiographic findings of Afl include an atrial deflection with rapid regular undulations that gives rise to a sawtooth appearance, mainly in the inferior leads (6). The atrial rate is usually between 250 and 350 beats/minute.

A major limitation of the currently published guidelines for management of patients with AF and Afl is its complexity, the fact that official guidelines are published separately for each of these arrhythmias, and that they were published several years ago. To address these deficiencies, we have developed a novel pathway (Fig. 19-1) (7) for management of AF and Afl at St. Luke's-Roosevelt Hospital Center (SLRHC), a university hospital of Columbia University College of Physicians and Surgeons.

The necessity to develop such a pathway at our institution was compelling, yet typical of the need at many other large medical centers, where it has become increasingly difficult for all house staff to grasp all the subtleties in the management of AF and Afl and to rapidly, efficiently, and accurately implement clinical protocols. It should be emphasized that this pathway is the opinion of our group and may differ somewhat from the published guidelines. The pathway has been designated with the acronym of RACE, which reflects the three main components in patient management: Rate control, Anti-Coagulation therapy, and Electrophysiology/anti-arrhythmic medication.

This pathway is an attempt to incorporate, in a user-friendly format, the keys to the initial diagnosis and management of these prevalent arrhythmias. This is followed by a comprehensive guideline for therapy.

GOALS AND STRATEGIES IN MANAGING PATIENTS WITH ATRIAL FIBRILLATION AND ATRIAL FLUTTER BASED ON THE RACE PATHWAY

Initial Assessment

All patients should have undergone an initial assessment (Fig. 19-2) on presentation to the emergency department (ED), including 12-lead ECG (to be done within 10 minutes after arrival to the ED), history, and physician exam. Patients should be considered for evaluation of acute coronary syndrome by obtaining a blood specimen for cardiac markers and also should be considered for evaluation for acute heart failure by obtaining a BNP (β-type natriutretic peptide) level if diagnosis is uncertain. If the BNP level exceeds 500 pg/mL, patients should be treated for acute heart failure. It has been shown in multiple clinical trials that the prevalence of AF increased relative to the New York Heart Association heart failure class (8). Acute coronary syndrome and acute heart failure should be treated respectively per published guidelines and pathways (9,10).

Additional initial laboratory tests should include a basic metabolic panel, complete blood count, magnesium level, thyroid function tests, and coagulation panel. All patients should have a chest x-ray.

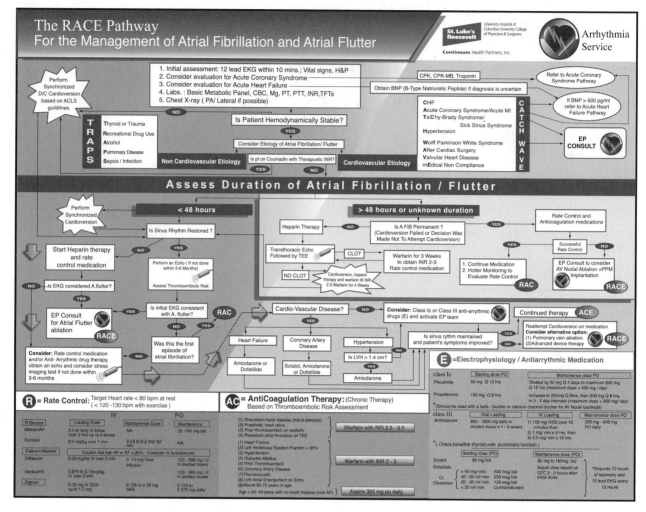

FIGURE 19-1. The RACE pathway for the management of atrial fibrillation and atrial flutter.

Assessment of Patient Hemodynamic Stability

All patients should be assessed for hemodynamic stability (Fig. 19-3) as defined by advanced cardiac life support (ACLS) guidelines (11). If patients are unstable, emergency synchronized D/C cardioversion should be performed.

Defining the Etiology and Pathophysiology of Atrial Fibrillation and Atrial Flutter

We have developed a systematic approach to the pathophysiology of AF and Afl (Fig. 19-4) by using acronyms that can easily be remembered by physicians, nurses, and other health care personnel:

(a) Noncardiovascular etiology: <u>**TRAPS**</u>
  T—Thyroid disease
  R—Recreational drug use
  A—Alcohol
  P—Pulmonary disease
  S—Sepsis/infection
(b) Cardiovascular etiology: <u>**CATCH WAVE**</u>
  C—Congestive heart failure
  A—Acute coronary syndrome/acute myocardial infarction (MI)
  TC—TaChy-brady syndrome (sick sinus syndrome)
  H—Hypertension
  W—Wolff-Parkinson-White syndrome
  A—After cardiac surgery
  V—Valvular heart disease
  E—mEdical noncompliance

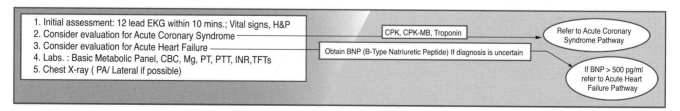

FIGURE 19-2. Initial assessment of patients with atrial fibrillation and atrial flutter.

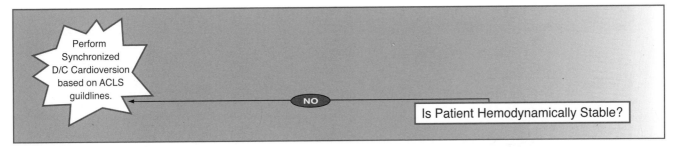

FIGURE 19-3. Rapid assessment of patients' stability as defined by ACLS guidelines.

Assessment of Duration of Atrial Fibrillation and Atrial Flutter

Timing the duration of atrial fibrillation and atrial flutter is sometimes difficult if the patient cannot pinpoint the starting time of their arrhythmia. It is well accepted that patients whose arrhythmia is less than 48 hours in duration can safely have a cardioversion performed (Fig. 19-5), and those with arrhythmia >48 hours may have developed atrial thrombus, which increases the risk of thromboembolic events postcardioversion.

Restoring Sinus Rhythm-Cardioversion, Electrical or Pharmacologic

Transthoracic electrical cardioversion is more successful than pharmacologic cardioversion, with an overall success rate of 75% to 93%, inversely related to the duration of AF, chest wall impedance, and left atrial size (12–14). The success rate for pharmacologic cardioversion in selected patients approaches 70% at best (15), and there is a risk of proarrhythmia. For this reason, we recommend electrical cardioversion.

There are two conventional positions for the electrode placement: anterior-lateral and anterio-posterior. Several studies have shown that less energy is required and a higher success rate is achieved with electrodes in the anteroposterior position (16,17). For this reason, we recommend the anteroposterior location. The energy required for cardioversion of AF is often >200 joules (18). More energy is required in obese patients and for long-standing AF. The initial energy used depends in part on the waveform of the current delivered by the defibrillation. Biphasic devices have been shown to be more effective and require less energy than monophasic devices (19).

Management of Patients with Atrial Fibrillation and Atrial Flutter of More Than 48 Hours or of an Unknown Duration

When the onset of AF cannot be accurately determined or if AF is longer than 48 hours, anticoagulation should always be administered (Fig. 19-6).

The conventional approach was to recommend anticoagulation with a therapeutic international normalized ratio (INR) (2.0 to 3.0) for 3 weeks before and 4 weeks after cardioversion.

Anticoagulation prior to cardioversion can be shortened if transesophageal echo (TEE) is done and indicates the absence of thrombus in the left atrium or the left atrial appendage. The TEE guided approach has been evaluated in the Assessment of Cardioversion Utilizing Echocardiography (ACUTE) trial (20,21). With this approach, which we often employ, heparin is given immediately and concurrently with warfarin, and heparin is continued until the INR is therapeutic. Cardioversion is done immediately when the TEE suggests that there is no evidence of thrombus; warfarin is continued for at least 4 weeks depending on long-term risk.

Either intravenous unfractionated heparin or subcutaneous low-molecular-weight heparin may be used (22). Consideration of discontinuation of warfarin after 4 weeks can be made when there is no recurrence of AF and there are no stroke risk factors.

Management of Permanent Atrial Fibrillation

The nomenclature used to classify AF has been diverse (23). The published guidelines (4) suggest the classification of first detected, paroxysmal (self-terminating), persistent (not self-terminating), and permanent (Fig. 19-7).

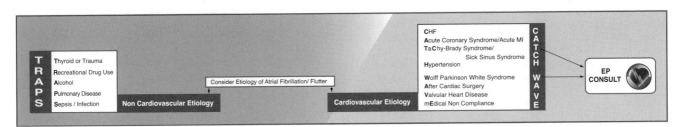

FIGURE 19-4. Pathophysiology of atrial fibrillation and atrial flutter based on cardiovascular and noncardiovascular etiology.

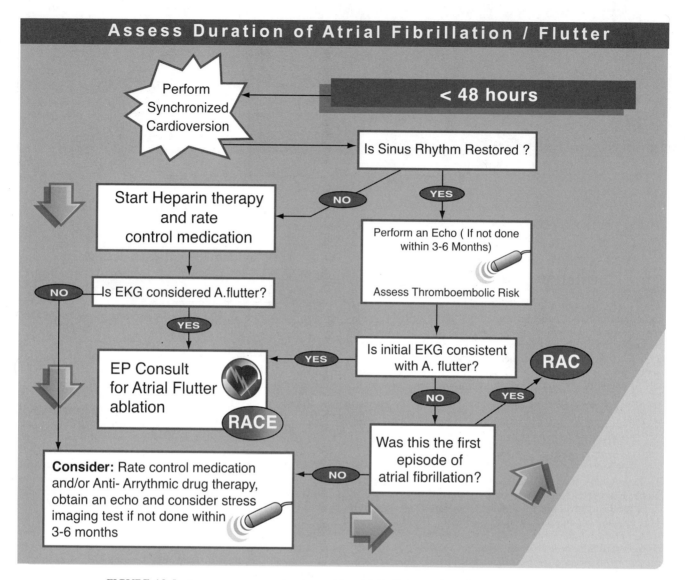

Assess Duration of Atrial Fibrillation / Flutter

< 48 hours

Perform Synchronized Cardioversion

Is Sinus Rhythm Restored ?

Start Heparin therapy and rate control medication

NO

YES

Perform an Echo (If not done within 3-6 Months)

Assess Thromboembolic Risk

NO

Is EKG considered A.flutter?

YES

EP Consult for Atrial Flutter ablation

RACE

Is initial EKG consistent with A. flutter?

YES

RAC

NO

YES

Was this the first episode of atrial fibrillation?

NO

Consider: Rate control medication and/or Anti- Arrythmic drug therapy, obtain an echo and consider stress imaging test if not done within 3-6 months

FIGURE 19-5. Acute management of patients with atrial fibrillation and atrial flutter of <48 hours.

In this regard we define permanent AF as continuous AF of longer than 7 days, with failed cardioversion or when a decision has been made not to attempt cardioversion. A patient with permanent AF will be managed with rate control and anticoagulation medication. Holter monitoring can be used to evaluate rate control. Patients whose rate control is unsuccessful should have an electrophysiology (EP) consult to consider atrioventricular (AV) nodal ablation and permanent pacemaker implantation.

Management of Atrial Flutter

The RACE pathway published in September 2005 (7) was the first one to include both AF and Afl in a single pathway. Because both arrhythmias will require anticoagulation and rate control medication, the initial assessment and management is similar. However, if the ECG is consistently Afl, we highly recommend consulting the EP team for consideration for Afl ablation, as shown in Figure 19-5.

Electrophysiological studies have shown that Afl results from tachycardia using a re-entry circuit. The re-entry circuit occupies large areas of the atrium and is referred to as "macro-re-entrant." The classic type of Afl (typical flutter) is dependent

on the cavotricuspid isthmus (5). Catheter ablation of the cavotricuspid isthmus for isthmus-dependent flutter had been proven to be successful in 80% to 100% (24,25), and is superior to antiarrhythmic therapy (26).

Our recommendation is to consult the EP team for all patients with Afl for consideration of ablation. If medically treated, Afl resumes in the vast majority of patients within 6 months (25).

Cardiac Imaging for Patients with Atrial Fibrillation and Atrial Flutter

Echocardiography is essential in the evaluation of patients with AF and Afl. As discussed earlier, TEE plays a major role in the acute management of patients with AF and with Afl when longer than 48 hours or of an unknown duration. Echocardiography is crucial for the assessment of thromboembolic risk, which will define anticoagulation therapy (Fig. 19-8). Also, the selection of antiarrhythmic drugs in Figure 19-10 is based on the existence of cardiovascular diseases (hypertension, coronary artery disease, and heart failure) for which the key is the echocardiographic exam.

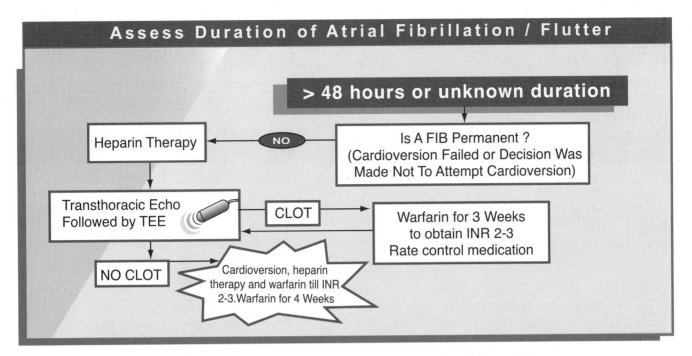

FIGURE 19-6. Acute management of patients with atrial fibrillation and atrial flutter >48 hours, or of unknown duration.

We recommend performing echocardiographs in all patients with AF and Afl, if not done within the last 3 to 6 months (Fig. 19-5).

Prevention of Embolic Stroke with Anticoagulation Therapy Based on Thromboembolic Risk Assessment

AF is thought to be responsible for approximately 15% to 25% of ischemic strokes (27–31). The stroke rate varies from 0.5% per year for young patients without structural heart disease, to 12% per year for patients with AF who have had a previous stroke (30,32–35). The pathophysiology of AF-associated stroke is complex, but it appears to arise as a result of the embolization of a thrombus formed within the dysfunctioning left atrium, especially the left atrial appendage (36). Clot formations are more likely under the conditions of stasis accompanying impaired atrial contraction.

Anticoagulation with warfarin is the current recommended treatment in patients with AF and Afl. Warfarin is associated with a small but significant risk of hemorrhage, making close monitoring mandatory (37).

Stratification of thromboembolic risk is central to the current recommendation from the American College of Chest Physicians (ACCP) (38) and the ACC/AHA/ESC Guidelines for anticoagulation of patients with AF (4). We summarize these recommendations in Figure 19-8. Patients at a very high risk are those with rheumatic heart disease, prosthetic heart valve, and prior thromboemboli on warfarin and persistent atrial

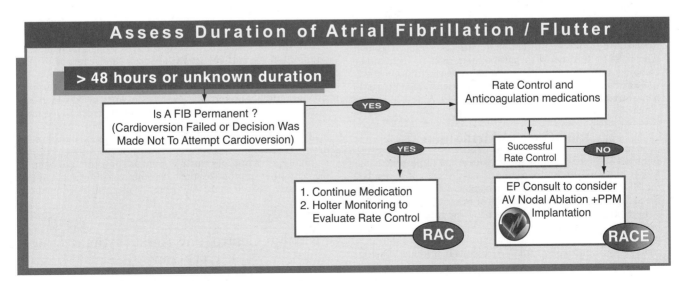

FIGURE 19-7. Management of permanent atrial fibrillation.

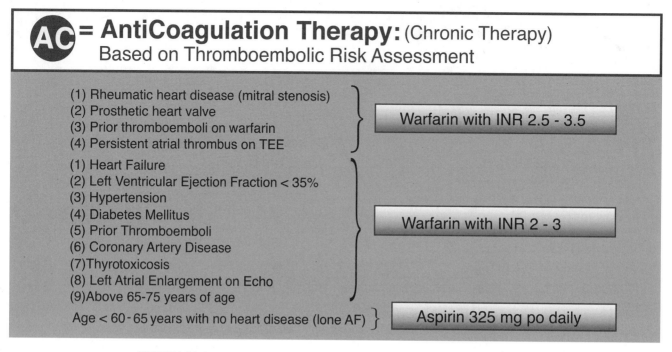

FIGURE 19-8. Anticoagulation therapy based on thromboembolic risk assessment.

thrombus on TEE. These patients will benefit from warfarin treatment with a higher target INR of 2.5 to 3.5.

Patients with heart failure, left ventricular ejection fraction of less than 35%, hypertension, diabetes mellitus, coronary artery disease, thyrotoxicosis, left atrial enlargement on echo, and age above 65 to 75 years old will benefit from anticoagulation with warfarin with a target INR of 2 to 3.

Patients younger than 60 to 65 years with no evidence of heart disease ("lone" AF) can be treated with aspirin alone.

Meta-analyses, pooling trial data from large numbers of patients, have re-examined the relative efficacies of oral anticoagulants and antiplatelet drugs in the prevention of AF-associated thromboembolism (38,39). Reviewing six trials with a total of 2,900 patients has shown that warfarin, dose adjusted on the basis of INR, reduced the risk of stroke by 62% (39).

Warfarin has a narrow therapeutic window and complex and variable pharmacodynamics and pharmacokinetics. It also interacts with many drugs and foods and requires regular blood level monitoring. As a result, there has been much interest in finding agents to replace warfarin. Ximelagatran, the first oral direct thrombin inhibitor, has been shown to be noninferior to warfarin for stroke prevention in patients with nonvalvular AF (40–42). It appears to have similar risks of intracranial bleeding and major bleeding relative to warfarin but a lower risk of minor hemorrhage (41,42). Because of a small risk of hepatotoxicity, the drug has not attained FDA approval.

Rate Control Medication

In about 60% to 70% of patients with AF, a rapid ventricular rate is observed, and symptoms are usually present depending on the rapidity of the ventricular response, the length of time the arrhythmia is sustained, and the presence and type of underlying heart disease (43). Acute ventricular rate control is the primary goal initially because patients' symptoms are chiefly governed by the rapid ventricular rate (44,45). In addition, a reduction in ventricular rate in AF results in a longer diastolic filling period and higher ventricular stroke volume. Acute ventricular rate control in AF can be achieved by pharmacotherapy, nonpharmacologic therapy, and early cardioversion to

sinus rhythm. In addition, correction of precipitating factors often helps in controlling ventricular rates in addition to enhancing the chances for conversion to sinus rhythm.

We have defined rate control in AF as a resting ventricular rate of less than 80 beats per minute and less than 120 to 130 beats per minute with exercise (depending on the patient's age).

Atrioventricular node blocking agents including beta-adrenergic blockers, nondihydropyridine calcium channel blockers, and digoxin are usually effective in controlling ventricular rate in AF and Afl. Intravenous beta-blocker and nondihydropyridine calcium channel blockers are equally effective in rapidly controlling the ventricular rate. The addition of digoxin to the regimen is helpful, but digoxin as a single agent is generally less effective. Magnesium and amiodarone have also been used for acute ventricular rate control in AF. The agent of first choice is usually individualized depending on the clinical situation. Beta-blockers are preferable in patients with myocardial ischemia, myocardial infarction, and hyperthyroidism and in a postoperative state, but should be avoided in patients with bronchial asthma and chronic obstructive pulmonary disease, when nondihydropyridine calcium channels blockers are preferred. Beta-blockers are preferred in AF during pregnancy. In addition, in AF with Wolff-Parkinson-White syndrome, beta-blockers, calcium channel blockers, and digoxin should be avoided, as these drugs are selective AV node blockers without slowing conduction through the accessory pathway, which can lead to increased transmission of impulses preferentially through the accessory pathway and precipitate ventricular fibrillation. The drug of choice for AF in pre-excitation syndrome is procainamide.

Figure 19-9 outlines our recommendation for rate control medication. It summarizes the intravenous loading and maintenance dose, as well as the oral dose for recommended medications.

Rhythm Control and Antiarrhythmic Drug Therapy

Over the past decades various antiarrhythmic drugs have been investigated for maintenance of sinus rhythm in patients with

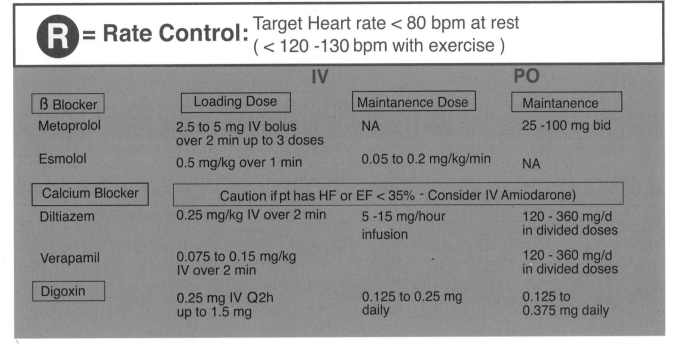

R = Rate Control: Target Heart rate < 80 bpm at rest (< 120 -130 bpm with exercise)

	IV		PO
ß Blocker	**Loading Dose**	**Maintanence Dose**	**Maintanence**
Metoprolol	2.5 to 5 mg IV bolus over 2 min up to 3 doses	NA	25 -100 mg bid
Esmolol	0.5 mg/kg over 1 min	0.05 to 0.2 mg/kg/min	NA
Calcium Blocker	Caution if pt has HF or EF < 35% - Consider IV Amiodarone)		
Diltiazem	0.25 mg/kg IV over 2 min	5 -15 mg/hour infusion	120 - 360 mg/d in divided doses
Verapamil	0.075 to 0.15 mg/kg IV over 2 min		120 - 360 mg/d in divided doses
Digoxin	0.25 mg IV Q2h up to 1.5 mg	0.125 to 0.25 mg daily	0.125 to 0.375 mg daily

FIGURE 19-9. Optimal dosing of intravenous and oral rate control medication.

AF. Their efficacy and safety has been comprehensively reviewed (46,47).

The inefficacy and adverse effects of antiarrhythmic drugs, coupled with the efficacy of warfarin, led to question whether or not a rhythm control strategy and selective anticoagulation should be the primary approach compared to a rate control strategy and anticoagulation.

The AFFIRM trial (48) is the largest of these trials, with 4,060 AF (paroxysmal and persistent) patients randomized to rate control using drugs and anticoagulation or rhythm control with the most effective and best tolerated of several approved antiarrhythmic drug therapies. Treatment was frequently changed based on the patients' clinical status. Patients had to be at least 65 years of age or have other risks factors for stroke or death and with no contraindications to anticoagulation. All patients were initially anticoagulated, but those in the rhythm control strategy who were thought to have maintained sinus rhythm for at least 3 months could come off warfarin. After a mean follow-up of 3.5 years, there was a trend ($P = 0.06$) toward a lower incidence of death with rate control (21.3% versus 23.8%) (49). There was a trend toward a higher risk of ischemic stroke with the rhythm control approach, and the majority of strokes in both groups occurred in patients receiving no or suboptimal anticoagulation. The number of patients requiring hospitalization during follow-up was significantly lower in the rate control group than the rhythm control group.

The RACE trial (50) randomized 522 patients (mean age 65 years) with recurrent persistent AF that had been previously electrically cardioverted to rate control (beta-blocker, calcium channel blocker, or AV junction ablation) or rhythm control (sotalol, flecainide, propafenone.) There was a protocol-determined sequence for changing antiarrhythmic drugs and repeat electrical cardioversion in the rhythm control arm. After a mean follow-up of 2.3 years, there was a trend toward a lower incidence of the primary composite endpoint (cardiovascular death, admission for heart failure, thromboembolic events, severe bleeding, pacemaker implantation, or severe side effect from antiarrhythmic drugs) with rate control (17.2% versus 22.6% with rhythm control). There was no difference in cardiovascular mortality between the two groups.

In summary, the combined evidence of these trials has failed to confirm any of the presumed benefits of the pharmacologic rhythm control approach.

Figure 19-10 presents an abbreviated algorithm for selection of the most appropriate antiarrhythmic drug for maintaining sinus rhythm in selected categories of patients whereas Figure 19-11 lists selected doses of our recommended class Ic and class III antiarrhythmic medications.

If sinus rhythm is not maintained and there is no improvement in symptoms, patients should be considered for advanced device therapy or ablation of AF by targeting trigger pulmonary vein sites (Fig. 19-10).

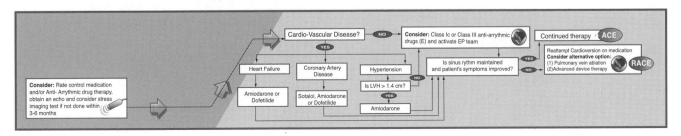

FIGURE 19-10. Antiarrhythmic therapy for patients with persistent or paroxysmal atrial fibrillation.

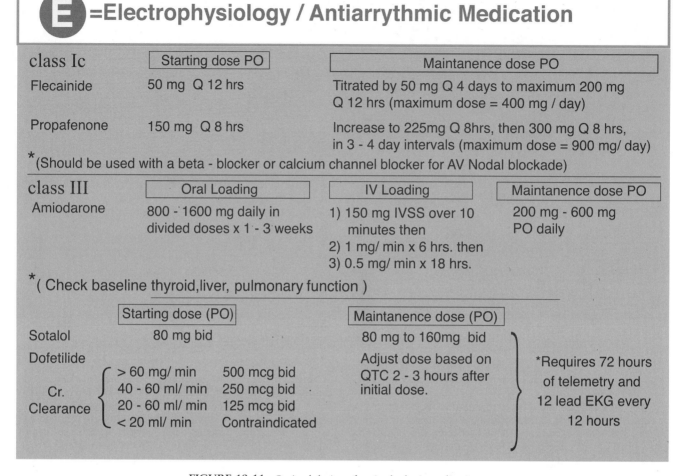

FIGURE 19-11. Optimal dosing of antiarrhythmic medication.

CONCLUSION

This chapter describes a newly developed novel pathway for management of AF and Afl. It incorporates a differential diagnosis into the mechanism and pathophysiology of AF and Afl. This chapter provides guidelines for therapy and incorporates them into an algorithm. Initiation of patient care is rapid and should start in the emergency department. The user categorizes the patient using the key concepts of patient stability and duration of symptoms. Appropriate care is then initiated and continued until the time of discharge.

References

1. Braunwald E, Zipes DP, Libby P. *Heart disease. a textbook of cardiovascular medicine*, 6th ed., Vol. 1. Philadelphia: Saunders; 2001:830–835.
2. Agarwal A, York M, Kantharia BK, et al. Atrial fibrillation: modern concepts and management. *Annu Rev Med* 2005;65:475–494.
3. Ganz, LI. *Management of atrial fibrillation*. Baltimore: Lippincott Williams & Wilkins; 2001:163–170.
4. Fuster V, Rydén LE, Asinger RW, et al. ACC/AHA/ESC pocket guidelines: management of patients with atrial fibrillation: a report of American College of Cardiology/American Heart Association Task Force on Practice Guidelines (Committee to Develop Guidelines for the Management of Patients with Atrial Fibrillation). *J Am Coll Cardiol* 2001;38(4):1266i–1266lxx.
5. Blomström-Lundqvist C, Scheinman MM, Aliot EM, et al. ACC/AHA/ESC guidelines for the management of patients with supraventricular arrhythmias. *J Am Coll Cardiol* 2003;42(8):1493–1531.
6. Chou, T. *Electrocardiography in clinical practice: adult and pediatric*, 4th ed. Philadelphia: WB Saunders; 1996:351–361.
7. Herzog E, Fischer A, Steinberg J. The rate control, anticoagulation therapy, and electrophysiology/antiarrhythmic medication pathway for the management of atrial fibrillation and atrial flutter. *Crit Pathways in Cardiol* 2005; 4(3):121–126.
8. Maisel W, Stevenson LW. Atrial fibrillation in heart failure: epidemiology, pathophysiology, and rational for therapy. *Am J Cardiol* 2003;91:2D–8D.
9. Herzog E, Saint-Jacques H, Rozanski A. The PAIN pathway as a tool to bridge the gap between evidence and management of acute coronary syndrome. *Crit Pathways in Cardiol* 2004;3:20–24.
10. Herzog E, Varley C, Kukin M: Pathway for the management of acute heart failure. *Crit Pathways in Cardiol* 2005;4:37–42.
11. Hazinski MF, Cummins RO, Field JM. *2000 handbook of emergency cardiovascular care for healthcare providers*. Dallas, TX: American Heart Association; 2000.
12. Gallagher MM, Guo XH, Poloniecki JD, et al. Initial energy sitting, outcome and efficiency in direct current cardioversion of atrial fibrillation. *J Am Coll Cardiol* 2001;38:1498–1504.
13. Lundstrom T, Ryden L. Chronic atrial fibrillation: long term results of direct current cardioversion. *Acta Med Scand* 1988;223:53–59.
14. Dalzell GW, Anderson J, Adgey AA. Factors determining success and energy requirement for cardioversion of atrial fibrillation. *Q J Med* 1990;76: 903–913.
15. Boriani G, Diemberger I, Biffi M, et al. Pharmacological cardioversion of atrial fibrillation: current management and treatment options. *Drugs* 2004; 64:2741–2762.
16. Kirchhof O, Eckardt L, Loh P, et al. Anterior-posterior versus anterior-lateral electrode positions for external cardioversion of atrial fibrillation. *Lancet* 2002;360:1275–1279.
17. Myerburg RJ, Castellanos A. Electrode positioning for cardioversion of atrial fibrillation. *Lancet* 2002;360:1263–1264.
18. Ricard P, Levy S, Trigamo J, et al. Prospective assessment of the minimum energy needed for external cardioversion of atrial fibrillation. *Am J Cardiol* 1997;79:815–816.

19. Page RL, Kerber RE, Russell JK, et al. Biphasic versus monophasic shock waveform for conversion of atrial fibrillation. The result of an international randomized, double-blind multicenter trial. *J Am Coll Cardial* 2002;39: 1956–1963.

20. Klein AL, Grimm RA, Black IW, et al. Cardioversion guided by transesophageal echocardiography: the ACUTE Pilot Study. *Ann Intern Med* 1997;126: 200–209.

21. Klein AL, Grimm RA, Murray RD, et al. Use of transesophageal echocardiography to guide cardioversion in patients with atrial fibrillation. *N Engl J Med* 2001;344:1411–1420.

22. Stellbrink C, Nixdorff U, Hofmann T, et al. Safety and efficacy of enoxaparin compared with unfractionated heperain and oral anticoagulation for prevention of thromboembolic complications in cardioversion of nonvascular atrial fibrillation: the anticoagulation in cardioversion using enoxaparin (ACE) trial. *Circulation* 2004;109:997–1003.

23. Iqbal MB, Taneja AK, Lip GYH, et al. Recent developments in atrial fibrillation. *BMJ* 2005;330:238–243.

24. William S, Weiss C, Ventura R, et al. Catheter ablation of atrial flutter guided by electroanatomic mapping (CARTO): a randomized comparison to the conventional approach. *J Cardiovasc Electrophysiol* 2000;11: 1223–230.

25. Babaev A, Suma V, Tita C, et al. Recurrence rate of atrial flutter after initial presentation in patients on drug treatment. *Am J Cardiol* 2003;92: 1122–1124.

26. Natale A, Newby KH, Pisano E, et al. Prospective randomized comparison of antiarrhythmic therapy versus first-line radiofrequency ablation in patients with atrial flutter. *J Am Coll Cardial* 2000;35:1898–1904.

27. Hersi A, Wyse DG. Management of atrial fibrillation: *Curr Probl Cardiol* 2005;30:175–234.

28. Kannel WB, Abbott RD, Savage DD, et al. Epidemiologic features of chronic atrial fibrillation the Framingham study. *N Engl J Med* 1982;306: 1018–1022.

29. Freidman GD, Loveland DB, Ehrlich SP Jr. Relationship of stroke to other cardiovascular disease. *Circulation* 1968;38:533–541.

30. Wolf PA, Abbott RD, Kannel WB. Atrial fibrillation: a major contributor to stroke in the elderly. The Framingham study. *Arch Intern Med* 1987; 147:1561–1564.

31. Atrial Fibrillation Investigators. Risk factor for stroke and efficacy of antithrombotic therapy in atrial fibrillation: analysis of pooled data from five randomized controlled trials. *Arch Intern Med* 1994;154:1449–1457.

32. Kopecky SL, Gersh BJ, McGoon MD, et al. The natural history of lone atrial fibrillation. A population based study over three decades. *N Engl J Med* 1987;317:669–674.

33. EAFT (European Atrial Fibrillation Trial) Study Group. Secondary prevention in non-rheumatic atrial fibrillation after transient ischemic attack or minor stroke. *Lancet* 1993;342:1255–1262.

34. The SPAF III Investigators. Adjusted-dose warfarin versus low intensity fixed-dose warfarin plus aspirin for high-risk patients with atrial fibrillation. Stroke Prevention Trial in Atrial Fibrillation III randomized clinical trial. *Lancet* 1996;348:633–638.

35. Hart RG, Pearce LA, McBride R, et al. Factors associated with ischemic stroke during aspirin therapy in atrial fibrillation: analysis of 2012 participant in the SPA I-III clinical trials. The stroke prevention in atrial fibrillation (SPAF) investigators. *Stroke* 1999;30:1223–1229.

36. Nixdorff U. Antithrombotic strategies for the management of non-valvular atrial fibrillation. *I J Card* 2005;100:191–198.

37. Lamassa M, Di Carlo A, Pracucci G, et al. Characteristics, outcome, and care of stroke associated with atrial fibrillation in Europe: data from a multicenter multinational hospital based registry (The European Community Stroke Project). *Stroke* 2001;32:392–398.

38. Albers GW, Dalen JE, Laupacis A, et al. Antithrombotic therapy in atrial fibrillation. *Chest* 2001;119:194S–206S.

39. Hart RG, Benavente O, McBride R, et al. Antithrombotic therapy to prevent stroke in patients with atrial fibrillation: a meta-analysis. *Ann Intern Med* 1999;131:492–501.

40. Olsson SB on behalf of the SPORTIF III Investigators. Stroke prevention with the oral direct thrombin inhibitor ximelagatran compares with warfarin in patients with non-vascular atrial fibrillation (SPORTIF III): randomized controlled trial. *Lancet* 2003;362:1691–1698.

41. Halperin JL. Ximelagatran: oral direct thrombin inhibition as anticoagulant therapy in atrial fibrillation. *J Am Coll Cardiol* 2005;45:1–9.

42. SPORTIF V Investigators. Ximelagatran vs warfarin for stroke prevention in patients with nonvalvular atrial fibrillation. *JAMA* 2005;293:690–698.

43. Khan IA, Nair CK, Singh N, et al. Acute ventricular rate control in atrial fibrillation and atrial flutter. *I J Card* 2004;97:7–13.

44. Benjamin JE, Wolf PA, D'Agostino BR, et al. Impact of atrial fibrillation on the risk of death: the Framingham heart study. *Circulation* 1998;98: 946–952.

45. Tavel ME, Sopher SM, Camm AJ. Atrial fibrillation: problem in management. *Chest* 1996;110:1089–1091.

46. Miller MR, McNamara RL, Segal JB, et al. Efficacy of agents for pharmacological conversion of atrial fibrillation and subsequent maintenance of sinus rhythm: a meta-analysis of clinical trials. *J Fran Pract* 2000;49;1033–1046.

47. Nichol G, McAlister F, Pham B, et al. Meta-analysis of randomized controlled trials of the effectiveness of antiarrhythmic agents at promoting sinus rhythm in patients with atrial fibrillation. *Heart* 2002;87:535–549.

48. Wyse DG, Waldo AL, DiMarco JP, et al. A comparison of rate control and rhythm control in patients with atrial fibrillation. *N Engl J Med* 2002;347: 1825–1833.

49. Steinberg JS, Sadaniantz A, Kron J, et al. Analysis of cause-specific mortality of the Atrial Fibrillation Investigation Follow-up Investigation of Rhythm Management Trial. *Circulation* 2004;109:1973–1980.

50. Van Gelder IC, Hagnes VE, Bosker HA, et al. A comparison of rate control and rhythm control in patients with recurrent persistent atrial fibrillation. *N Engl J Med* 2002;347:1834–1840.

CHAPTER 20 ■ HEART FAILURE

GREGG C. FONAROW

UNDERUTILIZATION OF STANDARD-OF-CARE
   THERAPIES IN HEART FAILURE
IN-HOSPITAL INITIATION OF THERAPY
Risk-Treatment Mismatch
CRITICAL PATHWAY TOOLS
Success of Critical Pathways
OPTIMAL HF TREATMENT USING DOSING CHARTS
   AND ALGORITHMS
Pharmacological Agents That Decrease Morbidity and Mortality
Pharmacology for Patients with Preserved Systolic Function and
   HF
Nonpharmacologic Therapy
Symptomatic Treatments
PATIENT EDUCATION
NEXT STEPS
CONCLUSIONS

Heart failure (HF) affects 5 million Americans, and 550,000 new diagnoses are made each year (1). HF results in approximately 1 million hospitalizations, which translates into an annual estimated cost of nearly $23 billion. Prognosis is poor once a patient has been hospitalized with HF; the mortality risk after HF hospitalization is 11.3% at 30 days, 33.1% at 1 year, and well over 50% within 5 years (2). Heart failure is also the only major cardiovascular condition that is increasing in both its incidence and prevalence, which places a significant burden on the health care system. The almost 1 million hospital discharges due to HF in 2002 represents a 152% increase since 1972. Therefore, both high risks and costs are associated with HF hospitalization (3–5). In addition to the risk of mortality, patients diagnosed with HF have an increased risk of rehospitalization. In a study of almost 18,000 Medicare recipients, approximately 44% were rehospitalized at least once in the year following their index hospitalization. Nearly 20% of patients are rehospitalized twice for the same condition (6), and a number of studies indicate that a significant proportion of rehospitalizations for HF appear to be preventable (7–9). These statistics emphasize the need to develop and implement strategies to improve HF care.

UNDERUTILIZATION OF STANDARD-OF-CARE THERAPIES IN HEART FAILURE

Prior studies have shown that evidence-based, guideline-recommended therapies are significantly underutilized, and there is substantial variation in adherence to performance measures among hospitals caring for patients with HF (10–14). A well-documented treatment gap exists between national HF guidelines and the clinical management of HF. This HF treatment gap results from a variety of complex issues, including a lack of systems and disease management programs.

Despite the favorable effect on morbidity and mortality that has been demonstrated by the use of angiotensin-converting enzyme (ACE) inhibitors, studies indicate that only 48% of patients with previous HF were receiving these agents at the time of hospitalization (13), and that only 60% to 70% of eligible HF patients received ACE inhibitors at discharge (15,16). The Acute Decompensated Heart Failure National Registry (ADHERE) reported a similar statistic, with only 47% of chronic HF patients with previously diagnosed systolic dysfunction receiving a β-blocker on an outpatient basis before admission to the hospital (13).

Evidence-based clinical practice guidelines have been developed for the treatment of patients with HF (3,17–19), and components of these guidelines have been adapted by the Joint Commission on Accreditation of Healthcare Organizations (JCAHO) to create core performance measures for patients hospitalized with HF (Table 20-1) (20–22).

However, adherence to JCAHO core measures is variable. Data from more than 80,000 HF admissions to academic and nonacademic hospitals in the United States participating in the ADHERE registry were analyzed to determine the rates of conformity with the four core performance measures: discharge instructions (HF-1), assessment of left ventricular function (HF-2), use of ACE inhibitors in patients with left ventricular systolic dysfunction (LVSD) (HF-3), and smoking cessation counseling (HF-4) (23). Across all hospitals, the median rates of conformity with HF-1, HF-2, HF-3, and HF-4 were 24.0%, 86.2%, 72.0%, and 43.2%, respectively. Rates of conformity at individual hospitals varied from 0% to 100%, with statistically significant differences between academic and nonacademic hospitals. Figure 20-1 depicts the frequency distribution of conformity rates by hospital (23). For each measure, there were substantial clinically relevant differences in performance between hospitals at different percentile levels. These differences were most notable for the measures with the lowest overall conformity. For HF-1, there was a 100-fold difference in conformity between hospitals at the 10th and 90th percentiles. For HF-4, there was an 11.2-fold difference in conformity at these percentiles. In contrast, there was a 1.3- and a 1.5-fold difference in conformity between hospitals at the 10th and 90th percentiles for HF-2 and HF-3, respectively (23).

Median hospital length of stay varied from 2.3 to 9.5 days, and in-hospital mortality varied from 0% to 11.1%. Among the hospitals enrolled in ADHERE, there was significant individual variability in conformity to quality-of-care indicators and clinical outcomes and a substantial gap in overall performance. Academic and nonacademic hospitals differed in their conformity with the four performance measures. Nonacademic hospitals demonstrated significantly better median conformity with HF-1 than academic hospitals, whereas academic hospitals demonstrated slightly better median conformity than nonacademic hospitals with HF-2 and HF-3 (23).

The gaps in care that currently exist in the hospital suggest that new efforts targeting education and effective patient

TABLE 20-1

JCAHO CORE PERFORMANCE MEASURES FOR HEART FAILURE

Performance Measure	Criterion Met or Acceptable Alternative
HF-1: Discharged patients with heart failure with written instructions or education materials given to the patient or caregiver at discharge or during the hospital stay that address all of the following: • Activity level • Diet • Discharge medications • Follow-up appointment • Weight monitoring • What to do if symptoms worsen	*Discharge instructions.* For discharge patients with or without home health services, documentation of written instructions or educational materials given to the patient or caregiver must address all of the following: • Activity level after discharge • Diet and fluid intake after discharge • Names of all discharge medications • Follow-up with a physician, nurse practitioner, or physician assistant after discharge • Weight monitoring after discharge • What to do if heart failure symptoms worsen after discharge
HF-2: Patients with heart failure with documentation in the hospital record that LV function was assessed before arrival or during hospitalization or that it is planned for after discharge	*LV function assessment.* In cases in which there is no reason documented by a physician, nurse practitioner, or physician assistant for not assessing LV function there must be: • Documentation that an echocardiogram, appropriate nuclear medicine test, or cardiac catheterization with a left ventriculogram was performed during this hospital stay OR • Documentation that one of the above diagnostic tests was performed anytime before arrival OR • Documentation of LV function, either as an ejection fraction or as a narrative qualitative description (e.g., "Patient admitted with severe LV dysfunction") OR • Documentation of a plan to assess LV function after discharge
HF-3: Patients with heart failure with LVSD and without ACE inhibitor contraindications who are prescribed an ACE inhibitor at hospital discharge	*ACE inhibitor.* Documentation that an ACE inhibitor was prescribed at discharge in patients with LVSD who are not participating in an ACE inhibitor alternative clinical trial at the time of discharge and where there is no documentation of a potential contraindication or reason for not prescribing an ACE inhibitor at discharge (e.g., ACE inhibitor allergy, moderate or severe aortic stenosis, or another reason documented by a physician, nurse practitioner, or physician assistant). LVSD is defined as documentation of an LV ejection fraction <40% or a narrative description of LV function consistent with moderate and severe systolic dysfunction. Where there are ≥2 documented LV functional studies, the LV function study closest to discharge is used.
HF-4: Patients with heart failure with a history of smoking cigarettes who are given smoking cessation advice or counseling during the hospital stay	*Adult smoking cessation advice or counseling.* Documentation of smoking cessation advice or counseling in patients with a history of smoking cigarettes anytime during the year before hospital arrival. Smoking cessation advice or counseling includes prescription of a cessation aid.

ACE, angiotensin-converting enzyme; JCAHO, Joint Commission on Accreditation of Healthcare Organizations; LV, left ventricular; LVSD, left ventricular systolic dysfunction.
Reprinted from Joint Commission on Accreditation of Healthcare Organizations. Specification manual for national implementation of hospital core measures: Version 2.0—implementation to begin with July 2004 discharges. Oakbrook Terrace, IL: Joint Commission on Accreditation of Healthcare Organizations, 2004, with permission.

intervention should be investigated to improve the overall quality of care for patients with HF. Hospital-based systems for HF have been demonstrated to improve the provision of evidence-based care. Previous studies have demonstrated the importance of hospital-based systems and in-hospital initiation of cardiovascular protective therapies for improving treatment rates and clinical outcomes in patients with atherosclerosis (12,24).

IN-HOSPITAL INITIATION OF THERAPY

The setting in which HF therapy is initiated is an important factor influencing treatment and compliance/adherence rates. The care of HF patients while hospitalized is critical to their outcome. Therapy that is initiated in the hospital is likely to

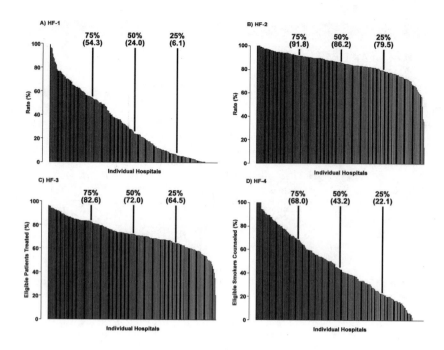

FIGURE 20-1. Frequency distribution of conformity rates by hospital for Joint Commission on Accreditation of Healthcare Organizations core performance measures: (**A**) HF-1 (eligible patients provided discharge instructions or guidance); (**B**) HF-2 (left ventricular function documentation obtained or scheduled); (**C**) HF-3 (angiotensin-converting enzyme inhibitor prescribed at discharge for left ventricular systolic dysfunction); (**D**) HF-4 (smoking cessation counseling, if needed). Each bar represents an individual hospital; vertical lines above bars indicate the 25th, 50th, and 75th percentiles. (Adapted from Fonarow GC, Yancy CW, Heywood JT. Adherence to heart failure quality-of-care indicators in US hospitals: analysis of the ADHERE registry. *Arch Intern Med* 2005;165: 1469–1477, with permission.)

have higher adherence rates due to both patient and physician behavior: the hospital is a patient "capture point." Therapy recommended in the hospital carries more weight with the patient and will be viewed as a necessary, lifesaving medication. The hospital setting also provides a teachable moment, where the physician has the attention of both the patient and family members. Other physicians, nurses, and health care workers are also available to answer questions. The hospital structure can also provide a better setting for initiation of therapy, because the patient is monitored closely, and the physician uses standard protocols and guidelines for treatment.

The importance of initiating therapy before a patient is discharged cannot be overemphasized. The implementation of comprehensive in-hospital HF disease management programs, which include management of medications, patient education, and medical staff guidelines, results in improvements in medication dosing and decreased hospitalization for HF patients (12). The Duke Heart Failure Program, for example, showed a significant increase in both the use of β-blockers and the percentage of patients reaching target doses of β-blockers and a decrease in cost of care throughout the hospital system (12).

Various hospitals have developed a number of tools to encourage physicians to initiate as many lifesaving therapies as possible before patient discharge. The use of preprinted orders, care maps, discharge forms, physician/nursing education, and treatment utilization reports may facilitate the implementation of therapy. These tools are designed to help health care providers identify and initiate guideline-recommended treatments in appropriate HF patients without contraindications. The tools also provide guidance in identifying and managing factors that may exacerbate HF, major comorbidities, and concomitant risk factors (e.g., sudden death risk, lipids, diabetes, anemia, chronic obstructive pulmonary disease, and depression). These critical pathways also aim to enhance patient education, assessment of social support, discharge planning, follow-up, and outpatient monitoring.

Risk-Treatment Mismatch

Unfortunately, there is a risk-treatment mismatch in HF: patients with severe HF or those with the highest risk of morbidity

and mortality are less likely to receive therapy than those with lower risk. In a recent study of HF drug administration rates at hospital discharge and 90 days after discharge, the highest-risk HF patients were much less likely to receive lifesaving therapies (25). Low-risk patients were more likely to receive ACE inhibitors or angiotensin-receptor blockers (ARBs) (adjusted hazard ratio [HR], 1.61; 95% confidence interval [CI], 1.49 to 1.74) and β-receptor antagonists (HR, 1.80; 95% CI, 1.60 to 2.01) compared with high-risk patients (both $P < 0.001$) (Fig. 20-2) (25).

The highest-risk patients, those who have the greatest risk of death due to comorbidities, the lowest ejection fraction (EF), and other indicators of poor outcomes during hospitalization for HF, are the ones who would derive the greatest benefit from treatment. Because drug administration is currently inversely associated with risk, the potential benefit of HF pharmacotherapy will not be realized if current patterns continue. Greater quality improvement efforts aimed at increasing use of HF drugs in higher-risk patients are needed (25).

In addition, recognition of the patients at highest risk is important to the use of optimal therapy. Achieving the most accurate estimation of risk for poor outcomes after patients have been hospitalized for HF may help clinicians guide the type and intensity of therapy. Recent registries and clinical trials have identified markers of poor outcomes in hospitalized HF patients.

The Outcomes of a Prospective Trial of Intravenous Milrinone for Exacerbations of Chronic Heart Failure (OPTIME-CHF) study found that in 949 patients with decompensated HF, the variables at presentation that predicted death at 60 days were older age, lower systolic blood pressure, New York Heart Association (NYHA) class IV symptoms, elevated blood urea nitrogen (BUN), and decreased sodium (26). In a study of 988 patients with HF and preserved EF enrolled in the Digitalis Investigation Group (DIG) trial, among 18 variables considered, the strongest independent predictors of death were glomerular filtration rate, NYHA functional class III or IV, male gender, and older age (27).

The ADHERE program of more than 30,000 patients developed and validated a practical and user-friendly method of risk stratification for in-hospital mortality among patients

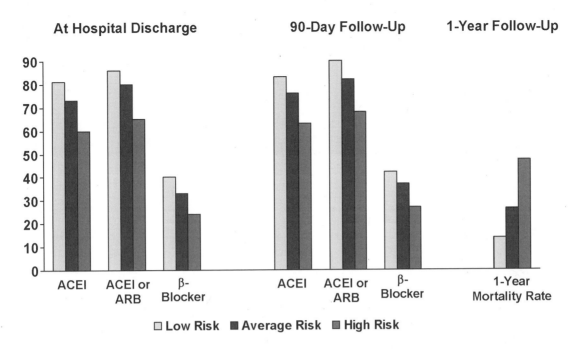

At Hospital Discharge   90-Day Follow-Up   1-Year Follow-Up

□ Low Risk   ■ Average Risk   ■ High Risk

FIGURE 20-2. Risk-treatment mismatch in heart failure: use rates of medications in absence of contrain-dications. For all drug classes, *P* <0.001 for trend. ACEI, angiotensin-converting enzyme inhibitor; ARB, angiotensin II receptor blocker. (From Lee DS, Tu JV, Juurlink DN, et al. Risk-treatment mismatch in the pharmacotherapy of heart failure. *JAMA* 2005;294:1240–1247.)

admitted with HF that could be applicable to the bedside (28). High-risk patients could be identified to determine in which patients resource-intensive interventions designed to improve outcomes may be justified. Of 39 variables in AD-HERE, the following were independent predictors of high risk for in-hospital mortality in classification and regression tree (CART) analysis: BUN level of 43 mg/dL or higher, serum creatinine level of 2.75 mg/dL or higher, and systolic blood pressure (SBP) of less than 115 mm Hg. In this multi-variate analysis, blood pressure (BP), heart rate, serum creati-nine, serum sodium, and liver disease were highly predictive of in-hospital mortality. Acutely decompensated HF patients at low, intermediate, and high risk for in-hospital mortality can be easily identified using vital signs and laboratory data obtained on hospital admission. The ADHERE risk tree pro-vides clinicians with a validated, practical bedside tool for mortality risk stratification (Fig. 20-3) (28).

CRITICAL PATHWAY TOOLS

The continued persistence of suboptimal compliance in all hospitals and the significant variability between hospitals in both compliance and outcome variables provide a compelling rationale for the implementation of critical pathway tools that may improve hospital performance.

It is important to recognize why therapy is suboptimal in order to devise effective strategies to improve it. Some of the barriers that prevent the implementation of cardioprotec-tive therapies in patients with HF are time constraints; lack of physician training, including inadequate appreciation of benefits and lack of prescription experience; a lack of re-sources; and lack of communication between specialists and generalists. In addition, the adherence to old guidelines that call for delaying initiation of therapy and including multiple steps, time points, and too many treatment options may

deter physicians from using optimal care. The use of HF critical pathway tools that simplify care and clarify the roles of each caregiver may break down some of these barriers. Use of these tools may also eliminate the variability in care between hospitals and improve the overall treatment of hospi-talized HF patients. The structure and education that these tools provide, in addition to improving coordination of care among staff in the hospital, make process-of-care programs invaluable.

Process-of-care programs are designed to implement a number of tools to check the treatment of the hospitalized HF patient at various stages, from admission, throughout hospital stay, and at discharge. An example of an HF admis-sion checklist is shown in Figure 20-4. This tool will aid in diagnosis, prompt the appropriate laboratory work, and re-mind the physician of the importance of an echocardiogram in HF patients to evaluate EF. Use of this checklist can help the physician more accurately assess a patient's needs for indicated therapy as well as facilitate identification of patients with contraindications to one or more therapies.

An example of standardized orders for HF is shown in Figure 20-5. This easy-to-read form serves as a guide for the physician, nurse, and other caregivers and allows each of them to follow standard HF treatment protocols and indicate each guideline-recommended therapy that has been initiated. These preprinted order sets can facilitate the identi-fication of patients with contraindications to one or more therapies and thus enhance patient safety, provide standard medication dosing, emphasize the need for monitoring certain laboratory tests, and help avoid medical errors of omission. The sets can also facilitate consultation and collaborative care.

In addition, a comprehensive HF critical pathway tool may be used throughout the patient's hospitalization to moni-tor care (Fig. 20-6). This tool may help the physician recog-nize the signs of poor outcomes, higher in-hospital mortality, and rehospitalization. Deviations from the critical pathway

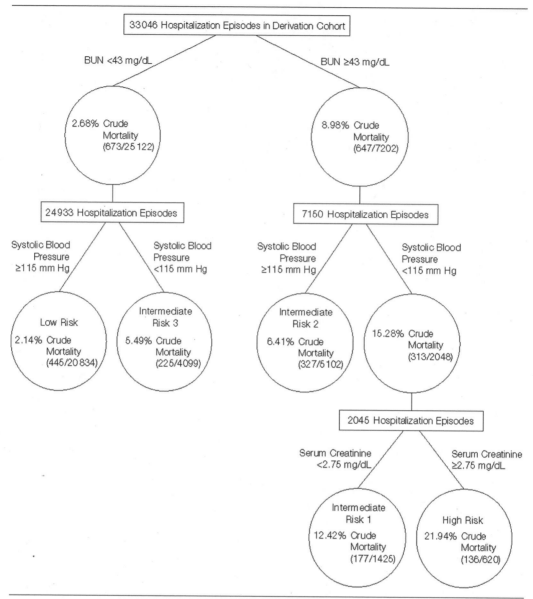

Each node is based on available data from registry patient hospitalizations for each predictive variable presented. BUN indicates blood urea nitrogen. To convert BUN to mmol/L, multiply by 0.357; creatinine to µmol/L, multiply by 88.4.

FIGURE 20-3. The Acute Decompensated Heart Failure National Registry (ADHERE) mortality risk stratification tree. (Reprinted from Fonarow GC, Adams KF Jr., Abraham WT, et al. Risk stratification for in-hospital mortality in acutely decompensated heart failure: classification and regression tree analysis. *JAMA* 2005;293:572–580, with permission.)

HEART FAILURE ADMISSION CHECKLIST

Patient name: _____

Admit date: _____

Admitting diagnosis: _____

Admitting physician: _____

Designated cardiologist: _____

BRIEF HISTORY: _____

Were the following assessments performed?	Y	N	Initials	Date Performed	Comments
Vital signs	☐	☐			
Weight taken	☐	☐			
History taken (for comorbidity)	☐	☐			
Physical examination (for comorbidity)	☐	☐			
Medical history taken	☐	☐			
Allergy history taken	☐	☐			
Risk stratification (good, fair, guarded)	☐	☐			
Advance directives	☐	☐			

Was the following lab work performed?	Y	N	Initials	Date Performed	Comments
12-lead ECG	☐	☐			
Echocardiogram/Doppler (MUGA)	☐	☐			
Chest X-ray	☐	☐			
INR, PTT	☐	☐			
Electrolytes, BUN, Cr	☐	☐			
CBC w/diff, Platelets	☐	☐			
Cardiac Enzymes (Troponins and/or CK-MB)	☐	☐			
Liver function tests	☐	☐			
BNP	☐	☐			
TFTs, iron, TIBC, RUA (if indicated)	☐	☐			
Pulse oximetry	☐	☐			

Was the following performed/discussed with the patient?	Cont'd as Before	D/C	Initiated	Not Used	Initials	Date	Comments
I + O totals	☐	☐	☐	☐			
Daily weight	☐	☐	☐	☐			
2000-mg Na diet	☐	☐	☐	☐			
Fluid restriction (if indicated)	☐	☐	☐	☐			
Heart failure patient education sheet	☐	☐	☐	☐			

FIGURE 20-4. Heart failure hospital admission checklist. (*continues*)

HEART FAILURE ADMISSION CHECKLIST (PAGE 2)

Check the appropriate box for each HF medication.	Cont'd as Before	D/C	Initiated	Not Used	Initials	Date	Comments
ACE inhibitor	❑	❑	❑	❑			
Angiotensin receptor blocker (if ACEI intolerant or in addition to ACEI)	❑	❑	❑	❑			
β-Blocker	❑	❑	❑	❑			
Aldosterone antagonist	❑	❑	❑	❑			
Loop diuretic	❑	❑	❑	❑			
Digoxin	❑	❑	❑	❑			
Supplemental oxygen	❑	❑	❑	❑			
Electrolyte supplement (K, Mg as needed)	❑	❑	❑	❑			
Warfarin (for atrial fibrillation)	❑	❑	❑	❑			
Antiplatelet (CAD, CVD, PVD, diabetes)	❑	❑	❑	❑			
Statins (CAD, CVD, PVD, diabetes)	❑	❑	❑	❑			
Diabetes control:	❑	❑	❑	❑			
Pain control:	❑	❑	❑	❑			
Antiarrhythmics (specific indications):	❑	❑	❑	❑			
Other:	❑	❑	❑	❑			
Other:	❑	❑	❑	❑			
Other:	❑	❑	❑	❑			

Were the following interventions or testing procedures performed/planned?	Performed	Planned	Not Applicable	Initials	Date Performed/ Planned	Comments
Echocardiography/Doppler	❑	❑	❑			
Stress testing – pharmacologic ❑ or	❑	❑	❑			
exercise ❑	❑	❑	❑			
Angiography/catheterization for possible revascularization	❑	❑	❑			
PCI (PTCA, balloon, stent)	❑	❑	❑			
CABG	❑	❑	❑			
Electrophysiology (sudden death risk assessment) • Biventricular pacing • Implantable cardioverter/defibrillator	❑	❑	❑			
Other cardiac imaging:	❑	❑	❑			

Were the following secondary prevention measures performed/initiated?	Performed	Planned	Not Applicable	Initials	Date Performed/ Planned	Comments
Lipid profile (total C, HDL-C, LDL-C, triglycerides)	❑	❑	❑			
Blood pressure control	❑	❑	❑			
Smoker? If yes: smoking cessation booklet and refer to program	❑	❑	❑			
Diabetic? If yes: HbA$_{1c}$, glucose, sliding scale insulin	❑	❑	❑			
Atrial fibrillation? If yes: EP consult, dietitian, anticoagulation clinic	❑	❑	❑			
Physical therapy/Cardiac rehab	❑	❑	❑			
Other:	❑	❑	❑			

FIGURE 20-4. (continued)

STANDARD ORDERS for HEART FAILURE

Date _____   Time _____

Intern _____
       LAST NAME   FIRST NAME   BEEPER

Resident _____
         LAST NAME   FIRST NAME   BEEPER

Attending _____
          LAST NAME   FIRST NAME   BEEPER

Patient _____
        LAST NAME   FIRST NAME   MI

Etiology _____

Reason for admission ☐ New HF ☐ Noncompliance, meds ☐ Noncompliance, diet
(Check all that apply) ☐ Volume overloaded ☐ Exacerbation of HF ☐ Refractory HF
                       ☐ Arrhythmias ☐ Over-diuresis ☐ Other _____

ACC/AHA Stage   ☐ C ☐ D
NYHA Class   ☐ I ☐ II ☐ III ☐ IV
Condition   ☐ Good ☐ Fair ☐ Guarded

Check/Initial/Date

☐ ___ /___   Allergies: _____

☐ ___ /___   Diet ☐ 2000 mg Na with 1500 cc by mouth fluid restriction
                    ☐ 2000 mg Na with 1900 cc (2 quarts) by mouth fluid restriction
                    ☐ 2000 mg Na; low cholesterol with _____ cc by mouth fluid restriction
                    ☐ Other _____

NURSING

☐ ___ /___   Vital signs (call House Officer if: SBP <80 or >150; HR <60 or >110; RR <10 or >24; T >38.5°C)

☐ ___ /___ O_2 _____ L/min nasal cannula for CP, SOB, SaO_2 <93%

☐ ___ /___   Cardiac monitor

☐ ___ /___   I+O totals q _____ h

☐ ___ /___   Daily AM weights

☐ ___ /___   Encourage progressive ambulation

FIGURE 20-5. Standard orders for heart failure.

can be documented and later analyzed to better understand variations and patterns to facilitate the quality improvement process.

In addition to all the tools contained in this chapter, a number of critical pathway aids should be used in all hospitals to improve the quality of care. Algorithms, care paths, standing orders, and patient education materials can all aid the physician in the hospital. A discharge summary checklist may be an important component, as it forces physicians to evaluate the therapy on which a patient is discharged and—in light of data that show increased adherence to medications that are prescribed before discharge—may cause them to initiate additional therapy (Fig. 20-7). As discussed previously, patients that are discharged on therapy are more likely to remain on therapy.

Success of Critical Pathways

The benefits of a hospital-based system to improve the use of ACE inhibitors before hospital discharge were demonstrated

by an analysis of more than 19,000 patients discharged after an HF-related hospitalization at a ten-hospital integrated health care system (29). Comparisons were made between patients discharged before ($n = 11,038$) and after ($n = 8,045$) the implementation of an HF discharge medication program. As a result of the program, the use of ACE inhibitors increased from 65% to 95%. The program also resulted in a reduction in the rate of readmission from 46.5% to 38.4% ($P < 0.0001$) and in the rate of mortality from 22.7% to 17.8% ($P < 0.0001$) at 1 year (29). Similar significant improvements were seen in a comprehensive HF management program involving 214 patients (NYHA class III or IV) who were candidates for heart transplantation (24). The program included modifications in drug therapy, patient education, and regular follow-up with the HF team. When data were compared for the 6-month period before initiation of the program with those from the 6 months following implementation, it was found that ACE inhibitor use increased by 18% (from 77% to 95%, $P = 0.05$) and hospital admission declined by 85% ($P < 0.0001$) (24).

The Initiation Management Predischarge: Process for Assessment of Carvedilol Therapy for Heart Failure (IMPACT-

198 Part III: Critical Pathways in the Hospital

Indicators	ED Day 1	Card/Med Unit Day 2	Card/Med Unit Day 3	Card/Med Unit Day 4
Consult/Evals	• Heart failure service or cardiology consult • Heart failure nurse coordinator • Assess need for additional consults, ie, neural, GI • Advance Directives	• Social worker • Dietary • Arrhythmia service (if indicated) • Physical therapy/cardiac rehab	• Reassessment by HP nurse coordinator • Ongoing eval and need for other consults	• Reassessment by HF nurse coordinator
MD/APN	• H+P • Initiate and/or titrate meds • CAD, HTN, diabetes assessment • Reversible causes of heart failure	• Change diet order per dietician/RN recommendations • Echo if previously not obtained • Evaluate for revascularization if indicated	• Begin formulating discharge medication regimen	• D/C regimen + prescriptions • Follow-up with PMD/cardiology in 1 wk or sooner • Follow-up testing/consults • Discharge note
Nursing Tx	• Cardiac monitor • I+O totals q12h • Admit weight • Diuretics, K dosing plan	• Cardiac monitor • I+O • Daily AM weights • Call MD if ↓ UO, hypertension, arrhythmias • Follow diuretic + K replacement protocol • Initiate medication teaching • Encourage early ambulation	• Cardiac monitor • I+O • Daily AM weights • Orthostatic BP prior to ambulating pt Q shift • Peripheral IV line • Medication teaching	• Cardiac monitor • I+O • Daily AM weights • Orthostatic BP prior to discharge • D/C med schedule to review with patients • Patient discharge declaration
Diet	• 2000-mg NA diet • Fluid restriction for volume overload • Evaluate additional restrictions for ↑ chol, DM, obesity, etc.	• 2000-mg NA diet • Fluid restriction for volume overload	• 2000-mg NA diet • Fluid restriction for volume overload	• 2000-mg NA diet • Fluid restriction for volume overload • Review discharge diet
Lab/Tests	• Echocardiogram to document LVEF if not previously done • CXR, EKG • Electrolytes, BUN, Cr, CBC w/ diff, PT, PTT, TFTs, Mg, UA, liver function tests, lipid panel • Glycosylated Hb (PRN) • Glucose • BNP	• Electrolytes, BUN, Cr	• Chemistry panel, electrolytes, BUN, Cr • PT if on warfarin	• Electrolytes, BUN/Cr • PT if on warfarin • BNP (if indicated)

FIGURE 20-6. Heart failure critical pathways grid.

HEART FAILURE DISCHARGE SUMMARY CHECKLIST

Patient name: _____

Discharge date: _____

Designated cardiologist: _____

BRIEF HISTORY: _____

Check duration of medication for each agent

Were the following discharge medications prescribed?	Y	N	Agent Prescribed	Contraindication? Y	N	Reason for Not Prescribing /Indicate Code Letter/Comments	Initials
ACE inhibitor	☐	☐		☐	☐		
ARB (if ACEI intolerant or in addition to ACEI)	☐	☐		☐	☐		
β-Blocker	☐	☐		☐	☐		
Loop diuretic	☐	☐		☐	☐		
Thiazide diuretic	☐	☐		☐	☐		
Digoxin (if atrial fibrillation or refractory symptoms)	☐	☐		☐	☐		
Aldosterone antagonist	☐	☐		☐	☐		
Nitrates (specify PRN, prescribed indef., or both)	☐	☐		☐	☐		
Warfarin (specify INR in comments)	☐	☐		☐	☐		
ASA	☐	☐		☐	☐		
Lipid-lowering agents	☐	☐		☐	☐		
Other	☐	☐		☐	☐		
Other	☐	☐		☐	☐		
Other	☐	☐		☐	☐		

Were the following interventions and counseling measures addressed?	Y	N	Initials	Date Performed	Initials	Comments
Treatment and adherence education	☐	☐				
Risk-modification counseling (general)	☐	☐				
Blood pressure controlled	☐	☐				
Diabetes controlled	☐	☐				
Smoking cessation recommended	☐	☐				
Dietitian/nutritionist interview	☐	☐				
Cardiac rehabilitation interview and enrollment	☐	☐				
Physical activity counseling	☐	☐				

Which follow-up services were scheduled?	Y	N	Initials	Date Scheduled	Comments
Cardiologist follow-up	☐	☐			
Primary care follow-up	☐	☐			
Cardiac rehabilitation	☐	☐			Begins:
Stress test follow-up	☐	☐			
Electrophysiology follow-up	☐	☐			
Lipid profile follow-up	☐	☐			
Anticoagulation service follow-up	☐	☐			
Other	☐	☐			
Clinical summary and patient education record faxed to appropriate physicians	☐	☐			

FIGURE 20-7. Heart failure hospital discharge summary checklist.

HF) was a multicenter, open-label trial involving 363 HF patients with left ventricular ejection fraction (LVEF) ≤40% who were admitted for an episode of HF decompensation (30). Patients were randomized to receive initiation of carvedilol therapy before hospital discharge (once the HF decompensation was treated successfully) or to usual care (initiation of any β-blocker 2 to 4 weeks after hospitalization and when the patient became stable). At the end of 60 days, 91% of the predischarge initiation patients were on carvedilol; in contrast, only 73% of patients in the postdischarge, physician-discretion initiation group (P <0.0001) were receiving any β-blocker. In the carvedilol initiation group, the mean percentage of target dose achieved was 36.3%; in the postdischarge initiation arm, it was 28.6% (P = 0.02). The median length of stay for patients did not increase with predischarge initiation, and there was no increased risk of serious adverse events (30).

The Organized Program to Initiate Lifesaving Treatment in Hospitalized Patients with Heart Failure (OPTIMIZE-HF) is the first national, hospital-based program designed to improve medical care and education of hospitalized HF patients and to accelerate the use of evidence-based, guideline-recommended therapies by in-hospital initiation (31). OPTIMIZE-HF has two main components designed to achieve its objectives: a Web-based registry and a process-of-care improvement plan. The registry tracked the use of lifesaving therapies before and after initiation as well as hospital progress and discharge planning. The Web site provided real-time reports and benchmark comparisons among institutions, both regionally and nationally, allowing them to share best practices. The registry also captured outcome data for patients at 60 to 90 days after enrollment. Data on the use of ACE inhibitors and angiotensin-receptor antagonists in systolic HF patients were collected, as were data on the use of evidence-based β-blockers. This provided hospitals with a greater ability to understand practice patterns and current quality of care than they would have obtained using a limited number of static performance measures.

The process-of-care improvement component of OPTIMIZE-HF focused on assisting hospitals in improving their systems with regard to the management of HF patients (31). The critical pathway from admission to discharge was managed with the use of a hospital "tool kit" that provided evidence-based best-practices algorithms, critical pathways, standardized orders, discharge checklists, pocket cards, chart stickers, and a variety of other elements to assist hospitals in improving HF management. OPTIMIZE-HF provided algorithms and dosing guides to facilitate the initiation and titration of guideline-recommended HF therapy based on American College of Cardiology/American Heart Association (ACC/AHA) HF guidelines, recent clinical trials, and the collective expertise of the OPTIMIZE-HF Steering Committee members.

The OPTIMIZE-HF In-Hospital Heart Failure Management Algorithm is shown in Figure 20-8 (31). Results from OPTIMIZE indicate that the use of critical pathways in the hospital can improve the quality of care. The percent of patients that received the JCAHO HF performance measures, plotted over time, is shown in Figure 20-9 (OPTIMIZE-HF registry database, final data report; Duke Clinical Research Institute, July 2005). Frequency of smoking-cessation counseling and the use of discharge instructions improved greatly with the program.

Hospital-based HF quality improvement is feasible on a national scale using largely pre-existing resources. OPTIMIZE-HF provides further evidence that the use of in-hospital process-of-care improvement programs and critical pathways can increase the use of lifesaving medications and adherence to quality measures. Hospital teams should work to implement processes such as those in OPTIMIZE-HF to insure the use of evidence-based therapies in their eligible HF patients prior to hospital discharge.

OPTIMAL HF TREATMENT USING DOSING CHARTS AND ALGORITHMS

The optimal management of HF is based on the following steps: (a) establish a diagnosis with history, physical examination, brain natriuretic peptide (BNP), and echocardiography; (b) determine the etiology; (c) characterize the syndrome (systolic versus diastolic); (d) analyze and correct precipitating factors; (e) evaluate and correct ischemia; (f) initiate pharmacological therapy (ACE inhibitors or ARBs, β-blockers, aldosterone antagonists, and diuretics); and (g) assess the patient's response to therapy. The use of inotropes outside the setting of cardiogenic shock is associated with increased mortality and should be avoided.

Pharmacological Agents That Decrease Morbidity and Mortality

A wealth of clinical data exists showing that the risk of morbidity and mortality associated with HF can be delayed and/or prevented with the use of pharmacologic agents. Numerous landmark clinical trials have demonstrated that treatment with ACE inhibitors and β-blockers significantly reduces morbidity, mortality, and hospitalizations in HF patients (32–37). Professional HF society guidelines recommend their use in all HF patients without contraindications or intolerance (3,38,39).

ACE Inhibitors

Several studies have established that ACE inhibitors can improve hemodynamics and clinical status as well as reduce symptoms and the risks of morbidity and mortality in patients with chronic HF. These benefits have been noted across the spectrum of patients with mild, moderate, or severe HF (36,40,41). Table 20-2 lists the commonly used ACE inhibitors and their initial and target doses; Table 20-3 shows an overview of the initiation and maintenance of ACE inhibitors; and Table 20-4 provides important information including contraindications and how to appropriately monitor patients. These types of tables can easily be incorporated into critical pathway tools for the management of HF.

Use of Angiotensin II Receptor Blockers

In several clinical settings and in placebo-controlled clinical trials of patients with chronic HF, ARBs produced hemodynamic, neurohormonal, and clinical effects similar to those obtained with ACE inhibitors (42–46). ACC/AHA guidelines recommend that ARBs should be used as alternative first-line therapy if a patient is intolerant to ACE inhibitors with symptomatic left ventricular dysfunction (3). The combination of an ARB, an ACE inhibitor, and aldosterone is not recommended because of the risk of adverse effects. When starting therapy with an ARB, it is important to begin with the minimal dose and then double it. Blood pressure, potassium, and renal function should be assessed within 2 weeks after the beginning of therapy. Recommended ARBs and their dosing can be found in Table 20-5.

β-Blockers

β-Blockers have traditionally been viewed as contraindicated in patients with LVSD. The 1999 Heart Failure Society of America (HFSA) guidelines suggested that, to maximize safety, patients should experience a period of clinical stability on standard therapy before β-blockers are introduced, and that β-blocker initiation in HF patients requires a careful baseline

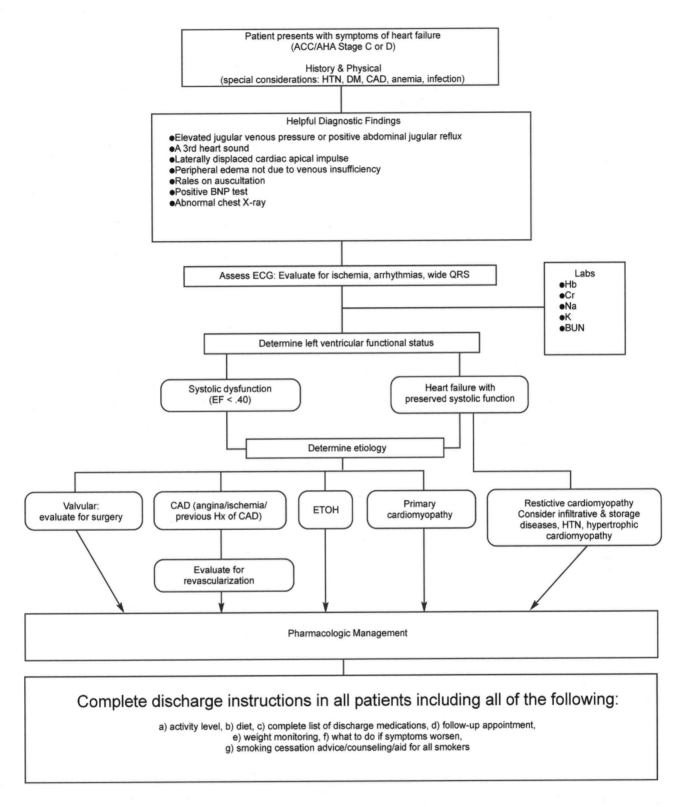

FIGURE 20-8. The Organized Program to Initiate Lifesaving Treatment in Hospitalized Patients with Heart Failure (OPTIMIZE-HF) in-hospital heart failure management algorithm.

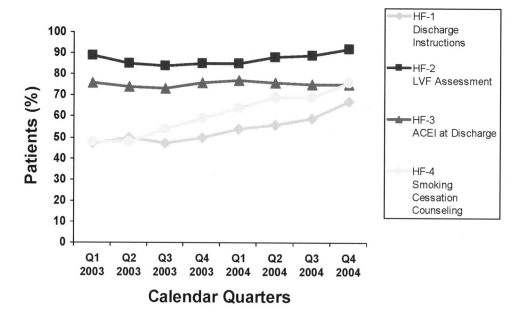

FIGURE 20-9. Joint Commission on Accreditation of Healthcare Organizations performance measures in the Organized Program to Initiate Lifesaving Treatment in Hospitalized Patients with Heart Failure (OPTIMIZE-HF) over time. ACEI, angiotensin-converting enzyme inhibitors; LVF, left ventricular function.

evaluation of clinical status (38). Because these guidelines were based on early, large-scale trials in which patients with chronic HF were treated with standard therapy consisting of ACE inhibitors, digoxin, and a diuretic for at least 2 months before starting β-blocker therapy, this recommendation led to many HF clinicians postponing β-blocker therapy for at least 2 to 4 weeks until stability was achieved. This plays into the concern of many practitioners that starting β-blockade in HF patients will necessarily worsen HF during the titration period. In the Carvedilol Prospective Randomized Cumulative Survival (COPERNICUS) study, significantly fewer patients on carvedilol experienced serious adverse events than on placebo (P <0.002) (47). This trial showed that the adverse event of utmost concern to clinicians regarding the initiation of β-blockers, worsening HF, occurred less frequently with carvedilol

than with placebo (47,48). COPERNICUS, in effect, indicates that the early initiation of lifesaving therapies should be approached with a sense of urgency and provides a mandate for expediting the administration of β-blocker therapy in HF patients. When comparing predischarge with postdischarge initiation for tolerability and safety in the IMPACT-HF study, it was found that there were no significant differences between the groups in either the occurrence of serious adverse events (bradycardia, hypotension, and worsening HF) or the occurrence of these events leading to the permanent withdrawal of the β-blocker. Fewer patients experienced worsening of HF in the predischarge than in the postdischarge group (0.5% vs. 1.7%), and there was a lower rate of composite death and rehospitalization (30).

TABLE 20-2

RECOMMENDED ANGIOTENSIN-CONVERTING ENZYME INHIBITORS AND DOSES*

Drug	Initial Dose	Target Dose
Captopril	6.25 mg PO tid	50 mg PO tid
Enalapril	2.5 mg PO bid	20 mg PO bid
Lisinopril	2.5–5 mg PO qd	20–40 mg PO qd or bid
Fosinopril	5–10 mg PO qd	40 mg PO qd
Quinapril	10 mg PO bid	40 mg PO bid
Ramipril	1.25–2.5 PO qd	10 mg PO qd

*Treatment should be initiated at low doses followed by gradual increments if lower doses are tolerated. Renal function and serum potassium should be assessed within 1 to 2 weeks of initiation or sooner if patient has renal insufficiency and periodically thereafter.

TABLE 20-3

INITIATION AND MAINTENANCE OF ANGIOTENSIN-CONVERTING ENZYME INHIBITORS

Assess patient's volume status, serum electrolytes, and renal function before initiation of therapy.

Do not start therapy in patients with symptomatic hypotension, hyperkalemia, or severe renal failure.

Initiate at a low dose and gradually up-titrate over 2–4 weeks to an optimal dose if lower doses are tolerated.

Repeat measurement of electrolytes (serum potassium) and renal function (BUN, Cr) after initiation of therapy (within 1–2 weeks) or dose change and after optimal dosing regimen has been achieved.

Repeat measurement of renal function and serum potassium within 1 week of initiation if patient has renal insufficiency.

TABLE 20-4

IMPORTANT ISSUES REGARDING ANGIOTENSIN-CONVERTING ENZYME INHIBITORS

Benefits are likely a class effect.

Contraindications include cardiogenic shock, angioneurotic edema, and hyperkalemia.

Renal insufficiency is not a contraindication; start at a low dose and monitor renal function closely.

Heart failure patients with severe renal insufficiency and on dialysis should be treated.

TABLE 20-6

RECOMMENDED β-BLOCKERS AND DOSES

Drug	Initial Dose	Target Dose
Bisoprolol[a]	1.25 mg PO qd	10 mg PO qd
Carvedilol	3.125 mg PO bid	25 mg PO bid[b]
Metoprolol succinate	25 mg PO qd[c]	200 mg PO qd

[a]Not approved for heart failure in the United States by the Food and Drug Administration.
[b]A maximum dose of 50 mg bid has been administered to patients with mild to moderate heart failure who weigh over 85 kg (187 lb).
[c]12.5 mg may be used in severe heart failure; one tablet cut in half.

These major trials clearly refute the common practices and perceptions regarding β-blocker therapy for HF that lead to unnecessary delays in treatment and deny patients the established benefits of this therapy. Specifically, the results of these studies challenge the beliefs commonly held by many clinicians that initiation of β-blockade is characterized by an unfavorable benefit–risk ratio, that survival curves do not diverge in favor of β-blockers for many months, and that early initiation necessarily carries the risk of worsening HF or intolerance leading to withdrawal of treatment. In contrast, these studies clearly demonstrate the high degree of tolerability for β-blockers and show that there is in fact a lower relative rate of discontinuation with β-blockers than with placebo.

Among the β-blockers that have established efficacy in HF—carvedilol, bisoprolol, and metoprolol—there are pharmacological differences that may alter the clinical responses to these agents in HF (49) and may have an impact on in-hospital initiation of therapy. β₁-specific blockers may decrease cardiac output, increase vascular resistance, or decrease renal blood flow, all of which can contribute to worsening HF (50). β-blockers with α-blockade, such as carvedilol, increase cardiac output while decreasing vascular resistance. The vasodilatory activity due to α₁-blockade offsets myocardial depression due to β-blockade, and the broad-based sympathetic antagonism may protect the patient from worsening HF in the early stages of initiation (50). In the Metoprolol Controlled-Release Randomised Intervention Trial in Congestive Heart Failure (MERIT-HF) of NYHA class III and IV patients, use of metoprolol, a β₁-specific blocker, showed a decrease in mortality; however, the metoprolol-treated group had a higher rate of withdrawal in the first 90 days (8.1%) than the placebo-treated group (5.9%) (P = NS) (51). Data from COPERNICUS showed that the carvedilol-treated group had a lower rate of worsening HF (5.1%) than the placebo group (6.4%) during

the initiation phase (7). In IMPACT-HF, only 0.5% of patients withdrew due to worsening HF if they were initiated with carvedilol before discharge, compared with 1.7% of patients that were initiated postdischarge with a β-blocker of the physician's choice (30). These considerations may make carvedilol a better choice of agent when initiating β-blocker therapy in the hospital setting.

β-blockers should be initiated in all compensated patients without contraindications. Patients requiring intravenous vasodilators or inotropic agents should have β-blocker therapy deferred until they are stabilized. The appropriate dosing for β-blockers is shown in Table 20-6, and contraindications to therapy are listed in Table 20-7. β-blocker dosage should be increased at 2-week intervals as tolerated until the target dose is achieved. To titrate patients to the highest dose tolerable, a number of techniques are helpful (Table 20-8). Significant issues such as timing of β-blocker up-titration and the importance of educating patients about short- and long-term effects are listed in Table 20-9. The use of an in-hospital algorithm for the initiation and titration of β-blockers may prove helpful as an aid for management of β-blocker therapy. An overall algorithm for the treatment of HF patients with β-blockers is presented in Figure 20-10.

Aldosterone Antagonists

Aldosterone receptor antagonists have also been demonstrated to reduce the risk of mortality in patients with severe HF and

TABLE 20-5

RECOMMENDED ANGIOTENSIN II RECEPTOR BLOCKERS AND DOSES

Drug	Initial Dose	Target Dose
Candesartan	8 mg PO qd	32 mg PO qd
Irbesartan	75 mg PO qd	300 mg PO qd
Losartan	25 mg PO qd	100 mg PO qd
Valsartan	80 mg PO qd	320 mg PO qd
Telmisartan	20 mg PO qd	80 mg PO qd

TABLE 20-7

CONTRAINDICATIONS TO β-BLOCKER USE

Symptomatic bradycardia

Hypotension (systolic blood pressure <80 mm Hg)

Signs of peripheral hypoperfusion (cold clammy skin, cyanosis, oliguria, impaired mental status)

Cardiogenic shock

Acute pulmonary edema

Advanced heart block (without pacemaker)

Reactive airway disease

Note that diabetes, peripheral vascular disease, asymptomatic bradycardia, mild to moderate asthma, and chronic obstructive pulmonary disease are not contraindications. Patients should be monitored for symptomatic hypotension or symptomatic bradycardia.

TABLE 20-8

MANAGEMENT OF MOST COMMON SIDE EFFECTS OF β-BLOCKERS IN HEART FAILURE PATIENTS

Side Effect	Strategy
Lightheadedness, hypotension	Instruct patients to take ACE inhibitor and β-blocker at different times (at least 2 hours apart)
	Take with meals
	Reduce or discontinue non-ACE inhibitor vasodilators
	Reduce diuretic dose in euvolemic, stable patients
	Reduce ACE inhibitor dose (temporarily)
Worsening congestive signs/symptoms	Assess patient's compliance and determine if other conditions known to worsen heart failure are present
	Increase diuretics
	Decrease β-blocker dose if above are not successful
Bradycardia	Decrease digoxin (or calcium channel blocker) dose
	Reduce β-blocker dose
	Consider pacemaker

ACE, angiotensin-converting enzyme.

TABLE 20-9

IMPORTANT ISSUES REGARDING β-BLOCKERS

The ACC/AHA guidelines recommend using only those agents and doses proven to be effective in heart failure.

If a patient is currently on one β-blocker, consider appropriate switching to one that has been shown to be effective in large clinical trials. Only carvedilol and extended-release metoprolol are FDA-approved for use in heart failure.

Explain early potential/expected side effects (increased fatigue, shortness of breath, weight gain, dizziness) so that patients understand when to contact their caregiver for treatment (diuretics are the first line of treatment for signs/symptoms of fluid overload).

β-blockade should be up-titrated slowly (i.e., q 2 weeks or longer).

Explain the late benefits (improved NYHA class, ejection fraction) of treatment, which may begin within weeks to several months.

ACC/AHA, American College of Cardiology/American Heart Association; FDA, Food and Drug Administration; NYHA, New York Heart Association.

more mild HF symptoms after myocardial infarction (3,52,53). The recommended agents and dosing for aldosterone antagonists are listed in Table 20-10, followed by important issues regarding their use in Table 20-11.

Pharmacology for Patients with Preserved Systolic Function and HF

Although there are no randomized clinical trials available to guide therapy for HF patients with preserved systolic function, these patients have similar etiologies, neurohumoral activation, functional impairment, and hemodynamics as patients with systolic dysfunction. Observational studies have suggested that ACE inhibitor and β-blocker use is associated with reduced morbidity and mortality in patients with HF and preserved systolic function (54).

In addition, these patients frequently have comorbid conditions such as hypertension and/or coronary artery disease, for which ACE inhibitors and β-blockers have shown proven benefit. It is recommended, based on pathophysiology, observational data, and expert opinion, that HF patients with preserved systolic function be treated with the same medical regimen recommended for HF with systolic dysfunction (ACE inhibitors, β-blockers, diuretics for volume control, and digoxin as needed for atrial fibrillation rate control or symptoms). Note that the in-hospital HF management algorithm shown in Figure 20-8 is a guide for treatment of this type of patient.

Nonpharmacologic Therapy

The Sudden Cardiac Death in Heart Failure Trial (SCD-HeFT) investigated the use of implantable cardioverter defibrillators (ICDs) in NYHA class II or III HF (LVEF <35%) patients with both ischemic and nonischemic etiologies (55). Seventy percent of patients were in NYHA class II, 96% were taking ACE inhibitors or ARBs, and 69% were on β-blocker therapy. SCD-HeFT extended the potential benefit of ICD therapy to patients with nonischemic cardiomyopathy by showing that patients on ICD therapy had a 23% mortality risk reduction compared with patients on placebo (P = 0.007). ICD therapy improved survival, especially in certain subgroups: patients in NYHA class II derived a 46% risk reduction versus placebo, and patients with a lower LVEF (≤30%) and those on β-blockers also benefited to a greater degree. This suggests that ICDs are effective in preventing sudden cardiac death in less-sick patients but do little to change mortality in patients with more advanced HF who may die due to worsening "pump" failure. The data on biventricular pacemakers have focused on stage C patients with NYHA class II and III HF. Biventricular pacemakers have been shown to promote significant positive remodeling of the ventricle (56).

Symptomatic Treatments

Treatment of the symptoms of HF may not reduce mortality; however, agents that reduce symptoms are an integral part of therapy (Table 20-12).

Diuretics

Several trials have demonstrated the ability of diuretics to decrease signs of fluid retention in patients with HF. Appropriate administration of diuretics is crucial for the success of the other drugs being used. The 2005 ACC/AHA guidelines (3) recommend that diuretics be prescribed to all patients who have evi-

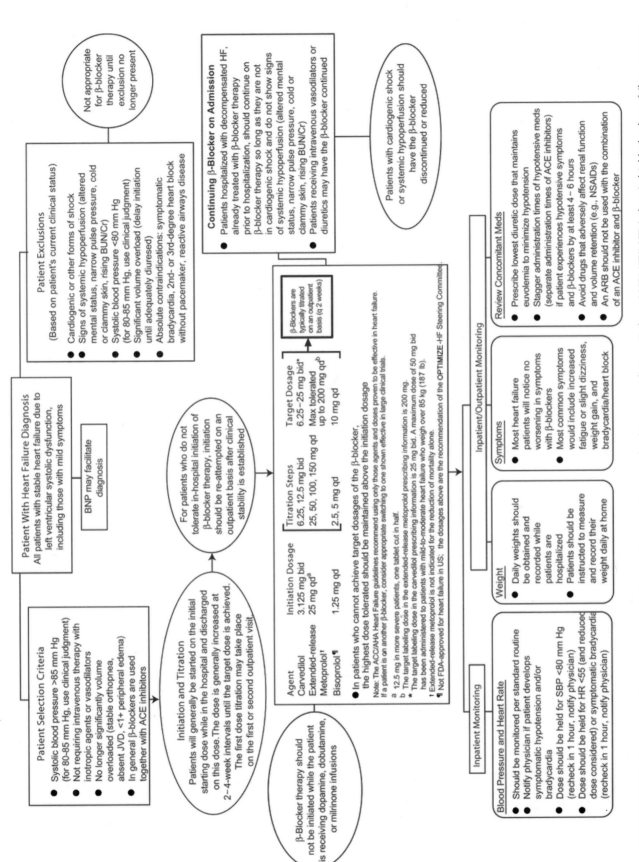

FIGURE 20-10. The Organized Program to Initiate Lifesaving Treatment in Hospitalized Patients with Heart Failure (OPTIMIZE-HF) in-hospital β-blocker heart failure treatment algorithm. CR/XL, controlled release/extended release; FDA, Food and Drug Administration; HR, heart rate; JVD, jugular venous distension; q, once. (Reprinted from Fonarow GC, Abraham WT, Albert NM, et al. Organized Program to Initiate Lifesaving Treatment in Hospitalized Patients with Heart Failure (OPTIMIZE-HF): rationale and design. *Am Heart J* 2004;148:43–51, with permission.)

TABLE 20-10

RECOMMENDED ALDOSTERONE ANTAGONISTS AND DOSES

Drug	Initial Dose	Target Dose
Spironolactone	6.25 mg qd	25 mg qd
Eplerenone	25 mg qd	50 mg qd

dence of fluid retention, and that they should be combined with an ACE inhibitor and a β-blocker (and usually digoxin). The inclusion and exclusion criteria for diuretic use are listed in Table 20-13. Therapy should be initiated with low doses that are then increased until urine output increases and weight decreases, generally by 0.5 to 1.0 kg/day. Once fluid retention has resolved, treatment with the diuretic should be maintained to prevent the recurrence of volume overload. The dose should be adjusted periodically, allowing the patient to make changes in dose if his or her weight increases or decreases beyond a specified range. Important issues to regard when using diuretics are listed in Table 20-14.

Digoxin

Digoxin may be used early to reduce HF symptoms in patients who have been started on, but have not yet responded symptomatically to, treatment with an ACE inhibitor or a β-blocker. Alternatively, treatment with digoxin may be delayed until the patient's response to their ACE inhibitor and β-blocker has been defined and used only in patients who remain symptom-

TABLE 20-11

IMPORTANT ISSUES REGARDING ALDOSTERONE ANTAGONISTS

Patients' serum potassium level should be <5 mmol/L, and their serum creatinine level should be <2.5 mg/dL before initiation of therapy. Closely monitor renal function and serum K levels. Renal function and serum potassium should be assessed within 1–2 weeks of initiation or sooner in patients with baseline renal insufficiency and periodically thereafter.

Spironolactone should be discontinued if serious hyperkalemia or painful gynecomastia develops.

Dosages above 25 mg/d of spironolactone may be associated with risk of hyperkalemia.

Eplerenone is contraindicated in patients with the following conditions: serum potassium >5.0 mEq/L and creatinine clearance ≤30 mL/min.

The principal risk of eplerenone use is hyperkalemia, which can be minimized by assessing creatinine clearance and baseline serum potassium concentration prior to initiation of eplerenone therapy. Periodic monitoring is recommended in patients at risk for the development of hyperkalemia; during the clinical trials, serum potassium levels were monitored every 2 weeks for the first 1–2 months and then monthly thereafter. Consider discontinuing potassium supplementation when serum potassium is 4.5 mEq/L or higher. Monitor renal function with any change in dose.

atic despite therapy. It is recommended that in patients with atrial fibrillation with rapid ventricular response and HF, digoxin should be combined with β-blockers. Patients should not be given digoxin if they have significant sinus or atrioventricular block unless treated with a permanent pacemaker. In the case of atrial fibrillation with a rapid ventricular rate, the β-blocker dose rather than the digoxin dose should be increased, because higher serum digoxin concentrations are associated with increased risk for adverse events. Digitalis toxicity is commonly associated with serum digoxin levels >2 ng/mL, but may occur with lower digoxin levels, especially if hypokalemia, hypomagnesemia, or hypothyroidism is present.

PATIENT EDUCATION

Physicians treating patients with HF must advocate education for their patients to achieve optimal care. Patient education is recognized by JCAHO as important and one of the core measures for successful treatment of hospitalized HF patients. At discharge or during the hospital stay, HF patients and/or their caregivers should be given written instructions or educational materials addressing all of the following six components of education: activity level, diet, discharge medications, follow-up appointment, weight monitoring, and what to do if symptoms worsen. Educating HF patients and their families is critical. Patient noncompliance with physician's instructions is often the cause of rehospitalization.

Previous studies evaluating the effect of HF patient discharge education combined with various postdischarge support programs have demonstrated benefit in reductions in number of hospitalizations and costs (57–60). Comprehensive patient care programs have shown dramatic results: rehospitalizations were decreased by 85% with a management program that included adjustment of medication and an increase in patient education (24). An education and support intervention without medical management components reduced readmissions and in-hospital costs among patients with HF (60). These intervention patients also exhibited significantly longer readmission-free survival. Reductions of nearly 40% in total readmissions and nearly 50% in HF readmissions were achieved with this in-hospital program that focused on patient empowerment through education about managing chronic illness and through support for seeking appropriate care (60). A randomized, controlled trial of 223 systolic HF patients compared the effects of a 1-hour, one-on-one teaching session with a nurse educator to the standard discharge process (58). Subjects who received the teaching session ($n = 107$) had fewer days hospitalized or dead in the follow-up period compared with controls ($P = 0.009$) and a 35% lower risk of rehospitalization or death ($P = 0.018$).

Important factors related to rehospitalization are premature discharge and noncompliance. To prevent readmission, interventions should be employed in the areas of discharge planning, patient education, and follow-up. The use of preprinted care instructions and educational materials would increase the number of patients that received education prior to discharge. From the ADHERE registry, we know that there is large variability in the percentage of patients that are discharged with instructions; in academic hospitals, the percent of patients discharged with instructions was only 21%, whereas at nonacademic hospitals 34% of patients received discharge instructions (15). Both percentages are far too low, but it is especially disappointing that academic teaching hospitals have shown poor patient care in this regard. A process-of-care improvement program that includes critical pathways for the physician must also include patient education materials to be successful.

TABLE 20-12

AGENTS THAT REDUCE SYMPTOMS OF HEART FAILURE

Drug	Dosing	Notes
Vasodilators	Hydralazine up to 100 mg qd Isordil up to 80 mg tid Doxazosin up to 4–8 mg bid	Administer if blood pressure remains increased despite maximum dose of ACE inhibitor.
Digoxin	0.125 mg/day	Digitalis toxicity is commonly associated with serum digoxin levels >2 ng/mL, but may occur with lower digoxin levels, especially if hypokalemia, hypomagnesemia, or hypothyroidism is present.
Diuretics	Initiate with low doses and increase until urine output increases and weight decreases, generally by 0.5–1.0 kg/day.	Loop diuretics with potassium supplementation. Flexible regimen with doubled dose for 2-lb weight gain and PRN metolazone.

ACE, angiotensin-converting enzyme.

NEXT STEPS

The gaps and variation in care that currently exist in the nation's hospitals suggest that efforts that target education and effective patient intervention, such as those initiated by OPTI-MIZE-HF, will be necessary to improve the overall quality of care for patients with HF. The Get With the Guidelines initiative, a hospital-based quality improvement program conceived by the AHA and the American Stroke Association, aims to standardize care using the most updated evidence-based guidelines. Recent data demonstrate that Get With the Guidelines is an effective tool for improving hospital care. In a large, multicenter evaluation, significant improvements relative to baseline were seen in all ten quality-of-care measures for coronary artery disease by the third quarter of Get With the Guidelines implementation (61). These improvements occurred equally at both academic and nonacademic institutions (62). The ACC Guidelines Applied in Practice (GAP) program showed similar improvements (63).

Thus, implementation of a hospital-based system for HF should enhance adherence to established guidelines and core performance measures, reducing the treatment variability between hospitals. As a result, overall quality of care should improve significantly, reducing the morbidity, mortality, and economic cost associated with this disorder.

CONCLUSIONS

There is an urgent need for effective strategies to improve the use of the evidence-based therapies outlined in this chapter. In-hospital initiation of ACE inhibitors and β-blockers has been demonstrated to improve treatment rates, long-term patient adherence, and clinical outcomes. The adoption of in-hospital critical pathways and tools for the care of patients with HF has been shown to increase the initiation of evidence-based HF therapies and could substantially improve treatment rates, decrease the risk of future hospitalizations, and prolong life in the large number of patients who are hospitalized each year for HF. There is significant individual variability among hospitals providing care for HF in their conformity to quality-of-care indicators, plus a substantial gap in overall performance. Establishing educational initiatives and quality improvement systems to reduce this variability and eliminate this gap would be expected to substantially improve the care of these patients.

TABLE 20-13

INCLUSION AND EXCLUSION CRITERIA FOR DIURETIC USE

Inclusion Criteria	Exclusion Criteria
HF patients with evidence of volume overload in whom diuresis with intravenous diuretics is clinically indicated. HF patients admitted with any of the following baseline levels: —blood pressure ≥80 mm Hg —potassium ≥3.5 or ≤5.0 mmol/L —creatinine ≤2.0 mg/dL	Advanced HF patients admitted with any of the following baseline levels:* —blood pressure <80 mm Hg —potassium <3.5 or >5.0 mmol/L —creatinine >2.0 mg/dL

*Individualize care for these patients.

TABLE 20-14

IMPORTANT ISSUES REGARDING DIURETIC THERAPY

Loop diuretics have emerged as the preferred diuretic agents for use in most HF patients.

Diuretics should generally be combined with an ACE inhibitor and a β-blocker (and usually digoxin). Diuretics should not be used alone in the treatment of HF.

The use of inappropriately low doses of diuretics will cause fluid retention, which can diminish the response to ACE inhibitors and increase the risk of treatment with β-blockers. Conversely, the use of inappropriately high doses of diuretics will lead to volume contraction, which can increase the risk of hypotension with ACE inhibitors and ARBs.

Patients may become unresponsive to high doses of diuretic drugs if they:
—consume large amounts of dietary sodium
—take agents that can block the effects of diuretics (e.g., NSAIDs, including COX-2 inhibitors)
—have significant impairment of renal function or perfusion.

Adverse effects of diuretics include hypotension and/or diminished renal perfusion, leading to the development of prerenal azotemia or acute intrinsic renal failure that may resolve by decreasing the diuretic dose.

Hypokalemia and hypomagnesemia may increase the risk of life-threatening ventricular arrhythmias in patients with HF and may contribute to the incidence of sudden death, particularly during treatment with digoxin. Usually, use in combination with ACE inhibitors and, if appropriate, spironolactone, will minimize potassium loss. Magnesium and/or potassium supplements can be given as needed. If hypotension or azotemia is observed, the rapidity of diuresis could be reduced, but diuresis should be maintained until fluid retention is eliminated.

Diuretics may also cause metabolic alkalosis, carbohydrate intolerance, hyperuricemia, hypersensitivity reactions, and acute pancreatitis. It is prudent to use the lowest dose of diuretic that helps control congestion and perhaps use torsemide, which has a more predictable bioavailability and may be safer than furosemide.

ACE, angiotensin-converting enzyme; ARB, angiotensin II receptor antagonist; HF, heart failure; NSAID, nonsteroidal anti-inflammatory drug.

Thus, implementation of critical pathways for HF should enhance the adherence to established guidelines and core performance measures, reducing the treatment variability from one hospital to the next. As a result, overall quality of care should improve substantially, reducing the morbidity, mortality, and economic cost associated with this disorder. Use of hospital-based health care provider education materials, process-of-care materials, and patient education materials can improve the standard of care in patients with HF in both the hospital and outpatient settings, increase the utilization of evidence-based therapies, and save lives.

REFERENCES

1. American Heart Association. Heart disease and stroke statistics—2006 update. Dallas, TX: American Heart Association, 2006.
2. American Heart Association. African Americans and cardiovascular diseases—statistics. Dallas, TX: American Heart Association, 2005.
3. Hunt, SA, Abraham, WT, Chin, MH, et al. ACC/AHA 2005 guideline update for the diagnosis and management of chronic heart failure in the adult: a report of the American College of Cardiology/American Heart Association Task Force on Practice Guidelines (writing committee to update the 2001 guidelines for the evaluation and management of heart failure). Available at: http://www.acc.org/clinical/guidelines/failure/index.pdf; Accessed November 30, 2005.
4. O'Connell JB. The economic burden of heart failure. Clin Cardiol 2000;23: III6–10.
5. Lee WC, Chavez YE, Baker T, et al. Economic burden of heart failure: a summary of recent literature. Heart Lung 2004;33:362–371.
6. Krumholz HM, Parent EM, Tu N, et al. Readmission after hospitalization for congestive heart failure among Medicare beneficiaries. Arch Intern Med 1997;157:99–104.
7. Krum H, Roecker EB, Mohacsi P, et al. Effects of initiating carvedilol in patients with severe chronic heart failure: results from the COPERNICUS Study. JAMA 2003;289:712–718.
8. Gattis WA, O'Connor CM. Predischarge initiation of carvedilol in patients hospitalized for decompensated heart failure. Am J Cardiol 2004;93:74–76.
9. Franciosa JA, Massie BM, Lukas MA, et al. Beta-blocker therapy for heart failure outside the clinical trial setting: Findings of a community-based registry. Am Heart J 2004;148:718–726.
10. Bart BA, Ertl G, Held P, et al. Contemporary management of patients with left ventricular systolic dysfunction. Results from the Study of Patients Intolerant of Converting Enzyme Inhibitors (SPICE) Registry. Eur Heart J 1999; 20:1182–1190.
11. Cohn JN, Tognoni G. A randomized trial of the angiotensin-receptor blocker valsartan in chronic heart failure. N Engl J Med 2001;345: 1667–1675.
12. Whellan DJ, Gaulden L, Gattis WA, et al. The benefit of implementing a heart failure disease management program. Arch Intern Med 2001;161: 2223–2228.
13. Fonarow GC, Adams K, Strausser BP. ADHERE (Acute Decompensated Heart Failure National Registry): rationale, design, and subject population [abstr]. J Card Fail 2002;8:S49.
14. Cleland JG, Cohen-Solal A, Aguilar JC, et al. Management of heart failure in primary care (the IMPROVEMENT of Heart Failure Programme): an international survey. Lancet 2002;360:1631–1639.
15. Fonarow GC, Yancy CW, Chang SF. Variation in heart failure quality of care indicators among U.S. hospitals: analysis of 230 hospitals in ADHERE. Presented at the American Heart Association Scientific Session 2003; November 9–12, 2003; Orlando, FL [Abstract 2057]. Circulation 2003;108 Suppl IV:IV–447.
16. Yancy CW, Chang SF, for the ADHERE Scientific Advisory Committee and Investigators. Clinical Characteristics and outcomes in patients admitted

with heart failure with preserved systolic function: a report from the AD-HERE database. *J Card Fail* 2003;9:S84.

17. American College of Cardiology, American Heart Association Task Force. Guidelines for the evaluation and management of heart failure. Report of the American College of Cardiology/American Heart Association Task Force on Practice Guidelines (Committee on Evaluation and Management of Heart Failure). *Circulation* 1995;92:2764–2784.

18. Hunt SA, Baker DW, Chin MH, et al. ACC/AHA guidelines for the evaluation and management of chronic heart failure in the adult: executive summary. A report of the American College of Cardiology/American Heart Association Task Force on Practice Guidelines (Committee to revise the 1995 Guidelines for the Evaluation and Management of Heart Failure). *J Am Coll Cardiol* 2001;38:2101–2113.

19. DiDomenico RJ, Park HY, Southworth MR, et al. Guidelines for acute decompensated heart failure treatment. *Ann Pharmacother* 2004;38:649–660.

20. Krumholz HM, Baker DW, Ashton CM, et al. Evaluating quality of care for patients with heart failure. *Circulation* 2000;101:E122–E140.

21. Centers for Medicare & Medicaid Services. *Medicare quality improvement priorities.* Version 1.0 ed. Baltimore: U.S. Department of Health and Human Services, 2003.

22. Joint Commission on Accreditation of Healthcare Organizations. Specification manual for national implementation of hospital core measures: Version 2.0—implementation to begin with July 2004 discharges. Oakbrook Terrace, IL: Joint Commission on Accreditation of Healthcare Organizations, 2004.

23. Fonarow GC, Yancy CW, Heywood JT. Adherence to heart failure quality-of-care indicators in US hospitals: analysis of the ADHERE registry. *Arch Intern Med* 2005;165:1469–1477.

24. Fonarow GC, Stevenson LW, Walden JA, et al. Impact of a comprehensive heart failure management program on hospital readmission and functional status of patients with advanced heart failure. *J Am Coll Cardiol* 1997;30:725–732.

25. Lee DS, Tu JV, Juurlink DN, et al. Risk-treatment mismatch in the pharmacotherapy of heart failure. *JAMA* 2005;294:1240–1247.

26. Klein L, O'Connor CM, Leimberger JD, et al. Lower serum sodium is associated with increased short-term mortality in hospitalized patients with worsening heart failure: results from the Outcomes of a Prospective Trial of Intravenous Milrinone for Exacerbations of Chronic Heart Failure (OPTIME-CHF) study. *Circulation* 2005;111:2454–2460.

27. Jones RC, Francis GS, Lauer MS. Predictors of mortality in patients with heart failure and preserved systolic function in the Digitalis Investigation Group trial. *J Am Coll Cardiol* 2004;44:1025–1029.

28. Fonarow GC, Adams KF Jr., Abraham WT, et al. Risk stratification for in-hospital mortality in acutely decompensated heart failure: classification and regression tree analysis. *JAMA* 2005;293:572–580.

29. Pearson TA, Horne BD, Maycock CA, et al. An institutional heart failure discharge medication program reduces future cardiovascular readmissions and mortality: an analysis of 19,083 heart failure patients. *Circulation* 2001;104(Suppl II):II-838.

30. Gattis WA, O'Connor CM, Gallup DS, et al. Predischarge initiation of carvedilol in patients hospitalized for decompensated heart failure: results of the Initiation Management Predischarge: Process for Assessment of Carvedilol Therapy in Heart Failure (IMPACT-HF) trial. *J Am Coll Cardiol* 2004;43:1534–1541.

31. Fonarow GC, Abraham WT, Albert NM, et al. Organized Program to Initiate Lifesaving Treatment in Hospitalized Patients with Heart Failure (OPTIMIZE-HF): rationale and design. *Am Heart J* 2004;148:43–51.

32. Packer M, Bristow MR, Cohn JN, et al. The effect of carvedilol on morbidity and mortality in patients with chronic heart failure. U.S. Carvedilol Heart Failure Study Group. *N Engl J Med* 1996;334:1349–1355.

33. MERIT-HF Investigators. Effect of metoprolol CR/XL in chronic heart failure: Metoprolol CR/XL Randomised Intervention Trial in Congestive Heart Failure (MERIT-HF). *Lancet* 1999;353:2001–2007.

34. CIBIS-II Investigators. The Cardiac Insufficiency Bisoprolol Study II (CIBIS-II): a randomised trial. *Lancet* 1999;353:9–13.

35. Packer M, Coats AJ, Fowler MB, et al. Effect of carvedilol on survival in severe chronic heart failure. *N Engl J Med* 2001;344:1651–1658.

36. CONSENSUS Trial Study Group. Effects of enalapril on mortality in severe congestive heart failure. Results of the Cooperative North Scandinavian Enalapril Survival Study (CONSENSUS). The CONSENSUS Trial Study Group. *N Engl J Med* 1987;316:1429–1435.

37. SOLVD Investigators. Effect of enalapril on survival in patients with reduced left ventricular ejection fractions and congestive heart failure. The SOLVD Investigators. *N Engl J Med* 1991;325:293–302.

38. Heart Failure Society of America. Heart Failure Society of America (HFSA) practice guidelines. HFSA guidelines for management of patients with heart failure caused by left ventricular systolic dysfunction—pharmacological approaches. *J Card Fail* 1999;5:357–382.

39. Packer M, Cohn JN. Consensus recommendations for the management of chronic heart failure. *Am J Cardiol* 1999;83:1A–38A.

40. Jong P, Yusuf S, Rousseau MF, et al. Effect of enalapril on 12-year survival and life expectancy in patients with left ventricular systolic dysfunction: a follow-up study. *Lancet* 2003;361:1843–1848.

41. SOLVD Investigators. Effect of enalapril on mortality and the development of heart failure in asymptomatic patients with reduced left ventricular ejection fractions. The SOLVD Investigators. *N Engl J Med* 1992;327:685–691.

42. Cohn JN. Improving outcomes in congestive heart failure: Valsartan in Heart Failure Trial. *Cardiology* 1999;91(Suppl 1):19–22.

43. Krum H, Carson P, Farsang C, et al. Effect of valsartan added to background ACE inhibitor therapy in patients with heart failure: results from Val-HeFT. *Eur J Heart Fail* 2004;6:937–945.

44. Yusuf S, Pfeffer MA, Swedberg K, et al. Effects of candesartan in patients with chronic heart failure and preserved left-ventricular ejection fraction: the CHARM-Preserved Trial. *Lancet* 2003;362:777–781.

45. Granger CB, McMurray JJ, Yusuf S, et al. Effects of candesartan in patients with chronic heart failure and reduced left-ventricular systolic function intolerant to angiotensin-converting-enzyme inhibitors: the CHARM-Alternative trial. *Lancet* 2003;362:772–776.

46. McMurray JJ, Ostergren J, Swedberg K, et al. Effects of candesartan in patients with chronic heart failure and reduced left-ventricular systolic function taking angiotensin-converting-enzyme inhibitors: the CHARM-Added trial. *Lancet* 2003;362:767–771.

47. Packer M, Fowler MB, Roecker EB, et al. Effect of carvedilol on the morbidity of patients with severe chronic heart failure: results of the Carvedilol Prospective Randomized Cumulative Survival (COPERNICUS) Study. *Circulation* 2002;106:2194–2199.

48. Krum H, Roecker EB, Mohacsi P, et al. Efficacy and safety of initiating carvedilol in patients with severe chronic heart failure: results of Copernicus study. Presented at American Heart Association 75th Scientific Sessions; November 17–20, 2002; Chicago, IL [abstr]. *Circulation* 2002;106:II-612.

49. Packer M, Colucci WS, Sackner-Bernstein JD, et al. Double-blind, placebo-controlled study of the effects of carvedilol in patients with moderate to severe heart failure. THE PRECISE Trial. Prospective Randomized Evaluation of Carvedilol on Symptoms and Exercise. *Circulation* 1996;94:2793–2799.

50. Bristow MR. Mechanism of action of beta-blocking agents in heart failure. *Am J Cardiol* 1997;80:26L–40L.

51. Gottlieb SS, Fisher ML, Kjekshus J, et al. Tolerability of beta-blocker initiation and titration in the Metoprolol CR/XL Randomized Intervention Trial in Congestive Heart Failure (MERIT-HF). *Circulation* 2002;105:1182–1188.

52. Pitt B, Williams G, Remme W, et al. The EPHESUS trial: eplerenone in patients with heart failure due to systolic dysfunction complicating acute myocardial infarction. Eplerenone Post-AMI Heart Failure Efficacy and Survival Study. *Cardiovasc Drugs Ther* 2001;15:79–87.

53. Pitt B, Zannad F, Remme WJ, et al. The effect of spironolactone on morbidity and mortality in patients with severe heart failure. Randomized Aldactone Evaluation Study Investigators. *N Engl J Med* 1999;341:709–717.

54. Chen HH, Lainchbury JG, Senni M, et al. Diastolic heart failure in the community: clinical profile, natural history, therapy, and impact of proposed diagnostic criteria. *J Card Fail* 2002;8:279–287.

55. Bardy GH, Lee KL, Mark DB, et al. Amiodarone or an implantable cardioverter-defibrillator for congestive heart failure. *N Engl J Med* 2005;352:225–237.

56. St. John Sutton MG, Plappert T, Abraham WT, et al. Effect of cardiac resynchronization therapy on left ventricular size and function in chronic heart failure. *Circulation* 2003;107:1985–1990.

57. Hanumanthu S, Butler J, Chomsky D, et al. Effect of a heart failure program on hospitalization frequency and exercise tolerance. *Circulation* 1997;96:2842–2848.

58. Koelling TM, Johnson ML, Cody RJ, et al. Discharge education improves clinical outcomes in patients with chronic heart failure. *Circulation* 2005;111:179–185.

59. Cline CM, Israelsson BY, Willenheimer RB, et al. Cost effective management programme for heart failure reduces hospitalisation. *Heart* 1998;80:442–446.

60. Krumholz HM, Amatruda J, Smith GL, et al. Randomized trial of an education and support intervention to prevent readmission of patients with heart failure. *J Am Coll Cardiol* 2002;39:83–89.

61. LaBresh KA, Ellrodt AG, Gliklich R, et al. Get with the guidelines for cardiovascular secondary prevention: pilot results. *Arch Intern Med* 2004;164:203–209.

62. Fonarow GC, Bonow RO, Tyler P, et al. Does the AHA "Get With the Guidelines" program improve the quality of care in hospitalized patients with coronary artery disease at both teaching and non-teaching hospitals? *Circulation* 2003;108:IV-721–IV-722.

63. Mehta RH, Montoye CK, Gallogly M, et al. Improving quality of care for acute myocardial infarction: The Guidelines Applied in Practice (GAP) Initiative. *JAMA* 2002;287:1269–1276.

CHAPTER 21 ■ DEVICE THERAPY IN HEART FAILURE: SELECTION OF PATIENTS FOR ICD AND CRT

ELI V. GELFAND AND PETER J. ZIMETBAUM

TYPES OF AVAILABLE DEVICES
ICD Components and Function
Device Implantation
DEVICE THERAPY IN SECONDARY PREVENTION OF SUDDEN CARDIAC DEATH
DEVICE THERAPY IN PRIMARY PREVENTION OF SUDDEN CARDIAC DEATH
DEVICE THERAPY FOR PRIMARY SUDDEN CARDIAC DEATH PREVENTION IN SPECIAL POPULATIONS
CARDIAC RESYNCHRONIZATION THERAPY
Cardiac Dyssynchrony
Biventricular Pacemaker Design and Implantation
Trials of Cardiac Resynchronization
NONINVASIVE IMAGING OF PATIENTS UNDERGOING CRT
Echocardiography for Assessment of Dyssynchrony
Echocardiography to Aid Optimization of Biventricular Devices Following Implantation
Multislice Computed Tomography
Cardiovascular Magnetic Resonance: A Comprehensive Noninvasive Modality

Heart failure (HF) currently represents a major public health problem in the United States. Superior treatment strategies for acute coronary syndromes have created a large population of acute myocardial infarction (MI) survivors with poor left ventricular (LV) function. The growing burden of diabetes mellitus and undertreated hypertension contribute to a rising prevalence of HF. As a result, HF is now the leading hospital discharge diagnosis and accounts for 15 million office visits in the United States (1).

A clinical diagnosis of HF portends an increased risk of ventricular arrhythmias and sudden cardiac death (SCD). However, even in absence of congestive symptoms, a dilated, hypocontractile left ventricle is a marker of an increased risk. Whereas for patients with advanced (New York Heart Association [NYHA] class III-IV) congestive heart failure (CHF), declining ventricular pump function, and organ failure due to hypoperfusion may represent the common mode of death, for patients with NYHA class II CHF, incidence of death from arrhythmia may dominate that from pump failure. The goals of device therapy in HF are to (a) prevent SCD, (b) reduce symptoms of heart failure, (c) attenuate or reverse cardiac remodeling, and (d) allow for a more aggressive pharmacologic therapy, proven to reduce mortality (Table 21-1).

Since the publication of secondary prevention clinical trials conducted in the 1990s, there has been little controversy over the use of implantable devices to prevent *recurrent* cardiac arrest or hemodynamically unstable ventricular arrhythmias. The major focus of recent investigations has been on primary prevention of sudden cardiac death from arrhythmia in patients with HF.

Concurrent with an ever-expanding body of data on device therapy, the device design itself has advanced at a rapid pace. In the 1970s, an implantable cardioverter defibrillator (ICD) was a relatively bulky device, which required a thoracotomy for implantation. Current-generation ICDs are microprocessor-driven units that weigh less than 60 g. They are implanted transvenously from a subcutaneous pocket and are capable not only of terminating a ventricular tachyarrhythmia by a direct-current countershock, but also of antitachycardia pacing, backup pacing for bradycardia, biventricular pacing, complex arrhythmia analysis, and electrogram storage. Improved battery design means that the life span of an average ICD has been extended to over 5 years. Driven largely by recent trial data, the number of device implants has skyrocketed in the United States in the late 1990s to the early 2000s (Fig. 21-1) (2).

The goal of this chapter is to suggest an evidence-based rationale for selection of patients with HF, for whom device therapy is indicated and appropriate. Also, it is our goal to aid the clinician with the selection of a proper device type for a particular patient population.

TYPES OF AVAILABLE DEVICES

ICD Components and Function

Implantable cardioverter defibrillators used in treatment of patients with HF are broadly divided into three types: single-chamber, dual-chamber, and biventricular (cardiac resynchronization therapy, CRT) ICDs. Most commercially available ICDs incorporate full pacemaker capabilities; however, detailed review of those features is outside the scope of this chapter. The basic components of any ICD system are similar (Fig. 21-2) and consist of a battery encased in a sealed titanium can, capacitors that store the energy prior to cardioversion/defibrillation, a microprocessor that analyzes the cardiac rhythm and governs the ICD function and a header, through which the leads are attached. The ICD leads function as both pacing electrodes, as well as defibrillation coils.

In a single-chamber defibrillator system (Fig. 21-2A), a single lead is implanted into the right ventricular apex or septum and thus is able to pace and defibrillate the ventricle. In a dual-chamber system (Fig. 21-2B), an atrial lead is added, which can track atrial activity and provide backup atrial pacing if necessary. A biventricular device (Fig. 21-2C) generally has three leads: an atrial pacing lead, a right ventricular pacing/

TABLE 21-1

RATIONALE FOR PURSUING DEVICE THERAPY IN PATIENTS WITH CONGESTIVE HEART FAILURE WITH DEPRESSED LEFT VENTRICULAR FUNCTION

Rationale	Type	Goal
Increased propensity for ventricular tachyarrhythmia	ICD	Primary and secondary prevention of SCD
Abnormal hemodynamic state • Decreased stroke volume and cardiac output • Loss of RV/LV synchrony • Loss of intraventricular LV synchrony • Prolonged AV delay, loss of AV synchrony • Functional mitral regurgitation	BiV pacing	• Restoration of AV, interventricular, and intraventricular synchrony • Optimizing atrial contribution to LV filling • Improving symptoms of congestion and low forward cardiac output • Reducing severity functional mitral regurgitation
Inability to tolerate increasing doses of β-blocker because of bradycardia	RV/BiV pacing	Prevention of symptomatic bradycardia

AV, atrioventricular; BiV, biventricular; ICD, implantable cardioverter defibrillators; LV, left ventricular; RV, right ventricular; SCD, sudden cardiac death.

defibrillation lead, and a LV pacing lead. The LV lead is placed via the coronary sinus into one of the lateral cardiac veins overlying the LV surface. Biventricular devices are available with and without defibrillator capability.

Device Implantation

Implantation of an ICD is typically performed under conscious sedation, in much the same way as a pacemaker insertion. Complications of implantation are uncommon, but include cardiac perforation with tamponade, venous trauma, bleeding into the device pocket, and lead dislodgment. Most important long-term complication of ICD therapy is device or lead infection. If device infection is diagnosed, prolonged antibiotic therapy is mandated, and device removal with lead explantation is often required. The latter is associated with an approximately 2.5% risk of serious complications, including central venous trauma, hemopericardium, and hemothorax (3).

DEVICE THERAPY IN SECONDARY PREVENTION OF SUDDEN CARDIAC DEATH

It is now recognized that in absence of a reversible cause of sudden cardiac death (e.g., acute ischemia causing ventricular tachycardia [VT] or ventricular fibrillation [VF]), the risk of SCD recurrence is high. Three important randomized, controlled clinical trials have demonstrated that when com-

*Numbers for 2004-2006 are estimates

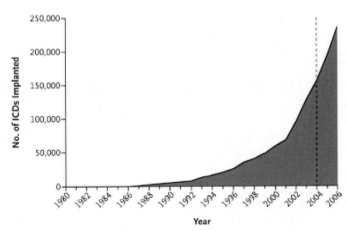

FIGURE 21-1. Growth in ICD implantation procedures in the United States 1980–2006. (Reproduced with permission from Jauhar S, Slotwiner DJ. The economics of ICDs. *N Engl J Med* 2004;351(24):2542–2544.)

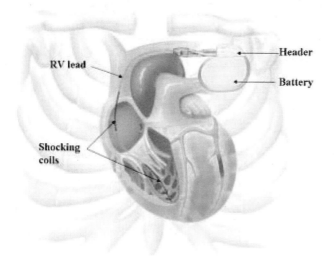

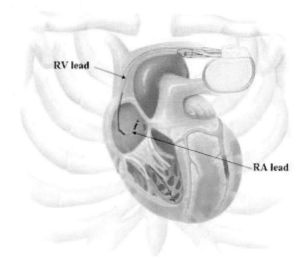

A

B

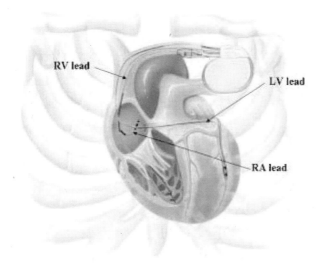

C

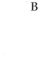

FIGURE 21-2. Basic components of commonly available heart failure devices. Images provided courtesy of Guidant Corp. (**A**) single-chamber ICD, (**B**) dual-chamber ICD, (**C**) biventricular ICD.

pared with antiarrhythmic therapy, ICD therapy is associated with a decrease in the incidence of recurrent SCD (Table 21-2) (4–6).

In the Antiarrhythmic Versus Implantable Defibrillator (AVID) trial (4), mortality after 2 years was 18.4% in the ICD group, and 25.3% in the antiarrhythmic group, yielding an approximately 30% relative decrease in all-cause mortality, which persisted through 3 years of follow-up. Most of the patients in the AVID antiarrhythmic group received amiodarone. These results were confirmed in the Canadian Implantable Defibrillator (CIDS) trial (5), in which patients were randomly assigned to receive amiodarone or an ICD. A 20% relative risk reduction in all-cause mortality over 3 years of follow-up was observed, although it did not reach statistical significance. Critique of AVID and CIDS included the more frequent use of β-blockers in the ICD arms of both trials, which may have biased the findings toward device therapy. An 11-year follow-up from a single-center subset of CIDS demonstrated that the benefit of ICD therapy over amiodarone increases over time (7). Additionally, the major-

ity of patients treated with amiodarone (82%) developed significant adverse effects from the medication, resulting in discontinuation in 50% of the patients. The third trial in the series was the Cardiac Arrest Study Hamburg (CASH) (6), in which patients were randomly assigned to receive a β-blocker metoprolol, amiodarone, or ICD. In this trial, ICD was again superior to antiarrhythmic therapy (both metoprolol and amiodarone), with an approximately 30% reduction in SCD mortality in the device group.

Meta-analysis of AVID, CIDS, and CASH (8) was published in 2005 and demonstrated that among survivors of SCD, defibrillator therapy was associated with a 28% relative risk reduction of all-cause mortality, which was almost entirely to a 50% reduction in the risk of recurrent SCD. Over the follow-up period of 6 years, ICD therapy prolonged patient survival by 4.4 months compared to antiarrhythmic therapy.

Based on the findings of these randomized trials, ICD therapy is a Class I recommendation (beneficial, useful, and effective treatment) for patients who suffered cardiac arrest from VT or VF, or had unstable/high risk VT (Table 21-3).

TABLE 21-2

SELECTED MAJOR CLINICAL TRIALS OF DEVICE THERAPY FOR SECONDARY PREVENTION OF SUDDEN CARDIAC DEATH

Type	Year	Population	Therapy	n	Major findings
AVID (4)	1997	SCD survivors	ICD vs. AAD	1,016	30% mortality decrease in ICD group (survival 75.4% vs. 64.1% at 3 years, $P < 0.02$). Notably, beta-blockers were used more frequently in the ICD group.
CASH (6)	2000	SCD survivors	ICD vs. AAD	349	Significant decrease in SCD in ICD group (13% vs. 33% for pooled drug Rx group, $P = 0.005$). Increase in SCD in propafenone group compared to ICD, no difference in SCD rates with amiodarone or BB compared to ICD. Trend toward reduced all-cause mortality with ICD.
CIDS (5)	2000	Survivors of SCD or unstable VT	ICD vs. AAD	259	ICD associated with a trend toward decreased mortality over 3 years (8.3% vs. 10.2% per year, 19.7% RRR, $P = 0.142$). Beta-blockers were used more frequently in the ICD group.

AAD, antiarrhythmic drugs; SCD, sudden cardiac death; RRR, relative risk reduction; Rx, pharmacologic therapy; VT, ventricular tachycardia.

DEVICE THERAPY IN PRIMARY PREVENTION OF SUDDEN CARDIAC DEATH

Survival from an out-of-hospital cardiac arrest remains low despite a significant investment in such effective public health measures as automated external defibrillators (AEDs) (9). Therefore, identification of patients at high risk for a first episode of SCD has been and remains an important scientific and public health priority. In an attempt to define such a population, randomized clinical trials enrolled progressively broader groups of patients and tested ICD therapy as means of primary prevention of SCD (Table 21-4).

Coronary disease in combination with poor ventricular function is thought to portend an especially high risk of malig-

TABLE 21-3

RECOMMENDATIONS FOR ICD THERAPY IN _SECONDARY_ PREVENTION OF SUDDEN CARDIAC DEATH

Patient characteristics	Strength of recommendation
Any one of the following: 1. Cardiac arrest due to VF or VT 2. VT requiring cardioversion 3. VT with LVEF <40%, and symptoms suggesting hemodynamic compromise due to arrhythmia (angina, heart failure, or near-syncope)	Class I

LVEF, left ventricular ejection fraction; VF, ventricular fibrillation.

nant ventricular arrhythmias. The first trial to demonstrate benefit of ICD over antiarrhythmic therapy was the small Multicenter Automatic Defibrillator Implantation Trial (MADIT) (10), which enrolled patients with a documented history of MI, ejection fraction (EF) ≤35%, and nonsustained ventricular tachycardia (NSVT). Patients underwent electrophysiological (EP) study, and if VT could be induced but not suppressed, they were randomized to antiarrhythmic therapy or ICD. Over the course of follow-up, patients in the ICD group benefitted from a 54% reduction in mortality compared to placebo. Based on the results of MADIT (and despite the small sample size of the study, as well as the more frequent use of β-blockers in the ICD group), ICD therapy was approved for this indication. A much larger Multicenter Unsustained Tachycardia Trial (MUSTT) (11) was a study comparing a medical approach with an electrophysiology-guided approach for primary prevention of SCD. Patients were enrolled if they had a history of MI, EF ≤40%, and NSVT. Though MUSTT was not designed as a "device trial," its protocol specified that a subset of patients in the EP-guided group have an ICD implanted. Comparison of this subpopulation with matched antiarrhythmic controls demonstrated a marked benefit to ICD therapy (a 76% decrease in the incidence of SCD), indirectly supporting the results of MADIT. In comparison with MADIT-I and MUSTT, the second MADIT trial (MADIT-II) markedly widened its enrollment criteria (12). It enrolled patients with a history of MI and EF ≤30%. No documentation of NSVT, or proof of VT inducibility in the EP lab was required. Over 1,200 patients were randomized to ICD or conventional therapy, and 31% mortality reduction with ICD therapy compared to control was observed beginning at 9 months after implantation (14.2% vs. 19.8%, $P = 0.016$). The study was stopped prematurely because of the marked benefit in the ICD group.

How early after the first determination of poor LV function is made should the ICD be implanted? Indeed, do patients with myocardial stunning and low LV EF early after MI represent appropriate candidates for ICD therapy? The DINAMIT trial (13) answered this question in a population of 674 patients with a recent (<40 days) MI and EF ≤35%. Desire to identify an even higher-risk group among this population led to ran-

TABLE 21-4

SELECTED MAJOR CLINICAL TRIALS OF DEVICE THERAPY FOR PRIMARY PREVENTION OF SUDDEN CARDIAC DEATH

Primary prevention of SCD					
Trial name	Year	Population enrollment	Therapy	n	Major findings
MADIT (10)	1996	NSVT, EF ≤35%, Documented MI, Nonsuppressible VT at EPS	ICD vs. AAD	196	54% reduction in mortality in the ICD group compared to drug therapy (HR 0.46, $P = 0.009$). Most of mortality benefit was due to a reduction in arrhythmic death.
MUSTT (11)	1999	NSVT, EF ≤40%, Documented MI	EPS-guided Rx vs. conventional Rx	2,202	Decrease in mortality at 2 and 5 years with EP-guided therapy. Though not technically a "device trial," it demonstrated that the mortality decrease in EP-guided therapy group was driven by the benefit of ICD therapy.
MADIT II (12)	2002	EF ≤30%, Documented MI	ICD vs. conventional Rx	1,232	31% mortality reduction with ICD therapy (14.2% vs 19.8%, $P = 0.016$). Mortality reduction observed beginning at 9 mo. after implantation. Study stopped prematurely because of survival benefit with ICD.
DINAMIT (13)	2004	EF ≤35%, *recent* (<40 days) MI, depressed HRV	ICD vs. conventional Rx	674	No difference in all-cause mortality after mean follow-up of 2.5 years.
DEFINITE (14)	2004	VPD or NSVT, nonischemic CMP, EF≤35%	ICD vs. conventional Rx	458	Significant reduction in SCD in ICD group (HR 0.20, $P = 0.006$). Nonsignificant trend toward lower all-cause mortality in ICD group.
SCD-HeFT (15)	2005	CMP of any etiology, EF ≤35%, Class II-III CHF for at least 3 mos.	ICD vs. amiodarone vs. placebo	2,521	Significant reduction in mortality with ICD vs. placebo (22% vs. 29%, $P = 0.007$) after a mean follow-up of 45.5 months. No overall mortality difference between amiodarone and placebo. Increased mortality with amiodarone vs. placebo for patients in NYHA class III CHF. Single-lead ICDs were used in this trial.

CRT, cardiac resynchronization therapy; CRT-D, cardiac resynchronization therapy with ICD; EPS, electrophysiological study; HRV, heart rate variability; LBBB, left bundle-branch block; MI, myocardial infarction; NSVT, nonsustained ventricular tachycardia; NYHA, New York Heart Association; VPD, ventricular premature depolarizations.

domization only of those patients who demonstrated abnormal heart rate variability—a marker of autonomic dysfunction. ICD therapy in this group, when compared to conventional treatment, demonstrated no benefit in reducing mortality after 2.5 years of follow-up.

In summary, results from MADIT-I, MUSTT, and MADIT-II demonstrated convincingly that among patients with a history of MI and poor ventricular function, implantation of an ICD, as compared with conventional medical therapy, results in a significant reduction in the risk of arrhythmic death. Based on the results from DINAMIT, decisions regarding ICD implantation should be made at least 40 days after the diagnosis of MI (Table 21-5).

Two recent important trials provided guidance regarding the use of ICD therapy among patients with cardiomyopathy from nonischemic causes (Table 21-4). The Defibrillators in Non Ischemic Cardiomyopathy Treatment Evaluation (DEFINITE) trial (14) randomized 458 patients with nonischemic cardiomyopathy, EF $\leq$35%, and ventricular ectopy/NSVT to ICD therapy, or conventional management. ICD therapy was associated with a significant reduction in SCD (heart rate 0.20, P = 0.006), and a trend toward decreased all-cause mortality. The Sudden Cardiac Death in Heart Failure (SCD-HeFT) was a larger trial, where 2,521 patients with cardiomyopathy of any etiology (approximately 50% with coronary artery disease [CAD]), EF $\leq$35%, and NYHA class II-III HF, were randomized to ICD therapy, conventional antiarrhythmic therapy with amiodarone, or placebo (15). Notably, the ICDs tested in SCD-HeFT were single-chamber devices, programmed only to provide defibrillation, and thus intended to treat rapid, sustained VT or VF. Dual-chamber or biventricular devices were prohibited by protocol. After a mean follow-up of 45.5 months, significant reduction in mortality was observed with ICD therapy compared to placebo (22% vs. 29%, respectively, P = 0.007). There was a significant benefit to ICD therapy in the whole population, whereas within the CAD subgroup this was only a strong trend. The trial also demonstrated no mortality benefit for amiodarone versus placebo.

Together, the results from DEFINITE and SCD-HeFT suggest that for selected patients with HF, in whom LV dysfunction persists despite optimal medical therapy with angiotensin-

converting enzyme (ACE) inhibitors and β-blockers, implantation of an ICD is associated with a decrease in mortality, compared to antiarrhythmic therapy or placebo (Table 21-5).

DEVICE THERAPY FOR PRIMARY SUDDEN CARDIAC DEATH PREVENTION IN SPECIAL POPULATIONS

Special HF populations where prophylactic use of ICDs should be considered include patients with hypertrophic cardiomyopathy (HCM) and arrhythmogenic right ventricular (RV) dysplasia/cardiomyopathy (ARVD/C). Implantation of an ICD for primary prevention of SCD in both of these disorders carries a class IIa indication (probably beneficial) from the ACC/AHA.

Patients with HCM are at a significantly increased risk of malignant ventricular arrhythmias and sudden death. Hypertrophic cardiomyopathy exhibits a heterogeneous phenotype, thus making clinical risk stratification possible. Patients at an increased risk of SCD are those with marked LV hypertrophy (wall thickness $\geq$30 mm), hypotensive response during treadmill exercise testing, NSVT on ambulatory monitoring or during exercise, unexplained syncope, or family history of premature sudden death. ICD implantation for primary prevention is usually reserved for these high-risk patients. Patients with HCM and a history of cardiac arrest should receive an ICD as part of the standard secondary prevention strategy.

Like HCM, arrhythmogenic RV dysplasia/cardiomyopathy is a disorder with a wide spectrum of clinical manifestations, from an incidental finding of asymptomatic RV dysfunction, to right-sided HF, ventricular arrhythmias, and sudden death. Patients at high risk for SCD are those with severe RF dysfunction and frequent ventricular ectopy/VT on ambulatory monitoring. Because there is a relatively small number of patients with ARVD/C, a randomized primary prevention trial is unlikely. Therefore, implantation of ICD in this population is largely individualized, with high-risk patients receiving the devices.

ICD therapy is also used in patients with idiopathic VF,

TABLE 21-5

RECOMMENDATIONS FOR *PRIMARY* PREVENTION OF SUDDEN CARDIAC DEATH IN PATIENTS WITH HEART FAILURE*

Patient characteristics LVEF	Other characteristics	Strength of recommendation
$\leq$35%	Cardiomyopathy from any cause, NYHA Class II-III on optimal medical therapy, expected survival >1 year	Class I
$\leq$35%	CAD, at least 40 days after MI, NYHA Class II–III on optimal medical therapy, expected survival >1 year	Class I
$\leq$35%	History of MI, NSVT, NYHA Class <IV, inducible and nonsuppressible VT/VF at EPS	Class I
$\leq$40%	Ischemic cardiomyopathy, NSVT, inducible VT/VF at EPS	Class I
>40%	Any	Not recommended

*Taking into consideration recent reimbursement recommendations by Centers for Medicare and Medicaid Services.

congenital long QT syndrome, and Brugada syndrome, but discussion of these intrinsic electrical disorders is beyond the scope of this chapter.

CARDIAC RESYNCHRONIZATION THERAPY

Cardiac Dyssynchrony

In patients with advanced LV systolic dysfunction and HF, conduction defects are common and lead to cardiac mechanical dyssynchrony. At least three distinct types of dyssynchrony are recognized. Atrioventricular (AV) dyssynchrony is the result of an abnormally delayed AV conduction, indicated by a prolonged PR interval on the electrocardiogram (ECG). Clinically, AV dyssynchrony is often associated with an ineffective ventricular filling, diastolic mitral regurgitation, and decreased cardiac output. Interventricular dyssynchrony is represented by an abnormally prolonged delay between the contraction of right and left ventricles. Intraventricular dyssynchrony is a regional contractile phase delay between the different LV walls and develops as a result of the remodeling in the cardiac conduction system. Intraventricular dyssynchrony is associated with an impairment in systolic function, reduction in cardiac output, worsening mitral regurgitation, and increase in wall stress (16). Observational studies show that patients with HF and intraventricular dyssynchrony marked by left bundle branch block (LBBB) or intraventricular conduction delay (IVCD) have worsening of the NYHA symptom class and a higher incidence of sudden death, when compared to patients without such markers (16,17). In addition, pacing of the right ventricle before the left ventricle may have deleterious effects on ventricular function and may worsen clinical HF (18). This likely occurs because RV pacing simulates LBBB, and results in hemodynamic effects similar to an intrinsically dyssynchronous heart.

Conversely, in many patients with HF, ventricular resynchronization has a number of desirable effects (Table 21-6). A number of studies discussed further in this chapter have shown that CRT is associated with decreased morbidity and mortality and leads to beneficial cardiac remodeling. The latter is manifested by a reduction in cardiac size and ventricular mass, as well as attenuation of functional mitral regurgitation.

Biventricular Pacemaker Design and Implantation

Device therapy may be used to moderate all three types of cardiac dyssynchrony in HF. Dual-chamber (atrial and ventricular) sequential pacing has been available for over 30 years and enhances the contribution of atrial systole and maximizes LV filling. Biventricular (BiV) pacing uses multilead devices capable of simultaneous pacing of right ventricle via stimulation of either the RV apex or septum and left ventricle via stimulation of the lateral wall epicardium. Biventricular devices that incorporate a full-function ICD are widely available.

The atrial and RV leads of a BiV device are implanted identically to a standard dual-chamber pacemaker or ICD. Implantation of an LV lead is often more challenging and involves insertion of a guidewire into the os of the coronary sinus and advancement of the lead to a distal cardiac vein under fluoroscopic guidance. Human coronary vein anatomy is highly variable, therefore contrast coronary venography is typically performed prior to lead insertion. Presence of a suitable coronary vein that overlies the lateral cardiac wall is then confirmed. In

TABLE 21-6

BENEFICIAL EFFECTS OF RESYNCHRONIZATION THERAPY

Effects of CRT	Specific Evidence
• Decreased mortality	COMPANION (25) CARE-HF (26)
• Reduction in heart failure symptoms • Reduction in NYHA heart failure class • Reduction in hospitalizations • Increased 6-minute walked distance • Enhanced quality of life	MIRACLE (22) MIRACLE-ICD (23) COMPANION (25) MUSTIC-SR (21) CARE-HF (26)
• Improvement in contractile function • Increased LVEF • Increased systolic blood pressure • Decreased plasma nt-proBNP levels • Increase in cardiac output • Reduction in pulmonary capillary wedge pressure • Increase in myocardial energy efficiency • Increased peak O_2 consumption (MVO_2)	PATH-CHF (20) CONTAK CD (24) MIRACLE (22) MIRACLE-ICD (23) CARE-HF (26) Ukkonen et al (38)
• Reverse cardiac remodeling • Decrease in LV dimensions • Decrease in LV mass • Decrease in LA mass • Reduction in severity of mitral regurgitation	MIRACLE (22) Saxon et al (39) Yu et al (40)

approximately 10% of cases, a suitable lateral vein is absent, and surgical placement of an epicardial LV lead is then recommended. Recently, multislice computed tomography (MSCT) has been proposed as an alternative to anatomic mapping of coronary veins (19). Use of MSCT for this application may potentially reduce the frequency of BiV device implantation procedures, which have to be aborted because of unsuitable vein anatomy.

Once the LV lead is implanted, its location determines the degree to which intraventricular dyssynchrony is reduced. Recent developments in device software have allowed the operator to manually adjust the delay between the RV and LV activation. Thus, interventricular dyssynchrony can be reduced, allowing for maximal cardiac output. Atrioventricular dyssynchrony is minimized via programming of the AV delay in devices with an atrial lead.

Trials of Cardiac Resynchronization

At least seven major randomized controlled clinical trials addressing CRT have been published to date (Table 21-7). The trials differ with respect to their specific inclusion criteria, type

SELECTED MAJOR CLINICAL TRIALS OF CARDIAC RESYNCHRONIZATION THERAPY FOR CONGESTIVE HEART FAILURE

Trial name	Year	Population	Number	Dyssynchrony mark	Therapy	Failed implant rate	Major findings
PATH-CHF (20)	2001	Mean EF 22% Class III or IV HF Sinus rhythm >55 bpm PR >150 msec	42	QRS >120 ms	CRT vs. RV pacing	N/A	CRT but not RV pacing associated with an increase in LVEF (from 22±7% to 26±9%, $P = 0.03$), decrease in LV volumes and dimensions after 6 months
MUSTIC-SR (21)	2001	EF ≤35% Class III HF LVEDD ≥60 mm	67	QRS >150 ms	CRT: active vs. backup pacing (crossover)	8.0%	Active BiV pacing associated with 23% higher 6-minute walking distance, (399 ± 100 vs. 326 ± 134 m, $P <0.001$), slightly higher peak O_2 consumption (16.2 vs. 15.0 mL/kg/min, $P = 0.03$), and an improved quality of life score
MIRACLE (Pacing Study) (22)	2002	EF ≤35% Class III–IV HF, LVEDD ≥55 mm 6-minute walking distance of ≤450 m	453	QRS ≥130 ms	CRT vs. medical Rx	8.0%	CRT associated with improved 6-min walk distance (+39 vs. +10 m, $P = 0.005$), improved HF by ≥1 NYHA class (68% vs. 38%, $P <0.001$), quality of life, and ejection fraction (+4.6% vs. −0.2%, $P <0.001$). CRT also associated with a significantly improved peak O_2 consumption (+1.1 vs. +0.2 mL/kg/min, $P = 0.009$)
MIRACLE-ICD (23)	2002	EF ≤35% Class III–IV HF ICD indications	555	QRS ≥130 ms	CRT-D vs. ICD	7.8%	CRT associated with HF improvement by ≥1 class ($P = 0.007$), and quality of life, but not 6-min walk test. No mortality benefit to CRT found in this trial. Device implantation unsuccessful in 50 patients (not randomized)

(continues)

TABLE 21-7

CONTINUED

Trial name	Year	Population	Number	Dyssynchrony mark	Therapy	Failed implant rate	Major findings
CONTAK CD (24)	2003	EF ≤35% Class II–IV HF VT/VF	490	QRS ≥120 ms	CRT-D vs. ICD		Overall, CRT associated with a nonsignificant trend toward reduction in HF progression. CRT associated with significant increase in peak O_2 consumption and 6-min walk test. In pts with Class III or IV HF, there was improvement in functional status
COMPANION (25)	2004	EF ≤35% Class III–IV HF with recent hospitalization	1,520	QRS ≥120 ms PR >150 ms	CRT-D vs. ICD vs. medical Rx	CRT: 13% CRT-D: 9%	CRT or CRT-D associated with lower combined endpoint of all-cause mortality and all-cause hospitalizations at a median follow-up of 14 mos (HR ~ 0.8, P <0.02) for both vs. medRx
MIRACLE-ICD II (41)	2004	EF ≤35% Class II HF ICD indications	186	QRS ≥130 ms	CRT-D vs. ICD		CRT associated with significant improvements in LV volumes and ejection fraction, and NYHA class after 6 months. No difference in quality of life, or 6-minute walk distance
CARE-HF (26)	2005	EF ≤35% Class III–IV HF sinus rhythm	813	QRS ≥150 ms; QRS 120–149 ms with echo signs of dyssynchrony	CRT vs. medical Rx	5%	CRT associated with a decrease in all-cause mortality or hospitalization for a major cardiovascular event (39% vs. 55% for placebo, HR 0.63, P <0.001) after median follow-up of 29.4 mos

LVEDD, left ventricular end-diastolic dimension; QRS, QRS complex width; PR, PR segment duration.

of device studied, and length of follow-up, although in general, they recruited similar populations. Patients enrolled in these trials generally had NYHA class III or IV HF on the basis of ischemic or nonischemic dilated cardiomyopathy, were in sinus rhythm, and demonstrated wide QRS complex on ECG. Most were treated optimally for HF with standard pharmacotherapy, including β-blockers, ACE inhibitors or angiotensin-receptor blockers, and diuretics.

The Pacing Therapies in Congestive Heart Failure (PATH-CHF) trial (20) compared CRT with RV pacing and demonstrated evidence of beneficial cardiac remodeling with CRT.

The Multisite Stimulation in Cardiomyopathies (MUSTIC)-SR trial (21) published the same year and utilized a crossover design, where patients with dilated cardiomyopathy (left ventricular end-diastolic dimension [LVEDD] ≥60 mm) and very wide QRS complex (>150 ms) were randomized to active versus backup BiV pacing. It showed that CRT is associated with an improvement in HF symptoms and quality of life, as well as with objective improvements in peak O_2 consumption and 6-minute walking distance.

These small trials were followed by the much larger MIRACLE (22) and MIRACLE-ICD (23) studies, in which CRT was compared with medical therapy or with ICD therapy alone, respectively. Both studies showed that CRT was associated with the improvement in HF class and quality of life. There was no mortality benefit to CRT in either trial. These results were supported by the findings of the CONTAK CD trial (24), although in that trial, the endpoint of reduction in HF progression did not reach statistical significance.

Important mortality data with CRT were provided by the Comparison of Medical Therapy, Pacing, and Defibrillation in Heart Failure (COMPANION) trial (25). More than 1,500 patients with moderate or severe HF and dyssynchrony evidenced by wide QRS complex and prolonged PR interval, were enrolled and randomized to CRT with defibrillator, ICD alone, or medical therapy. When compared to medical therapy, CRT with or without defibrillation was associated with a lower combined endpoint of all-cause mortality and all-cause hospitalizations (20% reduction at 14 months, $P < 0.02$).

Cardiac Resynchronization in Heart Failure (CARE-HF) (26) trial was unique in its utilization of advanced echocardiographic methods for inclusion. Patients with moderately wide increased QRS (120 to 149 ms) were required to have additional echocardiographic evidence of ventricular dyssynchrony (see later in this section). Those with markedly wide increased QRS ($\geq$150 ms) were included without such echocardiographic requirements. Results from CARE-HF demonstrated that CRT was associated with a 37% relative decrease in combined all-cause mortality, or unplanned cardiovascular hospitalization. Heart failure hospitalizations were reduced, and quality of life scores were also improved.

In summary, inclusion criteria and results from several randomized clinical trials demonstrate that CRT is appropriate for patients with systolic dysfunction (EF $\leq$35%), class III to IV HF despite maximal medical management, sinus rhythm, and QRS width $\geq$120 ms (Table 21-8). One suggested algorithm for selecting candidates for CRT-D is given in Figure 21-3.

NONINVASIVE IMAGING OF PATIENTS UNDERGOING CRT

Based on the early clinical experience with CRT, several important issues emerged. First, a significant proportion of CRT device implantations was unsuccessful. In trials, this proportion was 5% to 13%, and may have been initially higher in the routine clinical setting. Second, anatomic variations in the coronary veins precluded advancement of the lead into a lateral vein in many patients. These patients benefitted from cardiothoracic surgery referral for epicardial lead placement. Third,

TABLE 21-8

RECOMMENDATIONS FOR USE OF CARDIAC RESYNCHRONIZATION THERAPY IN PATIENTS WITH CONGESTIVE HEART FAILURE

Patient Characteristics
NYHA class III or IV heart failure, receiving optimal medical therapy
LVEF $\leq$35%
Stable sinus rhythm
QRS duration $\geq$130 ms
LV end-diastolic diameter $\geq$55 mm
No expected improvement from coronary revascularization or valve surgery

although many patients enjoyed improvement in their HF symptoms following CRT, up to 30% of patients failed to improve (27), and thus require reprogramming of their device and/or escalation of medical therapy. Therefore, the current goals of noninvasive imaging prior to CRT implantation are (a) to identify patients in whom transvenous approach to CRT is precluded by anatomy, (b) to reduce the number of unnecessary implants by identifying potential "nonresponders" to CRT prior to the procedure, (c) to guide optimization of device programming following device implantation, and (d) to identify reasons for failure to improve following device implantation. Another future goal may be identification of patients who are not candidates for CRT based on the electrocardiographic criteria, but in whom significant mechanical dyssynchrony may nevertheless be present.

Echocardiography for Assessment of Dyssynchrony

The most basic manifestation of ventricular dyssynchrony is a wide QRS complex on a surface ECG. Nevertheless, the sensitivity of QRS width to predict a benefit for BiV pacing in an individual patient is low (28).

Echocardiography has emerged as a relatively simple, noninvasive tool for assessment of ventricular dyssynchrony (Table 21-9). Using M-mode imaging, delayed activation of the inferolateral LV wall is identified as septal-to-posterior wall motion delay $\geq$130 ms (29). Aortic pre-ejection period (PEP_{ao}) is defined as the time between the onset of QRS on ECG to aortic valve opening, and is considered abnormal when it exceeds 140 ms (26). Pulmonic PEP (PEP_{pulm}) measurement is analogous to that of PEP_{ao}. Difference between PEP_{pulm} and PEP_{ao} of >40 ms is termed interventricular mechanical delay (IVMD), indicates a delayed activation of right ventricle, and is a convenient measure of interventricular dyssynchrony (26).

Tissue synchronization imaging (TSI) is a newer echocardiographic modality, which utilizes low-velocity tissue Doppler information. Using TSI, segments of myocardium are color-coded according to time-to-peak tissue systolic velocities. These temporal data are superimposed on 2D echo images, and segments of dyssynchrony are thus visualized in real time. Delay in contraction between any two segments of myocardium can be easily demonstrated and quantified (Fig. 21-4). In particular, opposing wall delay of >64 ms has been used as a marker of intraventricular dyssynchrony (30). Finally, a more comprehensive "Global Asynchrony Index" (GAI) uses information from 12 myocardial segments to derive a standard deviation of contraction delay. A GAI of >33 ms has been shown to predict improvement in reverse LV remodeling, NYHA HF class, and quality of life following CRT (31).

Of all the large clinical trials of CRT to date, only CARE-HF used echocardiography to enroll patients with dyssynchrony. To be enrolled in that trial, patients with QRS width 120 to 149 ms had to satisfy at least two of three dyssynchrony criteria: (a) PEP_{ao} >140 ms, (b) IVMD >40 ms, and (c) delayed activation of the inferolateral LV wall (30).

Echocardiography to Aid Optimization of Biventricular Devices Following Implantation

Optimal AV interval in a patient with an implanted HF device should permit ventricular systole to occur following maximum, undisturbed ventricular diastole. Optimal AV delay is noted on echocardiography, when the end of transmitral A-wave coincides with the complete mitral valve closure. If AV interval is too short, "cannon A-waves" may result, whereas inappro-

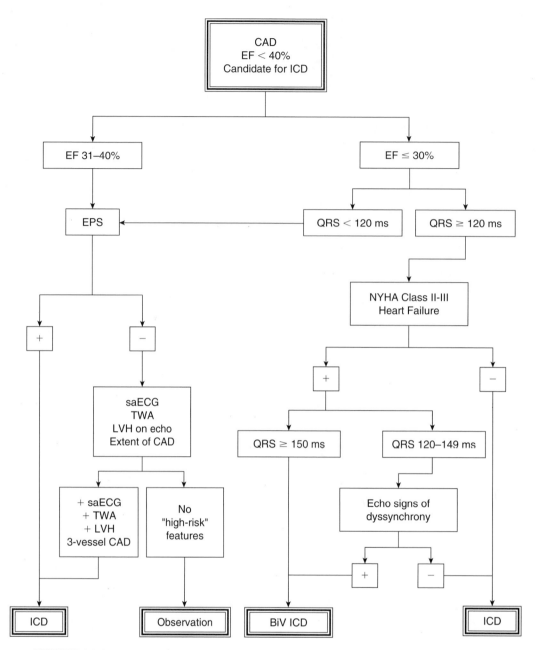

FIGURE 21-3. A sample decision tree regarding implantation of ICD or CRT device in a patient with an established ischemic cardiomyopathy. BiV, biventricular; CAD, coronary artery disease; echo, echocardiogram; LVH, left ventricular hypertrophy; saECG, signal-averaged ECG; TWA, microvolt T-wave alternans.

TABLE 21-9

SELECTED ECHOCARDIOGRAPHIC SIGNS OF VENTRICULAR DYSSYNCHRONY

Parameter	Echocardiographic sign	Abnormal value
Septal to posterior wall motion delay (29)	M-mode	≥130 ms
Peak opposing wall delay (30)	Tissue synchronization imaging	>64 ms
Global 12-segment asynchrony index (40)	Tissue synchronization imaging	>33 ms
Aortic pre-ejection interval (26)	Doppler imaging	>140 ms
Interventricular mechanical delay (26)	Doppler imaging	>40 ms

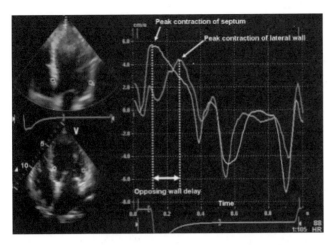

FIGURE 21-4. Tissue synchronization imaging (TSI). Shown is a fragment of a still frame of the left ventricle, taken in the apical four-chamber view. Delayed contraction of the lateral wall as compared to the inferior septum is visually apparent as an area of different color. Opposing wall contraction delay is then quantitatively demonstrated as the difference in time-to-peak systolic velocities between the lateral wall and septum.

priately long AV intervals produce diastolicmitral regurgitation and worsen symptoms of HF. Modified Ritter method of AV optimization calls for temporary programming of the device to a long AV interval (AVlong >250 ms) (32,33). Interval t is then measured from transmitral continuous wave Doppler as time between the end of A-wave and the beginning of mitral regurgitation. "Optimal" AV interval is then programmed as AVopt = AVlong − t.

Optimization of RV/LV contraction sequence is less well defined (34), and further prospective studies are necessary before definite recommendations are given. One echocardiography-guided approach includes trials of RV and LV preactivation, with measurement of transaortic time-velocity integral (TVIao, a surrogate of cardiac output) 2 to 3 minutes following each programming change. A setting that results in the highest TVIao is then considered "optimal."

Multislice Computed Tomography

Recent reports demonstrate feasibility of using multislice (16-slice) computed tomography (MSCT) to image coronary vein anatomy (19,35). Using this technique, one could identify obstruction within the cardiac veins, such as ostial coronary sinus narrowing by a thebesian valve, and presence or absence of suitable venous tributaries overlying the site of latest LV activation. This technique has the limitations of requiring iodinated

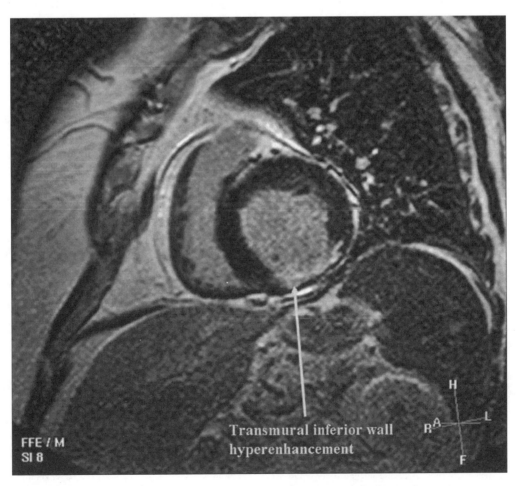

FIGURE 21-5. Myocardial scar demonstration by contrast-enhanced cardiovascular magnetic resonance. Gadolinium contrast is injected intravenously, and images are obtained 10 to 15 minutes later. With this technique, normal myocardium appears dark, whereas scar tissue demonstrates high signal intensity.

contrast and exposing the patient to additional ionizing radiation beyond that expected during fluoroscopy-guided device implantation.

Cardiovascular Magnetic Resonance: A Comprehensive Noninvasive Modality

Success of resynchronization therapy depends on the ability of the ventricular myocardium at the site of latest intrinsic activation to respond to the pacing stimulus. If that area is extensively scarred, usually as a result of a previous transmural MI, resynchronization may not be achieved. Gadolinium-enhanced cardiovascular magnetic resonance (CMR) is able to provide precise information on the location and transmurality of the scar Fig. 21-5) (36). It does so noninvasively, without the use of iodinated contrast or ionizing radiation. In addition, CMR is a noninvasive gold standard for assessment of LV volumes, dimensions, function, and ventricular mass and is an excellent modality for imaging patients with regional LV dysfunction. Strain-encoded MRI (SENC) requires little image processing and provides instantaneous information on longitudinal and radial ventricular strain (37). Ultimately, CMR may prove to be the single modality for comprehensive assessment of HF patients, who may be candidates for CRT. Limitations of CMR include relatively long image acquisition times and its inability to image patients with the current generation of implanted devices.

References

1. Hunt SA, Abraham WT, Chin MH, et al. ACC/AHA 2005 Guideline Update for the Diagnosis and Management of Chronic Heart Failure in the Adult: a report of the American College of Cardiology/American Heart Association Task Force on Practice Guidelines (Writing Committee to Update the 2001 Guidelines for the Evaluation and Management of Heart Failure): developed in collaboration with the American College of Chest Physicians and the International Society for Heart and Lung Transplantation: endorsed by the Heart Rhythm Society. Circulation 2005;112:154–235.
2. Jauhar S, Slotwiner DJ. The economics of ICDs. N Engl J Med 2004;351:2542–2544.
3. Smith HJ, Fearnot NE, Byrd CL, et al. Five-years experience with intravascular lead extraction. U.S. Lead Extraction Database. Pacing Clin Electrophysiol 1994;17:2016–2020.
4. The Antiarrhythmics versus Implantable Defibrillators (AVID) Investigators. A comparison of antiarrhythmic-drug therapy with implantable defibrillators in patients resuscitated from near-fatal ventricular arrhythmias. N Engl J Med 1997;337:1576–1584.
5. Connolly SJ, Gent M, Roberts RS, et al. Canadian implantable defibrillator study (CIDS): a randomized trial of the implantable cardioverter defibrillator against amiodarone. Circulation 2000;101:1297–1302.
6. Kuck KH, Cappato R, Siebels J, et al. Randomized comparison of antiarrhythmic drug therapy with implantable defibrillators in patients resuscitated from cardiac arrest: the Cardiac Arrest Study Hamburg (CASH). Circulation 2000;102:748–754.
7. Bokhari F, Newman D, Greene M, et al. Long-term comparison of the implantable cardioverter defibrillator versus amiodarone: eleven-year follow-up of a subset of patients in the Canadian Implantable Defibrillator Study (CIDS). Circulation 2004;110:112–116.
8. Connolly SJ, Hallstrom AP, Cappato R, et al. Meta-analysis of the implantable cardioverter defibrillator secondary prevention trials. AVID, CASH and CIDS studies. Antiarrhythmics vs implantable defibrillator study. Cardiac Arrest Study Hamburg. Canadian Implantable Defibrillator Study. Eur Heart J 2000;21:2071–2078.
9. Caffrey SL, Willoughby PJ, Pepe PE, et al. Public use of automated external defibrillators. N Engl J Med 2002;347:1242–1247.
10. Moss AJ, Hall WJ, Cannom DS, et al. Improved survival with an implanted defibrillator in patients with coronary disease at high risk for ventricular arrhythmia. Multicenter Automatic Defibrillator Implantation Trial Investigators. N Engl J Med 1996;335:1933–1940.
11. Buxton AE, Lee KL, Fisher JD, et al. A randomized study of the prevention of sudden death in patients with coronary artery disease. Multicenter Unsustained Tachycardia Trial Investigators. N Engl J Med 1999;341:1882–1890.
12. Moss AJ, Zareba W, Hall WJ, et al. Prophylactic implantation of a defibrillator in patients with myocardial infarction and reduced ejection fraction. N Engl J Med 2002;346:877–883.
13. Hohnloser SH, Kuck KH, Dorian P, et al. Prophylactic use of an implantable cardioverter-defibrillator after acute myocardial infarction. N Engl J Med 2004;351:2481–2488.
14. Kadish A, Dyer A, Daubert JP, et al. Prophylactic defibrillator implantation in patients with nonischemic dilated cardiomyopathy. N Engl J Med 2004;350:2151–2158.
15. Bardy GH, Lee KL, Mark DB, et al. Amiodarone or an implantable cardioverter-defibrillator for congestive heart failure. N Engl J Med 2005;352:225–237.
16. Shamim W, Francis DP, Yousufuddin M, et al. Intraventricular conduction delay: a prognostic marker in chronic heart failure. Int J Cardiol 1999;70:171–178.
17. Baldasseroni S, Opasich C, Gorini M, et al. Left bundle-branch block is associated with increased 1-year sudden and total mortality rate in 5517 outpatients with congestive heart failure: a report from the Italian network on congestive heart failure. Am Heart J 2002;143:398–405.
18. Wilkoff BL, Cook JR, Epstein AE, et al. Dual-chamber pacing or ventricular backup pacing in patients with an implantable defibrillator: the Dual Chamber and VVI Implantable Defibrillator (DAVID) Trial. JAMA 2002;288:3115–323.
19. Jongbloed MR, Lamb HJ, Bax JJ, et al. Noninvasive visualization of the cardiac venous system using multislice computed tomography. J Am Coll Cardiol 2005;45:749–753.
20. Stellbrink C, Breithardt OA, Franke A, et al. Impact of cardiac resynchronization therapy using hemodynamically optimized pacing on left ventricular remodeling in patients with congestive heart failure and ventricular conduction disturbances. J Am Coll Cardiol 2001;38:1957–1965.
21. Cazeau S, Leclercq C, Lavergne T, et al. Effects of multisite biventricular pacing in patients with heart failure and intraventricular conduction delay. N Engl J Med 2001;344:873–880.
22. Abraham WT, Fisher WG, Smith AL, et al. Cardiac resynchronization in chronic heart failure. N Engl J Med 2002;346:1845–1853.
23. Young JB, Abraham WT, Smith AL, et al. Combined cardiac resynchronization and implantable cardioversion defibrillation in advanced chronic heart failure: the MIRACLE ICD Trial. JAMA 2003;289:2685–2694.
24. Higgins SL, Hummel JD, Niazi IK, et al. Cardiac resynchronization therapy for the treatment of heart failure in patients with intraventricular conduction delay and malignant ventricular tachyarrhythmias. J Am Coll Cardiol 2003;42:1454–1459.
25. Bristow MR, Saxon LA, Boehmer J, et al. Cardiac-resynchronization therapy with or without an implantable defibrillator in advanced chronic heart failure. N Engl J Med 2004;350:2140–2150.
26. Cleland JG, Daubert JC, Erdmann E, et al. The effect of cardiac resynchronization on morbidity and mortality in heart failure. N Engl J Med 2005;352:1539–1549.
27. Kass DA. Ventricular resynchronization: pathophysiology and identification of responders. Rev Cardiovasc Med 2003;4(Suppl 2):S3–S13.
28. Ansalone G, Giannantoni P, Ricci R, et al. Biventricular pacing in heart failure: back to basics in the pathophysiology of left bundle branch block to reduce the number of nonresponders. Am J Cardiol 2003;91:55F–61F.
29. Pitzalis MV, Iacoviello M, Romito R, et al. Ventricular asynchrony predicts a better outcome in patients with chronic heart failure receiving cardiac resynchronization therapy. J Am Coll Cardiol 2005;45:65–69.
30. Gorcsan J 3rd, Kanzaki H, Bazaz R, et al. Usefulness of echocardiographic tissue synchronization imaging to predict acute response to cardiac resynchronization therapy. Am J Cardiol 2004;93:1178–1181.
31. Yu CM, Fung WH, Lin H, et al. Predictors of left ventricular reverse remodeling after cardiac resynchronization therapy for heart failure secondary to idiopathic dilated or ischemic cardiomyopathy. Am J Cardiol 2003;91:684–688.
32. Ritter P, Dib JC, Lelievre T. Quick determination of the optimal AV delay at rest in patients paced in DDD mode for complete AV block. (abstract). Eur J CPE 1994;4:A163.
33. Meluzin J, Novak M, Mullerova J, et al. A fast and simple echocardiographic method of determination of the optimal atrioventricular delay in patients after biventricular stimulation. Pacing Clin Electrophysiol 2004;27:58–64.
34. Porciani MC, Dondina C, Macioce R, et al. Echocardiographic examination of atrioventricular and interventricular delay optimization in cardiac resynchronization therapy. Am J Cardiol 2005;95:1108–1110.
35. Abbara S, Cury RC, Nieman K, et al. Noninvasive evaluation of cardiac veins with 16-MDCT angiography. AJR Am J Roentgenol 2005;185:1001–1006.
36. Kim RJ, Wu E, Rafael A, et al. The use of contrast-enhanced magnetic resonance imaging to identify reversible myocardial dysfunction. N Engl J Med 2000;343:1445–1453.
37. Osman NF, Sampath S, Atalar E, et al. Imaging longitudinal cardiac strain on short-axis images using strain-encoded MRI. Magn Reson Med 2001;46:324–334.

38. Ukkonen H, Beanlands RS, Burwash IG, et al. Effect of cardiac resynchronization on myocardial efficiency and regional oxidative metabolism. *Circulation* 2003;107:28–31.

39. Saxon LA, De Marco T, Schafer J, et al. Effects of long-term biventricular stimulation for resynchronization on echocardiographic measures of remodeling. *Circulation* 2002;105:1304–1310.

40. Yu CM, Chau E, Sanderson JE, et al. Tissue Doppler echocardiographic evidence of reverse remodeling and improved synchronicity by simultaneously delaying regional contraction after biventricular pacing therapy in heart failure. *Circulation* 2002;105:438–445.

41. Abraham WT, Young JB, Leon AR, et al. Effects of cardiac resynchronization on disease progression in patients with left ventricular systolic dysfunction, an indication for an implantable cardioverter-defibrillator, and mildly symptomatic chronic heart failure. *Circulation* 2004;110:2864–2868.

CHAPTER 22 ■ VENOUS THROMBOEMBOLISM

SAMUEL Z. GOLDHABER

EPIDEMIOLOGY
DIAGNOSIS
Deep Vein Thrombosis
Pulmonary Embolism
INITIAL THERAPY
Deep Vein Thrombosis
Pulmonary Embolism
Embolectomy
ORAL ANTICOAGULANT THERAPY
Warfarin
PREVENTION
CONCLUSIONS

Venous thromboembolism (VTE) encompasses both deep vein thrombosis (DVT) and pulmonary embolism (PE). Diagnosis, management, and prevention of VTE can be standardized and adapted to critical pathways.

Cardiologists need to be adept in detecting DVT and in managing complicated cases that require catheter-directed thrombolysis, mechanical thrombectomy, or placement of an inferior vena caval filter. Furthermore, cardiologists should set the standard for recommending and implementing prophylaxis among their hospitalized patients and among patients on whom they consult preoperatively.

Cardiologists are often summoned to help diagnose suspected PE because of their familiarity with the differential diagnosis of chest pain and dyspnea, their ability to recognize clinical manifestations of acute pulmonary hypertension, and their facility with echocardiography for risk stratification. The cardiologist is often the specialist asked to manage high-risk patients with thrombolysis and, if necessary, suction catheter embolectomy. The cardiologist may also serve as the liaison with the cardiac surgeon who is summoned to perform urgent open surgical embolectomy.

EPIDEMIOLOGY

VTE is the third most common cardiovascular disease, after acute coronary syndrome and stroke (1). VTE spans a wide age range, from teenagers to the elderly. It strikes all socioeconomic groups in developed Western countries. However, rates of VTE in Japan are quickly catching up to those in North America and Europe (2).

Factor V Leiden is an autosomal dominant single-point genetic mutation that increases the likelihood of developing DVT or PE (3,4). This mutation also contributes to placental vein thrombosis and is associated with otherwise unexplained first trimester pregnancy losses (5). Racially, factor V Leiden is most commonly found in Caucasians, especially Northern Europe-

ans (6). The mutation expresses itself with clinical venous thrombosis more frequently as patients age (7). Although factor V Leiden is the most thoroughly studied hereditary thrombophilia, other mutations with similar effects have been described, such as the prothrombin gene mutation (8–10).

Acquired risk factors warrant attention (11). These include long-haul air travel, women's health issues (oral contraceptives, pregnancy, and hormone replacement therapy), obesity, cigarette smoking, hypertension, increasing age, and cancer. Certain combinations of genetic and acquired risk factors lead to a markedly increased likelihood of thrombosis, such as oral contraceptives in the setting of factor V Leiden.

Sorting out the contributions of heredity versus environment remains challenging. Widespread genetic testing will rarely change the management of patients with thromboembolic disease. Future studies will define more precisely the interaction between genetic thrombophilia and acquired risk factors for thrombosis.

For those who survive, DVT may result in lifelong disability with painful and disfiguring venous insufficiency of the legs. Chronic leg swelling, bulging varicose veins, and occasional ulceration may ensue, along with brownish skin discoloration at the medial malleolus. Venous insufficiency is surprisingly common. It can develop in as many as one-third of patients who have DVT. Often, it becomes apparent as a late complication, years after the initial thrombotic event.

Acute PE patients may develop chronic thromboembolic pulmonary hypertension within 6 weeks to several years. Chronic thromboembolic disease develops about 4% of the time (12). This is an upward revision from previous estimates of 1 in 500 cases. This devastating complication can cause profound dyspnea and lifestyle limitation that precludes ordinary walking and working outside the home. Patients with pulmonary hypertension are susceptible to sudden cardiac death and must cope with dyspnea at rest as well as with exertion.

There is also a huge psychological burden for many patients with VTE. They often are young and appear otherwise healthy. Yet their lifestyle is impaired by the constraints of long-term anticoagulation. They wonder whether their children or siblings will suddenly develop DVT or PE. Also, for those who discontinue anticoagulation, they can never be certain about whether VTE will recur.

VTE is underdiagnosed because it is often asymptomatic. The best clue to detection may be the clinical setting and assessment of predisposing risk factors (13). These include: "medical risk factors" such as prior VTE, cancer, surgery, trauma, bedrest, or immobilization, which are beyond control of the patient (Table 22-1), as well as "environmental factors," such as obesity, cigarette smoking, hypertension, oral contraceptives, pregnancy, hormone replacement therapy, and long-haul air travel (Table 22-2).

VTE is often a chronic illness. Overall, about 30% will suf-

TABLE 22-1

MEDICAL RISK FACTORS

1. Prior venous thromboembolism
2. Cancer and/or cancer chemotherapy
3. Surgery or trauma
4. Bedrest or immobilization

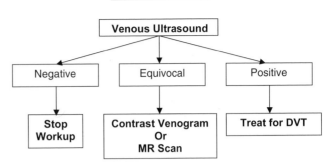

FIGURE 22-1. DVT diagnosis.

fer recurrence over the ensuing 10 years unless anticoagulation is continued.

DIAGNOSIS

Deep Vein Thrombosis

Figure 22-1 summarizes a critical pathway for DVT diagnosis. For DVT patients, the most common chief complaint is a cramp or "charley horse" in the lower calf that does not abate and gradually worsens after several days. Discomfort, at first intermittent, becomes persistent. Swelling may then ensue. Occasionally, erythema accompanies the leg edema. Erythema often suggests concomitant superficial venous phlebitis with saphenous vein involvement or coexisting cellulitis.

Unexplained arm edema may herald the presence of upper extremity DVT (14,15). This condition occurs most commonly in two divergent and contrasting populations: (a) as a complication of a chronic indwelling central venous catheter, or (b) in otherwise healthy individuals who have been exerting themselves with activities such as weight lifting.

Do not immediately jump to the diagnosis of DVT. Keep in mind the need to maintain a differential diagnosis (Table 22-3). Sudden, excruciating calf discomfort is most likely due to a ruptured Baker's cyst. Fever and chills usually suggest cellulitis rather than DVT, though DVT may be present concomitantly.

When detected early after onset, the physical findings of DVT may be minimal, consisting of mild palpation discomfort in the lower calf. If the DVT propagates proximally because it is not recognized at an early stage, one might find massive thigh swelling and marked tenderness when palpating the inguinal area over the course of the femoral vein. Such patients often have difficulty walking and may require a cane, crutches, or a walker. If a patient has upper-extremity venous thrombosis, there may be asymmetry in the supraclavicular fossae or in the girth of the upper arms. There may also be a prominent superficial venous pattern over the anterior chest wall.

If the leg is diffusely edematous, DVT is unlikely. Much more common is an acute exacerbation of venous insufficiency due to postphlebitic syndrome.

When DVT is suspected, it is useful to estimate the clinical likelihood that DVT will be the final diagnosis. Clinical probability can be estimated using the formal Wells DVT Scoring System (16), but this approach is rarely used. Much more common is to estimate the likelihood by *gestalt*.

A few institutions, especially in Europe, favor stopping the DVT workup if the clinical probability is low and a D-dimer enzyme-linked immunosorbent assay (ELISA) is normal and not elevated. However, at most institutions in the United States, including Brigham and Women's Hospital (BWH), we image with venous ultrasonography virtually all patients suspected of DVT. Of particular importance is proper interpretation of the ultrasound report. Unfortunately, the distal portion of the deep femoral vein is called the "superficial femoral vein." Even though **superficial** is part of the name of this vein, it is a **deep vein**, and patients with **superficial femoral vein thrombosis** should be treated for DVT. They should not be discharged home with the misdiagnosis of superficial thrombophlebitis. "Superficial femoral vein thrombosis" can be a lethal misnomer (17).

Usually, the venous ultrasound examination is definitive in detecting or excluding DVT in the large upper extremity veins as well as the deep veins from the common femoral proximally to the calf veins distally (18). Occasionally, the imaging test is equivocal because of the patient's body habitus, recent leg trauma or surgery, or profound edema that limits compression of vascular structures. Under these circumstances, consider pursuing other imaging (19).

Magnetic resonance imaging (MRI) can provide surprisingly precise, detailed information about the venous system. MRI is especially useful in assessing suspected pelvic vein thrombosis and in defining the extent of upper extremity vein

TABLE 22-2

ENVIRONMENTAL RISK FACTORS

1. Obesity
2. Cigarette smoking
3. Hypertension
4. Oral contraceptives, pregnancy, hormone replacement therapy
5. Long-haul air travel

TABLE 22-3

DIFFERENTIAL DIAGNOSIS OF DVT

1. DVT
2. Superficial thrombophlebitis
3. Ruptured Baker's cyst
4. Cellulitis
5. Venous insufficiency/postphlebitic syndrome

thrombosis (20). MRI can also help estimate the age of thrombus based on various "spin" characteristics of the image (21).

Invasive contrast venography (22) is rarely performed nowadays as a diagnostic test. Of necessity, invasive contrast venography is the first step when catheter intervention is planned with catheter-directed thrombolysis, suction embolectomy, angioplasty, or stenting.

Pulmonary Embolism

Figure 22-2 summarizes a critical pathway for PE diagnosis. Unexplained dyspnea and chest pain, often pleuritic, are the most common symptoms of PE. The Wells Scoring System for PE enjoys more popularity than the DVT Scoring System. However, I have never had a patient presented to me with incorporation of the Wells Scoring System unless I asked for it to be included. This Canadian system is used for clinical research purposes, so it is worth knowing. Nevertheless, *gestalt* is by far the most common way that clinical probability of PE is estimated.

The Wells Scoring System (23) is a point system where low probability for PE is less than 2 points, moderate probability is 2 to 6 points, and high probability is greater than 6 points. Seven variables comprised the point score: (a) clinical symptoms of DVT (3 points), (b) no alternative diagnosis (3 points), (c) heart rate greater than 100 beats per minute (1.5 points), (d) immobilization or surgery within the prior 4 weeks (1.5 points), (e) previous DVT or PE (1.5 points), (f) hemoptysis (1 point), and (g) cancer (1 point). The variable "no alternative diagnosis" is controversial because it is subjective, not objective, and is the "driving force" that makes the Wells Score an accurate predictor of the presence of absence of PE (24).

In a prospective observational study at BWH's Emergency Department, there was a trend toward increasing accuracy of PE diagnosis with increasing clinical experience (25). However, the difference was not as great between an intern and an attending physician as one might have expected. Physicians were asked whether they thought PE was the most likely diagnosis. The frequency of true-positive assessments was 17% for interns and 25% for attending physicians.

Keep in mind that only about 10% of patients who undergo emergency imaging for PE actually have PE. Therefore, the astute clinician will formulate a differential diagnosis (Table 22-4), even when the manifestations of PE seem obvious.

The "classic findings" such as tachycardia, tachypnea, or hypotension actually represent unusual patients with extensive PE and impaired compensatory mechanisms. With improved imaging modalities, PE is with increasing frequency identified in normotensive patients who may appear anxious, but whose heart rate is less than 100 beats per minute and whose respiratory rate, if actually counted inconspicuously, is less than 16 breaths per minute.

TABLE 22-4

ADJUNCTIVE MEASURES FOR DVT MANAGEMENT

1. Obtain family history and consider hypercoagulable workup.
2. Prescribe below-knee vascular compression stockings, 20 to 30 or 30 to 40 mm Hg, to prevent venous insufficiency.
3. Provide emotional support.
4. Educate re: LMWH and warfarin.
5. Offer Web addresses of educational sites: www.preventdvt.org.
6. Explain controversy concerning optimal duration of anticoagulation.

Electrocardiography

All patients suspected of PE undergo electrocardiography (26). Although new-onset atrial fibrillation/flutter and a new "S1Q3T3" sign are often cited as helpful clues, these findings are rare. The most common manifestation of right heart strain is T wave inversion in leads V1 to V4 (27).

Chest X-Ray

The chest x-ray (28) is useful for establishing alternative diagnoses such as pneumonia, congestive heart failure, or pneumothorax. PE patients may, however, present with an entirely normal chest x-ray.

Blood Tests

Arterial blood gases are unreliable and can be misleading (29,30). Specifically, patients who are otherwise healthy can present with large PE and yet maintain a high arterial PO_2 and a normal arterial-alveolar oxygen gradient.

The only useful blood screening test is the plasma D-dimer ELISA (31). D-dimers are released in the presence of PE because

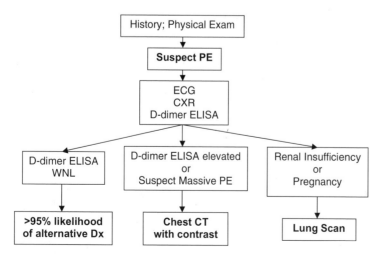

FIGURE 22-2. PE diagnosis.

of endogenous fibrinolysis. Plasmin dissolves some of the fibrin clot from PE, and subsequently, D-dimers are released into the plasma. The D-dimers can be recognized by commercially available monoclonal antibodies. The D-dimer ELISA has a high negative predictive value for PE. This means that if the D-dimer ELISA is normal, it is extremely unlikely that PE is present (32).

D-dimers are highly sensitive for the diagnosis of PE. This high sensitivity is crucially important in a screening test. However, D-dimers are nonspecific and will often be elevated in conditions that mimic PE such as acute myocardial infarction or pneumonia. They are also elevated in patients with cancer, in second or third trimester pregnancy, and in the postoperative state. Plasma D-dimer levels are usually elevated in hospitalized patients. Therefore, their contribution to diagnosis is greatest in outpatients suspected of PE; their use among hospitalized patients is minimal because the test results are rarely normal.

Imaging Tests

If the D-dimer ELISA is elevated, the next step is to order computed tomographic (CT) scanning of the chest. Chest CT scanning has revolutionized our diagnostic approach to suspected PE. By 2001, CT scanning was being used more often than lung scanning to investigate suspected PE (33). The clinical validity of using a CT scan to rule out PE is similar to that reported for conventional pulmonary angiography (34). This technology has evolved rapidly. The latest generation of scanners can diagnose submillimeter PE in sixth-order vessels. These thrombi are so tiny that their clinical significance is uncertain (35).

Chest CT scanning provides a satisfying dichotomous "yes" or "no" answer to whether PE is present. The CT examination can help identify the source of the clots in the legs, pelvis, or upper extremity. When PE is not present, the CT scan can help diagnose alternative pulmonary illnesses such as pneumonia, cancer, and interstitial lung diseases not apparent on the chest x-ray. The major limitation of chest CT scanning is the need to administer intravenous contrast.

Lung scanning has been the standard noninvasive imaging test for patients suspected of PE. It is highly specific when there is high probability for PE but it is not sensitive. Based on the Prospective Investigation of Pulmonary Embolism Diagnosis (PIOPED), more than half of the patients with PE proven by angiography had non-high probability lung scans (36). The principal disadvantage of lung scanning is that the majority of the scans are of intermediate probability for PE and frustrate the clinician because they do not provide a clear-cut answer to the diagnostic dilemma of whether PE is present.

When the lung scan is equivocal, leg vein ultrasonography may be helpful. If the venous ultrasound demonstrates DVT, this usually suffices as a surrogate for PE and the diagnostic workup can stop at this point. However, it is crucial to understand that as many as half of patients with PE will have no evidence of DVT, probably because the clot has already embolized to the lungs (37).

With a multislice CT scanner and a technologically adequate examination, the diagnosis of PE should be considered "ruled out" if the chest CT is negative (38). If a single-slice CT scanner shows no evidence of PE, it is still possible that multiple subsegmental PEs are present. Therefore, if clinical suspicion remains high, and if there is no access to a multislice CT scanner, and if a lung scan is equivocal, then invasive contrast pulmonary angiography should be considered (39).

MRI (40) is promising because it can combine imaging of the pulmonary arteries with functional and structural assessment of the right ventricle. MRI is also an excellent alternative among patients who are poor candidates for receiving intravenous contrast agent because of renal insufficiency or contrast

dye allergy. For now, though, this technology is not sufficiently "mature" to be placed on a diagnosis critical pathway.

INITIAL THERAPY

Deep Vein Thrombosis

The treatment of DVT has changed dramatically. DVT management used to require a 5-day hospitalization with intravenous unfractionated heparin administered as a bridge to warfarin. The administration of intravenous heparin required an initial intravenous bolus followed by a continuous infusion. The dose was titrated to achieve an activated partial thromboplastin time (aPTT) two to three times control (41). Generally, this corresponded to an aPTT between 60 and 80 seconds.

This standard approach to therapy was problematic. First, most patients were underdosed with heparin so that it required 24 to 48 hours to achieve therapeutic levels. There would be multiple changes in the dose of the continuous intravenous heparin infusion, based on emergency ("STAT") aPTT values. These changes in dosing often led to medication errors (42). They were also extremely inconvenient and required additional physician and nurse time, often in the middle of the night. Although a robotic dosing system has been successfully tested (43), the need for traditional heparin appears to be limited to patients who are massively obese or in renal failure or who have an abhorrence of injections. Exposure to unfractionated heparin also increased the possibility of developing heparin-induced thrombocytopenia (44).

Now, however, most patients receive acute DVT treatment as outpatients or with an overnight hospital stay. In the United States, immediate anticoagulation is usually achieved with the low-molecular-weight heparin enoxaparin. This strategy is safe (45) and cost effective (46). Other U.S. Food and Drug Administration (FDA)-approved regimens include the low-molecular-weight heparin tinzaparin and the anti-Xa pentasaccharide fondaparinux.

Enoxaparin has received FDA approval for DVT treatment, as a "bridge" to warfarin because of its superior efficacy and safety compared with unfractionated heparin. Low-molecular-weight heparin is administered as a fixed dose according to weight (1 mg/kg twice daily or, among hospitalized patients, 1.5 mg/kg once daily) and is cost effective because no routine laboratory testing is required. It has become the foundation of anticoagulation of DVT patients and can facilitate complete outpatient treatment of this disease among properly selected patients.

Like low-molecular-weight heparin, fondaparinux is administered by subcutaneous injection, and no laboratory monitoring is required (47). Fondaparinux requires a once daily subcutaneous injection, requires only one of three possible doses based on weight, and has never been reported to cause heparin-induced thrombocytopenia. For fondaparinux, patients weighing less than 50 kg receive 5 mg, 50-kg to 100-kg patients receive 7.5 mg, and patients weighing more than 100 kg receive 10 mg. The drug is available in prefilled syringes of 5 mg, 7.5 mg, or 10 mg.

Even those patients who require prolonged hospitalization (Fig. 22-3) can usually be managed with low-molecular-weight heparin or fondaparinux until they achieve a stable and therapeutic level of warfarin, based upon a target International Normalized Ratio (INR) of 2.0 to 3.0. Overlap with the "bridging" anticoagulant should continue until two INRs are obtained in the therapeutic range. The success of an anticoagulation critical pathway depends primarily on reliable dosing and monitoring of warfarin. However, adjunctive measures for DVT management are also of paramount importance (Table 22-4).

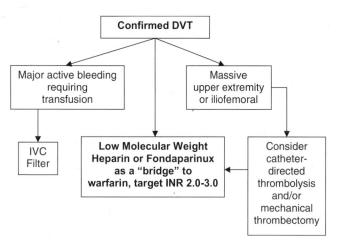

FIGURE 22-3. DVT treatment.

Direct Thrombin Inhibitors

For patients with suspected or proven heparin-induced thrombocytopenia, neither unfractionated heparin nor low-molecular-weight heparin can be safely administered. The only FDA-approved alternative is the use of direct thrombin inhibitors, either argatroban or lepirudin (48). Argatroban, metabolized primarily by the liver, is particularly useful for patients with renal insufficiency. Lepirudin, metabolized primarily by the kidneys, is particularly useful for patients with hepatic dysfunction.

Catheter-Directed Interventions

The indications for DVT thrombolysis are uncertain and controversial (49). DVT thrombolysis should theoretically restore venous valve patency and function, thereby preventing the development of venous insufficiency and the postthrombotic syndrome. However, this hypothesis has not been proven. In addition, DVT thrombolysis may be especially useful in patients who have developed an upper-extremity thrombosis due to a long-term indwelling central venous catheter. For example, a patient may require completion of additional courses of chemotherapy or may need intravenous hyperalimentation.

At BWH, we advise DVT catheter-directed thrombolysis for young, otherwise healthy patients who have massive iliofemoral DVT with marked leg swelling, leg tenderness, and difficulty walking (Fig. 22-3). For patients with large DVT who require intervention in addition to anticoagulation, a combina-

tion of catheter-directed thrombolysis and catheter-assisted thrombectomy is usually utilized.

Chronic Venous Insufficiency

Venous insufficiency can first become clinically apparent several years after the initial DVT (50). The pathophysiological explanation is damage to the venous valves of the legs. Late onset of venous insufficiency is a separate problem from recurrent DVT. Wearing 30- to 40-mm Hg below-knee vascular compression stockings while ambulatory has proved effective in randomized clinical trials (51). Prescribing vascular compression stockings will halve the rate of subsequent venous insufficiency.

Emotional Support

Many patients with VTE will appear healthy and fit. They may be burdened with fear about the possible genetic implications of DVT or PE. They will often feel overwhelmed when advised to continue lifelong anticoagulation. Patients in whom anticoagulation is discontinued after 3 to 6 months of therapy may feel vulnerable to a future recurrent VTE. In addition, family, friends, and peers might not understand the implications of DVT or PE. My nurse and I help provide emotional support by running a support group one evening every third week. We and our patients have also written responses to Frequently Asked Questions, which we posted on the following Web site: http://web.mit.edu/karen/www/faq.html.

Pulmonary Embolism

Risk Stratification

The clinical spectrum and severity of PE is wide. Prompt and accurate risk stratification are of paramount importance. After the diagnosis of PE is established, critical pathways are utilized to streamline, standardize, and optimize therapy (Fig. 22-4).

Most patients with PE will remain hemodynamically stable and will not suffer recurrent PE or develop chronic pulmonary hypertension as long as they receive adequate anticoagulation. If the PE is anatomically small, involving less than 30% of the lungs, then it is likely that right ventricular (RV) function will not be impaired (52), especially if there is no underlying cardiopulmonary disease.

Cardiac Biomarkers

Imaging the right ventricle is probably not necessary if the patient appears clinically stable and has normal levels of cardiac

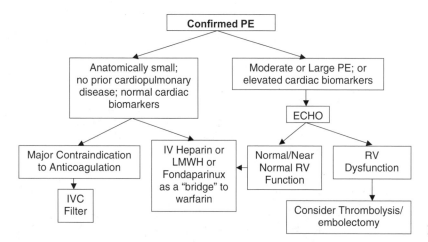

FIGURE 22-4. PE risk stratification.

biomarkers (53). Cardiac troponins are sensitive and specific biomarkers of myocardial cell damage. Elevations of troponin in PE patients are mild and of short duration compared with acute coronary syndromes. In acute PE, troponin levels correlate well with the extent of RV dysfunction (54).

Natriuretic peptides represent another class of cardiac biomarkers. The principal stimulus for synthesis and secretion of brain natriuretic peptide (BNP) is ventricular cardiomyocyte stretch (55). The prohormone, proBNP, has 108 amino acids. The biologically active BNP is a 32-amino acid peptide, with a plasma half life of 20 minutes. The remaining part of the prohormone, N-terminal (NT)-proBNP, has 76 amino acids and a half life of 60 to 120 minutes. The major role of cardiac biomarkers in risk stratification is to identify low-risk patients who do not require imaging of the right ventricle. Patients with normal levels of troponin and BNP are low risk. A simple risk stratification algorithm for PE patients is to employ either troponin or NT-proBNP testing as an initial step. Echocardiography should then be obtained if elevated biomarker levels are found (56). Echocardiography is not needed if both troponin and BNP (or pro-BNP) are normal.

Echocardiography

Classic risk stratification used to rely primarily on frequent assessment of systemic arterial pressure and heart rate. When patients became dependent on pressors to maintain a systolic blood pressure greater than 90 mm Hg, they were labeled as "high risk." This strategy delayed intervention with thrombolysis or embolectomy until patients were developing multisystem organ failure due to evolving cardiogenic shock. By that point, the response to aggressive intervention with thrombolysis or embolectomy was often disappointing.

Our approach to risk stratification has changed markedly. We now believe that among normotensive patients, assessment of RV function is pivotal to prognosticate accurately after PE is diagnosed (57). This assessment can at times be accomplished by finding normal cardiac biomarkers. However, patients who develop worsening RV function despite adequate anticoagulation have an ominous prognosis and are at high risk of in-hospital complications, including recurrent PE, respiratory failure, and death.

The International Cooperative Pulmonary Embolism Registry (ICOPER) enrolled 2,454 patients from 52 hospitals in 7 countries and is the largest PE registry that has ever been published (58). In ICOPER, age greater than 70 years increased the likelihood of death by 60%. Six other risk factors independently increased the likelihood of mortality by a factor of twofold to threefold: cancer, clinical congestive heart failure, chronic obstructive pulmonary disease, systemic arterial hypotension with a systolic blood pressure of <90 mm Hg, tachypnea (defined as >20 breaths per minute), and RV hypokinesis on echocardiogram, an especially useful sign to identify high-risk patients who might be suitable for aggressive interventions such as thrombolysis or embolectomy.

It is important to emphasize that RV dysfunction on echocardiogram is an important predictor of prognosis, even in patients with a systolic blood pressure greater than 90 mm Hg (59). Among this population in ICOPER, the 30-day survival rate was 91% in patients without RV hypokinesis compared with 84% in those with RV hypokinesis on baseline echocardiography (P <0.001).

Combined Biomarkers and Echocardiography

The combination of elevated biomarkers and moderate or severe RV dysfunction can portend a lethal outcome (60). At BWH, the combination of echocardiographic RV enlargement and elevated troponin significantly increased the 30-day mortality (38%) compared with patients with elevated troponin alone (23%), RV dilation alone (9%), and neither (5%).

Chest CT

Among patients with PE on chest CT scan, RV enlargement, defined as a reconstructed RV to left ventricular (LV) dimension ratio greater than 0.9, correlates with an unstable hospital course (61). In 431 consecutive patients, RV enlargement predicted 30-day death with a hazard ratio of 5.2, after multivariable analysis (62). This approach to prognosis has not been as widely verified as RV dysfunction on echocardiography.

Thrombolysis

For patients with massive PE (63) or smaller PE accompanied by moderate or severe RV dysfunction, anticoagulation alone may not yield a clinically successful outcome (64). When considering thrombolysis, careful screening for potential contraindications is necessary. Pay particular attention to a history of poorly controlled hypertension or presentation with PE and systemic hypertension. Patients should also be questioned about prior head trauma, seizures, or stroke.

The most feared complication from thrombolysis is intracranial bleeding. In ICOPER, 304 of the 2,454 patients received thrombolysis, and of these, 3% of the patients suffered intracranial hemorrhage.

In a separate registry of 312 patients receiving thrombolysis for PE in five clinical trials, there was a 1.9% risk (95% CI, 0.7% to 4.1%) of intracranial bleeding (65). Two of the six patients had pre-existing known intracranial disease and nonetheless received thrombolysis, in violation of the exclusion criteria listed in the clinical trial protocols. Two of the six intracranial hemorrhages probably were due to administration of heparin and not thrombolysis, because they occurred late, 62 and 157 hours after thrombolysis. Diastolic blood pressure on admission was elevated in patients who developed intracranial hemorrhage compared with those who did not (90.3 versus 77.6 mm Hg; P = 0.04). The mean age of patients with major bleeding was 63 years, whereas that of patients with no hemorrhagic complication was 56 years (P = 0.005). There was a 4% increased risk of bleeding for each additional year of age. Increasing body mass index and pulmonary angiography were also significant predictors of hemorrhage (66).

Predictors of Thrombolysis Efficacy

There is an inverse association between duration of symptoms and improvement on lung scan reperfusion after thrombolysis. We observed 0.8% less reperfusion on lung scanning per additional day of symptoms (95% CI, 0.2% to 1.4%; P = 0.008). After controlling for age and initial lung scan defect size, there was 0.7% less reperfusion per additional day of symptoms (95% CI, 0.2% to 1.2%; P = 0.007). Thus, delay in administering thrombolysis will attenuate efficacy. Nevertheless, thrombolysis is still useful in patients who have had symptoms for 6 to 14 days (67).

Practical Points

The FDA approved recombinant human tissue-type plasminogen activator (rt-PA) in 1990. Heparin is not coadministered, an important difference compared to thrombolysis for myocardial infarction. After administering thrombolysis, a partial thromboplastin time (PTT) should be obtained immediately. Usually, the PTT is less than 80 seconds, and intravenous unfractionated heparin can be initiated (or resumed) as a continuous intravenous infusion, without a loading dose. If the PTT exceeds 80 seconds, heparin should be withheld, and the test should be repeated every 4 hours until it drifts down to the recommended target (68). Substitution of low-molecular-weight heparin or fondaparinux for intravenous unfractionated heparin following thrombolysis has not been studied. Nevertheless, in clinical practice, it is quite common after a patient has stabilized to transition from intravenous unfractionated heparin to low-molecular-weight heparin, while initiating concurrent oral anticoagulation with warfarin.

Embolectomy

Catheter-Based Embolectomy

Greenfield demonstrated that transvenous catheter pulmonary embolectomy was feasible. He devised a steerable catheter with a distal radiopaque plastic cup. Syringe suction could be applied to aspirate a portion of the embolus into the cup, and a sustained vacuum by the syringe held the embolus as the catheter was withdrawn (69). This 12 French (F) double-lumen balloon-tipped catheter required femoral or jugular venotomy.

Interventional angiographers favor the "Meyerovitz technique" for aspiration; an 8 F or 9 F coronary guiding catheter without sideholes is placed through a 10 F arrow sheath; the clot is aspirated with a 60-mL syringe (70). Mechanical fragmentation and pulverization of thrombus can be accomplished with a rotating basket catheter, high-pressurized jets of normal saline, or a pigtail rotational catheter embolectomy. Mechanical fragmentation can also be combined with thrombolysis (71).

Recently, a new percutaneous catheter thrombectomy device has been tested for acute PE. The central part of the catheter system is a high-speed rotational coil within the catheter body that (a) creates negative pressure through an L-shaped aspiration port at the catheter tip, (b) macerates aspirated thrombus, and (c) removes macerated thrombus (72).

Surgical Embolectomy

Surgical embolectomy is best suited for patients with contraindications to thrombolysis, intracardiac thrombus, or both. Ideally, patients who have an adverse prognosis based on risk stratification with cardiac biomarkers and RV imaging will be referred prior to the onset of cardiogenic shock and multisystem organ failure.

At BWH, we have lowered our threshold for embolectomy. We use an aggressive multidisciplinary approach to triage patients with acute PE. We achieve rapid diagnosis with chest CT, which defines the clot burden and the surgical accessibility of thrombus. We assess RV function in patients with normal systemic arterial pressure. For those patients deemed at high risk, we consider surgical embolectomy if there are contraindications to thrombolytic therapy.

Surgical technique has improved (73). We avoid aortic cross clamping and operate on cardiopulmonary bypass with a warm, beating heart. We do not utilize intraoperative hypothermia. Blind instrumentation of the fragile pulmonary arteries is avoided. Extraction is limited to directly visible clot. In a series of 47 patients at BWH, there were three (6%) operative deaths, one with preoperative cardiac arrest. Actuarial survival at 1-year follow-up was 86% (74).

Pulmonary Thromboendarterectomy

Patients with chronic pulmonary hypertension due to prior PE may be virtually bedridden with breathlessness due to high pulmonary arterial pressures. Patients with chronic PE and cor pulmonale should receive lifelong anticoagulation and, in addition, may be candidates for lifelong continuous oxygen therapy. However, thromboendartectomy for chronic thromboembolic pulmonary hypertension will markedly reduce pulmonary artery pressures if successful. The operation is technically more demanding and riskier than embolectomy for acute PE (75,76).

The operation involves a median sternotomy incision, institution of cardiopulmonary bypass, and deep hypothermia with circulatory arrest periods. Incisions are made in both pulmonary arteries into the lower lobe branches. Pulmonary thromboendarterectomy is always bilateral, with removal of both organized thrombus and an endarterectomy plane that includes all involved vessels. When surgery is successful, one can expect a gradual decline in the pulmonary arterial pressures during the first few postoperative months, with a concomitant improvement in quality of life among patients previously debilitated from chronic pulmonary hypertension.

Among properly selected patients at experienced centers, the mortality rate from thromboendarterectomy is between 5% and 10%. The two major causes of mortality are: (a) inability to remove sufficient thrombotic material at surgery, resulting in persistent postoperative pulmonary hypertension and RV dysfunction; and (b) severe reperfusion lung injury. Thus, at designated centers, thromboendarterectomy can be performed with good results and at an acceptable risk to reduce debility from cor pulmonale due to PE.

Inferior Vena Caval Filters

Inferior vena caval filters are mechanical devices that are ordinarily placed below the renal veins to prevent embolization of thrombus from the pelvic or deep leg veins to the pulmonary arteries. The principal two indications for filter placement are (a) active bleeding (such as gastrointestinal hemorrhage requiring transfusion) that precludes anticoagulation, or (b) well-documented recurrence of PE despite therapeutic levels of anticoagulation. Other indications for PE are "soft" but might include situations such as preoperative insertion in a patient with recent PE who must undergo urgent or emergency surgery, such as hip fracture repair.

A review of the U.S. National Hospital Discharge Survey showed a 20-fold increase in inferior vena caval filter placement over the past two decades (77). Almost half the filters were placed in patients who had established DVT without pulmonary embolism. In the U.S. acute DVT registry of 5,451 patients, 14% of all patients underwent filter placement (78).

The largest trial of permanent vena caval filter placement followed patients for 8 years and found that filters reduced the risk of PE but increased the risk of DVT. Filters had no effect on survival (79).

Filters are almost always effective in preventing PE, but they do not halt the thrombotic process. Furthermore, filters appear to predispose to thrombosis and to DVT with the filter as the nidus for new clot formation (80). Therefore, in general, once a bleeding problem has been brought under control, anticoagulation should be initiated.

Retrievable vena caval filters (81) can be placed when it is uncertain that a patient will require a permanent filter. If not retrieved, the filter becomes a permanent filter. Such devices are especially suited for patients who have a transient risk factor for venous thrombosis or who are temporarily suffering from a bleeding problem that precludes anticoagulation.

Hospital Length of Stay

The FDA has not approved an abbreviated hospital length of stay for patients who present primarily with symptomatic PE. Some patients will be at such low risk that they can be managed as outpatients (82). The duration of hospitalization depends on risk assessment and clinical response to therapy. The hospital environment does have an important role for assessing response to therapy, ensuring resolution of symptoms of PE, such as shortness of breath, and providing education about PE and emotional support.

Outpatient Follow-Up

The initial office visit is ordinarily scheduled at about 2 weeks after the PE. The focus is on ensuring compliance with warfarin and discussing an optimal schedule for resumption of activities. For patients with an initial echocardiogram showing elevated pulmonary artery pressures, a repeat echocardiogram at 6 weeks may be useful. Patients with persistent moderate or severe pulmonary hypertension are susceptible to developing chronic thromboembolic pulmonary hypertension (83).

ORAL ANTICOAGULANT THERAPY

Under certain circumstances, long-term anticoagulation with low-molecular-weight heparin rather than warfarin will be appropriate. Extended enoxaparin monotherapy for acute symptomatic PE appears feasible and safe among properly selected patients (84). Consider this approach when the patient has underlying cancer, cannot tolerate warfarin because of rash or alopecia, or has great difficulty maintaining warfarin within the target therapeutic range.

In the CLOT Trial, 672 patients with cancer and acute DVT or PE were randomly assigned to dalteparin, a low-molecular-weight heparin, as a "bridge" to oral anticoagulation versus dalteparin as monotherapy for 6 months (85). During the study period, the probability of recurrent VTE was 17% in the oral anticoagulant group compared with 9% in the dalteparin monotherapy group ($P = 0.002$). There was no significant difference in the rate of major bleeding.

Warfarin

Warfarin is one of the most difficult drugs to dose and monitor because of marked patient-to-patient variability, drug–drug interactions, and drug–food interactions (86). Warfarin is not given in a fixed dose. Instead, it is administered in an adjusted dose to achieve a target prothrombin time expressed as an INR. For most patients, the target INR is between 2.0 and 3.0.

Beware that 1% to 3% of patients have a genetic mutation that delays metabolism of the S-racemer of warfarin. These patients become fully anticoagulated with tiny doses of warfarin, in the range of 1.0 to 1.5 mg daily (87,88).

Centralized anticoagulation services help patients receiving warfarin therapy to achieve better outcomes compared to the usual care provided by their personal physicians. This approach to anticoagulation management is rapidly gaining acceptance throughout North America and Europe as a strategy that maximizes patient safety. A centralized approach allows expert nurses, pharmacists, and physicians' assistants to develop expertise and coordinate efforts that minimize bleeding and clotting complications. The core philosophy is to achieve a coordinated and systematic approach.

A centralized telephonic model provides a setting for a small number of providers to manage a large patient population dispersed over a wide geographic area. Successful services require knowledgeable and experienced providers, reliable laboratory monitoring, and an organized system for timely patient follow-up.

A recent report (89) showed that a centralized, telephone-based anticoagulation service improved the time spent in a therapeutic range of anticoagulation. This resulted in fewer complications compared with usual care.

At BWH, we initiated an anticoagulation service in December 1996. Our volume increased from 72 patients staffed by 1 nurse and medical director to more than 1,900 patients staffed by 4 clinicians (nurses, physicians' assistants, and pharmacists), 1 administrator, and a medical director. Our mission statement (90) has six principles:

1. Careful monitoring and dosing of anticoagulants among hospitalized patients and outpatients
2. Facilitating and coordinating anticoagulation care among providers
3. Transitioning ("bridging") anticoagulation between the home and hospital settings
4. Educating patients, families, and professionals about the most recent developments in anticoagulation therapy
5. Continuous quality improvement to minimize thromboembolic and hemorrhaging complications, including tracking and critique of each complication that does occur
6. Organizing and participating in clinical research projects

We assessed our major bleeding complication rate in the BWH Anticoagulation Service in 2,460 patients with 3,684 years of warfarin exposure from 2000 to 2003. Eleven patients had 12 nonfatal major bleeding complications, with no fatal bleeds during the study. The average hospitalization cost per patient was $15,988, and the average length of hospitalization was 6.0 days. The incidence of major bleeding complications was 0.12% per year. There were 0.32 bleeds per 100 patient-years of coverage. Our bleeding rate was low compared with reports from other anticoagulation services, which had major bleeding complication rates from 1.1 to 2.1 per 100 patient-years of coverage (91).

An increasingly popular approach to warfarin dosing is self-management with a point-of-care machine that allows patients to self-test their INRs. Patients are taught how to adjust their own doses of warfarin, analogous to home testing and dose adjustment widely practiced by insulin-dependent diabetics. In a randomized trial of 737 patients allocated to self-management versus conventional anticoagulation clinic management, achieving INR goals was similar in both groups. However, major complications and minor hemorrhages were less common in the self-management group. The dropout rate during the 1-year study was 21% in the self-management group (92).

New Anticoagulants under Development

There is enormous interest in developing safer and more effective oral antithrombotic agents. Oral inhibitors of thrombin or factor Xa will have to be at least as effective, at least as safe, and yet require less laboratory monitoring. To achieve these goals, the compounds will need to have high and consistent oral bioavailability (93).

One promising approach is administration of oral heparin using a novel carrier that mediates passive gastrointestinal absorption of a noncovalent complex with heparin in a dose-dependent manner (94). Another strategy is use of a new oral direct thrombin inhibitor, such as dabigatran, that can be administered in a fixed dose without coagulation laboratory monitoring (95).

Optimal Duration of Anticoagulation

When consecutive patients with DVT receive time-limited anticoagulation, their risk of recurrence increases after anticoagulation is discontinued. A landmark cohort study by Prandoni and colleagues in Padua, Italy, followed 355 consecutive patients with a first episode of symptomatic DVT (96). The cumulative incidence of recurrent VTE was 18% after 2 years, 25% after 5 years, and 30% after 8 years. Those patients at lowest risk of recurrence had the initial DVT provoked by surgery, recent trauma, or fracture. Venous insufficiency (also known as post-thrombotic syndrome) developed in 23% after 2 years, 28% after 5 years, and 29% after 8 years. At the Mayo Clinic, VTE recurrence rates were similar with long-term follow-up: 30% at 10 years (97).

For uncertain reasons, the risk of recurrence is about three times higher in men than in women (98). In addition, patients with a first symptomatic PE have a higher risk of recurrent VTE than those who initially present with DVT alone (99).

Counterintuitively, testing for hereditary thrombophilia does not allow prediction of recurrent VTE after anticoagulant therapy is stopped (100). Assessment of clinical risk factors is much more helpful in predicting the likelihood of recurrence. Unprovoked VTE is much more likely to lead to recurrence after discontinuation of anticoagulation than VTE provoked by surgery, trauma, oral contraceptives, or hormone replacement therapy.

The optimal duration of anticoagulation remains the greatest challenge in long-term management of patients with VTE. There are two different strategic approaches. An epidemiologic approach focuses on the clinical circumstances when the DVT or PE was initially diagnosed. This probing of detailed clinical events ultimately leads to a recommendation of time-limited versus indefinite duration anticoagulation. The individual approach focuses more on each patient's coagulation status and residual venous thrombosis when considering whether to discontinue anticoagulation. Currently, most practitioners use the epidemiologic approach.

For unprovoked events, the standard duration of anticoagulation is 3 months for upper-extremity or isolated calf DVT and 6 months for proximal leg DVT or PE (Table 22.5). With 6 months of anticoagulation, the recurrence rate is halved compared with 6 weeks of anticoagulation (101). After a second episode of VTE, indefinite duration anticoagulation is a much better strategy than 6 months of repeated anticoagulation. With only 6 months of repeated anticoagulation, the risk of recurrence and a third VTE episode is eight times higher than with indefinite duration therapy. However, the major bleeding risk is three times higher with indefinite duration anticoagulation (102).

Epidemiologic Approach

Patients who receive extended anticoagulation are protected from recurrent VTE while receiving long-term therapy. In a meta-analysis of the duration of anticoagulation following VTE (103), the number of patients needed to treat to prevent one VTE event with lifelong anticoagulation is approximately nine. Patients with "idiopathic" VTE are especially likely to benefit from this strategy if their bleeding risk from anticoagulation is low (104–107).

Controversy exists over the optimal anticoagulation intensity for patients receiving indefinite duration anticoagulation. The Extended Low-Intensity Anticoagulation for Thrombo-Embolism (ELATE) Trial (108) demonstrated a remarkably low major bleeding rate of 1.1 events per 100 patient-years with standard anticoagulation, target INR between 2.0 and 3.0. Among patients receiving low-intensity anticoagulation, target INR between 1.5 and 1.9, the major bleeding rate was exactly the same as in the warfarin-PREVENT Trial of low-intensity anticoagulation (109), 0.9 events per 100 person-years.

My interpretation is that the remarkably low bleeding rate in the standard intensity ELATE patients is unprecedented in clinical trials (Table 22-6). It represents a combination of closer follow-up and monitoring that is difficult to achieve in the "real-world" setting plus the play of chance that favored these fortunate patients. The ELATE investigators observed a much higher major bleeding event rate of 3.8 per 100 person-years in their previous trial using standard intensity anticoagulation.

My biggest fear is that this controversy about warfarin intensity will dilute the principal message of these rigorous and well-executed trials—that warfarin should be prescribed for extended duration in most patients with idiopathic VTE.

The controversy is beneficial because it gives practicing health care providers a wide range of options. In our practice at BWH, our default strategy is low-intensity anticoagulation, target INR between 1.5 and 2.0, after 6 months of standard intensity warafin. However, in patients who appear to have an extraordinarily high risk of recurrence, we prescribe standard intensity anticoagulation as long as bleeding risk does not appear excessive. Overall, we find patients and referring physicians embrace the long-term strategy of lower intensity warfarin with its attendant reduction in the frequency of INR monitoring.

Individual Approach

The individual approach to determining whether indefinite anticoagulation should be prescribed relies on two strategies: (a) D-dimer determination after temporarily discontinuing warfarin, and (b) assessment of residual venous thrombosis after an initial treatment course of anticoagulation.

D-dimer is a global indicator of coagulation activation and fibrinolysis. In a study of 610 patients with unprovoked VTE (110), all of whom received at least 3 months of anticoagulation, D-dimer levels were measured on average 3 weeks after discontinuing oral anticoagulation. Those patients with a D-dimer ELISA less than 250 ng/mL had a very low risk of recurrent events. The total duration of follow-up was 1,945 patient-years. D-dimer served as a multifactorial assessment of thrombophilia. In the subset with low D-dimer levels, the cumulative probability of recurrent VTE after 2 years without anticoagulation was 3.7%. The recurrence rate was 11.5% for patients with higher D-dimer levels.

TABLE 22-5

ANTICOAGULATION DURATION FOR UNPROVOKED VTE

Isolated calf DVT:	3 months
Upper extremity DVT:	3 months
Proximal leg DVT:	6 months
Pelvic DVT:	6 months
Pulmonary Embolism:	6 months
Proximal DVT + PE:	6 months

TABLE 22-6

MAJOR BLEEDING COMPLICATION RATE ACCORDING TO INR INTENSITY

Trial	INR Range	Rate/100 Person-Years
Kearon 1999	2.0–3.0	3.8
Schulman 1997	2.0–2.85	2.4
Ridker 2003	1.5–2.0	0.9
Kearon 2003	2.0–3.0	0.9
Kearon 2003	1.5–1.9	1.1

In 313 consecutive outpatients with proximal DVT, all received anticoagulation for 3 months (111). After anticoagulation was discontinued, they underwent venous ultrasonography of the leg veins every 6 to 12 months for 3 years. Recurrent VTE was assessed over 6 years. The cumulative incidence of normal ultrasounds was 39% at 6 months, 58% at 12 months, 69% at 24 months, and 74% at 36 months. Of 58 recurrent episodes, 41 occurred in patients with residual venous thrombosis. The hazard ratio for recurrent VTE was 2.4 for patients with persistent residual venous thrombosis.

PREVENTION

To prevent postphlebitic syndrome, which is characterized by chronic leg swelling, calf aching, and occasionally ulceration at the medial malleolus, below-knee vascular compression stockings, 30 to 40 mm Hg, should be prescribed as soon as DVT is diagnosed. These stockings should be worn daily when out of bed. Occasionally, the stocking prescription will have to be deferred because of extreme leg pain and edema.

Effective pharmacological and mechanical measures have been proven to decrease asymptomatic DVT rates among hospitalized patients (112). Until recently, skeptics have questioned whether a decrease in asymptomatic DVT translates into a decrease in mortality.

A post hoc analysis of patients enrolled in the Prospective Evaluation of Dalteparin Efficacy for Prevention of VTE in Immobilized Patients Trial (dalteparin-PREVENT Trial, a different trial from the warfarin-PREVENT Trial) examined mortality rates in patients who developed asymptomatic DVT compared with those who did not develop DVT (113). Overall, 3,706 hospitalized medical service patients at risk for DVT were enrolled at 219 hospitals in 26 countries. They were randomized to dalteparin 5,000 units once daily versus placebo. Of asymptomatic patients alive on day 21, 1,738 had undergone technically adequate ultrasound examinations of both proximal and distal leg veins. These 1,738 patients constituted the study group for analysis of asymptomatic DVT. In this population, 1,540 had no DVT, 118 had calf DVT, and 80 had proximal DVT.

By day 90 of PREVENT, the death rate was 1.9% in the no DVT group, 3.4% in the calf DVT group, and 13.8% in the proximal DVT group. The hazard ratio for death in the asymptomatic proximal DVT group was 7.3 (95% CI = 3.8 to 15.3; $P <0.0001$) compared with the no DVT group. The association of asymptomatic proximal DVT with increased mortality remained highly significant after adjusting for differences in baseline demographics and clinical variables. The increased mortality rate in asymptomatic calf DVT compared with no DVT trended toward statistical significance. These findings underscore the clinical relevance of asymptomatic DVT and support the common practice of targeting asymptomatic DVT as an appropriate endpoint in clinical trials of thromboprophylaxis.

There appears to be gender bias against VTE prevention in women, who do not receive VTE prophylaxis as frequently as men (114). This finding is based on observations from the prospective U.S. registry of 5,451 patients with ultrasound-confirmed DVT. Men were 21% more likely than women to receive prophylaxis within 30 days prior to acute DVT (61% versus 56%; odds ratio, 1.21; $P = 0.017$). The observed gender difference was present in all age groups, in both academic and community hospitals and throughout all regions of the United States. The gender difference also persisted after multivariable analysis that adjusted for cancer, surgery, prior DVT, trauma, and age. These findings indicate that hospitalized women

TABLE 22-7

BARRIERS TO PROPHYLAXIS AGAINST VENOUS THROMBOEMBOLISM

1. Repetitive, mundane task: "boring"
2. Practitioners rarely witness fatal pulmonary embolism, so the risk may appear exaggerated
3. Concern about bleeding complications
4. Low priority task in a hospital environment that is increasingly rushed and pressured

should be included when considering pharmacological VTE prevention.

There are several barriers to VTE prophylaxis (Table 22-7). One barrier to consistent, universal prophylaxis among hospitalized patients may be the needlessly cumbersome and outdated classic approach to risk stratification. This strategy, which is not practical in contemporary clinical practice, categorizes patients into one of four risk groups and then prescribes differing prophylaxis regimens (or no prophylaxis) according to the degree of risk. This approach worked well in a previous era when low-risk patients were commonly hospitalized for prolonged lengths of stay. Nowadays, this time-consuming and often ambiguous scheme seems outdated. In modern practice, essentially all patients hospitalized for more than 1 night are at high risk of developing VTE (115).

Virtually every patient with an anticipated hospital stay of 48 hours or more warrants prophylaxis against VTE. The subtleties of distinguishing low risk from medium risk from high risk are distracting and impede focusing on the main task: effective and safe prophylaxis for all hospitalized patients with protocols that are routine, rapidly implemented, and practical.

Pharmacological prophylaxis should form the foundation for any VTE prevention program among hospitalized patients. For those with bleeding problems or whose risks of bleeding make this approach risky, mechanical prophylaxis should be utilized with graduated compression stockings, intermittent pneumatic compression devices, or both. Mechanical prophylaxis with graduated compression stockings or intermittent pneumatic compression devices has not been studied as extensively or rigorously as pharmacological prophylaxis. However, a meta-analysis of intermittent pneumatic compression devices in postoperative patients reviewed 2,270 patients in 15 eligible randomized controlled trials. In comparison to no device, those receiving intermittent pneumatic compression had a 60% reduction in the risk of DVT (116).

Low-dose unfractionated heparin, administered in a fixed dosing regimen of 5,000 units injected subcutaneously every 8 hours, can halve VTE rates. For surgical patients, the first dose is administered 2 hours before the skin incision. Prophylaxis should be continued for at least a week because the peak incidence of postoperative VTE is 5 to 10 days following surgery (117). In medical patients, heparin 5,000 units three times daily appears equivalent in efficacy and safety to low-molecular-weight heparin administered once daily (118).

Low-molecular-weight heparins and fondaparinux, an anti-Xa agent, provide the convenience of once-daily dosing. They are administered as fixed doses. In general, the concentration of drug needed to prevent VTE is about one-fourth the concentration needed to treat acute DVT or PE. Low-molecular-weight heparin and fondaparinux, in contrast to unfractionated heparin, also reduce the possible catastrophic side effect of heparin-induced thrombocytopenia. These agents are being used for VTE prevention in both surgical and medical patients.

With adherence to prophylaxis protocols, prevention of VTE can usually be achieved in the hospital setting. Primary prevention of VTE will be cost effective by avoiding the expenses associated with diagnosis and treatment of acute DVT and PE (119).

To achieve a true consensus on VTE prophylaxis, we must determine how to change physician behavior (Table 22-8). We can use protocols and consensus statements as a starting point, but the most challenging aspect remains devising strategies that translate evidence-based medicine into actual implementation in daily clinical practice. In the real world, the physician's orders on an individual patient are the real measure of whether the lessons about VTE prevention have been communicated effectively.

At BWH, we have an excellent educational network, and VTE management is a major clinical interest for many physicians. For the past decade, our computer has been programmed to suggest VTE prophylaxis if a computer order is entered for "bed rest." Nevertheless, audits of our own clinical practice reveal that many high-risk patients for VTE have not received prophylaxis orders. Therefore, we undertook a randomized clinical trial of high-risk patients who were not receiving VTE prophylaxis (120).

The primary endpoint of the trial was to reduce clinically diagnosed and objectively confirmed VTE. We worked closely with our Information Systems Department so that our hospital computers could identify high-risk patients and determine whether prophylaxis orders had been written. Our electronic alert trial was a test of changing physician behavior to improve implementation of prophylaxis. It was not a trial to test specific types of prophylaxis.

We devised a point score system to identify patients at high risk for VTE. We defined "high risk" as patients with 4 or more score points, and we assigned points as follows: prior VTE—3, cancer—3, hypercoagulability—3, major surgery—2, advanced age—1, obesity—1, bed rest—1, and hormone replacement therapy or oral contraceptives—1.

For those high-risk patients without prophylaxis orders, the computer randomized patients to an intervention group or to a control group. In the intervention group, the physician responsible for care of a high-risk patient not receiving prophy-

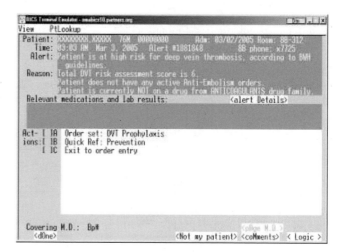

FIGURE 22-5. Electronic VTE prophylaxis alert.

laxis received an electronic alert suggesting prophylaxis (Fig. 22-5), whereas the physicians of patients in the control group received no electronic alert. In the intervention group, the responsible physician was required to acknowledge the alert and could then order or withhold prophylaxis.

During our trial, 2,506 patients at high risk for VTE and without prophylaxis orders were identified and enrolled—1,255 to the intervention group and 1,251 to the control group. Among these 2,506 high-risk patients not receiving prophylaxis, 83% were medical, 13% were surgical, and 4% were trauma. This finding emphasizes that failure to implement prophylaxis is mostly a problem on general medical and subspecialty medical services.

The primary endpoint of symptomatic and imaging-confirmed VTE occurred in 61 intervention-group and 103 control-group patients. At 90 days, the intervention strategy reduced the risk of VTE by 41%. There was no increase in major or minor bleeding in the intervention group. Thus, institution of an electronic alert system increased the use of VTE prophylaxis and markedly reduced the risk of symptomatic VTE (Table 22-9).

The beneficial effect of the electronic alert system can be replicated without computer support. A nurse or physician could round on all overnight admissions, review their charts, and determine whether specific patients are at high risk for developing VTE during hospitalization. They could then review the written physician orders to determine whether prophylaxis had been instituted. For high-risk patients not receiving prophylaxis, the reviewer could then page the responsible physician, point out the patient's high risk, note the absence of VTE prophylaxis orders, and suggest implementation of preventive measures. Within a few years, the voluntary aspects of

---

TABLE 22-8

CHANGING PHYSICIAN BEHAVIOR

1. Guidelines alone do not suffice.
2. Physician champions are crucial at the hospital level.
3. Individual hospital protocols should be written by consensus, implemented, and enforced.
4. Registries are useful to reflect "real-world" issues, at local, regional, and national levels.
5. Coalitions of health care providers and patients can provide impetus and momentum (such as the Coalition to Prevent DVT at www.preventdvt.org).
6. Medicolegal litigation against physicians can serve as a deterrent.
7. Electronic alerts to encourage prophylaxis in high-risk patients.

TABLE 22-9

ELECTRONIC VENOUS THROMBOEMBOLISM PREVENTION ALERTS

1. Detected patients at high risk of venous thromboembolism.
2. Increased prophylaxis rate to 33%.
3. Reduced symptomatic venous thromboembolism by 41%, without increased bleeding.

ordering VTE prophylaxis will disappear, as regulatory authorities and insurers demand that VTE prevention becomes obligatory.

CONCLUSIONS

VTE diagnosis, management, and prevention are suited to the development and implementation of critical pathways. D-dimer blood testing, venous ultrasonography, and chest CT scans have facilitated diagnosis. Rapid and accurate risk stratification is the key to optimal management. Most VTE that develops in the hospital can be avoided by instituting proven prophylaxis strategies.

References

1. Goldhaber SZ, Elliott CG. Acute pulmonary embolism: Part I—Epidemiology, pathophysiology, and diagnosis. *Circulation* 2003;108:2726–2729.
2. Nakamura M, Fujioka H, Yamada N, et al. Clinical characteristics of acute pulmonary thromboembolism in Japan: results of a multicenter registry in the Japanese Society of Pulmonary Embolism Research. *Clin Cardiol* 2001;24:132–138.
3. Middeldorp S, Meinardi JR, Koopman MM, et al. A prospective study of asymptomatic carriers of the factor V Leiden mutation to determine the incidence of venous thromboembolism. *Ann Intern Med* 2001;135:322–327.
4. Eichinger S, Weltermann A, Mannhalter C, et al. The risk of recurrent venous thromboembolism in heterozygous carriers of factor V Leiden and a first spontaneous venous thromboembolism. *Arch Intern Med* 2002;162:2357–2360.
5. Ridker PM, Miletich JP, Buring JE, et al. Factor V Leiden mutation as a risk factor for recurrent pregnancy loss. *Ann Intern Med* 1998;128:1000–1003.
6. Ridker PM, Miletich JP, Hennekens CH, Buring JE. Ethnic distribution of factor V Leiden in 4047 men and women. Implications for venous thromboembolism screening. *JAMA* 1997;277:1305–1307.
7. Ridker PM, Glynn RJ, Miletich JP, et al. Age-specific incidence rates of venous thromboembolism among heterozygous carriers of factor V Leiden mutation. *Ann Intern Med* 1997;126:528–531.
8. Ariens RA, de Lange M, Snieder H, et al. Activation markers of coagulation and fibrinolysis in twins: heritability of the prethrombotic state. *Lancet* 2002;359:667–671.
9. Joffe HV, Goldhaber SZ. Laboratory thrombophilias and venous thromboembolism. *Vasc Med* 2002;7:93–102.
10. Walker ID. Inherited thrombophilia. *Vasc Med* 2004;9:219–221.
11. Greaves M. Acquired thrombophilia. *Vasc Med* 2004;9:215–218.
12. Pengo V, Lensing AW, Prins MH, et al. Incidence of chronic thromboembolic pulmonary hypertension after pulmonary embolism. *N Engl J Med* 2004;350:2257–2264.
13. Heit JA. Venous thromboembolism: disease burden, outcomes and risk factors. *J Thromb Haemost* 2005;3:1611–1617.
14. Joffe HV, Goldhaber SZ. Upper extremity deep vein thrombosis. *Circulation* 2002;106:1874–1880.
15. Joffe HV, Kucher N, Tapson VF, et al. Upper-extremity deep vein thrombosis: A prospective registry of 592 patients. *Circulation* 2004;110:1605–1611.
16. Wells PS, Anderson DR, Bormanis J, et al. Value of assessment of pretest probability of deep-vein thrombosis in clinical management. *Lancet* 1997;350:1795–1798.
17. Bundens WP, Bergan JJ, Halasz NA, et al. The superficial femoral vein. A potentially lethal misnomer. *JAMA* 1995;274:1296–1298.
18. Stevens SM, Elliott CG, Chan KJ, et al. Withholding anticoagulation after a negative result on duplex ultrasonography for suspected symptomatic deep venous thrombosis. *Ann Intern Med* 2004;140:985–991.
19. Loud PA, Katz DS, Belfi L, et al. Imaging of deep venous thrombosis in suspected pulmonary embolism. *Semin Roentgenol* 2005;40:33–40.
20. Stern JB, Abehsera M, Grenet D, et al. Detection of pelvic vein thrombosis by magnetic resonance angiography in patients with acute pulmonary embolism and normal lower limb compression ultrasonography. *Chest* 2002;122:115–121.
21. Fraser DG, Moody AR, Morgan PS, et al. Diagnosis of lower-limb deep venous thrombosis: a prospective blinded study of magnetic resonance direct thrombus imaging. *Ann Intern Med* 2002;136:89–98.
22. Hull R, Hirsh J, Sackett DL, et al. Clinical validity of a negative venogram in patients with clinically suspected venous thrombosis. *Circulation* 1981;64:622–625.
23. Wells PS, Anderson DR, Rodger M, et al. Derivation of a simple clinical model to categorize patients probability of pulmonary embolism: increasing the models utility with the SimpliRED D-dimer. *Thromb Haemost* 2000;83:416–420.
24. Kabrhel C, McAfee AT, Goldhaber SZ. The contribution of the subjective component of the Canadian pulmonary embolism score to the overall score in emergency department patients. *Acad Emerg Med* 2005;12:915–920.
25. Kabrhel C, Camargo CA, Jr., Goldhaber SZ. Clinical gestalt and the diagnosis of pulmonary embolism: does experience matter? *Chest* 2005;127:1627–1630.
26. Kucher N, Walpoth N, Wustmann K, et al. QR in V1—an ECG sign associated with right ventricular strain and adverse clinical outcome in pulmonary embolism. *Eur Heart J* 2003;24:1113–1119.
27. Ferrari E, Imbert A, Chevalier T, et al. The ECG in pulmonary embolism: Predictive value of negative T waves in precordial leads—80 case reports. *Chest* 1997;111:537–543.
28. Elliott CG, Goldhaber SZ, Visani L, et al. Chest radiographs in acute pulmonary embolism. Results from the International Cooperative Pulmonary Embolism Registry. *Chest* 2000;118:33–38.
29. Stein PD, Goldhaber SZ, Henry JW. Alveolar-arterial oxygen gradient in the assessment of acute pulmonary embolism. *Chest* 1995;107:139–143.
30. Stein PD, Goldhaber SZ, Henry JW, et al. Arterial blood gas analysis in the assessment of suspected acute pulmonary embolism. *Chest* 1996;109:78–81.
31. Brown, MD, Rowe BH, Reeves MJ, et al. The accuracy of the enzyme-linked immunosorbent assay D-dimer test in the diagnosis of pulmonary embolism: A meta-analysis. *Ann Emerg Med* 2002;40:133–144.
32. Dunn KL, Wolf JP, Dorfman DM, et al. Normal D-dimer levels in emergency department patients suspected of acute pulmonary embolism. *J Am Coll Cardiol* 2002;40:1475–1478.
33. Stein PD, Kayali F, Olson RE. Trends in the use of diagnostic imaging in patients hospitalized with acute pulmonary embolism. *Am J Cardiol* 2004;93:1316–1317.
34. Quiroz R, Kucher N, Zou KH, et al. Clinical validity of a negative computed tomography scan in patients with suspected pulmonary embolism: a systematic review. *JAMA* 2005;293:2012–2017.
35. Schoepf UJ, Goldhaber SZ, Costello P. Spiral computed tomography for acute pulmonary embolism. *Circulation* 2004;109:2160–2167.
36. The PIOPED investigators. Value of the ventilation/perfusion scan in acute pulmonary embolism. *JAMA* 1990;263:2753–2759.
37. Turkstra F, Kuijer PMM, van Beek EJR, et al. Diagnostic utility of ultrasonography of leg veins in patients suspected of having pulmonary embolism. *Ann Intern Med* 1997;126:775–781.
38. Goldhaber SZ. Multislice computed tomography for pulmonary embolism—a technological marvel. *N Engl J Med* 2005;352:1812–1814.
39. Stein PD, Athanasoulis C, Alavi A, et al. Complications and validity of pulmonary angiography in acute pulmonary embolism. *Circulation* 1992;85:462–468.
40. Stein PD, Woodard PK, Hull RD, et al. Gadolinium-enhanced magnetic resonance angiography for detection of acute pulmonary embolism: an in-depth review. *Chest* 2003;124:2324–2328.
41. Raschke RA, Reilly BM, Guidry JR, et al. The weight-based heparin dosing nomogram compared with a "standard care" nomogram. A randomized controlled trial. *Ann Intern Med* 1993;119:874–881.
42. Fanikos J, Stapinski C, Koo S, et al. Medication errors associated with anticoagulation therapy in the hospital. *Am J Cardiol* 2004;94:532–535.
43. Cannon CP, Dingemanse J, Kleinbloesem CH, et al. Automated heparin-delivery system to control activated partial thromboplastin time: evaluation in normal volunteers. *Circulation* 1999;99:751–756.
44. Jang IK, Hursting MJ. When heparins promote thrombosis: review of heparin-induced thrombocytopenia. *Circulation* 2005;111:2671–2683.
45. Gould MK, Dembitzer AD, Doyle RL, et al. Low-molecular-weight heparins compared with unfractionated heparin for treatment of acute deep venous thrombosis. A meta-analysis of randomized, controlled trials. *Ann Intern Med* 1999;130:800–809.
46. Gould MK, Dembitzer AD, Sanders GD, et al. Low-molecular-weight heparins compared with unfractionated heparin for treatment of acute deep venous thrombosis: A cost-effectiveness analysis. *Ann Intern Med* 1999;130:789–799.
47. Buller HR, Davidson BL, Decousus H, et al. Fondaparinux or enoxaparin for the initial treatment of symptomatic deep venous thrombosis: a randomized trial. *Ann Intern Med* 2004;140:867–873.
48. Di Nisio M, Middeldorp S, Buller HR. Direct thrombin inhibitors. *N Engl J Med* 2005;353:1028–1040.
49. Watson LI, Armon MP. Thrombolysis for acute deep vein thrombosis. The Cochrane Database of Systematic Reviews 2004;3:CD002783.pub2.
50. Eberhardt RT, Raffetto JD. Chronic venous insufficiency. *Circulation* 2005;111:2398–2409.
51. Prandoni P, Lensing AW, Prins MH, et al. Below-knee elastic compression stockings to prevent the post-thrombotic syndrome: a randomized, controlled trial. *Ann Intern Med* 2004;141:249–256.
52. Wolfe MW, Lee RT, Feldstein ML, et al. Prognostic significance of right ventricular hypokinesis and perfusion lung scan defects in pulmonary embolism. *Am Heart J* 1994;127:1371–1375.

53. Kucher N, Goldhaber SZ. Cardiac biomarkers for risk stratification of patients with acute pulmonary embolism. *Circulation* 2003;108: 2191–2194.

54. Konstantinides S, Geibel A, Olschewski M, et al. Importance of cardiac troponins I and T in risk stratification of patients with acute pulmonary embolism. *Circulation* 2002;106:1263–1268.

55. Kucher N, Printzen G, Goldhaber SZ. Prognostic role of brain natriuretic peptide in acute pulmonary embolism. *Circulation* 2003;107:2545–2547.

56. Binder L, Pieske B, Olschewski M, et al. N-terminal pro-brain natriuretic peptide or troponin testing followed by echocardiography for risk stratification of acute pulmonary embolism. *Circulation* 2005;112:1573–1579.

57. Goldhaber SZ. Echocardiography in the management of pulmonary embolism. *Ann Intern Med* 2002;136:691–700.

58. Goldhaber SZ, Visani L, De Rosa M, for ICOPER. Acute pulmonary embolism: clinical outcomes in the International Cooperative Pulmonary Embolism Registry (ICOPER). *Lancet* 1999;353:1386–1389.

59. Kucher N, Rossi E, De Rosa M, et al. Prognostic role of echocardiography among patients with acute pulmonary embolism and a systolic arterial pressure of 90 mm Hg or higher. *Arch Intern Med* 2005;165:1777–1781.

60. Scridon T, Scridon C, Skali H, et al. Prognostic significance of troponin elevation and right ventricular enlargement in acute pulmonary embolism. *Am J Cardiol* 2005;96:303–305.

61. Quiroz R, Kucher N, Schoepf UJ, et al. Right ventricular enlargement on chest computed tomography: prognostic role in acute pulmonary embolism. *Circulation* 2004;109:2401–2404.

62. Schoepf UJ, Kucher N, Kipfmueller F, et al. Right ventricular enlargement on chest computed tomography: a predictor of early death in acute pulmonary embolism. *Circulation* 2004;110:3276–3280.

63. Kucher N, Goldhaber SZ. Management of massive pulmonary embolism. *Circulation* 2005;112:e28–e32.

64. Wan S, Quinlan DJ, Agnelli G, et al. Thrombolysis compared with heparin for the initial treatment of pulmonary embolism: a meta-analysis of the randomized controlled trials. *Circulation* 2004;110:744–749.

65. Kanter DS, Mikkola KM, Patel SR, et al. Thrombolytic therapy for pulmonary embolism. Frequency of intracranial hemorrhage and associated risk factors. *Chest* 1997;111:1241–1245.

66. Mikkola KM, Patel SR, Parker JA, et al. Increasing age is a major risk factor for hemorrhagic complications following pulmonary embolism thrombolysis. *Am Heart J* 1997;134:69–72.

67. Daniels LB, Parker JA, Patel SR, et al. Relation of duration of symptoms with response to thrombolytic therapy in pulmonary embolism. *Am J Cardiol* 1997;80:184–188.

68. Goldhaber SZ. A contemporary approach to thrombolytic therapy for pulmonary embolism. *Vasc Med* 2000;5:115–123.

69. Greenfield LJ, Proctor MC, Williams DM, et al. Long-term experience with transvenous catheter pulmonary embolectomy. *J Vasc Surg* 1993;18: 450–458.

70. Goldhaber SZ. Integration of catheter thrombectomy into our armamentarium to treat acute pulmonary embolism. *Chest* 1998;114:1237–1238.

71. De Gregorio MA, Gimeno MJ, Mainar A, et al. Mechanical and enzymatic thrombolysis for massive pulmonary embolism. *J Vasc Interv Radiol* 2002; 13:163–169.

72. Kucher N, Windecker S, Banz Y, et al. Percutaneous catheter thrombectomy device for acute pulmonary embolism: in vitro and in vivo testing. *Radiology* 2005;236:852–858.

73. Aklog L, Williams CS, Byrne JG, et al. Acute pulmonary embolectomy: a contemporary approach. *Circulation* 2002;105:1416–1419.

74. Leacche M, Unic D, Goldhaber SZ, et al. Modern surgical treatment of massive pulmonary embolism: results in 47 consecutive patients after rapid diagnosis and aggressive surgical approach. *J Thorac Cardiovasc Surg* 2005;129:1018–1023.

75. Fedullo PF, Auger WR, Kerr KM, et al. Chronic thromboembolic pulmonary hypertension. *N Engl J Med* 2001;345:1465–1472.

76. Jamieson SW, Kapelanski DP, Sakakibara N, et al. Pulmonary endarterectomy: experience and lessons learned in 1,500 cases. *Ann Thorac Surg* 2003;76:1457–1462; discussion 62–64.

77. Stein PD, Kayali F, Olson RE. Twenty-one year trends in the use of inferior vena cava filters. *Arch Intern Med* 2004;164:1541–1545.

78. Jaff MR, Goldhaber SZ, Tapson VF. High utilization rate of vena cava filters in deep vein thrombosis. *Thromb Haemost* 2005;93:1117–1119.

79. Eight-year follow-up of patients with permanent vena cava filters in the prevention of pulmonary embolism: the PREPIC (Prevention du Risque d'Embolie Pulmonaire par Interruption Cave) randomized study. *Circulation* 2005;112:416–422.

80. Decousus H, Leizorovicz A, Parent F, et al. A clinical trial of vena caval filters in the prevention of pulmonary embolism in patients with proximal deep-vein thrombosis. Prevention du Risque d'Embolie Pulmonaire par Interruption Cave Study Group. *N Engl J Med* 1998;338:409–415.

81. Stein PD, Alnas M, Skaf E, et al. Outcome and complications of retrievable inferior vena cava filters. *Am J Cardiol* 2004;94:1090–1093.

82. Beer JH, Burger M, Gretener S, et al. Outpatient treatment of pulmonary embolism is feasible and safe in a substantial proportion of patients. *J Thromb Haemost* 2002;1:186–187.

83. Ribeiro A, Lindmarker P, Johnsson H, et al. Pulmonary embolism: one

year follow-up with echocardiography Doppler and five-year survival analysis. *Circulation* 1999;99:1325–1330.

84. Kucher N, Quiroz R, McKean S, Sasahara AA, Goldhaber SZ. Extended enoxaparin monotherapy for acute symptomatic pulmonary embolism. *Vasc Med* 2005;10:251–256.

85. Lee AY, Levine MN, Baker RI, et al. Low-molecular-weight heparin versus a coumarin for the prevention of recurrent venous thromboembolism in patients with cancer. *N Engl J Med* 2003;349:146–153.

86. Schulman S. Care of patients receiving long-term anticoagulant therapy. *N Engl J Med* 2003;349:675–683.

87. Joffe HV, Xu R, Johnson FB, et al. Warfarin dosing and cytochrome P450 2C9 polymorphisms. *Thromb Haemost* 2004;91:1123–1128.

88. Voora D, Eby C, Linder MW, et al. Prospective dosing of warfarin based on cytochrome P-450 2C9 genotype. *Thromb Haemost* 2005;93:700–705.

89. Witt DM, Sadler MA, Shanahan RL, et al. Effect of a centralized clinical pharmacy anticoagulation service on the outcomes of anticoagulation therapy. *Chest* 2005;127:1515–1522.

90. Grasso-Correnti N, Goldszer RC, Goldhaber SZ. The critical pathways of an anticoagulation service. *Critical Pathways in Cardiology* 2003;1:41–45.

91. Fanikos J, Grasso-Correnti N, Shah R, et al. Major bleeding complications in a specialized anticoagulation service. *Am J Cardiol* 2005;96:595–598.

92. Menendez-Jandula B, Souto JC, Oliver A, et al. Comparing self-management of oral anticoagulation therapy with clinic management. A randomized trial. *Ann Intern Med* 2005;142:1–10.

93. Hirsh J, Weitz JI. New antithrombotic agents. *Lancet* 1999;353: 1431–1436.

94. Berkowitz SD, Marder VJ, Kosutic G, et al. Oral heparin administration with a novel drug delivery agent (SNAC) in healthy volunteers and patients undergoing elective total hip arthroplasty. *J Thromb Haemost* 2003;1: 1914–1919.

95. Eriksson BI, Dahl OE, Buller HR, et al. A new oral direct thrombin inhibitor, dabigatran etexilate, compared with enoxaparin for prevention of thromboembolic events following total hip or knee replacement: the BISTRO II randomized trial. *J Thromb Haemost* 2005;3:103–111.

96. Prandoni P, Lensing AW, Cogo A, et al. The long-term clinical course of acute deep venous thrombosis. *Ann Intern Med* 1996;125:1–7.

97. Heit JA, Mohr DN, Silverstein MD, et al. Predictors of recurrence after deep vein thrombosis and pulmonary embolism: a population-based cohort study. *Arch Intern Med* 2000;160:761–768.

98. Kyrle PA, Minar E, Bialonczyk C, et al. The risk of recurrent venous thromboembolism in men and women. *N Engl J Med* 2004;350:2558–2563.

99. Eichinger S, Weltermann A, Minar E, et al. Symptomatic pulmonary embolism and the risk of recurrent venous thromboembolism. *Arch Intern Med* 2004;164:92–96.

100. Baglin T, Luddington R, Brown K, et al. Incidence of recurrent venous thromboembolism in relation to clinical and thrombophilic risk factors: prospective cohort study. *Lancet* 2003;362:523–526.

101. Schulman S, Rhedin AS, Lindmarker P, et al. A comparison of six weeks with six months of oral anticoagulant therapy after a first episode of venous thromboembolism. Duration of Anticoagulation Trial Study Group. *N Engl J Med* 1995;332:1661–1665.

102. Schulman S, Granqvist S, Holmstrom M, et al. The duration of oral anticoagulant therapy after a second episode of venous thromboembolism. The Duration of Anticoagulation Trial Study Group. *N Engl J Med* 1997;336: 393–398.

103. Ost D, Tepper J, Mihara H, et al. Duration of anticoagulation following venous thromboembolism: a meta-analysis. *JAMA* 2005;294:706–715.

104. Kearon C, Gent M, Hirsh J, et al. A comparison of three months of anticoagulation with extended anticoagulation for a first episode of idiopathic venous thromboembolism. *N Engl J Med* 1999;340:901–907.

105. Agnelli G, Prandoni P, Santamaria MG, et al. Three months versus one year of oral anticoagulant therapy for idiopathic deep venous thrombosis. Warfarin Optimal Duration Italian Trial Investigators. *N Engl J Med* 2001; 345:165–169.

106. Agnelli G, Prandoni P, Becattini C, et al. Extended oral anticoagulant therapy after a first episode of pulmonary embolism. *Ann Intern Med* 2003; 139:19–25.

107. Schulman S, Wahlander K, Lundstrom T, et al. Secondary prevention of venous thromboembolism with the oral direct thrombin inhibitor ximelagatran. *N Engl J Med* 2003;349:1713–1721.

108. Kearon C, Ginsberg JS, Kovacs MJ, et al. Comparison of low-intensity warfarin therapy with conventional-intensity warfarin therapy for long-term prevention of recurrent venous thromboembolism. *N Engl J Med* 2003;349:631–639.

109. Ridker PM, Goldhaber SZ, Danielson E, et al. Long-term, low-intensity warfarin therapy for the prevention of recurrent venous thromboembolism. *N Engl J Med* 2003;348:1425–1434.

110. Eichinger S, Minar E, Bialonczyk C, et al. D-dimer levels and risk of recurrent venous thromboembolism. *JAMA* 2003;290:1071–1074.

111. Prandoni P, Lensing AW, Prins MH, et al. Residual venous thrombosis as a predictive factor of recurrent venous thromboembolism. *Ann Intern Med* 2002;137:955–960.

112. Goldhaber SZ, Turpie AG. Prevention of venous thromboembolism among hospitalized medical patients. *Circulation* 2005;111:e1–e3.

113. Vaitkus PT, Leizorovicz A, Cohen AT, et al. Mortality rates and risk factors

for asymptomatic deep vein thrombosis in medical patients. *Thromb Haemost* 2005;93:76–79.

114. Kucher N, Tapson VF, Quiroz R, et al. Gender differences in the administration of prophylaxis to prevent deep venous thrombosis. *Thromb Haemost* 2005;93:284–288.

115. ldhaber, SZ. Venous thromboembolism: An ounce of prevention. *Mayo Clinic Proceedings* 2005;80:725–726.

116. Urbankova J, Quiroz R, Kucher N, et al. Intermittent pneumatic compression and deep vein thrombosis prevention: A meta-analysis in postoperative patients. *Thromb Haemost* 2005;94:1181–1185.

117. Agnelli G. Prevention of venous thromboembolism in surgical patients. *Circulation* 2004;110:IV-4–IV-12.

118. Leizorovicz A, Mismetti P. Preventing venous thromboembolism in medical patients. *Circulation* 2004;IV-13–IV-19.

119. Avorn J, Winkelmayer WC. Comparing the costs, risks, and benefits of competing strategies for the primary prevention of venous thromboembolism. *Circulation* 2004;110:IV-25–IV-32.

120. Kucher N, Koo S, Quiroz R, et al. Electronic alerts to prevent venous thromboembolism among hospitalized patients. *N Engl J Med* 2005;352:969–977.

CHAPTER 23 ■ HYPERLIPIDEMIA

FREDERICK F. SAMAHA AND DANIEL J. RADER

OVERVIEW
RATIONALE FOR STRATEGIES FOR CHOLESTEROL
    LOWERING
BACKGROUND ABOUT THERAPY FOR LIPID DISORDERS
Nonpharmacologic Therapy
Pharmacologic Therapy
Pharmacologic Therapy for LDL Cholesterol Reduction
Pharmacologic Therapy for Atherogenic Dyslipidemia (Elevated
    Triglycerides and Low HDL-C)
HYPERTRIGLYCERIDEMIA
APPROACH TO PATIENTS WITH LOW HDL
    CHOLESTEROL

OVERVIEW

Large epidemiologic studies such as the Framingham Heart Study (1) and the Multiple Risk Factor Intervention Trial (MRFIT) (2) suggest a relationship between serum cholesterol and coronary heart disease (CHD). Subsequently, multiple prospective, randomized, controlled clinical trials have demonstrated the clinical benefit of cholesterol reduction, in both the secondary prevention and primary prevention of cardiovascular events (see later discussion). These trials have played an important role in the evolution of our treatment of hyperlipidemia.

The clinical management of patients with hyperlipidemia requires a general working knowledge of normal lipoprotein metabolism (3). Lipoproteins transport cholesterol and triglycerides within the blood. They contain a neutral lipid core consisting of triglycerides and cholesteryl esters surrounded by phospholipids and specialized proteins known as apolipoproteins. The five major families of lipoproteins are chylomicrons, very-low-density lipoproteins (VLDL), intermediate-density lipoproteins (IDL), low-density lipoproteins (LDL), and high-density lipoproteins (HDL). Chylomicrons are the largest and most lipid-rich lipoproteins, whereas HDL are the smallest lipoproteins and contain the least amount of lipid. Disorders of lipoprotein metabolism involve perturbations, which cause elevation or reduction of one or more lipoprotein classes. Many of these disorders increase risk of premature atherosclerotic cardiovascular disease. The remainder of this chapter will focus on the identification, diagnosis, and clinical management of patients with lipid disorders, especially regarding the prevention of atherosclerosis and its associated clinical events.

Apolipoproteins are required for the structural integrity of lipoproteins and direct their metabolic interactions with enzymes, lipid transport proteins, and cell surface receptors. Apolipoprotein B (apoB) is the major apolipoprotein in chylomicrons, VLDL, IDL, and LDL. Apolipoprotein A-I (apoA-I) is the major apolipoprotein in HDL. Lipoprotein receptors bind these apolipoproteins on the lipoprotein particles. The best understood lipoprotein receptor is the LDL receptor, which is responsible for the uptake and catabolism of LDL, as well as chylomicron and VLDL remnants (4). The level of LDL receptor expression in the liver plays a major role in regulating the plasma level of cholesterol. A second pathway for clearance of apoE-containing chylomicron and VLDL remnants is called the LDL receptor-related protein (LRP). This receptor is particularly important when there is a deficiency of LDL receptors (5).

Lipid modifying enzymes and lipid transport proteins also play a major role in lipoprotein metabolism and potentially in atherosclerosis. Lipoprotein lipase (LPL) is an enzyme that hydrolyzes triglycerides in chylomicrons and VLDL. It is bound to the surface of the capillary endothelium, especially in muscle and adipose tissue, and binds to the chylomicrons as they traverse the capillary bed. A required cofactor for LPL is apoC-II, which is found on the chylomicrons. The LPL-mediated hydrolysis of triglycerides generates free fatty acids when they enter the tissue to serve as a source of energy or fat storage. The resulting "chylomicron remnant" is released and eventually taken up by the liver. Hepatic lipase is synthesized primarily by the liver, where it is anchored to the vascular endothelium. It is involved in the hydrolyzing of triglycerides in chylomicron remnants, IDL, and HDL as well as phospholipids in HDL2 (6). Lecithin-cholesterol acyltransferase (LCAT) converts free cholesterol to cholesteryl ester on lipoproteins (especially HDL) by transferring fatty acids from phospholipids to cholesterol (7). The cholesteryl ester transfer protein (CETP) transfers cholesteryl esters and other lipids among lipoproteins (8). One major role is thought to be the transfer of cholesteryl esters from HDL (formed as a result of LCAT activity) to VLDL and IDL in exchange for triglycerides. This may be a major pathway by which cholesterol obtained from cells by HDL is eventually returned to the liver in a process that has been termed "reverse cholesterol transport." However, some cholesteryl esters are transferred by CETP to VLDL and LDL, and therefore CETP could promote atherogenesis; the relationship of CETP to atherosclerosis remains uncertain. In summary, these lipoprotein-modifying enzymes and lipid transport enzymes act in concert to modulate lipoprotein metabolism and probably have important effects on atherosclerosis.

RATIONALE FOR STRATEGIES FOR CHOLESTEROL LOWERING

Multiple randomized, controlled clinical trials have demonstrated the benefit of cholesterol reduction in the secondary prevention of cardiovascular events (i.e., in those who already have documented CHD or other atherosclerotic cardiovascular disease). The Coronary Drug Project demonstrated a modest benefit of niacin in reducing nonfatal myocardial infarction (MI) after 6 years of treatment (9) and in reducing total mortality after 15 years of follow-up (10). The POSCH trial employed the surgical technique of partial ileal bypass surgery to reduce LDL cholesterol levels and demonstrated a significant 35% relative reduction in fatal CHD and nonfatal MI, although not in total mortality (the primary endpoint of the trial) (11).

Three more recent secondary prevention trials utilized HMGCoA reductase inhibitors (statins). The Scandinavian Simvastatin Survival Study (4S) (12) was designed to address whether cholesterol reduction with simvastatin in people with CHD and elevated cholesterol would reduce total mortality. The trial enrolled 4,444 subjects with CHD whose total cholesterol levels were between 212 and 310 mg/dL, and who were randomized to placebo or simvastatin for a mean of 5.4 years. There was a highly significant 30% relative reduction in total mortality in the simvastatin-treated group ($P < 0.00001$). The relative risk of a major coronary event was reduced by 44%, and revascularization procedures were decreased by 34%. Importantly, the quartile with the lowest LDL cholesterol levels at baseline had proportionately as much benefit from treatment as the highest quartile (13). An economic analysis based on the 4S study concluded that the reduction in hospital costs alone as a result of the treatment would offset the cost of the medication (14).

The majority of patients with CHD, however, do not have such elevated cholesterol levels; in fact, approximately 35% of all people with CHD have total cholesterol levels less than 200 mg/dL (15). Therefore, another major trial, the Cholesterol and Recurrent Events (CARE) Study (16), addressed whether patients with prior MI and "average" cholesterol levels would benefit from further cholesterol reduction with pravastatin. In this trial, 4,159 patients who were 3 to 20 months post-MI and had total cholesterol levels <240 mg/dL were randomized to placebo or pravastatin 40 mg daily and followed for an average of 5 years. The mean baseline total cholesterol level was 209 mg/dL in each group, and the mean baseline LDL cholesterol level was only 139 mg/dL (range 115 to 174 mg/dL). After 5 years, there were 274 subjects in the placebo group who experienced a nonfatal MI or CHD death (the primary endpoint), compared with 212 subjects in the pravastatin-treated group, for a 24% reduction in relative risk ($P = 0.003$). Revascularization procedures were reduced by 27%. These results demonstrated that the benefit of cholesterol-lowering therapy extends even to those patients with CHD who have average cholesterol levels. The LIPID trial (17) was an even larger (9,014 patients) secondary prevention study of patients with CHD who had baseline cholesterol levels of 155 to 271 mg/dL. Subjects were randomized to placebo or pravastatin 40 mg and followed for an average of 6 years. Coronary heart disease mortality was reduced by 24% ($P < 0.001$) and overall mortality by 22% ($P < 0.001$), and there were significant reductions in other CHD events (MI, unstable angina, and need for revascularization), as well as strokes.

The benefit of therapies aimed at low HDL cholesterol in patients with CHD was recently addressed in the Veteran Affairs High-Density Lipoprotein Cholesterol Intervention Trial Study (VA-HIT) (18). Treatment with gemfibrozil (1,200 mg daily) in 2,531 patients with CHD, low HDL cholesterol (mean 32 mg/dL), and relatively low LDL cholesterol levels (mean 112 mg/dL) resulted in a 22% reduction in the primary endpoint (nonfatal MI and coronary death) compared to placebo ($P = 0.006$) after an average of 5.1 years. Notably, gemfibrozil resulted in a 6% increase in HDL cholesterol and a 31% decrease in triglycerides but no change in LDL cholesterol levels. This important study extends the indication for lipid-modifying drug therapy in patients with CHD to those with well-controlled LDL cholesterol but low HDL cholesterol.

Primary prevention of CHD is extremely important, as approximately one-quarter to one-third of first MIs result in death (19), precluding the opportunity for secondary preven-

tion. Randomized clinical trials support the use of cholesterol-lowering drug therapy in primary prevention as well. In the World Health Organization cooperative trial using clofibrate in hypercholesterolemic men (20), there was a 25% reduction in relative risk of nonfatal MI (the primary endpoint) after 5 years, although a substantial 47% increase in noncardiovascular deaths. In the Lipid Research Clinics (LRC) primary prevention trial with cholestyramine in hypercholesterolemic men (21,22), combined fatal CHD and nonfatal MI (the primary endpoint) were reduced by 19%. The Helsinki Heart Study (23) using gemfibrozil in men with elevated "non-HDL cholesterol" >200 mg/dL demonstrated a significant 34% reduction in combined fatal and nonfatal MI.

Two more recent trials with statins have confirmed the efficacy of cholesterol lowering in primary prevention. The West of Scotland Coronary Prevention Study (WOSCOPS) (24) was performed in 6,595 healthy Scottish men ages 45 to 64 with total cholesterol levels >252 mg/dL and LDL cholesterol levels 174 to 232 mg/dL. Subjects were randomized to pravastatin 40 mg/day versus placebo and followed for an average of 5 years. The primary endpoint of the study was nonfatal MI or CHD death. There were 248 such CHD events in the placebo group and 174 CHD events in the pravastatin group, resulting in a 31% reduction in relative risk of nonfatal MI or CHD death ($P < 0.001$). In addition, there was a significant 32% reduction in cardiovascular mortality and a 37% reduction in revascularization procedures. Importantly, the relative risk of death from any cause (total mortality) was reduced by 22% in the pravastatin-treated group. This trial clearly established that drug therapy for hypercholesterolemia decreases the risk of cardiovascular events and total mortality, even in people who do not have prior evidence of CHD.

The AFCAPS/TcxCAPS trials extended these findings for primary prevention into a population with average cholesterol levels (25). A total of 6,608 men and women without clinical cardiovascular disease, with an LDL cholesterol level of 130 to 190 mg/dL, and with HDL cholesterol levels <45 mg/dL in men and <47 mg/dL in women were randomized to lovastatin 20 mg or placebo for an average of 5.2 years. There was a 37% relative risk reduction ($P < 0.001$) in the primary endpoint (defined as either fatal or nonfatal MI, unstable angina, or sudden cardiac death) in the lovastatin-treated group. Revascularizations were also significantly reduced by 33%. Interestingly, only 17% of the subjects in this trial would have met current National Cholesterol Education Program (NCEP) guidelines for drug therapy. Therefore, the major clinical challenge in the use of drug therapy for cholesterol in primary prevention is the accurate identification of individuals who are likely to develop clinical CHD and who are therefore most likely to benefit from drug therapy.

One question that was generated by these prior statin trials was the potential merits of more intensive LDL cholesterol lowering. Findings from the Heart Protection Study provided preliminary evidence that this indeed might be the case. This study enrolled 20,536 patients with coronary artery disease (CAD), vascular disease, or diabetes and randomized them to simvastatin or placebo for 5 years. In the subgroup of patients with a baseline LDL cholesterol less than 117 mg/dL (6,793 patients), whose mean LDL cholesterol level was lowered to 70 mg/dL on simvastatin, there was still a 21% reduction in major vascular events (fatal or nonfatal MI, stroke, or revascularization) (26). More recently, the PROVE-IT trial compared intensive LDL cholesterol lowering with atorvastatin 80 mg to less-intensive LDL cholesterol lowering with pravastatin 40 mg in 4,162 patients who had just been hospitalized for an acute coronary syndrome. Those assigned to atorvastatin experienced a decrease in mean LDL cholesterol to 62 mg/dL versus a decrease to 95 mg/dL in the pravastatin group. The primary event rate (combined endpoint of all-cause death, nonfatal MI, unstable angina requiring hospitalization, revascularization within 30 days, or stroke) was 16% lower ($P = 0.005$) with more intensive LDL cholesterol lowering (27). Most recently the Treating to New Targets (TNT) trial addressed the issue of more- versus less-intensive LDL cholesterol lowering in stable patients with established CAD and an LDL cholesterol >130 mg/dL (28). This trial enrolled 10,001 patients with CHD randomized them to atorvastatin 80 mg or atorvastatin 10 mg, and followed them for a median of 4.9 years. Those assigned to 80 mg of atorvastatin experienced a decrease in LDL cholesterol to 77 mg/dL, as compared to 101 mg/dL in the group receiving the 10 mg of atorvastatin. More-intensive LDL cholesterol lowering in this trial led to a 22% lower ($P <0.001$) incidence of the primary endpoint (time to first major cardiovascular event, defined as CHD-death, nonfatal non-procedural-related MI, resuscitated cardiac arrest, and fatal and nonfatal stroke). Overall mortality, however, was not significantly different between groups.

In summary, the overall body of clinical data strongly supports the use of drug therapy for LDL cholesterol reduction in virtually all patients with established atherosclerotic vascular disease or diabetes and in certain higher risk groups without vascular disease. Aggressive cholesterol reduction in patients with CHD or other atherosclerotic disease is now the standard of care, as agreed on in a joint statement issued by the American Heart Association (AHA) and the American College of Cardiology (ACC) (29). A recent update to these AHA/ACC guidelines incorporated the findings from newer trials (30). With regard to intensive LDL cholesterol lowering, intensive LDL cholesterol lowering to achieve a level <70 mg/dL is now considered a therapeutic option for patients at very high risk, such as those with established cardiovascular disease plus (a) multiple risk factors (particularly diabetes), (b) severe and poorly controlled risk factors (especially continued cigarette smoking), (c) multiple features of the metabolic syndrome (particularly low HDL cholesterol and elevated triglycerides), and (d) a recent acute coronary syndrome.

BACKGROUND ABOUT THERAPY FOR LIPID DISORDERS

Nonpharmacologic Therapy

Dietary modification is an important component of the effective management of patients with lipid disorders. It is important for the physician to make a general assessment of the patient's diet, to provide suggestions for improvement, and to recognize whether a patient may benefit from referral to a dietician for more intensive counseling. The dietary approach depends on the type of hyperlipidemia. For predominant hypercholesterolemia, the major approach is restriction of saturated fat intake.

Current recommendations regarding total and saturated fat consumption are available from the NCEP Expert Panel (31), the AHA (32), and the U.S. Department of Health and Human Services (DHHS) and the U.S. Department of Agriculture (USDA) (33). The NCEP guidelines recommend that 25% to 35% of calories should be derived from fat, with <7% of calories from saturated fat. The AHA Dietary guidelines focus on the restriction of both saturated fat to <10% (or <7% for those with cardiovascular disease, diabetes, or elevated LDL cholesterol). The DHHS executive summary recommends consuming 20% to 35% of calories from fat, with <10% from saturated fats. All three of these guidelines also recommend the general restriction of trans fat because this is known to elevate total and LDL cholesterol while lowering HDL cholesterol.

The majority of patients have relatively modest (<10%) decreases in LDL cholesterol levels with restriction of saturated fat intake to <10% of total calories. If therapeutic goals for LDL cholesterol are not reached after 3 to 6 months with this degree of restriction, the patient may be counseled on further restriction in saturated fat to <7% of total calories. All patients with established atherosclerotic cardiovascular disease should be instructed directly in restricting saturated fat intake to <7%. Many people experience a decrease in HDL cholesterol when they decrease the amount of total and saturated fat in their diet. The clinical implications of this decrease in HDL-C are not clear, and patients should be reassured that a low-fat diet is nevertheless beneficial in terms of overall cardiovascular risk. Substituting unsaturated fat for saturated fat may lower LDL cholesterol without simultaneously lowering HDL cholesterol (34). This dietary principle partly underlies the Mediterranean style of diet, which has been associated with reduced cardiovascular event rates in two randomized controlled trials (35,36). The most recent guidelines from the NCEP have liberalized to a certain degree the intake of unsaturated fat (up to 10% polyunsaturated fat and up to 20% monounsaturated fat intake) (37). For patients with mild to moderate hypertriglyceridemia, dietary counseling should also include restriction of simple carbohydrates. Treatment of severe hypertriglyceridemia (>1,000 mg/dL) includes restriction of all fat intake, both saturated and unsaturated. Regular aerobic exercise can have a positive effect on lipids. Elevated triglycerides are especially sensitive to aerobic exercise, and people with hypertriglyceridemia can substantially lower their triglycerides by initiating an exercise program. The effect of exercise on LDL cholesterol levels is more modest. Although widely believed to be a method for raising HDL cholesterol, the effects of aerobic exercise on HDL are relatively modest in most individuals. Patients should also be reminded that aerobic exercise has cardiovascular benefits that extend well beyond its effect on lipid levels (38). Obesity is often associated with hyperlipidemia, especially with elevated triglycerides and low HDL cholesterol. In people who are overweight, weight loss can have a significant favorable impact on the lipid profile and should be actively encouraged. Along with counseling on other dietary issues, a dietician should also advise patients on the caloric restriction necessary for effective weight loss.

Hormone replacement therapy (HRT) decreases LDL cholesterol, raises HDL cholesterol, and decreases Lp(a) levels. However, HRT can raise triglycerides and is relatively contraindicated in women with triglycerides over 500 mg/dL. Although earlier observational studies suggested that estrogen replacement is associated with reduced cardiovascular risk (39), two subsequent prospective trials showed no such beneficial effect of HRT and perhaps an adverse effect. In the Heart and Estrogen/Progestin Replacement Study (HERS) of 2,763 postmenopausal women with CHD, HRT for an average of 4.1 years did not reduce the overall rate of nonfatal MI or CHD death (40). The Women's Health Initiative was a randomized controlled trial of 16,608 women aged 50 to 79, who were randomized to either conjugated equine estrogens, 0.625 mg/d, plus medroxyprogesterone acetate, 2.5 mg/d, or placebo (41). The primary outcome was CHD, defined as either nonfatal MI or CHD death, with invasive breast cancer as the primary adverse outcome. After a mean of 5.2 years of follow-up, the data and safety monitoring board recommended stopping the trial, because the test statistic for invasive breast cancer exceeded the stopping boundary for this adverse effect. The incidence of the primary outcome of CHD death or nonfatal MI was actually higher for those randomized to estrogen replacement, with a relative risk of 1.29 (1.02 to 1.63), whereas the incidence of invasive breast cancer was also higher, with a relative risk of 1.26 (1.00 to 1.59). Based on these findings, estrogen replacement therapy using this combination is not currently recommended.

Pharmacologic Therapy

Drug therapy for lipid disorders should be based on clinical trials indicating the benefit of treatment in decreasing the risk of cardiovascular morbidity and mortality. Low-density lipoprotein cholesterol levels are associated with increased risk of CHD, and abundant data exist that treatment to lower LDL decreases risk of clinical cardiovascular events in both secondary and primary prevention. Prior to initiating pharmacologic therapy for hyperlipidemia, the target LDL cholesterol level should be determined (see Fig. 23-1).

Pharmacologic Therapy for LDL Cholesterol Reduction

Inhibitors of 3-hydroxy-3-methylglutaryl coenzyme A (HMG-CoA reductase), the rate-limiting step in cholesterol biosynthesis, are known as statins and are first-line therapy for reducing LDL cholesterol levels. Six HMG-CoA reductase inhibitors are currently available: lovastatin (Mevacor), pravastatin (Pravachol), simvastatin (Zocor), fluvastatin (Lescol), atorvastatin (Lipitor), and rosuvastatin (Crestor). Statins are generally well tolerated, with gastrointestinal and musculoskeletal complaints the most common side effects. Severe myopathy and even rhabdomyolysis have been rarely reported. The incidence of rhabdomyolysis is increased by factors that lower volume of distribution (e.g., smaller body size) and that lower the metabolism of statins (e.g., older age, hepatic and renal dysfunction, hypothyroidism, and diabetes) (42). The majority of cases of rhabdomyolysis occur in patients taking drugs that affect the metabolism of statins, including fibrates, cyclosporine, macrolide antibiotics, warfarin, amiodarone, HIV protease inhibitors, and azole antifungals (42). The incidence of rhabdomyolysis can be minimized by avoiding whenever possible the concomitant therapy with these medications, using the lowest effective dose in achieving the lipid lowering target, and educating patients about the importance of stopping statins and reporting any unexplained muscle pains or discoloration of the urine. Overall, however, the risk of rhabdomyolysis is low, and creatine phosphokinase should not be monitored on a routine

basis. Liver transaminases should be monitored (after 6 to 8 weeks, then every 6 months thereafter), although significant elevation in transaminases is rare. Mild to moderate ($<3\times$ normal) elevation in transaminases in the absence of symptoms need not mandate discontinuing the medication.

Bile acid sequestrants include cholestyramine (Questran), colestipol (Colestid), and colesevelam (WelChol). They bind bile acids in the intestine, interrupt their enterohepatic circulation, and accelerate the loss of bile acids in the stool. The decreased intracellular cholesterol content results in upregulation of the hepatic LDL receptor and enhanced LDL clearance from the plasma. Thus bile acid sequestrants are especially effective in combination therapy with statins. These drugs should not, however, be prescribed for patients with elevated triglyceride levels because they exacerbate hypertriglyceridemia. The bile acid sequestrants are very safe drugs that are not systemically absorbed. However, they are often inconvenient and unpleasant to take. Most side effects are limited to the gastrointestinal tract; bloating and constipation are common and ultimately dose limiting. Colesevelam is a nonabsorbed polymer that has been specifically engineered to have high affinity for bile acids in the intestine and appears to be better tolerated than the other bile acid sequestrants (43). In addition, bile acid sequestrants may bind certain other drugs (e.g., statins, digoxin, and warfarin) and interfere with their absorption. For this reason, other medications should be taken at least 1 hour before or 4 hours after taking bile acid sequestrants.

Ezetimibe is the first in a new class of cholesterol-lowering drugs that inhibits the absorption of dietary and biliary cholesterol. This drug is used at a single oral dose of 10 mg and alone lowers LDL cholesterol by approximately 18%. The combination of ezetimibe with simvastatin, at doses of 10 mg to 80 mg, has been shown to lower LDL cholesterol by 44% to 59%, respectively (1,44,45). Vytorin is a formulation that combines ezetimibe 10 mg with the full range of simvastatin doses (i.e., 10 to 80 mg).

In summary, these drugs provide the armamentarium for the lowering of LDL cholesterol, and an algorithm for their use is given in Figure 23-2.

Pharmacologic Therapy for Atherogenic Dyslipidemia (Elevated Triglycerides and Low HDL-C)

Atherogenic dyslipidemia is most commonly observed in patients with the metabolic syndrome, currently defined as having at least three of the following abnormalities (37,46): (a) central obesity (waist size >40 inches in men and >35 inches in women), (b) fasting glucose >100 mg/dL, (c) fasting triglyceride levels >150 mg/dL or the requirement of drugs to lower triglycerides, (d) elevated blood pressure >130/85 or the requirement of antihypertensive medications, and (e) depressed HDL-C (<40 mg/dL in men and <50 mg/dL in women) or the use of drugs to raise HDL-C. Beyond metabolic syndrome, important lifestyle factors, concomitant drugs, and genetic abnormalities can give rise to elevated triglycerides and low HDL-C. The importance of atherogenic dyslipidemia in terms of cardiovascular disease and specific therapies for treating these lipid abnormalities is an evolving field. Elevated triglycerides may confer an increased risk of cardiovascular disease due to increased partially degraded VLDL or remnant lipoproteins that contain cholesterol (VLDL cholesterol). In patients with a triglyceride level >200 mg/dL, atherogenic risk is better estimated by adding together VLDL cholesterol + LDL cholesterol. This can be estimated by the non-HDL cholesterol = total cholesterol − HDL cholesterol. The goal for non-HDL cholesterol is set at 30 mg/dL higher than the LDL cholesterol goal (Fig. 23-1).

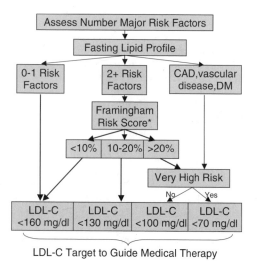

FIGURE 23-1. Algorithm for the initial evaluation of risk for major cardiovascular events and ascertainment of target LDL-C level.

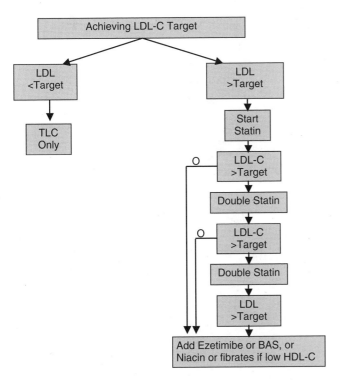

FIGURE 23-2. Algorithm for the medical therapy to obtain target LDL-C level.

HYPERTRIGLYCERIDEMIA

A large number of epidemiological studies have addressed the relationship between elevated serum triglyceride levels and cardiovascular risk (47–50). Although there is increasing recognition of triglycerides as an independent risk factor, some controversy still exists (51), partly due to the heterogenous metabolic disposition of triglycerides. In addition, triglycerides are transported in a number of different lipoprotein fractions that are known to have differing atherogenic potentials. Elevated triglycerides levels are associated with a number of other proatherogenic metabolic and physiological changes, such as a low HDL level, a procoagulant state, and increased small dense LDL particles. There are no clinical trial outcome data for drug therapy in patients with triglycerides greater than 400 to 500 mg/dL, as all the clinical trials discussed earlier excluded persons with triglycerides in this range.

Severe hypertriglyceridemia (fasting triglycerides >1,000 mg/dL) is always an indication of hyperchylomicronemia in the fasting state and points to an underlying genetic predisposition. The most common diagnosis in adults is type V hyperlipoproteinemia (HLP). The label of type V HLP is generally used for an adult with triglyceride levels over 1,000 mg/dL who does not have known familial chylomicronemia syndrome due to LPL or apoC-II deficiency (see earlier discussion). Type V HLP is also associated with risk of acute pancreatitis, which can be the initial presentation of this syndrome and is the major rationale for aggressive treatment of this condition. Type V HLP can also be associated with increased risk of cardiovascular disease, although some patients with type V do not appear to be at significantly increased risk. Type II diabetes mellitus or glucose intolerance frequently accompanies type V hyperlipidemia, but type V also occurs in people with normal glucose tolerance.

Another genetic lipid disorder associated with severe hypertriglyceridemia is type III hyperlipidemia, which is associated with elevated levels of remnant lipoproteins. This disorder is characterized by a defective form of apoE (apoE2) that results in impaired binding to hepatic receptors and hence markedly elevated serum total cholesterol and triglyceride levels (52). The apoE2 isoform differs from the most common apoE3 isoform by a single amino acid substitution and occurs with a surprisingly high allelic frequency of approximately 7%. Approximately 1% of the population is homozygous for the apoE2 (53). However, only 1 out of 50 individuals with the apoE2/E2 phenotype actually manifests type III hyperlipidemia, suggesting the need for additional environmental factors that increase remnant lipoprotein levels (e.g., weight gain, diabetes, or thyroid dysfunction) and/or drugs that further impair remnant lipoprotein uptake (e.g., certain HIV protease inhibitors) (52). Type III hyperlipidemia is associated with an increased risk for cardiovascular disease, but it is also typically amenable to intensive lifestyle and pharmacologic intervention.

The management of severe hypertriglyceridemia is first targeted to decreasing triglycerides to reduce the risk of pancreatitis, followed by further lipid lowering depending on future risk for cardiovascular events. Women taking estrogens and patients taking isotretinoin or etretinate should be encouraged to discontinue them if triglycerides are >1,000 mg/dL. Diabetes mellitus should be controlled as optimally as possible. In general, dietary management includes restriction of total fat as well as simple carbohydrates and alcohol in the diet. Regular aerobic exercise can significantly lower triglyceride levels and should be actively encouraged. If the patient is overweight, weight loss can help to decrease triglycerides as well.

Fibrates are agonists for the nuclear hormone receptor PPARα and have multiple effects on lipoprotein metabolism. Fibrates lower triglyceride levels effectively and raise HDL cholesterol levels modestly, but have limited ability to lower LDL cholesterol levels. In the United States, this class includes clofibrate (Atromid-S), gemfibrozil (Lopid), and micronized fenofibrate (TriCor). Fibrates are generally well tolerated; side effects include gastrointestinal upset and muscle pains. Elevated liver function tests can occur and should be monitored during therapy. Fibrates increase the lithogenicity of bile and therefore the risk of gallstones. Like niacin, fibrates potentiate the effect of warfarin. The most straightforward clinical roles of fibrates are in the treatment of significant hypertriglyceridemia. However, the VA-HIT study has extended the rationale for the use of fibrates to the prevention of cardiovascular events in patients with established CHD and low HDL cholesterol in the setting of a controlled LDL cholesterol level. There are two ongoing clinical trials comparing combination fibrate-statin therapy to statin monotherapy. The Fenofibrate Intervention and Event Lowering in Diabetes (FIELD) Study is examining the effects of long-term fenofibrate therapy versus placebo (in addition to usual care that may include statin therapy) on CHD event rates in 9,795 patients with type 2 diabetes mellitus (54). The results from this trial are anticipated in late 2005. The Action to Control Cardiovascular Risk in Diabetes (ACCORD) Trial will test whether adding fenofibrate to statin therapy reduces cardiovascular events more than statin monotherapy in patients with type II diabetes. Enrollment in this trial is expected to be complete by 2005, with follow-up projected to end in 2009.

Nicotinic acid, or niacin, is a B-complex vitamin that, in high doses, is an effective lipid-modifying drug. It reduces LDL cholesterol modestly (approximately 7% to 12%) (55,56) and more substantially when used in combination with statins (22% to 59%) (57,58). The recently discovered receptor for nicotinic acid (HM74A) is a G-protein coupled receptor that has β-hydroxybutyrate as its endogenous ligand (59–61). A major site of HM74A expression and action is in adipose tissue. When this receptor is activated by nicotinic acid, it inhibits adenylate cyclase, protein kinase A, and hormone sensitive li-

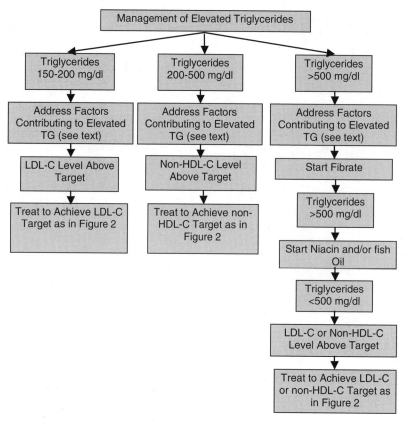

FIGURE 23-3. Algorithm for the management of hyperlipidemia in the setting of elevated triglyceride levels.

pase, thus reducing triglyceride lipolysis and free fatty flux from adipose. This mechanism most likely explains the 30% to 50% reduction in triglyceride levels with niacin therapy. Niacin also raises HDL-C by 20% to 35%, depending on the dose used. In contrast, it is unclear whether there is any relationship between this receptor and HDL cholesterol-raising effects of niacin.

The use of nicotinic acid has been traditionally limited because it commonly causes cutaneous flushing. However, Niaspan, an extended-release form of niacin that is administered once daily, is better tolerated than regular crystalline niacin, allowing greater patient adherence (62). Niacin can exacerbate glycemic control in people with diabetes, but can be safely used in patients with adequately controlled diabetes (56). It can cause elevations in uric acid and has been associated with precipitation of acute gout. Niacin has also been associated with exacerbation of peptic ulcer disease. Niacin potentiates the effect of warfarin and should be used cautiously in this setting. Mild elevation in liver transaminases (up to 2 to 3 times the upper limit of normal) can occur but does not necessarily mandate discontinuance of the niacin.

Fish oils are highly effective triglyceride-lowering agents and are useful for patients with severe hypertriglyceridemia resistant to or intolerant of gemfibrozil, fenofibrate, and niacin. They should not be used for hypercholesterolemia and have been reported to raise LDL cholesterol levels in some people. At least 6 grams/day is usually required for a substantial effect, and many patients require 9 to 12 grams day. Dyspepsia, diarrhea, and a fishy taste and fishy smell to the breath limit the use of fish oils in many patients. However, in patients with refractory hypertriglyceridemia and pancreatitis, fish oils can be exceptionally effective.

Once the triglycerides are adequately controlled, patients often remain significantly hypercholesterolemic. This often raises the issue of a second medication to better control the LDL cholesterol. In patients with CHD or who are at high risk for the development of CHD (such as patients with diabetes), the NCEP guidelines represent a useful guide to the decision to institute further drug therapy (37), as reviewed in Figure 23-3. Although there may be a small increased risk of myopathy when statins are combined with fibrates, this risk can be minimized by advising the patient to call the physician immediately in the event of generalized muscle pain. Overall, in the patient at high risk for future cardiovascular events, the significant benefit of further cholesterol lowering generally outweighs the very small risk of severe myositis associated with combination drug therapy. The FIELD Trial and ACCORD Trial should provide useful safety data on the combination of statins and fenofibrate.

APPROACH TO PATIENTS WITH LOW HDL CHOLESTEROL

High-density lipoproteins cholesterol levels are inversely associated with CHD independent of total and LDL cholesterol levels (63). However, formal guidelines for the approach to the patient with a low HDL cholesterol level (a condition often referred to as hypoalphalipoproteinemia) have not yet been developed. Many causes of low HDL cholesterol are secondary to other factors. Cigarette smoking, obesity, and physical inactivity contribute to low HDL cholesterol. Type II diabetes mellitus, end-stage renal disease, and hypertriglyceridemia from any cause are all associated with low HDL. Beta-blockers, thiazide diuretics, androgens, and progestins can all reduce HDL cholesterol levels. Importantly, a low-fat diet often results in a low level of HDL cholesterol; for example, most vegetarians have low levels of HDL cholesterol. In this case, the low HDL is not considered to be associated with an increased risk of CHD, as people who eat low-fat diets are at substantially reduced risk of premature CHD. However, many people with low HDL cholesterol levels have a genetic cause of hypoalphalipoproteinemia. Some genetic causes of low HDL include mutations in apoA-I, LCAT, and ABC1 (Tangier disease). However, most patients with low HDL do not have a currently identifiable mutation and have what is called primary or familial hypoalphalipoproteinemia (64,65). It is defined as an HDL cholesterol level below the 10th percentile in the setting of relatively normal cholesterol and triglyceride levels, no apparent secondary causes of low HDL, and no clinical signs of LCAT deficiency or Tangier disease. This syndrome is often referred to as "isolated low HDL." A family history of low HDL cholesterol facilitates the diagnosis of an inherited condition, which usually follows the pattern of an autosomal dominant trait.

There are no formal clinical practice guidelines for the management of patients with isolated low HDL cholesterol. However, some general guidelines can be proposed. Secondary factors should be sought and corrected when possible. Smoking should be discontinued, obese people should be encouraged to lose weight, and sedentary people should be encouraged to exercise. When possible, medications associated with reduced HDL cholesterol should be discontinued. Diabetes mellitus should be optimally controlled.

The difficult issue is whether pharmacologic intervention should be used to specifically raise the HDL cholesterol in healthy people. Niacin is the most effective among current FDA-approved drugs for raising HDL-C, and its effects on cardiovascular disease have been evaluated in a recent study. The HDL-Atherosclerosis Treatment Study (HATS) was a 3-year, double-blind study of 160 patients with low HDL cholesterol and normal LDL cholesterol, randomized to one of four regimens: simvastatin plus niacin, antioxidant therapy, combined simvastatin-niacin-antioxidant therapy, or placebo. The two primary endpoints of the study were change in average coronary artery stenosis and the frequency of cardiovascular events (death, MI, stroke, or revascularization). The HDL cholesterol increased by 26% in those receiving simvastatin-niacin, with an attenuated increase in those receiving simvastatin-niacin-antioxidant therapy. Those assigned to simvastatin-niacin experienced a small degree of regression in the average coronary stenosis, whereas each of the other three treatments resulted in significantly greater progression of average coronary stenosis (the primary endpoint of the study). Despite the small size of this study, the frequency of cardiovascular events was also significantly lower in those assigned to simvastatin-niacin (57). The potential benefits of combined statin-niacin therapy on major cardiovascular events will be more definitively tested in the Atherothrombosis Intervention in Metabolic Syndrome with Low HDL/High Triglycerides and Impact on Global Health Outcomes (AIM-HIGH) Trial. This trial, just now being initiated, will compare intensive LDL cholesterol lowering with simvastatin to combined intensive LDL cholesterol lowering and HDL cholesterol raising with simvastatin plus niacin-extended release in 3,300 patients with established vascular disease and atherogenic dyslipidemia. For now, low HDL cholesterol is considered a risk factor for cardiovascular disease, but not a therapeutic target, pending until the results of the FIELD Trial, ACCORD, and AIM-HIGH become available.

Another recent class of drugs are inhibitors of cholesteryl transferase protein (CETP-inhibitors). Cholesteryl transferase protein is a plasma glycoprotein that facilitates the transfer of cholesteryl esters from HDL cholesterol to apoB containing lipoproteins. These drugs provide an increase in HDL cholesterol from 34% (66) to 106% (67), depending on the formulation and dose. Ongoing clinical trials will evaluate whether the increase in HDL cholesterol with CETP inhibitors leads to improvement in coronary stenosis and cardiovascular outcomes.

References

1. Ballantyne CM, Abate N, Yuan Z, et al. Dose-comparison study of the combination of ezetimibe and simvastatin (Vytorin) versus atorvastatin in patients with hypercholesterolemia: The Vytorin Versus Atorvastatin (VYVA) Study. Am Heart J 2005;149(3):464–473.
2. Stamler J, Wentworth D, Neaton JD. Is relationship between serum cholesterol and risk of premature death from coronary heart disease continuous and graded? Findings in 356 222 primary screenees of the multiple risk factor intervention trial (MRFIT). JAMA 1986;256:2823–2828.
3. Rader DJ, Brewer HB. Lipids, apolipoproteins and lipoproteins. In: Goldbourt U, de Faire U. Berg K, eds. Genetic factors in coronary heart disease. Dordrecht: Kluwer Academic Publishers; 1994:83–103.
4. Brown MS, Goldstein JL. A receptor-mediated pathway for cholesterol homeostasis. Science 1986;232:34–47.
5. Beisiegel U. Receptors for triglyceride-rich lipoproteins and their role in lipoprotein metabolism. Curr Opin Lipidol 1995;6:117–122.
6. Santamarina-Fojo S, Haudenschild C, Amar M. The role of hepatic lipase in lipoprotein metabolism and atherosclerosis. Curr Opin Lipidol 1998;9: 211–219.
7. Rader DJ, Ikewaki K. Unravelling high density lipoprotein-apolipoprotein metabolism in human mutants and animal models. Curr Opin Lipidol 1996; 7:117–123.
8. Tall AR. Plasma high density lipoproteins. Metabolism and relationship to atherogenesis. J Clin Invest 1990;86:379–384.
9. The coronary drug project research group. Clofibrate and niacin in coronary heart disease. JAMA 1975;231:360–381.
10. Canner PL, Berge KG, Wenger NK, et al. Fifteen year mortality in Coronary Drug Project patients: long-term benefit with niacin. J Am Coll Cardiol 1986;8(6):1245–1255.
11. Buchwald H, Varco R, Matts J, et al. Effect of partial ileal bypass surgery on mortality and morbidity from coronary heart disease in patients with hypercholesterolemia—Report of the Program on the Surgical Control of the Hyperlipidemias (POSCH). N Engl J Med 1990;323:946–955.
12. Scandinavian Simvastatin Survival Study Group. Randomised trial of cholesterol lowering in 4444 patients with coronary heart disease: the Scandinavian Simvastatin Survival Study (4S). Lancet 1994;344:1383–1389.
13. Scandinavian Simvastatin Survival Study Group. Baseline serum cholesterol and treatment effect in the Scandinavian Simvastatin Survival Study (4S). Lancet 1995;345:1274–1275.
14. Pederson TR, Kjekshus J, Berg K, et al. Cholesterol lowering and the use of healthcare resources Results of the Scandinavian Simvastatin Survival Study. Circulation 1996;93:1796–1802.
15. Kannel WB. Range of serum cholesterol values in the population developing coronary artery disease. Am J Cardiol 1995;76:69C–77C.
16. Sacks FM, Pfeffer MA, Moye LA, et. al. The effect of pravastatin on coronary events after myocardial infarction in patients with average cholesterol levels. N Engl J Med 1996;335:1001–1009.
17. The Long-Term Intervention with Pravastatin in Ischaemic Disease (LIPID) Study Group. Prevention of cardiovascular events and death with pravastatin in patients with coronary heart disease and a broad range of initial cholesterol levels. N Engl J Med 1998;339:1349–1357.
18. Rubins HB, Robins SJ, Collins D, et al. Gemfibrozil for the Secondary Prevention of Coronary Heart Disease in Men with Low Levels of High-Density Lipoprotein Cholesterol. N Engl J Med 1999;341:410–418.
19. Kannel WB, Schatzkin A. Sudden death: lessons from subsets in population studies. J Am Coll Cardiol 1985;5:141b–149b.
20. Committee of Principal Investigators. A cooperative trial in the prevention of ischaemic heart disease using clofibrate. Br Heart J 1978;40:1069–1118.
21. Lipid Research Clinics Program. The lipid research clinics coronary primary prevention trial results. 1. Reduction in incidence of coronary heart disease. JAMA 1984;251:351–364.
22. Lipid Research Clinics Program. The lipid research clinics coronary primary prevention trial results: II. the relationship of reduction in incidence of coronary heart disease to cholesterol lowering. JAMA 1984;251:365–374.
23. Frick MH, Elo O, Haapa K, et al. Helsinki Heart Study: primary-prevention trial with gemfibrozil in middle-aged men with dyslipidemia. Safety of treatment, changes in risk factors, and incidence of coronary heart disease. N Engl J Med 1987;317:1237–1245.
24. Shepherd J, Cobbe SM, Ford I, et al. Prevention of coronary heart disease with pravastatin in men with hypercholesterolemia. N Engl J Med 1995; 333:1301–1307.
25. Downs JR, Clearfield M, Weis S, et al. Primary prevention of acute coronary events with lovastatin in men and women with average cholesterol levels: results of AFCAPS/TexCAPS. JAMA 1998;279:1615–1622.
26. Heart Protection Study Collaboration Group. MRC/BHF Heart Protection

Study of cholesterol lowering with simvastatin in 20 536 high-risk individuals: a randomised placebo-controlled trial. *Lancet* 2002;360:7–22.

27. Cannon CP, Braunwald E, McCabe CH, et al. the Pravastatin or Atorvastatin Evaluation and Infection Therapy-Thrombolysis in Myocardial Infarction 22 Investigators. Intensive versus moderate lipid lowering with statins after acute coronary syndromes. *N Engl J Med* 2004;350(15):1495–1504.

28. LaRosa JC, Grundy SM, Waters DD, et al. Intensive lipid lowering with atorvastatin in patients with stable coronary disease. *N Engl J Med* 2005; 352(14):1425–1435.

29. Smith J, Blair S, Criqui M, et al. Preventing heart attack and death in patients with coronary disease. *Circulation* 1995;92:2–4.

30. Grundy SM, Cleeman JI, Merz CN, et al. Implications of Recent Clinical Trials for the National Cholesterol Education Program Adult Treatment Panel III Guidelines. *Circulation* 2004;110:227–239.

31. National Cholesterol Education Program Expert Panel on Detection, Evaluation, and Treatment of High Blood Cholesterol in Adults (Adult Treatment Panel III) Final Report. *Circulation* 2002;106(25):3163–3223.

32. Krauss RM, Eckel RH, Howard B, et al. AHA dietary guidelines: revision 2000: a statement for healthcare professionals from the Nutrition Committee of the American Heart Association. *Circulation* 2000;102(18): 2284–2299.

33. U.S. Department of Health and Human Services. U.S. Department of Agriculture. Available at www.healthierus.gov/dietaryguidelines. Accessed June 6, 2006.

34. Mensink RP, Katan MB. Effect of monounsaturated fatty acids versus complex carbohydrates on high-density lipoproteins in healthy men and women. *Lancet* 1987;1:122–125.

35. de Lorgeril M, Salen P, Martin J-L, et al. Mediterranean diet, traditional risk factors, and the rate of cardiovascular complications after myocardial infarction: final report of the Lyon Diet Heart Study. *Circulation* 1999; 99(6):779–785.

36. Singh RB, Dubnov G, Niaz MA, et al. Effect of an Indo-Mediterranean diet on progression of coronary artery disease in high risk patients (Indo-Mediterranean Diet Heart Study): a randomised single-blind trial. *Lancet* 2002;360:1455–1461.

37. Expert Panel on Detection, Evaluation, and Treatment of High Blood Cholesterol in Adults. Executive Summary of the Third Report of the National Cholesterol Education Program (NCEP) Expert Panel on Detection, Evaluation, and Treatment of High Blood Cholesterol in Adults (Adult Treatment Panel III). *JAMA* 2001;285:2486–2497.

38. Fletcher GF. The antiatherosclerotic effect of exercise and development of an exercise prescription. *Cardiol Clin* 1996;14:85–95.

39. Kafonek SD. Postmenopausal hormone replacement therapy and cardiovascular risk reduction. A review. *Drugs* 1994;47:16–24.

40. Hulley S, Grady D, Bush T, et al. Randomized trial of estrogen plus progestin for secondary prevention of coronary heart disease in postmenopausal women. Heart and Estrogen/progestin Replacement Study (HERS) Research Group. *JAMA* 1998;280:605–613.

41. Rossouw JE, Anderson G, Prentice R, et al. Risks and benefits of estrogen plus progestin in healthy postmenopausal women. Principal results from the Women's Health Initiative Randomized Controlled Trial. *JAMA* 2002;288 (3):321–333.

42. Thompson PD, Clarkson P, Karas RH. Statin-associated myopathy. *JAMA* 2003;289:1681–1690.

43. Davidson MH, Dillon MA, Gordon B, et al. Colesevelam hydrochloride (Cholestagel): a new, potent bile acid sequestrant associated with a low incidence of gastrointestinal side effects. *Arch Intern Med* 1999;159(16): 1893–1900.

44. Goldberg AC, Sapre A, Liu J, et al. Efficacy and safety of ezetimibe coadministered with simvastatin in patients with primary hypercholesterolemia: a randomized double-blind, placebo-controlled trial. *Mayo Clin Proc* 2004; 79:620–629.

45. Davidson MH, McGarry T, Bettis R, et al. on behalf of the Ezetimibe Study Group. Ezetimibe coadministered with simvastatin in patients with primary hypercholesterolemia. *J Am Coll Cardiol* 2004;40(12):2125–2134.

46. Grundy SM, Cleeman JI, Daniels SR, et al. Diagnosis and management of the metabolic syndrome. An American Heart Association/National Heart, Lung, and Blood Institute Scientific Statement. Executive Summary. *Circulation* 2005;112(17):2735–2752.

47. Hokanson JE, Austin MA. Plasma triglyceride level is a risk factor for cardiovascular disease independent of high-density lipoprotein cholesterol level: a meta-analysis of population-based prospective studies. *J Cardiovasc Risk* 1996;3:213–219.

48. Castelli WP. Epidemiology of triglycerides: a view from Framingham. *Am J Cardiol* 1992;70:3H–9H.

49. Jeppesen J, Hein H, Suadicani P, et al. Triglyceride concentration and ischemic heart disease: an eight-year follow-up in the Copenhagen Male Study. *Circulation* 1998;97:1029–1036.

50. Miller M, Seidler A, Moalemi A, et al. Normal triglyceride levels and coronary artery disease events: the Baltimore Coronary Observational Long-Term Study. *J Am Coll Cardiol* 1998;31:1252–1257.

51. Bass KM, Newschaffer C, Klag M, et al. Plasma lipoprotein levels as predictors of cardiovascular death in women. *Arch Intern Med* 1993;153: 2209–2216.

52. Mahley RW, Huang Y, Rall SC Jr. Pathogenesis of type III hyperlipoproteinemia (dysbetalipoproteinemia): questions, quandaries, and paradoxes. *J Lipid Res* 1999;40(11):1933–1949.

53. Guyton JR. Treatment of Type III Hyperlipoproteinemia. *Am Heart J* 1999; 138:17–18.

54. Keech A. Fenofibrate Intervention and Event Lowering in Diabetes (FIELD) study: baseline characteristics and short-term effects of fenofibrate. *Cardiovasc Diabetol* 2005;4:13.

55. Grundy SM, Vega GL, McGovern ME, et al. Efficacy, safety, and tolerability of once-daily niacin for the treatment of dyslipidemia associated with type 2 diabetes: results of the Assessment of Diabetes Control and Evaluation of the Efficacy of Niaspan Trial. *Arch Intern Med* 2002;162(14):1568–1576.

56. Elam MB, Hunninghake DB, Davis KB, et al. Effect of niacin on lipid and lipoprotein levels and glycemic control in patients with diabetes and peripheral arterial disease: the ADMIT study: A randomized trial. Arterial Disease Multiple Intervention Trial. *JAMA* 2000;284(10):1263–1270.

57. Brown BG, Zhao X-Q, Chait A, et al. Simvastatin and niacin, antioxidant vitamins, or the combination for the prevention of coronary disease. *N Engl J Med* 2001;345(22):1583–1592.

58. Wolfe ML, Vartanian SF, Ross JL, et al. Safety and effectiveness of Niaspan when added sequentially to a statin for treatment of dyslipidemia. *Am J Cardiol* 2001;87:476–479.

59. Wise A, Foord SM, Fraser NJ, et al. Molecular identification of high and low affinity receptors for nicotinic acid. *J Biol Chem* 2003;278:9869–9874.

60. Taggart AKP, Kero J, Gan X, et al. (D)-β-hydroxybutyrate inhibits adipocyte lipolysis via the nicotinic acid receptor PUMA-G. *J Biol Chem* 2005; 280(29):26649–26652.

61. Soga T, Kamohara M, Takasaki J, et al. Molecular identification of nicotinic acid receptor. *Biochem Biophys Res Commun* 2003;303:364–369.

62. Morgan JM, Capuzzi D, Guyton J, et al. Treatment effect of Niaspan, a controlled-release niacin, in patients with hypercholesterolemia: a placebo-controlled trial. *J Cardiovasc Pharm Ther* 1996;1:195–202.

63. Gordon DJ, Rifkind BM. High-density lipoproteins—the clinical implications of recent studies. *N Engl J Med* 1989;321:1311–1316.

64. Third JL, Montag J, Flynn M, et al. Primary and familial hypoalphalipoproteinemia. *Metabolism* 1984;33:136–146.

65. Genest J, Bard J, Fruchart J, et al. Familial hypoalphalipoproteinemia in premature coronary artery disease. *Arterioscler Thromb Vasc Biol* 1993; 13:1728–1737.

66. de Grooth GJ, Kuivenhoven JA, Stalenhoef AFH, et al. Efficacy and safety of a novel cholesteryl ester transfer protein inhibitor, JTT-705, in humans: a randomized phase II dose-response study. *Circulation* 2002;105(18): 2159–2165.

67. Brousseau ME, Schaefer EJ, Wolfe ML, et al. Effects of an inhibitor of cholesteryl ester transfer protein on HDL cholesterol. *N Engl J Med* 2004; 350(15):1505–1515.

CHAPTER 24 ■ DIABETES AND METABOLIC SYNDROME

EMILY D. SZMUILOWICZ AND MERRI PENDERGRASS

GLUCOSE TOLERANCE CATEGORIES
Diabetes Mellitus
Prediabetes
METABOLIC SYNDROME
PREVENTION OF DIABETES
Prevention of T1DM
Prevention of T2DM
PREVENTION OF DIABETES COMPLICATIONS
TREATMENT OF HYPERGLYCEMIA
T1DM
T2DM
CONCLUSIONS

Diabetes mellitus and the "metabolic syndrome" are among the most challenging problems facing health care providers today. Over 18 million Americans, or about 9% of the adult population, are currently estimated to have diabetes (1). Approximately 50 million Americans, or 24% of adults, are estimated to have the metabolic syndrome (2). The metabolic syndrome refers to a constellation of interrelated cardiovascular risk factors that increase risk for the development of type 2 diabetes (T2DM) (3) and cardiovascular disease (4).

The morbidity and mortality associated with diabetes is profound. Diabetes is associated with multiple complications including heart disease, cerebrovascular disease, blindness, renal failure, neuropathy, lower extremity amputations, dental disease, and adverse pregnancy outcomes. Fortunately, complications can be reduced with glycemic control, cardiovascular risk reduction, and preventive care practices for eyes, kidneys, and feet. Unlike diabetes, for which there is widespread consensus regarding diagnostic criteria, metabolic syndrome is a poorly defined cluster of conditions. Furthermore, metabolic syndrome is not clearly associated with any risk beyond that attributable to its individual components. Because treatment currently involves nothing more than treating these individual components, the value of the diagnosis remains controversial.

The focus of this chapter will be on diabetes and hyperglycemia. We will begin by reviewing the various glucose tolerance categories. We will discuss the metabolic syndrome and its relationship to abnormal glucose tolerance and cardiovascular disease. Following a brief review of strategies to prevent diabetes, we will devote the remainder of the chapter to a discussion of therapeutic options for treating hyperglycemia. Other strategies to reduce cardiovascular disease (CVD) in diabetes, such as blood pressure control, treatment of hyperlipidemia, renin-angiotensin system blockade, antiplatelet therapy, and smoking cessation, are discussed in other chapters and will not be addressed here.

GLUCOSE TOLERANCE CATEGORIES

Diabetes Mellitus

Diabetes mellitus refers to a spectrum of metabolic diseases characterized by hyperglycemia that results from defects in insulin secretion, insulin action, or both. The American Diabetes Association (ADA) recognizes four categories of diabetes with different underlying pathophysiologic mechanisms, as shown in Table 24-1. There is frequent overlap between the various types, and many patients do not easily fit into a single class. It is therefore less important to label the particular type of diabetes than it is to understand the pathogenesis of the hyperglycemia and to treat it effectively.

Prediabetes

The ADA Expert Committee recognizes an intermediate group of people whose glucose levels, although not meeting criteria

TABLE 24-1

CATEGORIES OF DIABETES MELLITUS

Type of diabetes	Description
Type 1 diabetes mellitus	Pancreatic β-cell destruction (usually autoimmune) results in *absolute* insulin deficiency.
Type 2 diabetes mellitus	Combination of (1) insulin resistance (which results in decreased peripheral glucose uptake and increased hepatic gluconeogenesis) and (2) *relative* insulin deficiency.
Gestational diabetes mellitus	Any degree of glucose intolerance with onset or first recognition during pregnancy.
Other specific types	Heterogeneous group of disorders including genetic disorders of β-cell function or insulin action, exocrine pancreatic disorders, endocrinopathies, drug- or chemical-induced pancreatic processes, and infections.

Adapted from Diabetes Association. Diagnosis and classification of diabetes mellitus. *Diabetes Care* 2005;28(Suppl 1):S37–S42.

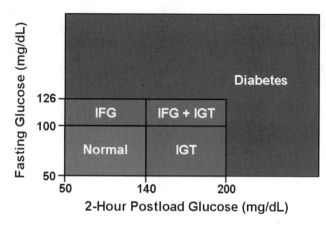

FIGURE 24-1. Categories of glucose tolerance.

for diabetes, are too high to be considered normal (5) (Fig. 24-1). These individuals have been categorized as having *impaired fasting glucose* (IFG) and/or *impaired glucose tolerance* (IGT). IFG and IGT are often referred to as "*prediabetes*," indicating the high risk for future development of T2DM. The annual rate of progression from prediabetes to T2DM is approximately 5% to 10% (6). Although this term may be useful in that it stresses the increased risk of diabetes associated with these conditions, it potentially excludes many people who are also at increased risk. Other important risk factors for diabetes include advanced age, excess adiposity, sedentary lifestyle, family history of diabetes, high-risk ethnic group, history of gestational diabetes, hypertension, dyslipidemia, polycystic ovarian syndrome, and history of vascular disease (7). Most individuals with prediabetes are euglycemic in their daily lives. They may experience transient elevation of the blood glucose during an acute illness, especially if amplified by certain drugs or intravenous glucose. This transient hyperglycemia, which likely indicates reduced insulin sensitivity or secretory capacity, is sometimes the first clue to incipient diabetes. Although the hyperglycemia may resolve immediately following resolution of the illness, it is important to recognize these patients as being at increased risk for T2DM. Regular screening for diabetes should be incorporated into their subsequent medical care.

Although there is increasing evidence that prediabetes increases risk for CVD and CVD mortality independent of traditional cardiovascular risk factors (8), there is no clear evidence that lowering glucose at this stage will reduce diabetes complications. On the other hand, because prediabetes is frequently associated with the metabolic syndrome (see following), components of the syndrome should be sought out and treated.

METABOLIC SYNDROME

The metabolic syndrome refers to a constellation of CVD risk factors that are associated with increased risk of diabetes and CVD (3,4,9). Over the past couple of decades, this cluster of clinical conditions has been referred to by several other names, including Syndrome X, the Dysmetabolic Syndrome, and the Insulin Resistance Syndrome. Key components of the syndrome include obesity, abnormal glucose metabo-lism, dyslipidemia, and hypertension. Insulin resistance and microalbuminuria are included in some, but not all, definitions. Although insulin resistance is widely considered to be the hallmark of the metabolic syndrome (9,10), it is not uniformly accepted to be the

primary pathophysiologic abnormality (11). Multiple sets of diagnostic criteria have been described, each with slightly different components and diagnostic cut points, as shown in Table 24-2 (10,12–15).

The metabolic syndrome has been associated with increased cardiovascular risk in patients without diabetes (16–18) and with T2DM (18). It has also been associated with increased risk of diabetic nephropathy and poor glycemic control in type 1 diabetes (T1DM) (19). Although there is no question that certain CVD risk factors are prone to cluster together, recent studies have questioned whether the metabolic syndrome predicts CVD better than established risk assessment models (16,20) or than the sum of its parts (11).

A recent joint statement by the ADA and the European Association for the Study of Diabetes challenged the prognostic and therapeutic utility of the metabolic syndrome as it is currently conceived (11). Although most clinicians are now aware of the metabolic syndrome, there is little consensus about its definition and significance. Different definitions are ambiguous and discordant. For example, obesity is defined by body mass index (BMI) in some definitions and by waist circumference in others. Furthermore, the dichotomous diagnostic cut points may not account for the spectrum of risk that is likely attributable to varying degrees of abnormality. The value of diagnosing this syndrome also has been questioned because no specific therapies (beyond those established for its individual components) have been deemed effective (11).

PREVENTION OF DIABETES

Prevention of T1DM

To date, trials aimed at preventing T1DM have not been successful. Treatments with parenteral insulin (21), oral insulin (22), and oral nicotinamide (23) have not been effective in preventing T1DM among relatives of patients with T1DM. Nevertheless, this remains an area of intense investigation. Multiple trials aimed to prevent T1DM or to delay the progressive loss of β-cell function in newly diagnosed patients are currently in progress.

Prevention of T2DM

It has been estimated that 20% to 60% of people with newly diagnosed T2DM already have a complication at the time of diagnosis (24,25). Consequently, there is intense interest in preventing diabetes, and many trials have studied whether the onset of T2DM can be avoided or delayed (6,26). The hope is that forestalling the development of T2DM would likewise reduce diabetic complications. However, the impact of diabetes prevention on diabetes complications is currently unknown. It is likely that diabetes prevention would reduce microvascular complications (retinopathy, nephropathy, and neuropathy), which are strongly associated with hyperglycemia (25). However, because people with prediabetes and metabolic syndrome have an increased risk for CVD even in the absence of overt hyperglycemia, preventing T2DM in these individuals may not significantly reduce cardiovascular risk.

The major diabetes prevention trials are outlined in Table 24-3. Lifestyle changes (27,28) and treatment with metformin (28), troglitazone (29,30), and acarbose (31) have all been shown to reduce rates of progression to T2DM among high-risk patients. It is still not known whether these interventions truly prevent diabetes or simply delay its inevitable diagnosis.

TABLE 24-2

COMPONENTS OF THE METABOLIC SYNDROME

Concepts Common to All Definitions	Specific Criteria Present in Some Definitions
• Obesity	• Waist circumference >40 inches for men, >35 inches for women (13) • Ethnic-specific values for increased waist circumference (14,15) • BMI >30 kg/m² (12) • BMI >25 kg/m² (10) • Waist-hip ratio >0.9 for men, >0.85 for women (12)
• Abnormal glucose metabolism	• IFG (10,12–15) • IGT (10,12) • T2DM (12,14) • Treatment for elevated glucose (15)
• Dyslipidemia (↓HDL and ↑TG)	• HDL <50 mg/dL for women, <40 mg/dL for men (10,13–15) • HDL <35 mg/dL for men, <39 mg/dL for women (12) • TG ≥150 mg/dL (10,12-14) • Treatment for dyslipidemia (14,15)
• Hypertension	• BP ≥130/85 mm Hg (10,13–15) • BP ≥ 140/90 mm Hg (12) • Treatment for hypertension (12,14,15)
• Other	• Albuminuria (12) • Insulin resistance (12)

BMI, body mass index; IFG, impaired fasting glucose; IGT, impaired glucose tolerance; T2DM, type 2 diabetes; HDL, high-density lipoprotein; TG, triglycerides; BP, blood pressure.

TABLE 24-3

MAJOR T2DM PREVENTION TRIALS

Study	Number of subjects	Entry criteria	Intervention(s)	Relative risk reduction
Finnish Diabetes Prevention Study (27)	522	IGT	Lifestyle modification	58%
Diabetes Prevention Program (DPP) (28)	3,234	IGT	1. Metformin 2. Lifestyle modification	1. Metformin: 31% 2. Lifestyle modification: 58%
Study To Prevent Noninsulin-Dependent Diabetes Mellitus (STOP-NIDDM) (31)	1,429	IGT	Acarbose	25%
Troglitazone in Prevention of Diabetes (TRIPOD) (30)	266	Hispanic women with history of GDM (70% with IGT)	Troglitazone	55%

T2DM, type 2 diabetes mellitus; IGT, impaired glucose tolerance; GDM, gestational diabetes mellitus.
Adapted from Padwal R, Majumdar SR, Johnson JA, et al. A systematic review of drug therapy to delay or prevent type 2 diabetes. *Diabetes Care* 2005;28(3):736–744.

Post-trial testing after discontinuation of metformin (32) and troglitazone (30) suggest persistent reductions in progression to diabetes, but further studies will be needed to establish that these treatments significantly alter the natural history of disease.

At this point in time, lifestyle modification remains the preferred approach to diabetes prevention. Weight loss and increased physical activity have beneficial effects on the entire cardiovascular risk profile (33–35) in addition to potential benefits in delaying the onset of diabetes. Unfortunately, lifestyle modification is difficult to achieve and maintain. Pharmacologic therapy to prevent T2DM may become an important therapeutic modality when lifestyle interventions are not sufficiently potent or are not feasible. Currently, there is insufficient evidence that pharmacologic therapy can produce sustained effects. Furthermore, its safety and cost-effectiveness are unknown.

PREVENTION OF DIABETES COMPLICATIONS

Because diabetes is considered a coronary heart disease risk equivalent (36), patients with diabetes should be treated with the same aggressive cardioprotective strategies that are recommended for nondiabetic patients with known CVD. These therapies are presented in detail in other chapters and will not be discussed here.

Glycemic control remains a central focus of treatment for diabetic patients. Hemoglobin A_{1c} (A1C), a measure of long-term glycemic control, is used to guide therapy. Although elevated A1C levels are strongly associated with microvascular disease (25,37), the role of glycemic control in the development of CVD has been more controversial. Prospective studies have clearly demonstrated reductions in microvascular complications with intensive glycemic control in both T1DM (37) and T2DM (25). Although reductions in CVD were not found in these studies, emerging prospective (38,39) and epidemiologic data (40,41) suggest that glycemic control may also reduce CVD risk.

In the Diabetes Control and Complications Trial (DCCT), intensive glycemic control in T1DM (A1C 7.2% vs. 9.1%) reduced the risk of retinopathy by 76%, the risk of microalbuminuria by 34%, and the risk of neuropathy by 69% (37). Although CVD event rates were not reduced in the initial study, observational follow-up studies of DCCT participants 6 to 10 years after completion of the initial trial revealed significant reductions in carotid intima-media thickness (38) and fewer CVD events (39) among the participants who had originally been assigned to intensive therapy. These data suggest a delayed effect of glycemic control on cardiovascular risk.

In the United Kingdom Prospective Diabetes Study (UKPDS) of patients with T2DM, a 1% reduction in A1C was associated with a 25% reduction in microvascular complications in the intensively treated group (median A1C = 7.0%) compared with the conventionally treated group (median A1C = 7.9%) after 10 years of follow-up ($P = 0.0099$) (25). There was a 16% reduction ($P = 0.052$) in myocardial infarction observed for the intensively treated group compared with the conventionally treated group. Although this difference did not reach statistical significance, these findings suggest that glycemic control may protect against CVD in T2DM.

Recently there has been increasing evidence suggesting that increased postprandial glucose values also play a role in the development of CVD. Furthermore, reducing postprandial hyperglycemia may decrease atherosclerotic risk. Reduction of postprandial hyperglycemia has been associated with carotid

intima-media thickness regression, reductions in inflammatory markers, and improved endothelial function (40–42).

In summary, good glycemic control clearly reduces microvascular complications. Its effect on macrovascular disease is not as well understood. Ongoing trials are prospectively studying the impact of specific antihyperglycemic therapies, more stringent glycemic control, and intervention earlier in disease course on cardiovascular outcomes (43,44,46–48). Future treatments will likely be designed to afford a combination of benefits, in addition to glucose control. In the meantime, treatment of CVD risk factors such as obesity, hypertension (49), and dyslipidemia (50,51) remains an essential component of diabetes management.

TREATMENT OF HYPERGLYCEMIA

Recommended glycemic goals for nonpregnant adults are shown in Table 24-4. These must be interpreted as general guidelines. Available data do not identify the optimal level of control for individual patients, and there may be large individual differences in the risks of hypoglycemia, weight gain, and other adverse effects of antihyperglycemic therapies. No clinical trial data are available on the effects of glycemic control in elderly patients or in patients with advanced complications. Less-stringent treatment goals may be appropriate for patients with limited life expectancies or comorbid conditions. For example, hypoglycemia may impose greater risk in those with underlying ischemic heart disease (52).

For the remainder of the chapter we will discuss treatment of hyperglycemia in nonpregnant adult patients. Treatment of diabetes in children and pregnant women is beyond the scope of this discussion. Treatment for secondary forms of diabetes should be targeted at the underlying cause. If this is not possible, treatment strategies are similar to those outlined here for T1DM and T2DM.

T1DM

Insulin

In T1DM (which is characterized by absolute insulin deficiency), insulin therapy is necessary at all times for prevention of both hyperglycemia and life-threatening ketoacidosis. Traditional insulin regimens have been limited by their inability to

TABLE 24-4

GLYCEMIC GOALS

Parameter	ADA	ACE
Premeal plasma glucose (mg/dL)	90–130	<110
Postprandial plasma glucose (mg/dL)		<140
HbA$_{1c}$ (%)	<7	<6.5

ADA, American Diabetes Association; ACE, American College of Endocrinology.
Adapted from American College of Endocrinology. American College of Endocrinology consensus statement on guidelines for glycemic control. *Endocr Pract* 2002;8(Suppl 1):5–11; American Diabetes Association. Standards of medical care in diabetes. *Diabetes Care* 2005;28(Suppl 1):S4–S36.

mimic normal physiologic insulin secretion. As the importance of tight glycemic control has become increasingly recognized, new insulin analogue preparations with pharmacokinetic profiles that more closely resemble patterns of endogenous insulin secretion (53) have been developed. The pharmacokinetic properties of the new insulin analogues are distinct from those of human insulins, and their onsets and durations of action range from rapid to prolonged (Table 24-5). The rapid-acting analogues are associated with improved postprandial glucose control and less risk of postprandial hypoglycemia. Long-acting insulin analogues have slightly longer durations of action and more consistent absorption and peaks of action than human insulins. These characteristics may reduce the number of injections necessary and the risk for between-meal hypoglycemia. The first inhaled insulin (which is a rapid-acting preparation) has recently been approved by the U.S. Food and Drug Administration (FDA) for use in T1DM and T2DM.

There are two main components of effective insulin regimens for patients with T1DM: *basal insulin* (to suppress hepatic glucose production in the fasting state and prior to meals) and *prandial insulin* (to control the hyperglycemia that results from nutritional sources). Basal insulin is best provided by an intermediate- (e.g., NPH) or long- (e.g., glargine, detemir) acting insulin preparation given once or twice daily. Prandial coverage is best provided by a rapid-acting analogue (e.g., lispro, aspart, or glulisine) administered immediately before meals. Insulin pump therapy can be used in lieu of injections. Insulin pumps provide basal coverage by delivering a continuous subcutaneous infusion of insulin at a predetermined, and often variable, rate. Prandial coverage is provided by patient-administered pump boluses before meals. Supplemental boluses also may be administered in response to hyperglycemia. The choice between insulin injection and pump therapy depends on multiple considerations, including cost, patient preference, and an individual's personal glycemic profile. Neither strategy can be considered superior for all patients.

The total daily dose (TDD) of insulin required for treatment of T1DM is highly variable. A person with T1DM typically requires approximately 0.5 to 0.7 units/kg/day of insulin. The TDD should be divided into its two main components: approximately half of the TDD should be given as basal insulin and approximately half of the TDD should be given as prandial insulin (with the prandial insulin divided among the different meals).

Frequent insulin adjustments based on fasting and premeal blood glucose values must be made to achieve and maintain euglycemia. Although postprandial hyperglycemia has been associated with adverse cardiovascular outcomes independent of fasting glucose (54), treatment of postprandial hyperglycemia has not yet been shown to improve clinical outcomes and is therefore not routinely recommended (outside pregnancy). It is reasonable to monitor and target postprandial blood glucose values if A1C values remain elevated despite normal premeal glucose levels.

Amylin Mimetics

Until recently, insulin was the only antihyperglycemic therapy approved for use in T1DM. Pramlintide was approved by the FDA on March 16, 2005, and is indicated for use in both T1DM and T2DM.

Pramlintide is a synthetic analogue of amylin, a hormone that is synthesized by pancreatic β-cells and cosecreted with insulin in response to a meal. Amylin slows gastric emptying, suppresses postprandial glucagon secretion, and increases satiety (55). Its secretion is diminished in T1DM and advanced T2DM (56), but its action is preserved. Because its predominant effect is to blunt postprandial hyperglycemia, it is given prior to each meal. Fixed-dose injections of pramlintide added to premeal insulin leads to mild reductions in A1C (~0.3%) and weight loss (55). Pramlintide does not cause hypoglycemia by itself, but it can increase the risk imparted by coadministered insulin. The main adverse effect is dose-dependent nausea.

TABLE 24-5

APPROXIMATE DURATION OF ACTION OF INSULINS AND INSULIN ANALOGUES

Insulin	Onset of Action	Peak Action	Effective Duration
Rapid-acting			
Insulin Aspart[a]	10–20 minutes	1–3 hours	3–5 hours
Insulin Lispro[a]	15–30 minutes	0.5–2.5 hours	3–6.5 hours
Insulin Glulisine[a] (FDA-approved, available soon)	10–15 minutes	1–1.5 hours	3–5 hours
Short-acting			
Regular insulin	30–60 minutes	1–5 hours	6–10 hours
Intermediate-acting			
NPH insulin	1–2 hours	6–14 hours	16–24 hours
Long-acting			
Insulin Glargine[a]	1–2 hours	None	24 hours
Insulin Detemir[a] (FDA-approved, available soon)	Data not available	6–8 hours	12–24 hours

[a]Insulin analogues.
Adapted from Comparison of insulins. *Pharmacist's Letter/Prescriber's Letter* 2005;21(8):210803.

T2DM

Type 2 diabetes is a heterogeneous disease manifested by hyperglycemia that results from multiple dysregulated biologic pathways. The two major metabolic abnormalities are (a) insulin resistance in skeletal muscle, liver, and adipocytes, and (b) a progressive decline in insulin production by pancreatic β-cells. Insulin resistance results from both environmental factors (predominantly obesity and physical inactivity) and genetic factors that have yet to be identified. Early in the natural history of T2DM, the insulin-resistant prediabetic individual compensates by secreting increased amounts of insulin. Hyperglycemia results when the capacity of the pancreas to secrete insulin deteriorates and endogenous insulin production becomes insufficient to overcome insulin resistance. Because β-cell failure is progressive, treatment interventions must be continuously monitored and advanced.

Diet, exercise, and attainment of ideal body weight (interventions that improve insulin sensitivity) are central components of any therapeutic regimen. Unfortunately, most patients are unable to achieve glycemic goals with these measures alone. Pharmacologic therapy becomes necessary when lifestyle treatment is ineffective at controlling hyperglycemia. Eight different classes of agents, in addition to insulin, are currently approved for treatment of hyperglycemia in T2DM. Additional classes are expected to become available soon. Most therapies directly target insulin resistance or insulin deficiency, the two major metabolic defects in T2DM. Some of the newer classes of agents target these defects indirectly.

The availability of multiple types of medications that can be used either alone or in many different combinations has made management of T2DM increasingly complicated. There are no studies directly comparing the efficacy of all available agents and combinations of agents. Data from multiple studies are summarized in Table 24-6. The progressive β-cell deterioration characteristic of T2DM mandates the stepwise addition of noninsulin agents and/or insulin over time. An agent that could halt the decline in β-cell function would be of tremendous benefit. Although the effect of different agents on preservation of β-cell function is the subject of intense investigation, no currently available agent is known to have this effect.

Insulin and Insulin Analogues

Whereas insulin therapy is required in T1DM, the decision of how and when to start insulin in T2DM can be more difficult. Insulin should be the initial therapy in cases of marked weight loss, severe hyperglycemia, or ketosis. In the absence of these features, insulin is usually added when glycemic goals are not met with multiple noninsulin agents or when glycemic goals are unlikely to be achieved with noninsulin therapy. A single daily dose of basal insulin may provide adequate glycemic control in up to 60% of patients (57). Patients with long-standing diabetes, particularly those who are nonobese, frequently become insulin deficient and may require multiple daily insulin injections, similar to the regimens used for T1DM. A common strategy is to start with a single bedtime dose of either NPH or insulin glargine and to titrate the dose until the fasting glucose is normal. Additional injections of insulin may be required if the fasting glucose normalizes but the A1C remains elevated.

Noninsulin Therapies

Tables 24-6 and 24-7 summarize the actions, side effects, and contraindications of the noninsulin therapies currently available for treatment of T2DM.

Insulin Secretagogues.

Sulfonylureas. Sulfonylureas (SUs) were initially developed in the 1950s and have remained a cornerstone of therapy ever since. SUs reduce blood glucose levels by stimulating insulin secretion in the pancreatic β-cells. The combination of their proven efficacy, low incidence of adverse events, and low cost has contributed to their success and continued use. Third generation SUs (which include glipizide, glyburide, and glimepiride) are frequently used as first-line agents for T2DM.

An early study, The University Group Diabetes Project (58), suggested increased cardiovascular mortality in patients randomized to SUs compared to other oral agents or insulin. This finding was not confirmed in the SU-treated cohort of the more recent UKPDS trial (25). On the contrary, the group treated with SUs alone in the UKPDS had significant reductions in microvascular complications as well as a trend for reduced cardiovascular complications.

Non-SU secretagogues. Since 1998, two new classes of insulin secretagogues have been introduced. These include the meglitinides (repaglinide) and the d-phenylalanine derivatives (nateglinide). Like SUs, they stimulate insulin secretion. Because of differences in pharmacokinetics, however, they have a more rapid onset and a shorter duration of action. They are taken just prior to meals and theoretically offer improved postprandial glucose control and reduced risk of late postprandial hypoglycemia. There are no long-term data available on the effects of non-SU secretagogues on diabetic complication rates. These agents are not used as commonly as the SUs, largely because of their higher cost, more frequent dosing, and reduced efficacy (nateglinide) compared to SUs.

Insulin Sensitizers.

Biguanides. Metformin, the only biguanide available in the United States, works primarily by decreasing hepatic glucose production. Metformin has surpassed the SUs as the most widely prescribed oral agent for T2DM in the United States. Although it is comparable to the SUs in reducing blood glucose concentrations, it has several advantages. Unlike the SUs, metformin is associated with weight loss. Because it does not increase insulin levels, it does not cause hypoglycemia. Because hyperinsulinemia has been shown to be an independent risk factor for ischemic heart disease (59), it has been postulated that agents that improve insulin sensitivity (and decrease insulin levels) may decrease cardiovascular risk independent of their effects on blood glucose. Consistent with this hypothesis, a secondary analysis of the obesity substudy of the UKPDS showed that use of metformin (the only insulin sensitizer studied) led to a 39% reduction in the risk of myocardial infarction ($P = 0.01$) and a 30% reduction in the risk of macrovascular disease ($P = 0.02$) (60). These benefits were not found in the group assigned to intensive control with either SUs or insulin. The cardiovascular benefits of metformin in the UKPDS need to be confirmed prospectively before metformin can be recommended for reduction of cardiovascular risk.

Thiazolidinediones. Two thiazolidinediones (TZDs), rosiglitazone and pioglitazone, are currently available in the United States. They improve glycemia primarily by increasing insulin-mediated glucose uptake in muscle and adipocytes. To a lesser extent, they decrease hepatic glucose production. The mechanism by which the TZDs exert their effects is not completely understood. They bind to one or more peroxisome proliferator activator receptors (PPARs), which regulate several genes involved in carbohydrate and lipid metabolism. Both pioglitazone and rosiglitazone stimulate PPAR-γ. Pioglitazone also has some PPAR-α effects, which may account for its more favorable effect on lipids. Fibric acid derivatives, which are used to treat dyslipidemia, also exert their effects by acting as PPAR-α agonists. Compared to rosiglitazone, pioglitazone use is associated with greater reductions in triglyceride levels, a greater increase in high-density lipoprotein levels, a smaller increase in low-density lipoprotein levels, and a greater increase in low-density lipoprotein particle size (61).

Compared to SUs and metformin, TZDs are somewhat less effective at lowering blood glucose. Like metformin, TZDs do

TABLE 24-6

MECHANISMS OF ACTION AND EFFECTS OF NONINSULIN THERAPIES FOR T2DM MELLITUS

Medication class agents (trade names)	Primary mechanism of action	Approximate decrease in FPG (mg/dL)[b]	Approximate decrease in A1C (%)[b]	Effect on body weight
2nd-generation sulfonylureas • Glyburide[a] (Micronase, DiaBeta) • Glipizide[a] (Glucotrol) • Glimepiride (Amaryl)	Increase pancreatic insulin secretion	60–70	1.5–2.0	↑
Meglitinides • Repaglinide (Prandin)		60–70	1.5–2.0	
D-phenylalanine derivatives • Nateglinide (Starlix)		12–20	0.4–1.0	
Biguanides • Metformin[a] (Glucophage)	Decrease hepatic glucose production (and increase peripheral glucose uptake)	60–70	1.5–2.0	↓
α-Glucosidase inhibitors • Acarbose (Precose) • Miglitol (Glyset)	Delay carbohydrate absorption from gut	20–30	0.5–1.0	↔
Thiazolidinediones • Pioglitazone (Actos) • Rosiglitazone (Avandia)	Increase peripheral glucose uptake (and decrease hepatic glucose production)	35–40	1.0–1.5	↑
Incretin mimetics • Exenatide (Byetta)	• Increase glucose-dependent insulin secretion • Decrease pancreatic glucagon secretion • Slow gastric emptying • Increase satiety	20–25	0.5–1.0	↓
Amylin mimetics • Pramlintide (Symlin)	• Slow gastric emptying • Decrease postprandial pancreatic glucagon secretion • Increase satiety	Data not available	0.3–0.5	↓

T2DM, type 2 diabetes mellitus; FPG, fasting plasma glucose; A1C, hemoglobin A_{1c}.
[a]Available as generic.
[b]Response to therapy depends on patient characteristics as well as previous and concurrent drug treatments.

not cause hypoglycemia when used as monotherapy. The major side effects of TZDs are weight gain and fluid retention. Fluid retention occurs more commonly with concurrent insulin use, pre-existing edema, diastolic dysfunction, and chronic renal failure (serum creatinine >2.0 mg/dL). Weight gain is due to both fluid retention and an increase in subcutaneous fat. Visceral fat, which is associated with more adverse metabolic effects than subcutaneous fat, is decreased or unchanged. In contrast to SUs and metformin (which begin working immediately), TZDs have a slow onset of action and may take weeks to months to achieve their full effect.

Although the impact of TZDs in reducing diabetes compli-

cations has not been studied, it is generally believed they will reduce microvascular complications due to their effect of controlling hyperglycemia. Multiple nonhypoglycemic effects associated with reduced cardiovascular risk also have been described (62). PPAR-γ agonists have been shown to improve endothelial function and to reduce surrogate markers of inflammation, abnormal fibrinolysis, and atherosclerosis (62–65). In a study of patients with T2DM who underwent coronary stent implantation, addition of rosiglitazone to conventional antidiabetic therapy significantly reduced rates of in-stent restenosis, independent of glycemic control (66). Although these results are intriguing, these agents cannot be

TABLE 24-7

ADVERSE EFFECTS OF NONINSULIN THERAPIES FOR T2DM MELLITUS

Medication class	Adverse effects (Most common)	Contraindications and precautions	Hypoglycemia when used as monotherapy?
Sulfonylurea, Meglitinides, Phenylalanine Derivatives	• Hypoglycemia	• Predisposition to hypoglycemia (hepatic or renal insufficiency, malnutrition, alcohol excess)	Yes
Biguanides	• Nausea • Abdominal pain • Diarrhea • Dyspepsia • Lactic acidosis (very rare)	• Serum creatinine >1.5 mg/dL (men), >1.4 mg/dL (women), or abnormal creatinine clearance (CrCl <60–70 mL/minute) • CHF requiring pharmacologic treatment • Predisposition to lactic acidosis (including hepatic or renal insufficiency, tissue hypoperfusion, hypotension, hypoxemia, dehydration, sepsis) • Alcohol excess • Metabolic acidosis • Withhold for acute illness, surgery, radiocontrast studies	No
α-Glucosidase inhibitors	• Flatulence • Abdominal pain • Diarrhea	• Gastrointestinal intolerance • Chronic intestinal disorders • Cirrhosis • Serum creatinine >2.0 mg/dl	No
Thiazolidinediones	• Edema • Anemia	• Hepatic insufficiency (ALT >2.5 times upper limit of normal) • CHF (NYHA class III or IV)	No
Incretin mimetics	• Nausea	• Severe renal insufficiency (CrCl <30 mL/min) • Severe gastrointestinal disease	No
Amylin mimetics	• Nausea	• Gastroparesis	No

T2DM, type 2 diabetes mellitus; CrCl, creatinine clearance; CHF, congestive heart failure; ALT, alanine transaminase; NYHA, New York Heart Association.

recommended for the purpose of reducing cardiovascular risk until the impact of TZDs on cardiovascular outcomes is known. The recently published PROactive trial found that pioglitazone treatment in subjects with T2DM and macrovascular disease did not significantly reduce the primary composite endpoint of all-cause mortality, nonfatal MI, stroke, ACS, endovascular or surgical intervention on coronary or leg arteries, or leg amputation, but did significantly reduce the secondary composite endpoint of all-cause mortality, nonfatal MI, or stroke (45). The results of ongoing trials studying the effects of TZDs on cardiovascular outcomes are anxiously awaited (44,48,67).

α-Glucosidase Inhibitors. Although abnormal carbohydrate absorption is not a feature of T2DM, delaying carbohydrate absorption has been found to be an effective strategy for reducing postprandial hyperglycemia. Acarbose and miglitol are members of the α-glucosidase inhibitor (AGI) class of oral antihyperglycemic compounds. AGIs inhibit the last step of carbohydrate digestion in the small intestinal epithelium. When used before meals, they delay the absorption of complex carbohydrates and blunt postprandial hyperglycemia. They modestly improve glycemic control without increasing the risk for weight

gain or hypoglycemia. AGIs are not widely used in the United States. The main limitations to their widespread use are the need for frequent dosing, gastrointestinal side effects, and less-potent antihyperglycemic effects than other available agents.

Amylin Mimetics. Pramlintide, which was described earlier in the section on treatment of T1DM, is also approved for use in T2DM. It is not currently being marketed for use in T2DM, however, because of its minimal effects on blood glucose and the requirement for three injections per day.

Incretin Mimetics. Exenatide is the first member of a new class of agents called incretin mimetics. Exenatide exhibits many of the same glycoregulatory properties of glucagon-like peptide 1 (GLP-1), a naturally occurring incretin hormone. GLP-1 is normally secreted by intestinal cells in response to a meal. Although GLP-1 secretion is reduced in patients with T2DM (56), its action is preserved. Exenatide enhances glucose-dependent insulin secretion, suppresses hepatic glucagon secretion, and slows gastric emptying (68). It is also associated with reduced food intake and improved insulin sensitivity (69). Intriguing results in animal studies suggest that exenatide may also preserve β-cell function (70).

Improvements in glycemic control have been demonstrated

with exenatide use in patients taking maximal doses of SUs (71), metformin (69), and combination sulfonylurea-metformin therapy (72). In contrast to SUs and insulin, exenatide use is not associated with weight gain or hypoglycemia.

Because exenatide only became available for routine clinical use in June 2005, it is too soon to predict its eventual role in clinical practice. The major limitations to its widespread use may be the associated dose-dependent nausea and the requirement for twice-daily injections (72). However, the ability of exenatide to improve glycemic control without causing weight gain or hypoglycemia makes it an attractive new option. Similar new agents in this class, including a preparation that will require only a single weekly injection, are currently being evaluated in clinical trials.

Future Therapies

DPP-IV Inhibitors. Although it possesses multiple favorable metabolic effects, GLP-1 is not an ideal agent because it cannot be administered orally. Furthermore, GLP-1 is very rapidly cleaved and inactivated by the enzyme dipeptidyl peptidase IV (DPP-IV). Oral DPP-IV inhibitors are currently being investigated in clinical trials in an effort to circumvent these limitations. Preliminary evidence suggests that they are effective in reducing fasting and postprandial glucose and are not associated with weight gain (56). Of major concern, however, is the theoretical risk of inhibiting DPP-IV, which is a ubiquitous enzyme. It is unclear what the long-term consequences of nonspecifically inhibiting degradation of more than 20 endogenous peptides would be.

Glitazars. The glitazars are dual α- and γ-PPAR agonists that combine increased insulin sensitization with lipid control. These agents are currently undergoing FDA review. Several clinical trials have compared these agents with TZDs, which are primarily PPAR-γ agonists. Glycemic control and triglyceride lowering appeared somewhat superior with glitazar treatment (73,74). However, side effects (including fluid retention and congestive heart failure) may be worse with glitazar therapy.

Combination Therapy

Because β-cell failure in T2DM is progressive, treatment interventions must be continuously monitored and advanced over time. Choice of therapy depends on multiple factors including cost, side effects, contraindications, dosing frequency, and acceptability to patients. Initial treatment for most patients is a single oral agent. Metformin, SUs, and TZDs are all commonly used as first-line therapy. From a practical standpoint, agents that specifically target postprandial hyperglycemia (i.e., non-SU insulin secretagogues and α-glucosidase inhibitors) and injectable medications (i.e., insulin, pramlintide, exenatide) are rarely used as first-line agents.

Even if oral agent monotherapy is initially effective, glycemic control is likely to deteriorate over time due to progressive loss of β-cell function in T2DM. Therapy can then be escalated by addition of either a second noninsulin agent (from a different class) or insulin. Changing from one oral agent to another is rarely effective because most available agents have comparable antihyperglycemic effects. If patients progress to the point where dual therapy does not provide adequate control, either a third noninsulin agent or insulin can be added. Many effective combinations of insulin and oral agents have been reported (75,76), and there is no consensus about the optimal timing or method of initiating insulin therapy. When insulin is added, insulin sensitizers (metformin and/or a thiazolidinedione) are typically continued, but other agents are stopped. Multiple studies have demonstrated that a single bedtime injection of basal insulin, in combination with oral agents, controls hyperglycemia in up to 60% of patients (57,77). A common strategy is to start with a single bedtime dose of either NPH or insulin glargine and to titrate the dose until the fasting glucose is normal. Additional injections of insulin may be required if the fasting glucose normalizes but the A1C remains elevated.

CONCLUSIONS

Over the past decade, there have been enormous advances in the understanding of diabetes and its complications. Multiple new antihyperglycemic medications have become available, and improved strategies for treating comorbidities have been identified. Despite these advances, there is still plenty of room and need for improvement.

The successful long-term management of diabetes requires an aggressive, comprehensive approach. This includes identification of high-risk individuals and intervention at the prediabetes stage. Once the disease is established, treatment for diabetes must be promptly initiated, carefully monitored, and advanced. Treatment for diabetes should not be limited to lowering the blood glucose. All components of the metabolic syndrome require serious attention and concomitant therapy. Preventive care practices for eyes, kidneys, and feet must be included in all management regimens.

It is anticipated that emerging agents, with higher degree of selectivity for their molecular targets, will have greater efficacy and safety. However, the complexity of diabetes and its complications will continue to present a formidable challenge for any pharmacological strategy. A primary focus for diabetes prevention and treatment must remain on promotion of a healthy lifestyle for people of all ages.

References

1. National Diabetes Fact Sheet. American Diabetes Association: Alexandria, VA; 2005. Available at http://www.diabetes.org/uedocuments/NationalDiabetesFactSheetRev.pdf. Accessed June 6, 2006.
2. Ford ES, Giles WH, Dietz WH. Prevalence of the metabolic syndrome among US adults: findings from the third National Health and Nutrition Examination Survey. *JAMA* 2002;287(3):356–359.
3. Ford ES. Risks for all-cause mortality, cardiovascular disease, and diabetes associated with the metabolic syndrome: a summary of the evidence. *Diabetes Care* 2005;28(7):1769–1778.
4. Dekker JM, Girman C, Rhodes T, et al. Metabolic syndrome and 10-year cardiovascular disease risk in the Hoorn Study. *Circulation* 2005;112(5):666–673.
5. American Diabetes Association. Diagnosis and classification of diabetes mellitus. *Diabetes Care* 2005;28(Suppl 1):S37–S42.
6. Inzucchi SE, Sherwin RS. The prevention of type 2 diabetes mellitus. *Endocrinol Metab Clin North Am* 2005;34(1):199–219, viii.
7. American Diabetes Association. Screening for type 2 diabetes. *Diabetes Care* 2004;27(Suppl 1):S11–S14.
8. Tominaga M, Eguchi H, Manaka H, et al. Impaired glucose tolerance is a risk factor for cardiovascular disease, but not impaired fasting glucose. The Funagata Diabetes Study. *Diabetes Care* 1999;22(6):920–924.
9. Reaven G. The metabolic syndrome or the insulin resistance syndrome? Different names, different concepts, and different goals. *Endocrinol Metab Clin North Am* 2004;33(2):283–303.
10. Einhorn D, Reaven GM, Cobin RH, et al. American College of Endocrinology position statement on the insulin resistance syndrome. *Endocr Pract* 2003;9(3):237–252.
11. Kahn RP, Buse JP, Ferrannini E, et al M. The metabolic syndrome: time for a critical appraisal: joint statement from the American Diabetes Association and the European Association for the Study of Diabetes. *Diabetes Care* 2005;28(9):2289–2304.
12. Alberti KG, Zimmet PZ. Definition, diagnosis and classification of diabetes mellitus and its complications. Part 1: diagnosis and classification of diabetes mellitus provisional report of a WHO consultation. *Diabet Med* 1998;15(7):539–553.
13. Expert Panel on Detection, Evaluation, and Treatment of High Blood Cholesterol in Adults. Executive Summary of The Third Report of The National Cholesterol Education Program (NCEP) Expert Panel on Detection, Evaluation, and Treatment of High Blood Cholesterol in Adults (Adult Treatment Panel III). *JAMA* 2001;285(19):2486–2497.
14. The IDF consensus worldwide definition of the metabolic syndrome. Available at http://www.idf.org/webdata/docs/IDF_Metasyndrome_definiti-

on.pdf. Accessed September 15, 2005. International Diabetes Federation, Brussels, Belgium, 2005.

15. Grundy SM, Cleeman JI, Daniels SR, et al. Diagnosis and management of the metabolic syndrome. An American Heart Association/National Heart, Lung, and Blood Institute Scientific Statement. Executive Summary. *Circulation* 2005;112(17):2735–2752.

16. McNeill AM, Rosamond WD, Girman CJ, et al. The metabolic syndrome and 11-year risk of incident cardiovascular disease in the atherosclerosis risk in communities study. *Diabetes Care* 2005;28(2):385–390.

17. Lakka HM, Laaksonen DE, Lakka TA, et al. The metabolic syndrome and total and cardiovascular disease mortality in middle-aged men. *JAMA* 2002; 288(21):2709–2716.

18. Alexander CM, Landsman PB, Teutsch SM, et al. NCEP-defined metabolic syndrome, diabetes, and prevalence of coronary heart disease among NHANES III participants age 50 years and older. *Diabetes* 2003;52(5): 1210–1214.

19. Thorn LM, Forsblom C, Fagerudd J, et al. Metabolic syndrome in type 1 diabetes: association with diabetic nephropathy and glycemic control (the FinnDiane study). *Diabetes Care* 2005;28(8):2019–2024.

20. Stern MP, Williams K, Gonzalez-Villalpando C, et al. Does the metabolic syndrome improve identification of individuals at risk of type 2 diabetes and/or cardiovascular disease? *Diabetes Care* 2004;27(11):2676–2681.

21. Diabetes Prevention Trial—Type 1 Diabetes Study Group. Effects of insulin in relatives of patients with type 1 diabetes mellitus. *N Engl J Med* 2002; 346(22):1685–1691.

22. Skyler JS, Krischer JP, Wolfsdorf J, et al. Effects of oral insulin in relatives of patients with type 1 diabetes: The Diabetes Prevention Trial—Type 1. *Diabetes Care* 2005;28(5):1068–1076.

23. Gale EA, Bingley PJ, Emmett CL, et al. European Nicotinamide Diabetes Intervention Trial (ENDIT): a randomised controlled trial of intervention before the onset of type 1 diabetes. *Lancet* 2004;363(9413):925–931.

24. Harris MI. Definition and classification of diabetes mellitus and the criteria for diagnosis. In: LeRoith D, Taylor SI, Olefsky JM, eds. *Diabetes mellitus: a fundamental and clinical text.* 3rd ed. Philadelphia: Lippincott Williams & Wilkins; 2004:457–467.

25. Intensive blood-glucose control with sulphonylureas or insulin compared with conventional treatment and risk of complications in patients with type 2 diabetes (UKPDS 33). UK Prospective Diabetes Study (UKPDS) Group. *Lancet* 1998;352(9131):837–853.

26. Padwal R, Majumdar SR, Johnson JA, et al. A systematic review of drug therapy to delay or prevent type 2 diabetes. *Diabetes Care* 2005;28(3): 736–744.

27. Tuomilehto J, Lindstrom J, Eriksson JG, et al. Prevention of type 2 diabetes mellitus by changes in lifestyle among subjects with impaired glucose tolerance. *N Engl J Med* 2001;344(18):1343–1350.

28. Knowler WC, Barrett-Connor E, Fowler SE, et al. Reduction in the incidence of type 2 diabetes with lifestyle intervention or metformin. *N Engl J Med* 2002;346(6):393–403.

29. Knowler WC, Hamman RF, Edelstein SL, et al. Prevention of type 2 diabetes with troglitazone in the Diabetes Prevention Program. *Diabetes* 2005;54(4): 1150–1156.

30. Buchanan TA, Xiang AH, Peters RK, et al. Preservation of pancreatic beta-cell function and prevention of type 2 diabetes by pharmacological treatment of insulin resistance in high-risk Hispanic women. *Diabetes* 2002;51(9): 2796–2803.

31. Chiasson JL, Josse RG, Gomis R, et al. Acarbose for prevention of type 2 diabetes mellitus: the STOP-NIDDM randomised trial. *Lancet* 2002; 359(9323):2072–2077.

32. Diabetes Prevention Program Research Group. Effects of withdrawal from metformin on the development of diabetes in the diabetes prevention program. *Diabetes Care* 2003;26(4):977–980.

33. Gregg EW, Gerzoff RB, Caspersen CJ, et al. Relationship of walking to mortality among US adults with diabetes. *Arch Intern Med* 2003;163(12): 1440–1447.

34. Ratner R, Goldberg R, Haffner S, et al. Impact of intensive lifestyle and metformin therapy on cardiovascular disease risk factors in the diabetes prevention program. *Diabetes Care* 2005;28(4):888–894.

35. Klein S, Burke LE, Bray GA, et al. Clinical implications of obesity with specific focus on cardiovascular disease: a statement for professionals from the American Heart Association Council on Nutrition, Physical Activity, and Metabolism: endorsed by the American College of Cardiology Foundation. *Circulation* 2004;110(18):2952–2967.

36. Haffner SM, Lehto S, Ronnemaa T, et al. Mortality from coronary heart disease in subjects with type 2 diabetes and in nondiabetic subjects with and without prior myocardial infarction. *N Engl J Med* 1998;339(4):229–234.

37. The effect of intensive treatment of diabetes on the development and progression of long-term complications in insulin-dependent diabetes mellitus. The Diabetes Control and Complications Trial Research Group. *N Engl J Med* 1993;329(14):977–986.

38. Nathan DM, Lachin J, Cleary P, et al. Intensive diabetes therapy and carotid intima-media thickness in type 1 diabetes mellitus. *N Engl J Med* 2003; 348(23):2294–2303.

39. National Institute of Diabetes and Digestive and Kidney Diseases. Tight Glucose Control Lowers CVD by About 50 Percent in Diabetes. National Institutes of Health: Bethesda, MD; 2005. Available at http://www.nih.gov/ news/pr/jun2005/niddk-12a.htm. Accessed August 30, 2005.

40. Selvin E, Marinopoulos S, Berkenblit G, et al. Meta-analysis: glycosylated hemoglobin and cardiovascular disease in diabetes mellitus. *Ann Intern Med* 2004;141(6):421–431.

41. Selvin E, Coresh J, Golden SH, et al. Glycemic control, atherosclerosis, and risk factors for cardiovascular disease in individuals with diabetes: the atherosclerosis risk in communities study. *Diabetes Care* 2005;28(8): 1965–1973.

42. Ceriello A. Postprandial hyperglycemia and diabetes complications: is it time to treat? *Diabetes* 2005;54(1):1–7.

43. The ORIGIN Trial (Outcome Reduction with Initial Glargine Intervention). Aventis Pharmaceuticals, Canada; 2005. Available at http://www.clinical trials.gov/ct/show/NCT00069784. Accessed August 30, 2005.

44. Home P, Gubb J. For the Record Study Steering Committee and Investigators. Rosiglitazone Evaluated for Cardiac Outcomes and Regulation of Glycemia in Diabetes (RECORD): A long-term cardiovascular outcome study. *Diabetes* 2002;51(Suppl 2):A487.

45. Dormandy JA, Charbonnel B, Eckland D, et al. Secondary prevention of macrovascular events in patients with type 2 diabetes in the PROactive Study (PROspective pioglit A-zone Clinical Trial in macroVascular events): a randomized controlled trial. *Lancet* 2005;366:1279–1289.

46. Sobel BE, Frye R, Detre KM, et al. Burgeoning dilemmas in the management of diabetes and cardiovascular disease: rationale for the Bypass Angioplasty Revascularization Investigation 2 Diabetes (BARI 2D) Trial. *Circulation* 2003;107(4):636–642.

47. Action to Control Cardiovascular Risk in Diabetes (ACCORD). National Heart, Lung, and Blood Institute, Bethesda, MD, 2005. Available at http:// www.clinicaltrials.gov/ct/show/NCT00000620. Accessed September 5, 2005.

48. Skyler JS. Effects of glycemic control on diabetes complications and on the prevention of diabetes. *Clin Diabetes* 2004;22(4):162–166.

49. Tight blood pressure control and risk of macrovascular and microvascular complications in type 2 diabetes: UKPDS 38. UK Prospective Diabetes Study Group. *BMJ* 1998;317(7160):703–713.

50. Collins R, Armitage J, Parish S, et al. MRC/BHF Heart Protection Study of cholesterol-lowering with simvastatin in 5963 people with diabetes: a randomised placebo-controlled trial. *Lancet* 2003;361(9374):2005–2016.

51. Colhoun HM, Betteridge DJ, Durrington PN, et al. Primary prevention of cardiovascular disease with atorvastatin in type 2 diabetes in the Collaborative Atorvastatin Diabetes Study (CARDS): multicentre randomised placebo-controlled trial. *Lancet* 2004;364(9435):685–696.

52. Desouza C, Salazar H, Cheong B, et al. Association of hypoglycemia and cardiac ischemia: a study based on continuous monitoring. *Diabetes Care* 2003;26(5):1485–1489.

53. Hirsch IB. Insulin analogues. *N Engl J Med* 2005;352(2):174–183.

54. DECODE Study Group, the European Diabetes Epidemiology Group. Glucose tolerance and cardiovascular mortality: comparison of fasting and 2-hour diagnostic criteria. *Arch Intern Med* 2001;161(3):397–405.

55. SYMLIN® (pramlintide acetate) Injection (package insert). Amylin Pharmaceuticals, Inc., San Diego, CA, 2005. Available at http://www.fda.gov/cder/ foi/label/2005/021332lbl.pdf. Accessed August 30, 2005.

56. Uwaifo GI, Ratner RE. Novel pharmacologic agents for type 2 diabetes. *Endocrinol Metab Clin North Am* 2005;34(1):155–197.

57. Riddle MC, Rosenstock J, Gerich J, et al. The treat-to-target trial: randomized addition of glargine or human NPH insulin to oral therapy of type 2 diabetic patients. *Diabetes Care* 2003;26(11):3080–3086.

58. Goldner MG, Knatterud GL, Prout TE. Effects of hypoglycemic agents on vascular complications in patients with adult-onset diabetes. 3. Clinical implications of UGDP results. *JAMA* 1971;218(9):1400–1410.

59. Despres JP, Lamarche B, Mauriege P, et al. Hyperinsulinemia as an independent risk factor for ischemic heart disease. *N Engl J Med* 1996;334(15): 952–957.

60. Effect of intensive blood-glucose control with metformin on complications in overweight patients with type 2 diabetes (UKPDS 34). UK Prospective Diabetes Study (UKPDS) Group. *Lancet* 1998;352(9131):854–865.

61. Goldberg RB, Kendall DM, Deeg MA, et al. A comparison of lipid and glycemic effects of pioglitazone and rosiglitazone in patients with type 2 diabetes and dyslipidemia. *Diabetes Care* 2005;28(7):1547–1554.

62. Kunhiraman BP, Jawa A, Fonseca VA. Potential cardiovascular benefits of insulin sensitizers. *Endocrinol Metab Clin North Am* 2005;34(1):117–135.

63. Raji A, Seely EW, Bekins SA, et al. Rosiglitazone improves insulin sensitivity and lowers blood pressure in hypertensive patients. *Diabetes Care* 2003; 26(1):172–178.

64. Minamikawa J, Tanaka S, Yamauchi M, et al. Potent inhibitory effect of troglitazone on carotid arterial wall thickness in type 2 diabetes. *J Clin Endocrinol Metab* 1998;83(5):1818–1820.

65. Koshiyama H, Shimono D, Kuwamura N, et al. Rapid communication: inhibitory effect of pioglitazone on carotid arterial wall thickness in type 2 diabetes. *J Clin Endocrinol Metab* 2001;86(7):3452–3456.

66. Choi D, Kim SK, Choi SH, et al. Preventative effects of rosiglitazone on restenosis after coronary stent implantation in patients with type 2 diabetes. *Diabetes Care* 2004;27(11):2654–2660.

67. Viberti G, Kahn SE, Greene DA, et al. A diabetes outcome progression trial (ADOPT): an international multicenter study of the comparative efficacy of rosiglitazone, glyburide, and metformin in recently diagnosed type 2 diabetes. *Diabetes Care* 2002;25(10):1737–1743.

68. BYETTA™ (exenatide) injection (package insert). Amylin Pharmaceuticals, Inc., San Diego, CA, 2005. Available at http://www.fda.gov/cder/foi/label/2005/021773lbl.pdf. Accessed August 30, 2005.
69. DeFronzo RA, Ratner RE, Han J, et al. Effects of exenatide (exendin-4) on glycemic control and weight over 30 weeks in metformin-treated patients with type 2 diabetes. *Diabetes Care* 2005;28(5):1092–1100.
70. Li Y, Hansotia T, Yusta B, et al. Glucagon-like peptide-1 receptor signaling modulates beta cell apoptosis. *J Biol Chem* 2003;278(1):471–478.
71. Buse JB, Henry RR, Han J, et al. Effects of exenatide (exendin-4) on glycemic control over 30 weeks in sulfonylurea-treated patients with type 2 diabetes. *Diabetes Care* 2004;27(11):2628–2635.
72. Kendall DM, Riddle MC, Rosenstock J, et al. Effects of exenatide (exendin-4) on glycemic control over 30 weeks in patients with type 2 diabetes treated with metformin and a sulfonylurea. *Diabetes Care* 2005;28(5):1083–1091.
73. Frederich R, Viraswami-Appanna K, Rubin CJ. Effects of long-term therapy (2-year) with muraglitazar, a novel dual PPAR alpha/gamma agonist, on diabetic dyslipidemia in patients with type 2 diabetes: a double-blind, randomized, parallel-group study. *Diabetes* 2005;54(Suppl 1):A236.
74. Rubin CJ, Mohideen P, Ledeine J, et al. Attainment of A1C goals with muraglitazar, a novel dual PPAR alpha/gamma agonist, in combination with metformin in patients with type 2 diabetes: a double-blind, randomized comparison with pioglitazone plus metformin. *Diabetes* 2005;54(Suppl 1):A509.
75. Yki-Jarvinen H. Combination therapies with insulin in type 2 diabetes. *Diabetes Care* 2001;24(4):758–767.
76. Inzucchi SE. Oral antihyperglycemic therapy for type 2 diabetes: scientific review. *JAMA* 2002;287(3):360–372.
77. Janka HU, Plewe G, Riddle MC, et al. Comparison of basal insulin added to oral agents versus twice-daily premixed insulin as initial insulin therapy for type 2 diabetes. *Diabetes Care* 2005;28(2):254–259.
78. American College of Endocrinology. American College of Endocrinology consensus statement on guidelines for glycemic control. *Endocr Pract* 2002;8(Suppl 1):5–11.
79. American Diabetes Association. Standards of medical care in diabetes. *Diabetes Care* 2005;28(Suppl 1):S4–S36.
80. Comparison of insulins. *Pharmacist's Letter/Prescriber's Letter* 2005;21(8):210803.

CHAPTER 25 ■ HYPERTENSION

MICHAEL A. WEBER

HISTORY
DEFINITIONS
The Blood Pressure Approach
Staging of Hypertension
The Risk Factor Approach and the Metabolic Syndrome
A More Fundamental Definition
EVALUATION OF THE HYPERTENSIVE PATIENT
Measuring the Blood Pressure
Laboratory and Other Tests
APPROACHES TO TREATMENT
Lifestyle Modifications
STARTING DRUG TREATMENT
The JNC 7 Algorithm
Compelling Indications
Starting Treatment in Stage 1 Hypertension
Starting Treatment in Stage 2 Hypertension
The Growing Use of Drug Combinations
Complex Combinations
ARE THERE REASONS TO FAVOR PARTICULAR
 ANTIHYPERTENSIVE AGENTS?
Calcium Channel Blockers
ACE Inhibitors
Angiotensin-Receptor Blockers
SPECIAL SITUATIONS
INADEQUATE TREATMENT RESPONSES
Inadequate Adherence
Inappropriate Drug Combinations
Conflicting Nonantihypertensive Drug
Secondary Hypertension
Hypertensive Emergencies and Urgencies
EFFECTIVENESS

Hypertension is the most common chronic condition dealt with by physicians in the United States. Even so, there is no agreement on a straightforward and accurate way to describe it. Most directly, hypertension could simply be described as the clinical finding of high blood pressure, but most experts now recognize that hypertension often is part of a complex set of cardiovascular, renal, and metabolic abnormalities. There is a great deal of variability in the phenotypic characteristics of hypertension, suggesting that high blood pressure may be a reflection of differing underlying abnormalities. On the positive side, the creation of effective pharmacologic and lifestyle strategies for reducing blood pressure has at least provided dependable tools for clinicians to manage hypertension and improve patient outcomes in their practices.

HISTORY

Over 4,000 years ago observers noted that the finding of a hard pulse, particularly in older people, was indicative of a poor prognosis (1). Perhaps the real origin of hypertension as a contemporary condition was the report by Bright in 1836 that patients with renal disease tended to suffer from major cardiovascular events and often died from strokes (2). To this day, the powerful connection between the kidney and the circulation, presumably mediated by high blood pressure and the activation of mechanisms such as the renin-angiotensin system, remains a fundamental part of our understanding of hypertension. The work by Korotkoff in the early part of the 20th century showing how vascular sounds are indicative of blood pressure values helped lead to practical methods for clinicians to measure blood pressure routinely (3).

In what is now becoming a familiar paradigm for medical progress, the next two major developments came from industry. The first came from the life insurance industry when the Actuarial Society of America reported the close relationship between blood pressure measurements and life expectancy (4). In some ways, these data, published over 80 years ago, provide the rationale for our current aggressive approach to managing hypertension. This approach, though, could not have been possible without the second contribution from industry, in particular the discovery of pharmacologic agents that could effectively reduce blood pressure in the clinical setting.

Among the earliest antihypertensive drugs were the diuretics, which first became available in the 1950s and are still indispensable. Much of our progress in treating hypertension during the past 50 years has depended on the progressive development of newer, more selective drugs that have expanded efficacy as well as becoming progressively more tolerable to patients. A brief but delightful summary of this fascinating process has been published recently (5). It is noteworthy that the writer of that review (Dr. Edward Freis) contributed in a meaningful fashion to the history of hypertension by reporting in 1967 on the first clinical trial in which drug treatment of hypertension, as compared with placebo, significantly reduced the incidence of major cardiovascular events and death (6).

DEFINITIONS

Hypertension can be defined in different fashions. First of all, it can be described almost entirely in terms of blood pressure; then, it can be defined as part of a syndrome of cardiovascular risk factors, including high blood pressure, and by evidence for underlying vascular abnormalities; and finally, it can be regarded empirically as a high-risk condition in which cardiovascular prognosis can be improved by the application of appropriate therapies.

The Blood Pressure Approach

Since the early actuarial data that showed the connection between blood pressure and cardiovascular events, prospective clinical observations have continued to support the importance of this relationship. For instance, long-term follow-up of a large cohort of young and middle-age men recruited for a study known as the Multiple Risk Factor Intervention Trial has shown that both systolic and diastolic blood pressures were highly predictive of subsequent strokes and cardiovascular outcomes (7). A particularly powerful observation, based on a meta-analysis of a million people, has defined the link between blood pressure and major outcomes in a precise fashion (8). As shown in Figure 25-1, regardless of age, blood pressure is clearly a major determinant of coronary and stroke mortality. For every 20 mm Hg increment in systolic blood pressure there is approximately a doubling of the risk of events. When considered on a population basis, blood pressure differences of only 1 mm Hg multiply out into meaningful effects on clinical outcomes. Using these same data (8), it has been stressed that age is also a major determinant of outcomes (9).

Clinical trials that have studied the importance of reducing blood pressure in high-risk hypertension have arrived at similar conclusions. For instance, in the Hypertension Optimal Treatment (HOT) trial (10), hypertensive patients treated with more-aggressive as compared with less-aggressive blood pressure-lowering therapy—particularly if they were also diabetic—had significantly fewer clinical events. Likewise, in the United Kingdom Prospective Diabetes Study (11), tighter as compared with less-tight control of blood pressure was significantly more effective at preventing cardiovascular and diabetic clinical endpoints. Indeed, meta-analysis of hypertension clinical trials in general could lead to the conclusion that the clinical effects of antihypertensive therapy could be explained mainly by the effects on blood pressure (12).

Most recently, the clinical effects of achieving a systolic blood pressure goal of less than 140 mm Hg were examined in the Valsartan (VALUE) trial (13). For treatments based on either valsartan or amlodipine, as shown in Figure 25-2, achieving this treatment goal—regardless of the drug regimen used—sharply reduced the incidence of cardiac events, stroke, and mortality.

Largely for these reasons, the most recent report of the Joint

National Committee on the Prevention, Detection and Treatment of High Blood Pressure (JNC 7) has taken very much a blood pressure-focused approach toward defining and caring for hypertension (14). The criteria recommended by this committee are summarized in Table 25-1 and should be considered carefully.

Staging of Hypertension

The JNC has recommended that a diagnosis of hypertension should be made when blood pressure is 140/90 mm Hg or higher. As long as either the systolic or diastolic criterion is met, the diagnosis is established. Hypertensive patients whose blood pressures are below 160/100 mm Hg are classified as Stage 1, whereas those at or above this level are classified as Stage 2. As discussed later, this has implications for how treatment should be started. It is noteworthy that the diagnosis and decision to treat are in general not affected by the age, other demographic features, or comorbidities of patients. Blood pressure, by and large, is the predominant criterion. The main exception to the 140/90 mm Hg threshold is for patients with diabetes or chronic kidney disease, in whom the diagnosis should be made and treatment begun if blood pressure is 130/80 mm Hg or higher.

This apparently simplistic approach does not mean that the JNC failed to recognize the important effects on global cardiovascular risk of the multiple cardiovascular findings that often accompany high blood pressure. Rather, it indicates the belief by the JNC that because hypertension generally is not well managed, and that a disturbingly large number of hypertensive patients are either not being treated or are being treated inadequately, straightforward recommendations based on blood pressures alone are most likely to be understood and lead to action by the clinical community. It should also be noted that the goal of treatment for most patients is to reduce their blood

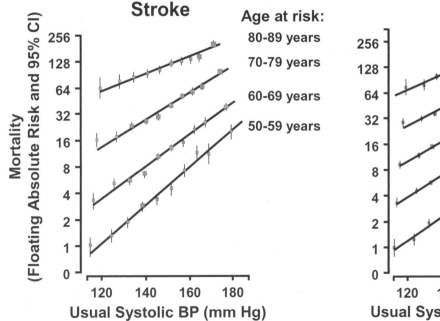
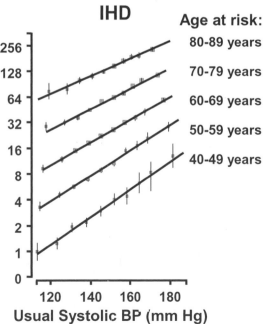

FIGURE 25-1. Relationships between systolic blood pressure and stroke or coronary heart disease mortality according to deciles of age derived from a meta-analysis of one million people. (From Lewington S, Clarke R, Qizilbash N, et al. Prospective Studies Collaboration. Age-specific relevance of usual BP to vascular mortality: a meta-analysis of individual data for one million adults in 60 prospective studies. *Lancet* 2002;14:1903–1913, with permission.)

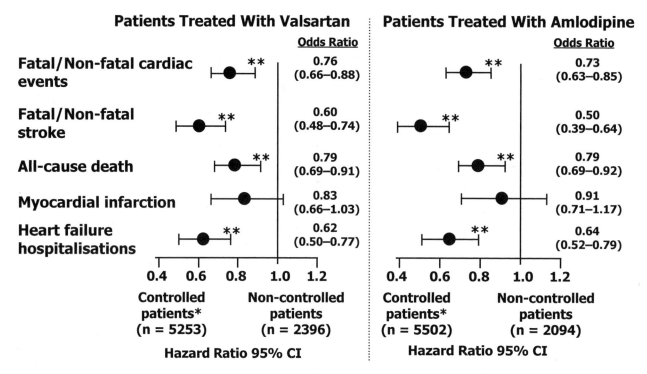

FIGURE 25-2. Effects on major clinical outcomes or mortality of blood pressure control (systolic BP <140 mm Hg) as compared with noncontrol in high-risk hypertensive patients treated with either valsartan or amlodipine-based antihypertensive therapy. (From Weber MA, Julius S, Kjeldsen SE, et al. Blood pressure dependent and independent effects of antihypertensive treatment on clinical events in the VALUE trial. *Lancet* 2004;363:2049–2051, with permission.)

TABLE 25-1

THE CHANGE IN CLASSIFICATION OF BLOOD PRESSURE BETWEEN THE TWO MOST RECENT REPORTS OF THE JNC, INDICATING THE RECENT ADOPTION OF A SIMPLIFIED CLASSIFICATION OF HYPERTENSION IN WHICH THE CONCEPT OF PREHYPERTENSION IS PROPOSED FOR THE FIRST TIME

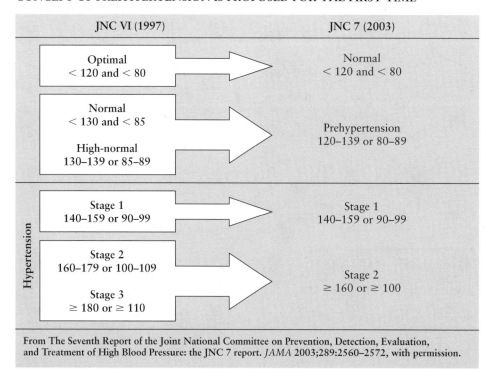

From The Seventh Report of the Joint National Committee on Prevention, Detection, Evaluation, and Treatment of High Blood Pressure: the JNC 7 report. *JAMA* 2003;289:2560–2572, with permission.

pressures to below 140/90 mm Hg, and in the case of those with diabetes or chronic kidney disease, below 130/80 mm Hg.

Why did the JNC choose these particular blood pressure criteria? After all, as shown in Figure 25-1, it is evident that prognosis is progressively better at levels of systolic blood pressure down to 115 mm Hg, or possibly even lower. Why, then, choose 140 mm Hg as a diagnostic criterion? Briefly, the JNC was guided by published evidence of clinical trials in which antihypertensive therapy reduced clinical events. However, most of this evidence so far has come from trials that used treatment criteria of around 140/90 mm Hg as their therapeutic blood pressure targets. Certainly, as shown in Figure 25-2, achieving a systolic goal of less than 140 mm Hg is associated with dramatic reductions in clinical events (13). Tempting as it may be to aim even lower, we still await clinical trial evidence that doing so will actually improve outcomes in hypertensive patients.

As an interim concept, the JNC (as shown in Table 25-1) has suggested the use of a category called prehypertension encompassing those patients with blood pressures between 120/80 and 139/89 mm Hg. And although not recommending treatment for such individuals (unless they are diabetic patients with renal disease) with therapeutic agents, they suggest the use of lifestyle modifications that could at least slow down the usual age-related increases in blood pressure and delay the onset of clinical hypertension.

The Risk Factor Approach and the Metabolic Syndrome

Hypertension commonly clusters with other cardiovascular risk factors, including lipid abnormalities, glucose intolerance, and obesity. This is sometimes referred to in terms such as the metabolic syndrome, syndrome X, and the hypertension syndrome (15). None of these descriptions is entirely satisfactory, for there is variability in the clinical picture. Moreover, because evidence for cardiovascular and renal changes are often part of this constellation of findings, limited terms such as "metabolic" do not really suffice.

It is interesting to note that evidence for this constellation of findings can appear early in life. It has been shown, for instance, that normotensive offspring of parents with hypertension can already exhibit evidence for early changes in metabolic findings and in such characteristics as microalbuminuria, early changes in the structure and function of the left ventricle, and stiffening of the arteries (15). It is not entirely certain whether these familial findings reflect a genetic tendency or simply the effects of a commonly shared environment. It should also be pointed out that because the definition of the metabolic syndrome is arbitrary (15), it may not truly represent a syndrome with a single underlying etiology (16).

Despite these controversies, there is no doubt that a number of metabolic, cardiovascular, and renal changes are commonly associated with hypertension and almost certainly affect total cardiovascular risk in such individuals. The official guidelines of the European Society of Hypertension (ESH) (17) differ quite sharply from the JNC guidelines in taking these comorbidities into account. Put simply, the European guidelines advocate earlier and more aggressive therapy in hypertensive patients who have concomitant risk factors, even if blood pressure is only modestly elevated and, at the same time, would allow a more deliberative and protracted period of observation before starting treatment in hypertensive patients who do not exhibit other risk factors.

One thing is clear. All the guidelines committees agree that every patient should be evaluated for all known cardiovascular risk factors, and when found, these risk factors should be dealt with in an effective fashion. One important example of this approach: there is compelling evidence that the use of statin therapy in hypertensive patients, even when their low-density lipoproteins (LDL) cholesterol levels do not reach the traditional criteria for such therapy, still contributes meaningful additional reductions in cardiovascular outcomes (18).

A More Fundamental Definition

A working group of the American Society of Hypertension has published a position paper on the definition of hypertension (19). The approach suggested in this report, as summarized in Table 25-2, is less empirical than those encompassed by the

TABLE 25-2

THE PROPOSED CLASSIFICATION OF HYPERTENSION BY A WORKING GROUP OF THE AMERICAN SOCIETY OF HYPERTENSION THAT, IN ADDITION TO BLOOD PRESSURE LEVELS, TAKES INTO ACCOUNT CONCOMITANT RISK FACTORS AS WELL AS EVIDENCE FOR CARDIOVASCULAR STRUCTURAL OR FUNCTIONAL CHANGES IN DETERMINING THE STATUS OF HYPERTENSIVE PATIENTS

Classification	Normal	Stage 1 Hypertension	Stage 2 Hypertension	Stage 3 Hypertension
BP pattern and CVD status	Normal BP or rare elevations AND no identifiable CVD	Occasional or intermittent BP elevations OR risk factors suggesting early CVD	Sustained BP elevations OR evidence of progressive CVD	Marked and sustained BP elevations OR evidence of advanced CVD
Cardiovascular risk factors	None	≥1 risk factor present	Multiple risk factors present	Multiple risk factors present
Early disease markers	None	0–1	≥2	≥2 present with evidence of CVD
Target organ damage	None	None	Early signs present	Overtly present with or without CVD events

From Giles TD, Berk BC, Black HR, et al. on behalf of the Hypertension Writing Group. Expanding the definition and classification of hypertension. *J Clin Hypertens* 2005;7:505–512, with permission.

JNC (14) or the ESH (17) and goes beyond the blood pressure and other clinical findings that characterize those definitions. Instead, this more fundamental paradigm sees hypertension as a disease affecting the structure and function of arteries and myocardium, together with other underlying abnormalities of renal and neuroendocrine mechanisms. In this construct of hypertension, clearly there is a heterogeneity of causes leading to the high blood pressure and an assumption that high blood pressure—although important—should also be interpreted as a diagnostic sign of underlying abnormalities.

There is good clinical evidence to support this protean view. Hypertensive patients can be differentiated on the basis of such phenotypes as their renin measurements, their age, and their body mass, and also by variations in the structure and function of such organs as the cardiac left ventricle, the degree of stiffness of small and large arteries, and characteristics of renal function (20). From a practical point of view, this definition does not provide the simplicity of the previous guidelines. On the other hand, this preliminary work sets the stage for anticipating that hypertension ultimately will be regarded as a set of varying conditions that, once carefully described, might respond optimally to different therapeutic strategies.

EVALUATION OF THE HYPERTENSIVE PATIENT

Evaluating and diagnosing a person who might have hypertension, though relatively straightforward, has lifelong implications for the patient. In general, an elevated blood pressure is all that is required to make a diagnosis, but the impact is considerable: quite apart from the costs and inconveniences of regular visits to clinicians, making lifestyle changes, and taking medications, there is also the issue of labeling a person with a lifelong diagnosis. In explaining to patients that they have hypertension, clinicians must describe cardiovascular events, strokes, and other serious outcomes that can result if the hypertension is not well treated. For many patients, this will be the first time that such serious events have been raised in the context of their own lives. So it is also critical to provide encouragement that this diagnosis should not affect their long-term outlook provided they make a sensible commitment to their own care. Because the published guidelines provide excellent detailed information on the comprehensive evaluation of hypertensive patients, only some brief comments are made here.

Measuring the Blood Pressure

In making a diagnosis of hypertension, the blood pressure readings should be confirmed on two or three occasions, preferably some days apart. Details of appropriate techniques are described in the guidelines (14). Some experts advocate the use of ambulatory blood pressure monitoring for patients in whom white coat hypertension—blood pressure that is high in the clinical setting but is normal at most other times—is suspected. This can be a useful test, though if other clinical findings provide an incentive to hypertensive therapy, particularly other risk factors or evidence for cardiovascular or renal changes, then it is probably not necessary to perform ambulatory monitoring to confirm the diagnosis. Home blood pressure readings by patients are interesting, but it should be remembered that typically blood pressures at home are lower than in the office because they are often taken at times of day when blood pressures are expected to be relatively low. It should also be remembered that our knowledge of the prognosis of hypertension is based on readings obtained in the clinical setting.

Laboratory and Other Tests

Because high blood pressure is often associated with other risk factors, laboratory studies should be carried out to evaluate findings such as lipids, glucose, electrolytes, renal function, and liver function. Fasting values should be used because they help in the diagnosis of diabetes and in calculating the lipid profile. Because it is an important predictive factor, microalbuminuria should be looked for; and likewise an electrocardiogram (or echocardiogram if feasible) should be performed to check for left ventricular hypertrophy or other evidence of cardiac involvement. All these tests are relevant because they can dictate the selection of antihypertensive drugs. Fuller recommendations can be found in published guidelines (14,17).

APPROACHES TO TREATMENT

After confirming the existence of high blood pressure, decisions must be made about how to initiate therapy. Although most patients will require antihypertensive drugs, there is evidence that some nonpharmacologic strategies—sometimes referred to as lifestyle modifications—are effective. With patients who are motivated to engage in lifestyle modifications and who have Stage 1 hypertension (between 140/90 and 159/99 mm Hg), a trial of up to 3 or even 6 months of nonpharmacologic strategies can be undertaken, though the JNC 7 guidelines would prefer a shorter period. At that point, depending on whether or not the blood pressure is controlled, a decision should be made regarding the start of drug therapy. Stage 2 patients require immediate drug therapy.

An alternative approach is to start drug treatment and lifestyle modification simultaneously, with a promise to the patient that successful implementation of the lifestyle strategies could enable the drug treatment to be reduced or even discontinued if blood pressure remains well controlled. This approach may be more positive than that of starting lifestyle modifications alone. After all, if lifestyle changes are unsuccessful in controlling blood pressure, starting drug treatment at that point could be interpreted by patients as a punitive response to their failure to adequately follow instructions. Regardless of which approach is used, appropriate dietary and other measures should be a continuing part of hypertension management.

Lifestyle Modifications

A summary of major lifestyle modifications that should be considered in the management of hypertension is shown in Table 25-3. The sources for this information are cited elsewhere (14). Perhaps the most compelling results in terms of blood pressure reduction occur in those overweight people who successfully lose weight. It is interesting that blood pressure will often start to fall after relatively small early weight reductions, suggesting that the metabolic and neuroendocrine factors that mediate the hypertension of obesity are almost immediately responsive to reduced calorie intake. The consequences and management of excess weight and obesity are discussed separately (21).

There has also been attention paid to the DASH diet. This strategy encompasses an increased intake of fruits and vegetables, with a reduction in dietary fats. This diet is effective in blood pressure reduction, particularly in African American patients, but may be difficult to follow in the home setting. The reports showing the benefit of this diet were based on studies in which meals were professionally prepackaged; it is not yet established whether the costs and effort involved in assembling such a diet privately will allow long-term adherence by hypertensive patients. A low-sodium diet likewise can reduce blood pressure. Interestingly, this may not be true for all patients, but for those who have some form of sodium sensitivity this

TABLE 25-3

RECOMMENDED NONPHARMACOLOGIC STRATEGIES THAT POTENTIALLY CAN PROVIDE MEANINGFUL BLOOD PRESSURE REDUCTIONS IN HYPERTENSIVE PATIENTS[a]

Modification	Approximate SBP reduction (range)
Weight reduction	5–20 mm Hg/10-kg weight loss
Adopt DASH eating plan	8–14 mm HG
Dietary sodium reduction	2–8 mm Hg
Physical activity	4–9 mm Hg
Moderation of alcohol consumption	2–4 mm Hg

[a]Citations for these differing approaches are listed in the JNC 7 report.
From The Seventh Report of the Joint National Committee on Prevention, Detection, Evaluation, and Treatment of High Blood Pressure: the JNC 7 report. *JAMA* 2003;289:2560–2572, with permission.

that those people who successfully take up an exercise program will often persist on a long-term basis. Moreover, those who exercise in a consistent fashion are more likely to follow other lifestyle strategies such as monitoring their caloric intake. One final strategy, albeit one that does not directly reduce blood pressure, should be mentioned: cigarette smoking. Many hypertensive patients smoke on a regular basis, a fact that dramatically increases their probability of experiencing cardiovascular complications. They should be strongly urged to stop.

STARTING DRUG TREATMENT

The object of antihypertensive therapy is to reduce blood pressure below 140/90 mm Hg in most hypertensive patients and below 130/80 mm Hg in high-risk groups such as those with diabetes or chronic kidney disease. Some of the recommended strategies for achieving these goals are straightforward; others complex or even contentious. There is no general agreement about which classes of drugs should be selected as initial therapy for many patients, though this may not be a critical issue because there is broad acknowledgement among experts that controlling blood pressure is not usually achieved by one drug alone. If combination therapies are to be used, which drug classes can be most effectively combined with each other to provide efficacious and well-tolerated blood pressure control? An algorithm proposed by the JNC 7 (Fig. 25-3) is often referred to, though even this approach differs from those recommended by other guideline committees and is debated by specialists in the field. Nevertheless, it provides some useful ideas.

The JNC 7 Algorithm

As shown in Figure 25-3, patients who satisfy the criteria for a diagnosis of hypertension, and for whom antihypertension

dietary modification helps. For people who consume large amounts of alcohol, a meaningful reduction results in blood pressure benefits. Although modest consumption of alcohol appears to be cardioprotective, amounts above two drinks a day often raise blood pressure, quite apart from other possible deleterious health effects.

Exercise, particularly of the aerobic type, is another useful way to reduce blood pressure. One virtue of this strategy is

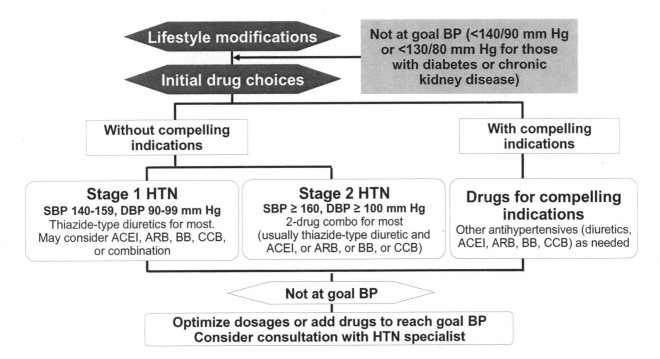

FIGURE 25-3. Recommendations of the Joint National Committee on the Prevention, Detection and Treatment of High Blood Pressure (JNC 7) for the diagnosis, setting of treatment goals, therapeutic strategies, and drug selection in patients with hypertension. (From The Seventh Report of the Joint National Committee on Prevention, Detection, Evaluation, and Treatment of High Blood Pressure: the JNC 7 report. *JAMA* 2003;289:2560–2572, with permission.)

therapy is to be started, can be divided into three groups. First are those with so-called compelling indications, which in essence are concomitant conditions that will dictate the use of certain drugs appropriate for those conditions as well as for hypertension. The next group is those with Stage 1 hypertension, with blood pressures between 140/90 and 159/99 mm Hg, and the final group is those with blood pressures of 160/100 mm Hg or higher. These designations lead to the following proposed strategies.

Compelling Indications

Hypertensive patients often have other conditions that require specific therapies. For example, hypertensive patients with diabetes or renal disease should receive blockers of the renin-angiotensin system like angiotensin-converting enzyme (ACE) inhibitors or angiotensin receptor blockers, which would then be the treatments of choice for both the concomitant condition and the hypertension. Likewise, agents such as beta-blockers or calcium channel blockers would be treatments of choice in patients with angina pectoris. Clearly, the choice of the blood pressure-lowering agent is dictated by the presence of these other conditions. A listing of major compelling indications and JNC 7-suggested drug types is provided in Table 25-4.

Starting Treatment in Stage 1 Hypertension

In general, the major guidelines recommend starting therapy with just one drug in such patients. The European Guidelines (17) and the guidelines for African American patients (22) are not prescriptive; they recommend that physicians choose an agent from any of the major available drug classes that appears to be appropriate. The JNC 7 guidelines (14), however, are somewhat biased in favor of thiazide diuretics, but even these guidelines acknowledge that other drug types can be considered. Even so, this recommendation continues to be debated and should not be blindly accepted.

The relative favor given to the thiazides in JNC 7 comes from clinical trials in which diuretics were found to be useful, compared with placebo, in preventing major clinical events. Most of the impetus, though, for this recommendation is based on the findings of one recent study, the Antihypertensive and Lipid Lowering to Prevent Heart Attack Trial (ALLHAT) (23). This prospective trial compared the effects of the thiazide-like diuretic, chlorthalidone, with the ACE inhibitor, lisinopril, and the calcium channel blocker, amlodipine, on clinical outcomes in high-risk hypertensive patients. Of note, there were no differences among the three drugs in their effects on the primary study endpoint—fatal and nonfatal coronary events—but the diuretic appeared to be better than the ACE inhibitor in preventing strokes and better than the calcium channel blocker in preventing heart failure. Because, as the authors of the ALLHAT report claimed, the diuretic is less costly than other agents (though this claim is based on purchase costs, not the overall costs of managing and monitoring patients on diuretics), this led to a recommendation that thiazides be considered as first-line drugs. Unfortunately, there were methodologic flaws in the conduct of this trial, resulting in unequal blood pressure effects in the three treatment arms that favored the diuretic. Moreover, the stroke benefit of the diuretic was seen only in African American patients when the diuretic was compared with the ACE inhibitor; these patients, predictably, had far poorer blood pressure responses when taking the ACE inhibitor. There was also debate concerning the diagnosis of heart failure, leading a number of experts to believe that the findings

TABLE 25-4

A SUMMARY OF POSSIBLE DRUG SELECTIONS IN HYPERTENSIVE PATIENTS WHOSE CONCOMITANT CARDIOVASCULAR OR OTHER CONDITIONS CAN BE TREATED WITH DRUGS THAT ARE ALSO APPROPRIATE FOR THE MANAGEMENT OF HIGH BLOOD PRESSURE[a]

Compelling Indication	Initial Therapy Options	Clinical Trial Basis
Heart failure	THIAZ, BB, ACEI, ARB, ALDO ANT	ACC/AHA Heart Failure Guideline, MERIT-HF, COPERNICUS, CIBIS, SOLVD, AIRE, TRACE, ValHEFT, RALES
Postmyocardial infarction	BB, ACEI, ALDO ANT	ACC/AHA Post-MI Guideline, BHAT, SAVE, Capricorn, EPHESUS
High CAD risk	THIAZ, BB, ACE, CCB	ALLHAT, HOPE, ANBP2, LIFE, CONVINCE
Diabetes	THIAZ, BB, ACE, ARB, CCB	NKF-ADA Guideline, UKPDS, ALLHAT
Chronic kidney disease	ACEI, ARB	NKF Guideline, Captopril Trial, RENAAL, IDNT, REIN, AASK
Recurrent stroke prevention	THIAZ, ACEI	PROGRESS

[a]Further details of the use of these drugs, and citations for the studies from which these recommendations are derived, are provided in the JNC 7 report.
From The Seventh Report of the Joint National Committee on Prevention, Detection, Evaluation, and Treatment of High Blood Pressure: the JNC 7 report. *JAMA* 2003;289:2560–2572, with permission.

of ALLHAT were far too tenuous to support meaningful recommendations on initial drug selection (24–26). Some practical reasons for choosing particular drug types are discussed later.

Starting Treatment in Stage 2 Hypertension

The major guidelines all agree that patients who will require reductions in blood pressures of at least 20/10 mm Hg should have their treatment started with combination therapy. This is a new development as compared with previous guidelines, where single therapy was generally preferred unless the hypertension was especially severe. The rationale for this recommendation is that, because most such patients will eventually require more than one drug, starting with a combination accelerates the treatment process and makes it more likely that patients will achieve blood pressure targets in a timely fashion. Evidence supporting a rapid approach to blood pressure control has come most recently from the VALUE trial (13) in which it was shown that the blood pressure responses measured after only 1 month of therapy were predictive of clinical outcomes during the following 5 years. The guidelines stop short of advising as to whether combination therapy should be composed of two separate formulations, or whether fixed combination products (containing both drugs in a single tablet or capsule) are preferred. Clearly, fixed combinations are more convenient for many patients, require taking fewer doses, and in many cases are more cost effective.

The Growing Use of Drug Combinations

Efficacy is not the only reason for using combinations of antihypertensive agents. Side effects or adverse events can also be reduced. There are two ways this can be done. First, because the dose-response characteristics of most antihypertensive agents provide much of their efficacy at relatively low doses, the combination of two agents in low doses can provide powerful blood pressure-lowering effects while minimizing adverse events. This is particularly relevant to such drugs as diuretics, beta-blockers, or centrally acting agents that have definite dose-dependent side effects.

The second way in which combination therapy can reduce adverse effects is to use drugs that counteract each other's unwanted actions. One example is the use of drugs like angiotensin-receptor blockers or ACE inhibitors in combination with diuretics. The blockers of the renin-angiotensin system are effective in reducing the unwanted actions of diuretics on potassium, glucose, and other metabolic findings. Another example is the use of ACE inhibitors or angiotensin-receptor blockers in combination with calcium channel blockers; the peripheral edema that can occur with calcium channel blockers, presumably reflecting the greater dilatory effect they have on the arterial than the venous circulation, can be largely offset by the blockers of the renin-angiotensin system, which equally dilate the venous and arterial circulations and so reduce peripheral fluid accumulation

At present, there are numerous fixed-dose combinations of both angiotensin-receptor blockers or ACE inhibitors in combination with low-dose thiazides, usually hydrochlorothiazide. Likewise, there are a number of beta-blockers/diuretic combinations available. The JNC 7 recommendations generally favor combinations containing low-dose thiazides, though the other guidelines are not so specific. Indeed, the combination of a calcium channel blocker with either an ACE inhibitor or an angiotensin-receptor blocker, quite apart from minimizing peripheral edema, provides powerful antihypertensive efficacy that is well tolerated in many patients.

Complex Combinations

Many patients will require more than two antihypertensive agents to reach their goals. Clinical trials that rigorously pursued appropriate levels of blood pressure control have indicated that typically between three and four drugs are required, particularly in older patients or those with a history with cardiovascular abnormalities. In general, a three-drug combination should be composed of a blocker of the renin-angiotensin system, a calcium channel blocker, and a diuretic. If a fourth drug is required, beta-blockers can be a useful addition. It should also be noted, as discussed earlier, that beta-blockers should be considered early in the antihypertensive regimen in patients who have an indication for their use, particularly those with a history of a myocardial infarction, current angina pectoris, or heart failure. Apart from centrally acting agents and some older drugs such as reserpine, it should be noted that the different types of calcium channel blockers can have additive effects. If the first calcium channel blocker used, for instance, is a dihydropyridine like amlodipine, then further efficacy can often be obtained by adding a nondihydropyridine such as verapamil or diltiazem.

ARE THERE REASONS TO FAVOR PARTICULAR ANTIHYPERTENSIVE AGENTS?

The abundance of antihypertensive agents can sometimes cause confusion. Several clinical trials have been completed in the last 3 or 4 years to compare the attributes of different drugs. Because the benefit of blood pressure reduction is so strongly established, none of these studies employed a placebo, but rather depended on comparing clinical endpoint benefits among different classes of active drugs. In general, these studies have lead to a conclusion that drugs that interrupt the renin-angiotensin system probably should be part of most antihypertensive regimens, though once again this belief should be tempered by the primacy of blood pressure reduction. In considering these trials, it should be noted that there is one evident bias: most research funding inevitably is focused in the newer classes, meaning that older agents are no longer being scrutinized with sufficient intensity to evaluate the full range of their potential attributes. Still, recent studies have cast useful light on drug selection.

Calcium Channel Blockers

Both dihydropyridine and nondihydropyridine agents have shown to be at least equal to other major drug classes in preventing major clinical outcomes and mortality (27,28). One recent trial studied amlodipine in patients with only minimally raised blood pressures (prehypertension), but with a history of coronary disease, and showed that this agent was particularly effective in reducing the need for coronary revascularization and hospitalization for angina (29). Also, in the VALUE trial (13) for equal blood pressure effects, amlodipine was as effective as an angiotensin-receptor blocker in preventing strokes, coronary events, and mortality, though less effective in preventing heart failure. In the ALLHAT trial (23), amlodipine-based therapy was at least as effective as diuretic or ACE inhibitor-based therapies in preventing coronary events, strokes, and mortality.

ACE Inhibitors

In hypertension, ACE inhibitors have been shown to be similar to other drug classes in preventing major clinical outcomes (30). It has never been completely established that the benefits of ACE inhibitors are independent of their blood pressure-lowering effects. In the ALLHAT study (23), an ACE inhibitor was equal to diuretic or calcium channel blocker regimens in preventing the primary endpoint of fatal and nonfatal coronary events, even though the study design put the ACE inhibitor at a disadvantage compared with the other agents in reducing blood pressure. Of note, in a major Australian trial in which an ACE inhibitor had virtually identical blood pressure effects to a thiazide diuretic, the ACE inhibitor appeared to have some outcomes advantages, particularly in preventing myocardial infarction (31).

Most recently, the Anglo Scandinavian Cardiac Outcomes Trial (ASCOT) has demonstrated (Fig. 25-4) that an ACE inhibitor added to a calcium channel blocker was significantly more effective than a traditional beta-blocker/diuretic combination in preventing mortality, coronary events, and strokes (32). Although the combination of the two newer drugs, the calcium channel blocker and the ACE inhibitor, was slightly more effective than the older agents in reducing blood pressure, detailed analyses of these data indicated that this could not explain the strong clinical outcomes advantages observed with the newer drugs (33).

Angiotensin-Receptor Blockers

These agents, the newest of the major classes, are effective in lowering blood pressure and are well tolerated. And, as shown in Figure 25-5, they are at least as effective as other antihypertensive drug classes in preventing major cardiovascular events (34). Like ACE inhibitors, they are also indicated for the treatment of congestive heart failure. Moreover, in patients with hypertension and diabetes with nephropathy, the angiotensin-receptor blockers (ARBs) have been shown to prevent progression to end-stage renal disease (35,36).

Two other areas in which these drugs might be beneficial have recently become apparent. In high-risk hypertensive patients (as evidenced by the presence of left ventricular hypertrophy on EKG), losartan was 25% more effective than a beta-blocker in reducing stroke (37). In a trial in patients who had already suffered ischemic strokes, eprosartan was shown to have identical blood pressure effects to a dihydropyridine but to reduce the incidence of recurrent stroke events by 25% (38).

Another area in which the ARBs might be differentiated from other antihypertensive drug classes is in the prevention of atrial fibrillation, though these data are still new. Again, when compared with a beta-blocker in hypertensive patients with left ventricular hypertrophy, losartan was significantly more effective in preventing new-onset atrial fibrillation despite equal blood pressure effects (39). Also, in patients with atrial fibrillation who were pharmacologically or electrically converted back to sinus rhythm and placed on amiodarone, the addition of irbesartan was more effective than placebo in preventing recurrence of the atrial fibrillation (40). Further evaluations of this potentially important action are required.

SPECIAL SITUATIONS

Because this chapter is focused primarily on essential or primary hypertension in adults, it will not deal with managing hypertension in pregnancy (which is best left to obstetricians trained in high-risk pregnancies or to credentialed hypertension specialists). Likewise, the management of hypertension in children, which has become an important subspecialty area, is be-

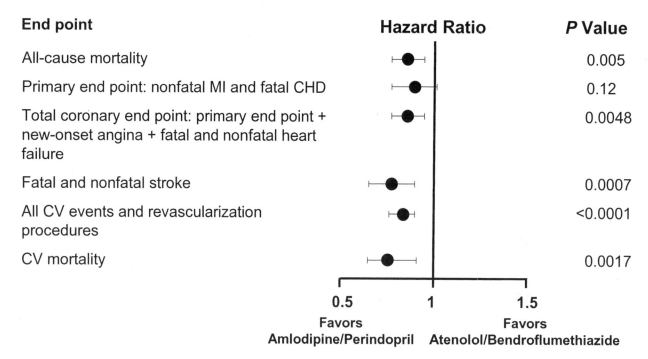

FIGURE 25-4. Hazard ratios (relative benefits) for major clinical outcomes and mortality in high-risk patients being treated with either an older antihypertensive drug combination (atenolol/thiazide) or a newer drug combination (amlodipine/perindopril) in high-risk hypertensive patients. (From Dahlof B, Sever PS, Poulter NR, et al. Prevention of cardiovascular events with an antihypertensive regimen of amlodipine adding perindopril as required versus atenolol adding bendroflumethiazide as required, in the Anglo-Scandinavian Cardiac Outcomes Trial-Blood Pressure Lowering Arm (ASCOT-BPLA): a multi-centre randomized controlled trial. *Lancet* 2005;366:895–906, with permission.)

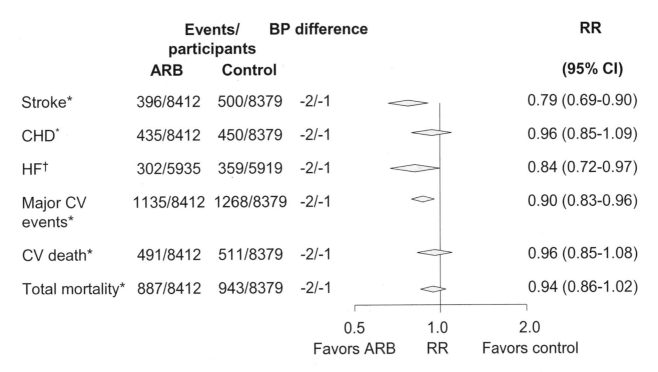

	Events/ participants		BP difference		RR
	ARB	Control			(95% CI)
Stroke*	396/8412	500/8379	-2/-1		0.79 (0.69-0.90)
CHD*	435/8412	450/8379	-2/-1		0.96 (0.85-1.09)
HF†	302/5935	359/5919	-2/-1		0.84 (0.72-0.97)
Major CV events*	1135/8412	1268/8379	-2/-1		0.90 (0.83-0.96)
CV death*	491/8412	511/8379	-2/-1		0.96 (0.85-1.08)
Total mortality*	887/8412	943/8379	-2/-1		0.94 (0.86-1.02)

FIGURE 25-5. A comparison of the effects of angiotensin-receptor blockers and control regimens (drugs other than ARBs or ACE inhibitors) on major clinical outcomes or mortality in hypertensive patients included in a large-scale meta-analysis. (From Blood Pressure Lowering Treatment Trialists' Collaboration. Effects of different blood pressure lowering regimens on major cardiovascular events: second cycle of prospectively designed overviews. *Lancet* 2003;362:1527–1535, with permission.)

yond the realm of this chapter. It should be noted, however, that the increasing prevalence of obesity and the metabolic syndrome in children and adolescents is inevitably increasing the incidence of hypertension in young people. Clinicians can make important contributions to resolving this problem by assertively dealing with the root causes—primarily reduced physical activity and increased caloric intake—of this troubling problem.

INADEQUATE TREATMENT RESPONSES

With the logical use of drug combinations it should be possible to achieve blood pressure goals in at least 80% of hypertensive patients. Admittedly, there are some patients who, despite such efforts, are still resistant to treatment. Although there are currently many available drugs, innovative products may still be necessary to optimize blood pressure results in a number of difficult-to-treat patients. In most cases, however, it should be possible to figure out why results are not optimal. The following is a brief checklist of possible explanations for poor results.

Inadequate Adherence

It is an unfortunate fact that some hypertensive patients simply do not even fill their drug prescriptions, and even when they do, there is often little if any attempt to remain with the recommended treatment regimen. Explanations for this so-called poor compliance are not entirely satisfactory; presumably some patients doubt the validity of their diagnosis or believe that subtle changes in lifestyle might eliminate their hypertension. Other patients may simply use mechanisms such as denial to avoid dealing with the implications of the diagnosis. Drug side effects certainly can be a factor in poor treatment compliance,

but the newer drug classes generally are very well tolerated. Cost also can be a reason why patients don't follow their treatment regimen; it should be noted, though, that in health systems where drugs are provided at minimal cost or completely free of charge, adherence to therapy is not much better than in the community in general. Certainly, in assessing a poor treatment response, clinicians should actively consider the possibility that the prescribed medications have not been taken.

Inappropriate Drug Combinations

It is important, as discussed earlier in this chapter, to use combinations of drugs that exhibit complementary mechanisms of action. Perhaps the single most common error made in putting together treatment combinations is the omission of a diuretic. Most patients eat diets containing excessive amounts of sodium, a factor that mitigates against the efficacy of many drug classes. Certainly in cases where patients will not modify their diets, a diuretic—for instance, hydrochlorothiazide in a dose of 25 mg daily—should be strongly considered.

Conflicting Nonantihypertensive Drug

A number of drug classes used for indications other than hypertension can raise blood pressure and interfere with the actions of blood pressure-lowering agents. Among the most common of these are the nonsteroidal anti-inflammatory drugs (NSAIDs). These drugs, which are frequently prescribed for arthritis and for the treatment of pain, often cause some degree sodium and water retention and produce increases in blood pressure. This applies both to the conventional drugs of this class as well as to the newer COX 2-selective inhibitors. Where it is necessary to use such drugs, it may be also necessary to add or increase the dose of a diuretic and certainly to try to reduce sodium intake to minimize this effect. Oral contraceptives are another type of commonly used therapy that can increase blood pressure. As well, a variety of cold remedies, particularly those containing sympathomimetic agents and antihistamines, can raise blood pressure. Usually such treatments are used only for symptomatic relief during the short term, and once they are discontinued, their adverse blood pressure effects should disappear fairly promptly. Some dietary agents also raise blood pressure and should be asked about in patients whose blood pressure responses to treatment seem inadequate.

Secondary Hypertension

If patients are not responding well to well-constructed treatment regimens and the more obvious explanations for this problem have been excluded, then it may be appropriate to consider secondary forms of hypertension. This is particularly worth considering in patients whose blood pressure control deteriorates rapidly as well as in those patients whose onset of hypertension, when it is first documented, is also rapid. The full workup and diagnosis of secondary forms of hypertension usually involve sophisticated laboratory and imaging techniques. For this reason, when a secondary form of hypertension is suspected, it is usually appropriate to refer the patient to a specialist in hypertension who has access to such resources. Table 25-5 provides a highly simplified summary of the approaches to some secondary forms of hypertension. Specialty texts should be consulted for more detailed descriptions.

Hypertensive Emergencies and Urgencies

True hypertensive emergencies generally require hospital care, and a detailed discussion of their management is beyond the scope of this chapter. A hypertensive emergency is not defined solely on the basis of high blood pressure, but requires evidence of acute blood pressure-related effects. Encephalopathy, pulmonary edema, and the appearance of hematuria are examples of such effects. This condition obviously requires closely monitored aggressive therapy, usually based on intravenous therapy selected according to the presumed underlying cause and clinical features of the crisis.

Very high blood pressure—systolic values above 180 mm Hg—without acute concomitant clinical findings is sometimes referred to as a hypertensive urgency and can be encountered in routine clinical practice. A few years ago it became popular to give such patients oral rapidly acting formulations of calcium channel blockers, which often restored blood pressure to near normal levels within minutes. Unfortunately, this short-term strategy often resulted in the return of severe hypertension after some hours, sometimes associated with strokes or major cardiac events. Today, oral treatment is still acceptable but should use drugs with long durations of action. Agents such as clonidine, ACE inhibitors, angiotensin-receptor blockers, beta-blockers, and long-acting calcium channel blockers will often bring blood pressure down to more acceptable levels within 1 to 4 hours. Using a combination of two agents should be strongly considered, but even if the initial result is gratifying patients should return for prompt follow-up visits to ensure that blood pressures remain at acceptable levels.

EFFECTIVENESS

Major public campaigns in the United States have acquainted people with the dangers of hypertension and encouraged its diagnosis and treatment. The National High Blood Pressure

TABLE 25-5

A HIGHLY SIMPLIFIED SCHEME FOR EVALUATING SOME OF THE MAIN FORMS OF SECONDARY HYPERTENSION

	Prevalence (% of all hypertension cases)	Initial diagnosis and screening tests	Confirmation
Intrinsic Renal Disease	5%	Urinalysis; routine blood chemistries	Renal biopsy; renal imaging
Renovascular Hypertension	1%	Sudden BP increase; treatment resistance; high or lateral abdominal bruit; captopril test (renins, renography)	Renal angiography
Primary Aldosteronism	1% (though recent claims of higher prevalence)	Hypokalemia; low plasma renin (R), high plasma aldosterone (A), high A:R ratio	Abdominal CT or MRI (also helps determine if adrenal ademona or bilateral hyperplasia)
Cushing's Syndrome	<1%	Typical facial and other physical findings; glucose and potassium changes	Basal plasma ACTH measurements; dexamethasone suppresion test
Pheochromocytoma	<1%	Paroxysmal hypertension, palpitations, sweatiness. Urinary metanephrines, plasma metanephrine and catecholamines	Clonidine suppression test; CT scan of adrenals and other potential locations
Coarctation of the Aorta	<1%	BP in arm > leg; ischemic symptoms in lower extremities; systolic flow murmur in thorax	Aortography; MRI; TE echo/Doppler

Education Program, which is sponsored by the National Institutes of Health, has been waging a successful campaign for many years. For this reason, hypertension management in the United States is probably more successful than in almost all other countries. Even so, data from the National Health and Nutrition Examination Survey (NHANES) indicates that our results are still somewhat disappointing (40). About three-quarters of all hypertensive people in this country know they have this condition, but only about half of all hypertensives are receiving some form of therapy, and barely one-third have blood pressures controlled to an acceptable level. A variety of social, emotional, and financial reasons have been studied to explain this result (41), but perhaps one of the most important explanations may lie with inadequate commitments by clinicians to ensure that blood pressure results in their patients are maximized.

As our population ages, a progressively higher number of people are requiring multiple therapies to deal with their growing number of ailments. Clearly, issues of complexity of drug regimens, the possibility of symptomatic or other side effects that are sometimes difficult to predict in patients receiving multiple agents, and again the question of cost can all at least partly explain the difficulties of achieving optimal results. Hypertension itself is a good case in point; we now know, based on our growing awareness, that high blood pressure is typically part of a broader syndrome and that many patients with this condition must also be treated for such associated problems as lipid abnormalities and diabetes.

As discussed earlier, in hypertensive patients with apparently normal or "usual" levels of LDL cholesterol, a low-dose statin was shown to significantly improve prognosis (42). In fact, compared with patients receiving conventional antihypertensive agents and not receiving a statin, those receiving more contemporary drugs in combination with a statin achieved a remarkable 48% reduction in major coronary events and a 44% reduction in strokes. From the point of view of prolonging life and reducing clinical events, this is good news; yet, at the same time, it adds to the challenges of dealing with this highly prevalent condition. From a practical point of view, optimal results in hypertension often require a team approach that provides sufficient resources and clinical interactions to deal with the complexities of this condition.

References

1. Nei Ching. Yellow Emperor's Classic of Internal Medicine, Books 2-9, Published between 2698 and 2598 bc.
2. Bright R. Cases and observations, illustrative of renal disease accompanied with the secretion of albuminous urine. *Guy's Hosp Rep* 1836;1:338–379.
3. Korotkov NS. A contribution to the problem of methods for the determination of blood pressure. *Rep ImperMil-Med Acca St. Petersburg* 1905;11:365–367.
4. Actuarial Society of America. *Blood pressure study of 1925.* New York: Actuarial Society of America and Association of Life Insurance Medical Directors, 1925.
5. Freis ED. A history of hypertension treatment. In: Oparil S, Weber MA, eds. *Hypertension: a companion to Brenner and Rector's the kidney,* 2nd ed. Philadelphia: Elsevier Saunders; 2005.
6. Veterans Administration Cooperative Study Group on Antihypertensive Agents. Effects of treatment on morbidity in hypertension: results in patients with diastolic blood pressure averaging 115 through 129 mm Hg. *JAMA* 1967;202:1028–1034.
7. Neaton JD, Wentworth D, for the Multiple Risk Factor Intervention Trial Research Group. Serum cholesterol, blood pressure, cigarette smoking, and death from coronary heart disease. Overall findings and differences by age for 316,099 white men. *Arch Intern Med* 1992;1S2:S6–64.
8. Lewington S, Clarke R, Qizilbash N, et al. Prospective Studies Collaboration. Age-specific relevance of usual BP to vascular mortality: a meta-analysis of individual data for one million adults in 60 prospective studies. *Lancet* 2002;14:1903–1913.
9. Weber MA. Is there more to life than blood pressure? *J Clin Hyperterns* 2005;7(3):149–151.
10. Hansson L, Zanchetti A, Carruthers S, et al. Effects of intensive blood-pressure lowering and low-dose aspirin in patients with hypertension: principal results of the Hypertension Optimal Treatment (HOT) randomized trial. *Lancet* 1998;351:1755–1762.
11. UK Prospective Diabetes Study Group. Tight blood pressure control and risk of macrovascular and microvascular complications in type 2 diabetes: UKPDS 38. *BMJ* 1998;317:703–713.
12. Staessen JA, Gasowski, Wang JG, et al. Risks of untreated and treated isolated systolic hypertension in the elderly meta-analysis of outcomes trials. *Lancet* 2000;104:865–872.
13. Weber MA, Julius S, Kjeldsen SE, et al. Blood pressure dependent and independent effects of antihypertensive treatment on clinical events in the VALUE trial. *Lancet* 2004;363:2049–2051.
14. The Seventh Report of the Joint National Committee on Prevention, Detection, Evaluation, and Treatment of High Blood Pressure: the JNC 7 report. *JAMA* 2003;289:2560–2572.
15. Weber MA. Cardiovascular and metabolic consequences of obesity. In: Topol EJ, ed., *Textbook of cardiovascular medicine,* 2nd ed. New York: Lippincott Williams & Wilkins; 2005.
16. Kahn R, Buse J, Ferrannini E, et al. The metabolic syndrome: time for a critical appraisal joint statement from the American Diabetes Association and the European Association for the Study of Diabetes. *Diabetologia* 2005; 48(9):1684–1699.
17. 2003 European Society of Hypertension. European Society of Cardiology guidelines for the management of arterial hypertension. *J Hypertens* 2003; 21:1011–1054.
18. Sever PS, Dahlof B, Poulter NR, et al for the ASCOT Investigators. Prevention of coronary and stroke events with atorvastatin in hypertensive patients who have average or lower-than-average cholesterol concentrations, in the Anglo-Scandinavian Cardiac Outcomes Trial-Lipid Lowering Arm (ASCOT-LLA): a multicentre randomized controlled trial. *Lancet* 2003;361: 1149–1158.
19. Giles TD, Berk BC, Black HR, et al. on behalf of the Hypertension Writing Group. Expanding the definition and classification of hypertension. *J Clin Hypertens* 2005;7:505–512.
20. Weber MA. Exploring a new definition of hypertension. *Rev Cardiov Med* 2005;6(3):164–172.
21. Weber MA. The metabolic syndrome. In: Antman EM, ed. *Cardiovascular therapeutics.* New York: Elsevier; 2005.
22. Douglas JG, Bakris GL, Epstein M, et al. Management of high blood pressure in African Americans: consensus statement of the Hypertension in African American Working Group of the International Society on Hypertension in Blacks. *Arch Intern Med* 2003;163:525–541.
23. The ALLHAT Officers and Coordinators for the ALLHAT Collaborative Research Group. Major outcomes in high-risk hypertensive patients randomized to angiotensin-converting enzyme inhibitor or calcium channel blocker vs diuretic. The Antihypertensive and Lipid-Lowering treatment to prevent Heart Attack Trial. (ALLHAT). *JAMA* 2002;288:2981–2997.
24. Weber MA. The ALLHAT Report: A case of information and misinformation. *J Clin Htn* 2003;5:9–13.
25. Julius S. The ALLHAT study: if you believe in evidence-based medicine, stick to it! *J Hypertens* 2003;21:453–454.
26. McInnes GT. Size isn't everything—ALLHAT in perspective. *J Hypertens* 2003;21:459–461.
27. Brown MJ, Palmer CR, Castaigne A, et al. Morbidity and mortality in patients randomized to double-blind treatment with a long-acting calcium-channel-blocker or diuretic in the International Nifedipine GITS study: Intervention as a Goal in Hypertension Treatment (INSIGHT). *Lancet* 2000; 356:366–372.
28. Vasan RS, Beiser A, Seshadri S, et al. Residual lifetime risk for developing hypertension in middle-aged women and men: The Framingham Heart Study. *JAMA* 2002;287:1003–1010.
29. Nissen SE, Tuzcu EM, Libby P, et al. Effect of antihypertensive agents on cardiovascular events in patients with coronary disease and normal blood pressure. The CAMELOT study: a randomized controlled trial. *JAMA* 2004; 292:2217–2226.
30. Blood Pressure Lowering Treatment Trialists' Collaboration. Effects of ACE inhibitors, calcium antagonists and other blood pressure lowering drugs: Results of prospectively designed overviews of randomized trials. *Lancet* 2000;355:1955–1964.
31. Wing LMH, Reid CM, Ryan P, et al. A comparison of outcomes with angiotensin-converting-enzyme inhibitors and diuretics for hypertension in the elderly. *N Engl J Med* 2003;348:583–592.
32. Dahlof B, Sever PS, Poulter NR, et al. Prevention of cardiovascular events with an antihypertensive regimen of amlodipine adding perindopril as required versus atenolol adding bendroflumethiazide as required, in the Anglo-Scandinavian Cardiac Outcomes Trial-Blood Pressure Lowering Arm (ASCOT-BPLA): a multicentre randomized controlled trial. *Lancet* 2005; 366:895–906.
33. Poulter NR, Wedel H, Dahlof B, et al. Role of blood pressure and other variables in the differential cardiovascular event rates noted in the Anglo-Scandinavian Cardiac Outcomes Trial-Blood Pressure Lowering Arm (ASCOT-BPLA). *Lancet* 2005;366:907–913.
34. Blood Pressure Lowering Treatment Trialists' Collaboration. Effects of different blood pressure lowering regimens on major cardiovascular events:

second cycle of prospectively designed overviews. *Lancet* 2003;362: 1527–1535.

35. Brenner BM, Cooper ME, DeZeeuw D, et als. Effects of losartan on renal and cardiovascular outcomes in patients with type 2 diabetes and nephropathy. *N Engl J Med* 2001;345:861–869.

36. Lewis EJ, Hunsicker LG, Clarke WR, et al. Renoprotective effect of the angiotensin-receptor antagonist irbesartan in patients with nephropathy due to type 2 diabetes. *N Engl J Med* 2001;345:851–860.

37. Lindholm LH, Ibsen H, Dahlof B, et al. Cardiovascular morbidity and mortality in patients with diabetes in the Losartan Intervention For Endpoint reduction in hypertension study (LIFE): a randomized trial against atenolol. *Lancet* 2002;359:1004–1010.

38. Schrader J, Luders S, Kulschewsli A, et al. Morbidity and mortality after stroke, eprosartan compared with nitrendipine for secondary prevention: principal results of a prospective randomized controlled study (MOSES). *Stroke* 2005;36:1218–1226.

39. Wachtell K, Lehto M, Gerdts E, et al. Angiotensin II receptor blockade reduces new-onset atrial fibrillation and subsequent stroke compared to atenolol: the Losartan Intervention for End Point Reduction in Hypertension (LIFE) study. *J Am Coll Cardiol* 2005;45:712–719.

40. Burt VL, Cutler JA, Higgins M, et al. Trends in the prevalence, awareness, treatment and control of hypertension in the adult US population. Data from the health examination surveys, 1960 to 1991. *Hypertension* 1995; 26:60–69.

41. Weir MR, Maibach EW; Bakris GL, et al. Implications of a healthy lifestyle and medication analysis for improving hypertension control. *Arch Int Med* 2000;160:481–490.

CHAPTER 26 ■ SMOKING CESSATION

BETH C. BOCK

EFFECTS OF SMOKING ON HEALTH
SMOKING CESSATION IN CARDIAC PATIENTS
PHYSICIAN INTERVENTIONS
TREATMENT APPROACHES
Ask
Advise
Assess
Assist
Arrange Follow-up
PHARMACOLOGIC THERAPIES
NICOTINE REPLACEMENT IN CARDIAC PATIENTS
PROGRAM REFERRAL
BOOKS AND OTHER SELF-HELP RESOURCES
Quitting
Relapse Prevention
Web Sites
SUMMARY AND CONCLUSIONS

EFFECTS OF SMOKING ON HEALTH

Cigarette smoking is the leading cause of preventable morbidity and mortality among all racial and ethnic groups in the United States (1,2). Tobacco use is the primary cause of lung cancer and is causally linked to other forms of cancer (3,4), heart disease, stroke (5), and chronic obstructive pulmonary disease (6,7), and it is responsible for more than $75 billion in annual health care expenditures (8). Each year in the United States, more than 438,000 deaths are linked to cigarette smoking, and one-third of deaths among former smokers are directly attributable to tobacco use (9). Moreover, environmental tobacco smoke or "secondhand smoke" has been strongly associated with respiratory illness in children and with both cancer and heart disease in adults living with smokers. Approximately 21.6% of U.S. adults are current smokers (10). Although this prevalence is lower than the 22.5% prevalence among U.S. adults in 2002 (11), the rate of decline is not sufficient to meet the national health objective for 2010.

SMOKING CESSATION IN CARDIAC PATIENTS

Coronary heart disease is the leading cause of mortality in the United States, accounting for nearly one-third of all deaths (12). Cigarette smoking greatly increases the risk of death from heart disease, and smoking cessation produces marked reductions in cardiovascular risk (6). The experience of hospitalization, particularly for cardiovascular disease, can result in smoking cessation even without intervention (13–15). However, cessation rates vary greatly, depending on the reason for hospitaliza-tion, length of stay, and the presence of depressive symp-

toms (16,17). For example, Rigotti et al found high cessation rates (58%) 1 year after hospitalization among patients having coronary bypass surgery, whereas other studies have shown low cessation rates among smokers immediately after hospitalization (13.7%) and at 1-year follow-up (9.2%) (18,19). Most individuals who quit smoking without intervention will relapse within 6 months (17,20).

PHYSICIAN INTERVENTIONS

Although 70% of smokers visit a physician each year, relatively few doctors use this opportunity to address the patient's smoking (21–23). Physicians practicing in specialties such as cardiology or emergency medicine are less likely to provide smoking cessation interventions than primary care physicians (24). Possible explanations cited for low physician intervention rates include lack of time, deficient training in counseling skills, and an absence of organizational supports (25–28). This is regrettable because multiple studies have shown that even a brief intervention lasting less than 3 minutes significantly increases the chance that the smoker will quit (22,29). Formal physician training, the use of cues or reminders, pharmacologic aids, follow-up visits, and supplemental educational materials all increase the effectiveness of physician-delivered interventions (22,30). Cardiologists seeing smokers with coronary artery disease, hypertension, or histories of recurrent chest pain can be especially effective because the patient's illness can be linked directly to smoking. The clinical encounter is an important opportunity to address smoking cessation and should not be missed (31). Many physicians, however, do not feel that they have the counseling skills or training to address the issue of smoking cessation effectively. This chapter provides a well-researched, effective, and simple approach that cardiologists can use to counsel their patients who smoke.

TREATMENT APPROACHES

Clinical guidelines have been developed through a joint collaboration between the Centers for Disease Control and the Agency for Healthcare Research and Quality (AHRQ) together with the National Cancer Institute, the National Heart, Lung, and Blood Institute, the National Institute on Drug Abuse, the Robert Wood Johnson Foundation, and the University of Wisconsin Medical School Center for Tobacco Research and Intervention (29). The recommendations made as a result of this extensive, systematic review and analysis of the extant peer-reviewed scientific literature form the basis of the approach taken in this chapter.

The key principles underlying these recommendations are

1. Physicians should identify all their patients who smoke.
2. Effective treatment is available for tobacco dependence.
3. Physicians should offer treatment to all their smoking patients who are ready to quit.

4. Physicians should offer treatment even to those smoking patients who are not yet ready or willing to quit because the physician's intervention has been shown to increase the smoker's readiness and motivation to quit.

5. The physician should understand that tobacco dependence is a chronic condition that typically requires repeated intervention before long-term success is achieved.

The best practice model for a brief intervention for smoking cessation is easily summarized by the mnemonic device of the "Five As" (Table 26-1). Each of these—Ask, Advise, Assess, Assist, and Arrange follow-up—is summarized in the following paragraphs (Fig. 26-1).

Ask

National guidelines recommend that physicians systematically determine the smoking status of all patients at every visit. This can be done by modifying the routine vital signs charting (Fig. 26-2).

Advise

Every tobacco user should be given clear, strong, and personalized advice to quit. Unfortunately, research has repeatedly shown that smoking counseling is not provided at most physician visits (26). Moreover, specialists are less likely to provide smoking counseling than primary care physicians (32).

Counseling does not need to be extensive to be effective. Brief, clear advice from a physician has been shown to **double** quit rates (29). For example, advice to a patient who is currently enrolled in cardiac rehabilitation might sound like this:

- **Clear:** "It is important for you to quit smoking."
- **Strong:** "Because you have already experienced heart disease (or specify condition), the most important thing you can do to avoid repeating this experience is to quit smoking."
- **Personal:** "Your exercise capacity and your ability to be physically active will improve much faster if you quit smoking."
- **Other phrases that work are:** "As your physician, I want you to know that the most important thing you can do to protect or improve your health is to quit smoking." "Quitting smoking is important for everyone who smokes, but for you its especially important because of (specify current health problem)."

Assess

Assess the patient's readiness to quit smoking and level of nicotine dependence.

Readiness to Quit Smoking

Readiness to quit smoking is a key determinant of the treatment approach (Fig. 26-3). Treatment for smokers who are ready to make a serious attempt to quit should be focused on behavioral strategies, including (a) selecting a target quit date, (b) reviewing and arranging appropriate pharmacologic therapies, and (c) referring to self-help or professional programs. Treatment for smokers who are not ready to quit should focus on helping the patient get ready to quit. Treatment for these smokers should focus on the psychological issues surrounding cessation, including reasons for quitting versus reasons for continued smoking, concerns about the cessation process, building the patient's self-confidence, and discussing family or social supports and barriers to quitting.

Motivation, or readiness to quit smoking, has most often been measured using Prochaska and DiClemente's stages of change model (33), which was developed for use in outpatient populations. Because smoking restrictions in the in-patient setting and hospitalization encourage serious thought about smoking habits, this algorithm may tend to misclassify hospitalized smokers as having more motivation to quit than they actually do. Research has shown that asking inpatients a single question regarding how likely it is that they will remain abstinent after hospital discharge may be more predictive of actual motivation (34).

Nicotine Dependence

The most widely used and validated measure of nicotine dependence is the *Fagerstrom Test for Nicotine Dependence* (Table 26-2). Patients scoring 6 or more are highly nicotine dependent. It is important to know the level of nicotine dependence because, although research shows that most smokers benefit from nicotine replacement therapy (NRT), providing NRT is especially important for highly dependent smokers. Overall, smokers who use nicotine replacement show double the success rates as those who do not (29,35). Highly nicotine-dependent smokers are three times more likely to be successful if they use nicotine replacement. Moreover, the physician should choose the initial dose of NRT after considering the patient's level of nicotine dependence.

Assist

Motivational Approaches

Many different types of smokers exist. To simplify, however, consider smokers as falling into one of two groups: those who are ready to quit and those who are not yet ready. Research studies have repeatedly shown that physicians who take a motivational approach to addressing smoking with their patients are more successful in helping these smokers to quit. Motivational approaches, including the "transtheoretical" or "stages of change" model and motivational interviewing, are widely used theoretical models of how people change health behaviors

TABLE 26-1

THE FIVE AS TO INTERVENTION IN SMOKING CESSATION

Ask	The physician should ask all patients if they smoke or have recently quit.
Advise	The physician should give every tobacco user clear, strong, and personalized advice to quit.
Assess	The physician should assess the patient's level of nicotine dependence and readiness to quit.
Assist	The physician should assist the patient in obtaining one or more of the effective treatments that exist for smoking cessation.
Arrange follow-up	The physician should arrange follow-up to reinforce successful efforts and to identify slips early so that barriers can be identified and motivation to try again is renewed.

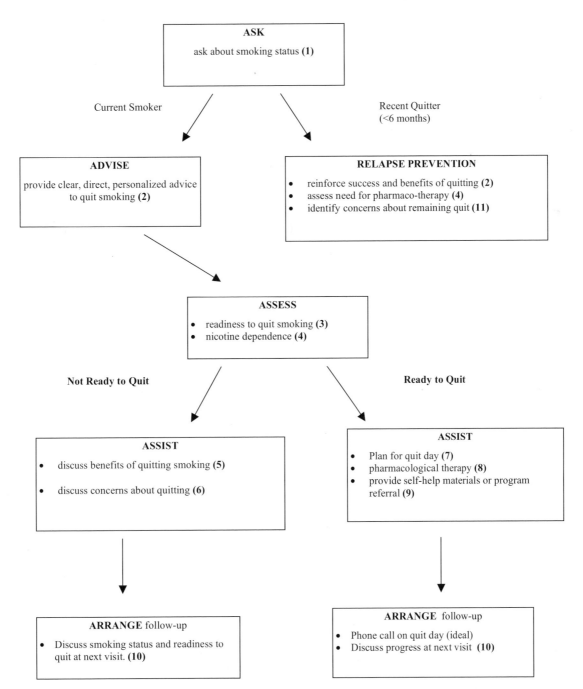

FIGURE 26-1. Summary of the "Five As."

VITAL SIGNS   Date of visit _____

Blood Pressure_____   Heart rate_____

Weight_____   Temperature_____   Respiration_____

Smoking Status: ☐ Current _____rate (cigarettes/day)

                  ☐ Former _____ date last smoked

                  ☐ Never

FIGURE 26-2. Sample routine vital sign charting.

ASSESS Readiness to Quit Smoking

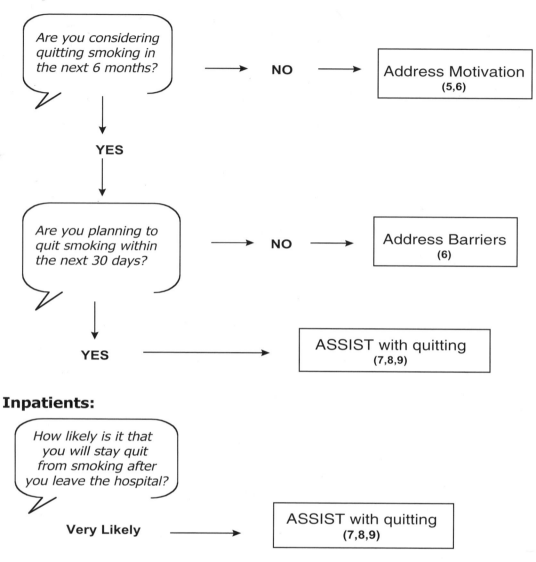

FIGURE 26-3. Assess readiness to quit smoking.

(33,36). Developed for use in outpatient populations, the basic tenet of these models is that individuals who are not yet ready to change behavior need to be approached differently than those who are ready to change. In practical terms, this means that treatment goals for smokers who are not yet ready to quit should focus on identifying reasons to quit, enhancing motivation for quitting, and identifying perceived barriers. Treatment for these smokers should avoid immediate behavioral goal setting (e.g., discussing quit dates or selecting pharmacologic treatments). Conversely, interventions for smokers who are ready to quit should focus on behavioral goals (e.g., choosing a target quit date and pharmacotherapy) and coping strategies.

Concerns about Quitting

Many patients are aware that they should quit smoking, but have concerns about the process of quitting or are discouraged from prior failed attempts. These patients may benefit by exploring their concerns about quitting. The decisional balance worksheet has been used in numerous smoking cessation trials to help smokers identify both their reasons for wanting to quit and perceived barriers to quitting (Table 26-3).

Not Ready to Quit

Patients who are not yet ready to quit need help identifying reasons to quit, improving their motivation and confidence in

TABLE 26-2

FAGERSTROM TEST FOR NICOTINE DEPENDENCE (FTND)

Points	0	1	2	3
How many cigarettes do you smoke per day?	≤10	11–20	21–30	≥30
Do you smoke more in the morning (or when you first wake up) compared to the rest of the day?	No	Yes		
Do you find it difficult to not smoke in places where smoking is not allowed, like church or the movies?	No	Yes		
How soon after waking do you smoke your first cigarette?	>60 min	31–60 min	6–30 min	<5 min
Do you smoke when you are so ill that you must stay in bed?	No	Yes		
Which cigarette of the day would you most hate to give up?	any other	the first		

From Heatherton TF, Kozlowski LT, Frecker RC, et al. The Fagerstrom test for nicotine dependence: a revision of the Fagerstrom Tolerance Questionnaire. *British Journal of Addiction* 1991;86:1119–1127, with permission.

their ability to quit, and identifying barriers to smoking cessation. These patients may lack, or believe they lack, the financial resources to afford NRT or pharmacologic aids to quitting or information about how smoking is affecting their health. They may have concerns about quitting—possibly related to prior failed attempts (38). The physician can intervene with these patients by providing relevant information that will help them identify barriers to quitting and find the resources necessary to support cessation. Motivational interventions are most successful when the physician is empathic, promotes patient autonomy (provides choices among options), supports the patient's sense of self-confidence, and avoids argumentation (39,40).

The "Good Reasons to Stop Smoking Now" and the "Benefits of Quitting Smoking" lists may be helpful (Table 26-3; Fig. 26-4).

Ready to Quit

Effective treatments exist for smoking cessation and should be provided to all smokers who are ready to quit. Effective treatment components include the following.

- Selecting a target quit day
- Reviewing pharmacologic therapies with the patient and selecting appropriate options
- Anticipating challenges (work schedules, stressors, social supports, and saboteurs)
- Offering referral to self-help materials or specialized programs and resources

Planning to Quit

Guidelines suggested to help those patients planning to quit include the following.

1. Select a target quit date, usually within 2 weeks of the office visit. Total abstinence as of this date is essential.

2. Prepare the environment. If possible, eliminate ashtrays, smoking paraphernalia, and cigarette supply.
3. Past experience. Review what worked and what caused prior relapses.
4. Plan the day. Patients need to consider how they will alter their usual routine to avoid smoking. Avoid alcohol. For a few days, the patient may need to avoid people and places associated with smoking. Patients should anticipate triggers and have a coping plan.
5. Recommend pharmacotherapy. Consider using medications if not contraindicated. Explain how these medications can reduce withdrawal symptoms and increase chances of success.
6. Suggest social support. Have the patient identify family, friends, or coworkers who will be helpful. Arrange for other household smokers to restrict their smoking near the patient.
7. Schedule a follow-up visit.

Arrange Follow-up

Follow-up Visits

Ideally, the first follow-up visit should occur within 1 week of the quit date. A phone contact on the quit day is helpful to most smokers. Congratulate and reinforce the patient's success. If the patient has smoked, identify circumstances surrounding slips; reframe slips as learning experiences—not as signs of failure; identify a new target quit day; reassess the need for pharmacotherapy; consider referral to a more intensive program. A second follow-up visit is recommended within 1 month.

Discuss Concerns About Remaining Quit

Nicotine dependence is a chronic and recurring condition, often requiring several serious quit attempts before permanent

TABLE 26-3

GOOD REASONS TO STOP SMOKING NOW

It's never too late to quit. The body begins to repair itself within minutes of the last cigarette.

Within 20 minutes of your last cigarette:
- Blood pressure begins to reduce
- Pulse drops to a more normal rate
- The temperature of hands and feet increases to normal

8 Hours:
- Carbon monoxide in the blood returns to normal
- Oxygen level in blood increases

24 Hours:
- Chance of heart attack decreases

48 Hours:
- Nerve endings start regrowing
- Your ability to smell and taste things is improved

72 Hours:
- Bronchial tubes relax, making breathing easier

2 Weeks to 3 Months:
- Circulation improves and walking becomes easier
- Lung function increases up to 30%

1 Month to 9 Months:
- Coughing, sinus congestion, fatigue, and shortness of breath all decrease
- Cilia regrow in the lungs, increasing your ability to handle mucus, clean the lungs, and reduce infection
- Your body's overall energy level increases

5 Years:
- The lung cancer death rate for the average smoker is cut in half

10 Years:
- Risk of lung cancer is almost as low as for those who never smoked
- Risk of other cancers (mouth, larynx, kidney, bladder, pancreas) all decrease.

From the American Cancer Society's FreshStart program.

success is achieved. Therefore, physicians should be prepared to address relapse prevention with any patient who has recently quit smoking (<6 months abstinence). Physicians should reinforce success and the benefits of quitting smoking and help patients identify any problems or concerns they may have about staying quit. Even patients who have recently quit smoking may be helped with pharmacotherapy or behavioral therapy and referrals (Table 26-4) (41,42).

Short-Term Coping Strategies

Short-term strategies the clinician can suggest to the patient include (a) remove all smoking-related paraphernalia (e.g., ash-trays, lighters) from the home, office, and car; (b) keep cigarettes out of easy reach (in an out-of-the-way kitchen cupboard, in the garage, in the trunk of the car); (c) be prepared to ask others to modify their behavior for a short while; (d) avoid alcohol; (e) exercise—brief walks during the day reduce stress and get the smoker out of the environment wherein smoking might be triggered; and (f) reward positive change.

PHARMACOLOGIC THERAPIES

All smokers who are ready to make a serious attempt to quit should be strongly encouraged to use pharmacotherapy to aid their quitting efforts, except where contraindicated (Table 26-5). As with other chronic disease conditions, nicotine dependence is best treated using multiple modalities. Physicians are advised to discourage patients from trying a single method and then switching to another single method only if the first approach fails. That strategy is likely to weaken the patient's resolve to quit before achieving success. Two first-line medications are effective for smoking cessation: bupropion and NRT. NRT is the most widely studied medication for managing nicotine dependence (29,43,44). Three primary mechanisms are responsible for NRTs efficacy: reduction of withdrawal symptoms, reducing the reinforcing value of tobacco products, and substituting positive effects obtained through smoking (e.g., mood enhancement, stress reduction). NRT is currently available in six different delivery formats: transdermal patch, gum, lozenge, sublingual tablet, nasal spray, and vapor inhaler. Bupropion (Zyban) was originally marketed as an antidepressant (Wellbutrin). It is chemically unrelated to the selective serotonin reuptake inhibitors (SSRIs) and tricyclic antidepressants. Although its mechanism of action is unknown, it is thought to act through noradrenergic or dopaminergic pathways. Bupropion has been shown to double quit rates compared to placebo among both men and women (45). Using either of these pharmacologic options (bupropion or NRT) increases the odds of successful cessation by 50% to 150% (32–34). NRT and bupropion can also be used simultaneously because they have different mechanisms of action. They are synergistic: using both entities together is more effective than using either alone.

Some clinical trials have begun to examine the use of combinations of different forms of NRT, the idea being to combine a passive form of nicotine delivery (patch) with a more acute, ad-libitum administration of medication when needed (e.g., gum). Results of these studies indicate that combination NRT may be more effective than either NRT product alone (46–49). Clonidine and nortriptyline have also shown some efficacy for smoking cessation, but they are not recommended as first-line treatment at present (50–52).

Key points related to pharmacologic therapy include the following.

- Use of pharmacotherapy approximately doubles quit rates and is safe for most patients.
- Pharmacotherapy is effective for a broad range of patients and should *not* be reserved only for "hard-core" smokers or heavy smokers.
- Different medication types (e.g., bupropion and NRT) can be combined to enhance chances of success.
- Combining the nicotine patch with self-administered forms of NRT (e.g., gum, inhaler) may be more effective than using a single form of NRT for some smokers.
- Long-term pharmacotherapy can reduce the risk of relapse.

BENEFITS OF QUITTING SMOKING

☺ Fresher breath.

☺ Cleaner smelling hair and clothes.

☺ Whiter teeth.

$ Saving money (a pack-a-day smoker will save almost $1,000 per year).

☺ Freedom from social restrictions and the demands of addiction.

→ no need to ensure continual cigarette supply.

☺ Improved circulation.

☺ Improved ability to exercise.

☺ Longer and better life.

☺ Less chance of having a heart attack, stroke, and cancer.

☺ Reduced risk of lung disease, fewer problems with existing respiratory disease.

☺ Improved health for the people you live with, especially your children.

☺ Better health: ex-smokers have fewer days of illness, fewer health complaints, better self-reported health status.

☺ After 10 years the risk of lung cancer for ex-smokers is cut in half.

☺ In about 10 years, the risk of stroke for ex-smokers is the same as for people who never smoked.

☺ For people with heart disease, quitting smoking reduces the risk of repeat heart attacks and death from heart disease by over 50%

FIGURE 26-4. Benefits of quitting smoking.

NICOTINE REPLACEMENT IN CARDIAC PATIENTS

When used in medical settings, NRT plus physician advice can produce impressive abstinence rates (53). However, soon after the nicotine patch was approved for use, the media reported a possible link between patch use and cardiovascular incidents. The use of NRT in cardiac patients has been of concern because some of the cardiotoxic effects of smoking are attributable to nicotine (54). Although nicotine does have sympathomimetic effects that increase heart rate and blood pressure and stimulate vasoconstriction, NRT use generally leads to significantly lower blood nicotine levels compared with smoking, even in patients who smoke during NRT treatment (55–60). NRT use is likely to result in fewer adverse cardiovascular effects than continued smoking. Anecdotal reports of adverse cardiac events have made physicians hesitant to prescribe NRT for cardiac patients (59–61). Systematic research over the past decade has found no reliable association between acute cardiovascular events and the use of the nicotine patch, even among patients who continue to smoke while using the patch (59–66).

Because cigarette smoking in general and nicotine ingestion in particular have cardiovascular effects, some caution is warranted regarding the safety of NRT among certain cardiac patients, such as those with (a) an immediate (within 2 to 4 weeks) history of myocardial infarction or other serious cardiovascular event, (b) serious arrhythmias, (c) uncontrolled hypertension, or (d) severe or unstable angina pectoris. Note that these are cautions, not contraindications. The physician must weigh the benefits of smoking cessation against any possible risk from nicotine replacement. Bupropion is generally well tolerated in cardiac patients, although rare reports have been made of exacerbation of hypertension.

PROGRAM REFERRAL

Most smoking cessation efforts are enhanced by behavioral supports. These can include self-help materials, telephone calls, support groups, and individual therapy for smoking cessation. Intervention intensity is positively associated with cessation success: essentially "more is better." Minimal interventions, such as brief (<3 minutes) counseling, from a physician increase the chance of successful cessation by approximately 30%, whereas high-intensity interventions such as individual counseling can more than double quit rates. Therefore, the more intervention resources the physician provides to the patient, the more likely the patient will quit smoking (Table 26-6).

BOOKS AND OTHER SELF-HELP RESOURCES

Numerous books and tapes are available as self-help aids for smokers who are attempting to quit. Most recently, a number of Internet Web sites have sprung up offering assistance to smokers who are trying to quit. Internet sites can be especially helpful to some smokers because chat rooms and other supports are available 24 hours a day. Many helpful books are available to patients who want to quit smoking. A few of these aids are listed following.

Quitting

The Stop Smoking Workbook: Your Guide to Healthy Quitting (Anita Maximin and Lori Stevic-Rust, New Harbinger Publications, 1995). This stop-smoking guide is out-

TABLE 26-4

FIRST-LINE PHARMACOLOGICAL THERAPIES

Medication	Contraindications	Precautions	Dosage/Use	Availability	Adverse Reactions	Comments
Bupropion (Zyban)	Seizure disorder, current bupropion use (e.g., Wellbutrin) or MAO inhibitors, anorexia or bulimia, allergy to bupropion.	Is usually well tolerated by patients with cardiovascular disease—infrequent reports of hypertension.	150 mg 1x day for 3 days, 150 mg twice per day for 7–12 weeks. Start 7–10 days prior to quit date.	Prescription	Dry mouth, insomnia.	May be used concurrently with nicotine replacement therapy. Treatment can be maintained for 6 months.
NRT	All: Allergy to nicotine.					
Patch	Severe eczema, allergy to adhesives or other skin disease.	Recent (2–4 weeks) myocardial infarction, severe arrhythmia, uncontrolled hypertension, severe angina pectoris.	Available in 7- to 21-mg doses. treatment usually lasts 4–12 weeks with dosage tapering.	OTC	Dizziness, headache, skin irritation (hydrocortisone cream/rotate patch sites); vivid dreams (avoid wearing during sleep).	Vary initial dose with smoking rate (e.g., <15 cigarettes/day should start at lower dosage. >35/day may need higher dose). May work best for regular-interval smokers.
Polacrilex (gum)	Severe temporo-mandibular joint disease, jaw problems, dentures.	Same as nicotine patch.	2 mg and 4 mg. One piece every 1–2 hours (24/day maximum).	OTC	Dizziness, headache, mouth soreness, hiccups, dyspepsia, jaw ache (review correct chewing technique).	May work especially well for light or irregular smokers. May help with oral substitution. Requires proper chewing technique
Inhaler	Allergy to menthol.	Same as nicotine patch. Use caution with patients who have asthma, wheezing, or other pulmonary disease.	4-mg cartridge (80 inhalations per cartridge). 6–16 cartridges per day. 3–6 months.	Prescription	Dizziness, headache, irritation of mouth, throat, coughing, rhinitis.	May work especially well for light or irregular smokers. May help with oral substitution.
Nasal Spray	Presence of asthma, rhinitis, nasal polyps, or sinusitis.	Same as nicotine patch. Use caution with patients who have asthma, wheezing, or other pulmonary disease.	1–2 doses per hour (5/hour and 40/day maximum). 3–6 months.	Prescription	Dizziness, headache, irritation in nose and throat, watering eyes, sneezing, and cough.	
Lozenge	Allergy to nicotine or to aspartame. Gastric and duodenal ulcers.	Same as nicotine patch.	Available in 2-mg and 4-mg doses. Not to exceed 20 lozenges per day.	Prescription	Heartburn, indigestion, nausea, hiccups, coughing, heartburn, headache, and flatulence.	Patients must suck (not chew) lozenge and move around mouth. Avoid excessive swallowing. Avoid biting or swallowing lozenge.

(continues)

TABLE 26-4

CONTINUED

Medication	Contraindications	Precautions	Dosage/Use	Availability	Adverse Reactions	Comments
Sublingual Tablet	Gastric and duodenal ulcers.	Same as nicotine patch.	Available in 2-mg and 4-mg doses. Not to exceed 60 mg/day.	Prescription	Heartburn, indigestion, Dizziness, headache, nausea, hiccups, sore mouth or throat, dry mouth, burning sensation in the mouth, rhinitis, palpitations.	Placed under tongue, dissolves in 30 minutes.

standing because of its comprehensive content and its inter-active workbook format. The practical exercises take smokers through a structured process that enables them to understand the realities of addiction and the different phases of quitting to help them make the changes in their lives that are necessary to quit for good.

No-Nag, No-Guilt: Do-It-Your-Own Way Guide to Quitting Smoking (Tom Ferguson, Random House, Inc., 1998). Dr. Ferguson is an experienced medical writer who avoids antismoking rhetoric. Instead, he offers a reasonable, practical program for smokers who want to quit.

American Cancer Society's "Fresh Start." This is a 21-day gradual smoking-reduction program that is helpful for smokers who wish to quit without using NRT. This book addresses coping with cigarette cravings, withdrawal symptoms, and the benefits of quitting smoking.

Quit Smoking for Good: A Supportive Program for Permanent Smoking Cessation (Andrea Baer, Crossing Press, 1998). This book focuses on making emotional and behavioral changes needed to prepare for permanent smoke-free living.

American Lung Association 7 Steps to a Smoke-Free Life (Edwin Fisher, Jr. and C. Everett Koop, John Wiley & Sons, 1998). Based on the American Lung Association's "Freedom from Smoking" program, this book helps smokers identify smoking triggers and develop coping strategies. Contains worksheets, checklists, and quick quit tips.

The Complete Idiot's Guide to Quitting Smoking (Lowell Kleinman, Deborah Messina-Kleinman, and Mitchell Nides, Macmillan Publishing, 2000). A solid, comprehensive guide to smoking cessation and pharmacotherapy.

When It Hurts Too Much to Quit: Smoking and Depression (Gerald Mayer, Desert City Press, 1997). This book presents information about the special challenges facing smokers who are trying to quit while experiencing clinical depression. It addresses the relationship between smoking and depression, the basics of brain chemistry, the essentials of effective treatment, and making choices about getting help.

Relapse Prevention

Out of the Ashes: Help for People Who Have Stopped Smoking (Peter Holmes & Peggy Holmes, Fairview Press, 1992). This book offers ex-smokers new ways to cope with the challenges of remaining smoke-free.

Web Sites

Many patients are familiar with computers and may have access at home or work to the Internet. This form of support can

TABLE 26-5

EFFICACY AND ESTIMATED ABSTINENCE RATES FOR INTERVENTION TYPES AND INTENSITIES

Level of Contact	Number of Studies	Estimated odds ratio (range)	Average abstinence rates
No intervention	39	1.0	10.9
Physician advice (3 minutes)	10	1.3 (1.1–1.6)	13.4
Self-help	93	1.2 (1.1–1.4)	12.3
Telephone counseling	26	1.2 (1.1–1.4)	13.1
Group counseling	52	1.3 (1.1–1.6)	13.9
Individual counseling	67	1.7 (1.4–2.0)	16.8

Adapted from Fiore MC, Bailey WC, Cohen SJ, et al. *Treating tobacco use and dependence. Clinical practice guideline.* Rockville, MD: US Department of Health and Human Services, Public Health Service; June 2000, with permission.

TABLE 26-6

PROBLEM SOLVING

Problem/Concern	Possible Solution
Strong, continued withdrawal symptoms or cravings.	NRT and/or Bupropion.
Depressive symptoms, negative mood	Provide counseling. Consider Bupropion. Refer to specialist.
Weight gain	Emphasize healthy diet (no strict dieting). Suggest increasing physical activity
Lack of support for quitting	Schedule follow-up visit. Identify social supports. Refer to organizations or groups for support.
Low motivation	Emphasize benefits of quitting. Elicit reasons for quitting from the patient

be particularly helpful to smokers who are having difficulty. They can access help and support on a 24-hour basis. The following is a list of smoking cessation support sites with a brief review of their contents. All site addresses (in bold) begin with http://www. except for the Nicotine Anonymous site.

QuitNet.com

The QuitNet Web site was developed in the 1990s by Dr. Nathan Cobb at Boston University School of Public Health. Today, QuitNet is an independent business with over 100,000 subscribers worldwide. QuitNet is a Web-based implementation of the surgeon general's guidelines of the best clinical practices for quitting smoking: (a) highly tailored individualized information; (b) diagnostic and quitting planning tools that lead to setting a quit date; (c) heavy doses of support that are delivered 24/7 through "buddies," chat rooms, and e-mail; (d) counseling delivered online; and (e) FDA-approved smoking cessation therapies. One of the key—and unique—features of QuitNet is its ability to provide extensive social support. It has a highly active online community of users. At any given moment, night or day, there are hundreds of people logged onto QuitNet, many of whom send and receive messages from one another cheering and encouraging each another on as they go through the stages of their quit. About 2,000 messages are posted in QuitNet public support forums every day. Thousands more are exchanged, privately, between buddies. And because QuitNet is available 24/7, it provides immediate access to other people who have been or are currently going through the same emotional, physical, and psychological challenges.

Quitsmoking.about.com

This site is part of the "About.com" network of health-related Web sites. The site contains a lot of information about smoking cessation methods, the "Ash Kickers" discussion forum, and links to many other resources.

Lungusa.org

The American Lung Association Web site featuring "Freedom From Smoking" and "7 Steps to a Smoke-Free Life" programs. This site offers help in both English and Spanish.

Nicorette.com

This GlaxoSmithKline Web site features Nicorette gum and the "Committed Quitters" program—a sound self-help cessation program for NRT gum users. Available in both English and Spanish.

Smokehelp.org

The "Smokers Helpline" Web site has general information about quitting smoking, the dangers of tobacco use, and so on. Caution: this site states that quitting cold turkey is the "best way" for most people to quit and discourages NRT use.

Cancer.org

This, the American Cancer Society Web site, is difficult to navigate and has only generalized informational pages about smoking-related issues, without providing much hands-on help. For example, clicking on their "Fresh Start" program brings up a single page telling you that "Fresh Start" is a program to help people quit smoking—with no content about the program, information, or links to any actual program.

http://nicotine-anonymous.org

The Nicotine Anonymous Web site has contacts for local chapters and instructions on setting up a Nicotine Anonymous (NA) group. NA follows a traditional 12-step model of addiction recovery. Caution: this site states that "Nicotine Anonymous accepts that nicotine is a toxic, addictive substance that endangers our quality of life," but goes on to say: "We neither endorse nor oppose such devices as nicotine gum or patches." This resource might be helpful to smokers who need group support, but the apparent bias against NRT and confusion between tobacco versus nicotine as toxic substances warrants caution.

SUMMARY AND CONCLUSIONS

Because 75% of all smokers will visit a physician at least once each year (1), smoking cessation interventions delivered in medical settings can reach a wide range of smokers who otherwise might not present for treatment (21). Medical settings can also provide a unique, teachable moment in which to influence patients' perception of risk from smoking-related illness and to enhance their motivation to quit (67,68).

Tobacco use is unique in that it constitutes a highly significant public health threat, for which clinicians tend not to intervene consistently, despite the presence of effective treatments. Specialists are even less likely to provide smoking counseling than primary care physicians (24,32). This is particularly unfortunate because smokers are more likely to quit when counseling is provided within the context of a sick visit (31). The reluctance of many physicians to provide counseling can be traced to many factors, including lack of counseling skills, inadequate training, time pressures (e.g., patients per hour), and absent organizational support. Large, multilayered hospital systems, third-party insurers, and administrative structures often create barriers to physicians trying to provide preventive health counseling. Physicians should not bear the entire blame for this unfortunate deficit in proactive preventive health intervention. However, physicians can and should always strive to address smoking with their patients with the same vigor with which they address hypertension. The guidelines for physician intervention presented in this chapter reflect recommendations for clinician intervention produced by the AHRQ and U.S. Public Health Service (29). These recommendations should become the standard of care for the millennium and be embraced by physicians, midlevel providers, and health care systems as they strive together to free their patients once and for all from the addiction to nicotine and the morbidity and mortality that inevitably surround tobacco use.

References

1. US Department of Health and Human Services. Cigarette smoking among adults—United States 1994. *MMWR* 1996;45:588–590.
2. USDHHS. Reducing tobacco use: A report of the surgeon general—executive summary. Atlanta, GA: U.S. Department of Health and Human Services, Centers for Disease Control and Prevention, National Center for Chronic Disease Prevention and Health Promotion, Office on Smoking and Health; 2000.
3. Kuper H, Boffetta P, Adami HO. Tobacco use and cancer causation: association by tumor type. *J Intern Med* 2002;170:1042–1043.
4. Vineis P, Alavanja M, Buffler P, et al. Tobacco and cancer: recent epidemiological evidence. *J Natl Cancer Inst* 2004;96(2);99–106.
5. Critchley J, Capewell S. Smoking cessation for the secondary prevention of coronary heart disease. *Cochrane Database Syst Rev* 2004;(1):CD003041.
6. US Department of Health and Human Services. *Health benefits of smoking cessation.* Report of the US Surgeon General. Washington, DC: US GPO DHHS Pub. No. (CDC) 90–8416, 1990.
7. Flaherty KR, Martinez FJ Cigarette smoking in interstitial lung disease: concepts for the internist. *Med Clin North Am* 2004;88(6):1643–1653.
8. CDC. *Smoking-attributable mortality, morbidity, and economic costs (SAMMEC): adult and maternal and child health software.* Atlanta, GA: US Department of Health and Human Services, CDC; 2004.
9. CDC. Annual smoking-attributable mortality, years of potential life lost, and productivity losses—United States, 1997–2001. *MMWR* 2005;54:625–628.
10. CDC. Cigarette smoking among adults–United States, 2003. *MMWR* 2005;54:509–513.
11. Centers for Disease Control and Prevention. Health objectives for the nation. Cigarette smoking among adults—United States, 1997. *MMWR* 1999a;48:993–996.
12. Hoyert DL, Kung HC, Smith BL. Deaths: Preliminary data from 2003. *Natl Vital Stat Rep* 2005;53:1–48.
13. Houston-Miller N, Smith PM, DeBusk RF, et al. Smoking cessation in hospitalized patients: results of a randomized trial. *Arch Intern Med* 1997;157:409–415.
14. Orleans CT, Ockene JK. Routine hospital-based quit-smoking treatment for the post myocardial infarction patient: an idea whose time has come. *J Am Coll Cariol* 1993;22:1703–1705.
15. Rigotti N, Arnsten JH, McKool KM, et al. Efficacy of a smoking cessation program for hospital patients. *Arch Intern Med* 1997;157:2653–2660.
16. Glasgow RE, Stevens VJ, Vogt TM, et al. Changes in smoking associated with hospitalization: quit rates, predictive variables, and intervention implications. *American Journal of Health Promotion* 1991;6:24–29.
17. Rigotti NA, Munafo MR, Murphy MF, et al. Interventions for smoking cessation in hospitalised patients. *Cochrane Database Syst Rev* 2001;(1):CD001837.
18. Rigotti N, McKool KM, Shiffman S. Predictors of smoking cessation after coronary artery bypass graft surgery. *Ann Intern Med* 1994;120:287–293.
19. Stevens VJ, O'Malley MS, Villagra VG, et al. A smoking cessation intervention for hospital patients. *Med Care* 1993;31:65–72.
20. Perkins K. Maintaining smoking abstinence after myocardial infarction. *J Subst Abuse* 1988;1:91–107.
21. Goldstein MG, Niaura R, Willey-Lessne C, et al. Physicians counseling smokers: a population-based survey of patient's perceptions of health care provider delivered smoking cessation interventions. *Arch Intern Med* 1997;157:1313–1319.
22. Lancaster T, Stead L. Physician advice for smoking cessation. *Cochrane Database Syst Rev* 2004;(Oct 18(4):CD000165.
23. Goldstein MG, Niaura R, Willey C, et al. An academic detailing intervention to disseminate physician-delivered smoking cessation counseling: smoking cessation outcomes of the Physicians Counseling Smokers Project. *Prev Med* 2003;36:185–196.
24. Thorndike AN, Rigotti NA, Stafford RS, et al. National patterns in the treatment of smokers by physicians. *JAMA* 1998;279:604–608.
25. Cohen SJ, Katz BP, Drook CA, et al. Encouraging primary care physicians to help smokers quit. A randomized controlled trial. *Ann Intern Med* 1989;61:822–830.
26. Cummings SR, Stein MJ, Hansen B, et al. Smoking counseling and preventive medicine. A survey of internists in private practices and health maintenance organizations. *Arch Intern Med* 1989;149:345–349.
27. Lewis CE, Clancy C, Leake B, et al. The counseling practices of internists. *Ann Intern Med* 1991;114:54–58.
28. Strecher VJ, O'Malley MS, Villagra VG, et al. Can residents be trained to counsel patients about quitting smoking? Results from a randomized trial. *J Gen Intern Med* 1991;6:9–17.
29. Fiore MC, Bailey WC, Cohen SJ, et al. *Treating tobacco use and dependence. Clinical practice guideline.* Rockville, MD: US Department of Health and Human Services, Public Health Service; June 2000.
30. Ockene JK, Kristeller J, Pbert L, et al. The physician-delivered smoking intervention projects: can short-term interventions produce long-term effects for a general outpatient population? *Health Psychol* 1994;13:278–281.
31. Daughton D, Susman J, Sitorius M, et al. Transdermal nicotine therapy and primary care: importance of counseling demographic and participant selection factors on 1-year quit rates. *Arch Fam Med* 1998;7:425–430.
32. Jaen CR, Stange KC, Tumiel LM, et al. Missed opportunities for prevention: smoking cessation counseling and the competing demands of practice. *J Fam Pract* 1997;45:348–354.
33. Prochaska JO, DiClemente CC. Stages and processes of self-change of smoking: toward an integrative model of change. *J Consult Clin Psychol* 1983;51:390–395.
34. Sciamanna CN, Hoch JS, Duke GC, et al. Comparison of five measures of motivation to quit smoking among a sample of hospitalized smokers. *J Gen Intern Med* 2000;15:16–23.
35. Leischow S, Muramoto ML, Cook G, et al. OTC nicotine patches: effectiveness alone and with brief physician intervention. *Am J Health Beh* 1999;23:61–69.
36. Miller W, Rollnick S. *Motivational interviewing: preparing people to change addictive behavior.* New York: Guilford; 1991.
37. Heatherton TF, Kozlowski LT, Frecker RC, et al. The Fagerstrom test for nicotine dependence: a revision of the Fagerstrom Tolerance Questionnaire. *Br J Addict* 1991;86:1119–1127.
38. Rundmo T, Smedslund G, Gotestam KG. Motivation for smoking cessation among the Norwegian public. *Addict Behav* 1997;22:377–386.
39. Colby SM, Barnett NP, Monti PM, et al. Brief motivational interviewing in a hospital setting for adolescent smoking: a preliminary study. *J Consult Clin Psychol* 1998;66:574–578.
40. Prochaska JO, Goldstein MG. Process of smoking cessation. Implications for clinicians. *Clin Chest Med* 1991;12:727–735.
41. Brandon TH, Tiffany ST, Obremski K, et al. Postcessation cigarette use: the process of relapse. *Addict Behav* 1990;15:105–114.
42. Hajek P, Stead LF, West R, et al. Relapse prevention interventions for smoking cessation. *Cochrane Database Syst Rev* 2005;25(1):CD003999
44. Henningfield JE, Fant RV, Buchhalter AR, et al. Pharmacotherapy for nicotine dependence. *CA Cancer J Clin* 2005;55:281–299.
43. American Psychiatric Association. Practice guideline for the treatment of patients with nicotine dependence. *Am J Psychiatry* 1996;153(10 suppl):1–31.
45. Scharf D, Shiffman S. Are there gender differences in smoking cessation, with and without bupropion? Pooled- and meta-analyses of clinical trials of Bupropion SR. *Addiction* 2004;99:1462–1469.
46. Fagerstrom KO, Schneider NG, Lunell E. Effectiveness of nicotine patch and nicotine gum as individual versus combined treatments of tobacco withdrawal symptoms. *Psychopharmacology* 1993;111:271–277.
47. Kornitzer M, Boutsen M, Dramaix M. Combined use of nicotine patch and gum in smoking cessation: a placebo-controlled clinical trial. *Prev Med* 1995;24:41–47.
48. Puska P, Korhonen HJ, Vartiainen EL, et al. Combined use of nicotine patch and gum compared with gum alone in smoking cessation—a clinical trial in North Karelia. *Tob Control* 1995;4:231–235.
49. Blondal T, Gudmundsson LJ, Olafsdottir I, et al. Nicotine nasal spray with nicotine patch for smoking cessation: randomised trial with six year follow up. *BMJ* 1999;318:285–289.
50. Hall SM, Reus VI, Munoz RF, et al. Nortriptyline and cognitive-behavioral therapy in the treatment of cigarette smoking. *Arch Gen Psychiatry* 1998;55:683–690.
51. Hughes J, Goldstein MG. Recent advances in the pharmacotherapy of smoking. *JAMA* 1999;281:72–76.
52. Wei H, Young D. Effect of clonidine on cigarette cessation and in the alleviation of withdrawal symptoms. *British Journal of Addiction* 1988;83:1221–1226.
53. Sachs DPL, Sawe U, Leischow SJ. Effectiveness of a 16-hour transdermal nicotine patch in a medical practice setting, without intensive group counseling. *Arch Intern Med* 1993;153:1881–1890.
54. Benowitz NL, Gourlay SG. Cardiovascular toxicity of nicotine: implications for nicotine replacement therapy. *J Am Coll Cardiol* 1997;29(7):1422–1431.
55. Benowitz NL. Pharmacologic aspects of cigarette smoking and nicotine addiction. *N Engl J Med* 1984;319:1318–1330.
56. Benowitz NL, Fitzgerald GA, Wilson M, et al. Nicotine effects on eicosanoid formation and hemostatic function: comparison of transdermal nicotine and cigarette smoking. *J Am Coll Cardiol* 1993;22:1159–1167.
57. Transdermal Nicotine Study Group. Transdermal nicotine for smoking cessation: six months results from two multi-center controlled clinical trials. *JAMA* 1991;266:3133–3138.
58. Joseph AM, Westman EC. Transdermal nicotine therapy for older medically ill patients: a pilot study. *J Gen Intern Med* 1995;10(Suppl):101.

59. McRobbie H, Hajek P. Nicotine replacement therapy in patients with cardiovascular disease: guidelines for health professionals. *Addiction* 2001;96: 1547–1551.

60. Ford CL, Zlabek JA. Nicotine replacement therapy and cardiovascular disease. *Mayo Clin Proc* 2005;80(5):652–656.

61. Warner JG Jr., Little WC. Myocardial infarction in a patient who smoked while wearing a nicotine patch. *Ann Intern Med* 1994;120:695.

62. Jackson M. Cerebral arterial narrowing with nicotine patch. *Lancet* 1993; 342:236–237.

63. Arnaot MR. Treating heart disease: nicotine patches may not be safe. *BMJ* 1995;310:663–664.

64. Benowitz NL, Gourlay SG. Cardiovascular toxicity of nicotine: implications for nicotine replacement therapy. *J Am Coll Cardiol* 1997;29:1422–1431.

65. Joseph AM, Norman SM, Ferry LH, et al. The safety of transdermal nicotine as an aid to smoking cessation in patients with cardiac disease. *N Engl J Med* 1996;335:1792–1798.

66. Mahmarian JJ, Moye LA, Nasser GA, et al. Nicotine patch therapy in smoking cessation reduces the extent of exercise-induced myocardial ischemia. *J Am Coll Cardiol* 1997;30:125–130.

67. Emmons K, Goldstein MG. Smokers who are hospitalized: a window of opportunity for cessation interventions. *Prev Med* 1992;21:262–269.

68. Bock BC, Becker B, Partridge R, et al. Physician intervention and patient attitudes among smokers with acute respiratory illness in the emergency department. *Prev Med* 2001;32:175–181.

CHAPTER 27 ■ SECONDARY PREVENTION OVERVIEW

SIDNEY C. SMITH, JR.

Secondary prevention therapies form an essential component of the treatment strategies for all patients with atherosclerotic vascular disease. Their benefits in reducing combined cardiovascular events have been shown to extend to all age groups and are observed for both men and women. Because their effects are additive, it is important to integrate the critical pathways discussed in the preceding sections on hyperlipidemia, diabetes and metabolic syndrome, hypertension, chronic kidney disease, and smoking cessation into an overall management plan for the patient. In many instances this is best done by coordinating the pathways in the various subspecialty clinics through a comprehensive cardiac rehabilitation program. For example, routine laboratory values can be obtained in association with visits for cardiac rehabilitation and sent to the appropriate subspecialty clinic for review with the patient by the health care provider. The results are then used for therapeutic recommendations arising from that clinic visit based on the appropriate clinical pathway.

The American Heart Association/American College of Cardiology (AHA/ACC) Guidelines for Secondary Prevention for Patients with Coronary and Other Atherosclerotic Vascular Disease (1) provides a valuable resource on which to develop critical pathways. The AHA "Get With the Guidelines" program uses performance measures developed from this guideline statement as a foundation for its outcomes measures. The statement provides a level of evidence for each classification of recommendation for a given secondary prevention therapy in an easily accessible table summary (Table 27-1). In the 2006 update (1), the recommendations from major practice guidelines from the ACC/AHA and the National Institutes of Health (2–24) were combined with new evidence from research studies (25–38) to develop a comprehensive integrated set of recommendations regarding secondary prevention guidelines for patients with coronary and other atherosclerotic vascular disease (ASVD).

The management of dyslipidemia remains a central focus for secondary prevention therapy. The current guidelines (1) (Table 27-1) recommend that low-density lipoprotein cholesterol (LDL-C) should be <100 mg/dL for all patients with ASVD including coronary heart disease (CHD). They further state that it is reasonable to treat to a target LDL-C of <70 mg/dL in these patients. The evidence is especially compelling for a lower target LDL-C among patients with recent acute coronary syndromes.

Antiplatelet therapy is a second major focus for secondary prevention therapy among patients with CHD and ASVD. The use of clopidogrel therapy has been proven to improve outcomes for patients with acute coronary syndromes and after stent implantation. The minimal duration of clopidogrel therapy varies from 1 month for those receiving bare metal stents, to 3 months for those with sirolimus-eluting stents, and 6 months for those receiving paclitaxel-eluting stents. The recommended dose of aspirin for chronic therapy of patients with CHD or other ASVD is 75 to 162 mg/d taken indefinitely.

This lower dosage has been recommended because of higher bleeding complications at higher doses without further benefit of reduction of cardiovascular events.

Considerable benefit has been demonstrated after treatment with medications that inhibit the renin-angiotensin-aldosterone system (RAAS) in patients with impaired left ventricular (LV) systolic function (LV ejection fraction ≤40%), and the use of these therapies received strong support in the 2006 update (1). For those with normal LV function, all should be considered for angiotensin-converting enzyme (ACE) inhibitor therapy; however, among those at lower risk with CHD with normal LV ejection fraction in whom other risk factors have been controlled and revascularization has been performed, the use of ACE inhibitors may be considered optional.

Behavioral modification remains a cornerstone of secondary prevention. Strategies to assist with smoking cessation, improve dietary habits and nutritional status, and increase physical activity should be a part of critical pathways for secondary prevention in the outpatient setting. The recommendation for physical activity is now 30 minutes on 7 days a week with a minimum of 5 days per week. Management of excess weight is important, and it is recommended that body mass index and/or waist circumference should be assessed on each clinic visit, with a waist circumference goal of <40 inches in men and <35 inches in women. Similarly, smoking status should be assessed on each visit with referral to special programs and use of pharmacotherapy for those unable to stop smoking.

Critical pathways for patients with chronic disorders of the cardiovascular system must consider the increased risk of complications from influenza. For this reason the 2006 update (1) recommends that all individuals with chronic disorders of the cardiovascular system receive vaccination with inactivated influenza vaccine. This is an important example of how critical pathways for patients with cardiovascular disease must anticipate and include therapies beyond those directed solely at the cardiovascular system.

It is important that critical pathways and other systems be implemented to ensure the broad use of secondary prevention therapies among patients with cardiovascular disease. Although the initiation of these therapies should occur prior to hospital discharge in most situations, their continuation and appropriate modification is a major responsibility of the health care providers seeing the patient in the outpatient setting. Unfortunately there still remain disparities in treatment received by various sociodemographic groups, especially the elderly where the risk from complications of cardiovascular disease is the highest and the benefit of secondary therapies is the greatest (39). The comprehensive application of critical pathways employing the current strategies for secondary prevention among all patients with cardiovascular disease holds tremendous potential to reverse these disparities and broadly improve cardiovascular outcomes.

TABLE 27-1

AHA/ACC SECONDARY PREVENTION FOR PATIENTS WITH CORONARY AND OTHER VASCULAR DISEASE*: 2006 UPDATE (1)

Intervention Recommendations with Class of Recommendation and Level of Evidence

SMOKING:

Goal

Complete cessation. No exposure to environmental tobacco smoke.
- Ask about tobacco use status at every visit. **I (B)**
- Advise every tobacco user to quit. **I (B)**
- Assess the tobacco user's willingness to quit. **I (B)**
- Assist by counseling and developing a plan for quitting. **I (B)**
- Arrange follow-up, referral to special programs, or pharmacotherapy (including nicotine replacement and bupropion). **I (B)**
- Urge avoidance of exposure to environmental tobacco smoke at work and home. **I (B)**

BLOOD PRESSURE CONTROL:

Goal

<140/90 mm Hg
or
<130/80 mm Hg if patient has diabetes or chronic kidney disease

For all patients:

- Initiate or maintain lifestyle modification—weight control; increased physical activity; alcohol moderation; sodium reduction; and emphasis on increased consumption of fresh fruits, vegetables, and low-fat dairy products. **I (B)**

For patients with blood pressure ≥140/90 mm Hg (or ≥130/80 mm Hg for individuals with chronic kidney disease or diabetes):

- As tolerated, add blood pressure medication, treating initially with β-blockers and/or ACE inhibitors, with addition of other drugs such as thiazides as needed to achieve goal blood pressure. **I (A)**

[For compelling indications for individual drug classes in specific vascular diseases, see Seventh Report of the Joint National Committee on Prevention, Detection, Evaluation, and Treatment of High Blood Pressure (JNC 7)] (4).

LIPID MANAGEMENT:

Goal

LDL-C <100 mg/dL

If triglycerides are ≥200 mg/dL, non-HDL-C should be <130 mg/dL†

For all patients:

- Start dietary therapy. Reduce intake of saturated fats (to <7% of total calories), *trans*-fatty acids, and cholesterol (to <200 mg/d). **I (B)**
- Adding plant stanol/sterols (2 g/d) and viscous fiber (>10 g/d) will further lower LDL-C.
- Promote daily physical activity and weight management. **I (B)**
- Encourage increased consumption of omega-3 fatty acids in the form of fish‡ or in capsule form (1 g/d) for risk reduction. For treatment of elevated triglycerides, higher doses are usually necessary for risk reduction. **IIb (B)**

(continued)

TABLE 27-1

CONTINUED

For lipid management:

Assess fasting lipid profile in all patients and within 24 hours of hospitalization for those with an acute cardiovascular or coronary event. For hospitalized patients, initiate lipid-lowering medication as recommended below before discharge according to the following schedule:

- LDL-C should be <100 mg/dL **I (A), and**
- Further reduction of LDL-C to <70 mg/dL is reasonable. **IIa (A)**
- If baseline LDL-C is ≥100 mg/dL, initiate LDL-lowering drug therapy.[§] **I (A)**
- If on-treatment LDL-C is ≥100 mg/dL, intensify LDL-lowering drug therapy (may require LDL-lowering drug combination[‖]). **I (A)**
- If baseline LDL-C is 70 to 100 mg/dL, it is reasonable to treat to LDL-C <70 mg/dL. **IIa (B)**
- If triglycerides are 200 to 499 mg/dL, non-HDL-C should be <130 mg/dL. **I (B), and**
- Further reduction of non-HDL-C to <100 mg/dL is reasonable. **IIa (B)**
- Therapeutic options to reduce non-HDL-C are:
  ⇒ More intense LDL-C–lowering therapy **I (B)**, or
  ⇒ Niacin[¶] (after LDL-C–lowering therapy) **IIa (B)**, or
  ⇒ Fibrate therapy[#] (after LDL-C–lowering therapy) **IIa (B)**
- If triglycerides are ≥500 mg/dL[#], therapeutic options to prevent pancreatitis are fibrate[¶] or niacin before LDL-lowering therapy; and treat LDL-C to goal after triglyceride-lowering therapy. Achieve non-HDL-C <130 mg/dL if possible. **I (C)**

PHYSICAL ACTIVITY:

Goal

30 minutes, 7 days per week (minimum 5 days per week)
- For all patients, assess risk with a physical activity history and/or an exercise test, to guide prescription. **I (B)**
- For all patients, encourage 30 to 60 minutes of moderate-intensity aerobic activity, such as brisk walking, on most, preferably all, days of the week, supplemented by an increase in daily lifestyle activities (e.g., walking breaks at work, gardening, household work). **I (B)**
- Encourage resistance training 2 days per week. **IIb (C)**
- Advise medically supervised programs for high-risk patients (e.g., recent acute coronary syndrome or revascularization, heart failure). **I (B)**

WEIGHT MANAGEMENT:

Goal

Body mass index: 18.5 to 24.9 kg/m^2

Waist circumference: men <40 inches, women <35 inches
- Assess body mass index and/or waist circumference on each visit and consistently encourage weight maintenance/reduction through an appropriate balance of physical activity, caloric intake, and formal behavioral programs when indicated to maintain/achieve a body mass index between 18.5 and 24.9 kg/m^2. **I (B)**
- If waist circumference (measured horizontally at the iliac crest) is ≥35 inches in women and ≥40 inches in men, initiate lifestyle changes and consider treatment strategies for metabolic syndrome as indicated. **I (B)**
- The initial goal of weight loss therapy should be to reduce body weight by approximately 10% from baseline.

With success, further weight loss can be attempted if indicated through further assessment. **I (B)**

DIABETES MANAGEMENT:

Goal

HbA$_{1c}$ <7%
- Initiate lifestyle and pharmacotherapy to achieve near-normal HbA$_{1c}$. **I (B)**
- Begin vigorous modification of other risk factors (e.g., physical activity, weight management, blood pressure control, and cholesterol management as recommended above). **I (B)**
- Coordinate diabetic care with patient's primary care physician or endocrinologist. **I (C)**

(continued)

TABLE 27-1

CONTINUED

ANTIPLATELET AGENTS/ANTICOAGULANTS:

- Start aspirin 75 to 162 mg/d and continue indefinitely in all patients unless contraindicated. I (A)
  ⇒ For patients undergoing coronary artery bypass grafting, aspirin should be started within 48 hours after surgery to reduce saphenous vein graft closure. Dosing regimens ranging from 100 to 325 mg/d appear to be efficacious. Doses higher than 162 mg/d can be continued for up to 1 year. I (B)
- Start and continue clopidogrel 75 mg/d in combination with aspirin for up to 12 months in patients after acute coronary syndrome or percutaneous coronary intervention with stent placement (≥1 month for bare metal stent, ≥3 months for sirolimus-eluting stent, and ≥6 months for paclitaxel-eluting stent). I (B)
  ⇒ Patients who have undergone percutaneous coronary intervention with stent placement should initially receive higher-dose aspirin at 325 mg/d for 1 month for bare metal stent, 3 months for sirolimus-eluting stent, and 6 months for paclitaxel-eluting stent. I (B)
- Manage warfarin to international normalized ratio = 2.0 to 3.0 for paroxysmal or chronic atrial fibrillation or flutter, and in post-myocardial infarction patients when clinically indicated (e.g., atrial fibrillation, left ventricular thrombus). I (A)
- Use of warfarin in conjunction with aspirin and/or clopidogrel is associated with increased risk of bleeding and should be monitored closely. I (B)

RENIN-ANGIOTENSIN-ALDOSTERONE SYSTEM BLOCKERS:

ACE inhibitors:

- Start and continue indefinitely in all patients with left ventricular ejection fraction ≤40% and in those with hypertension, diabetes, or chronic kidney disease, unless contraindicated. I (A)
- Consider for all other patients. I (B)
- Among lower-risk patients with normal left ventricular ejection fraction in whom cardiovascular risk factors are well controlled and revascularization has been performed, use of ACE inhibitors may be considered optional. IIa (B)

Angiotensin receptor blockers:

- Use in patients who are intolerant of ACE inhibitors and have heart failure or have had a myocardial infarction with left ventricular ejection fraction ≤40%. I (A)
- Consider in other patients who are ACE inhibitor intolerant. I (B)
- Consider use in combination with ACE inhibitors in systolic-dysfunction heart failure. IIb (B)

Aldosterone blockade:

- Use in post-myocardial infarction patients, without significant renal dysfunction** or hyperkalemia††, who are already receiving therapeutic doses of an ACE inhibitor and β-blocker, have a left ventricular ejection fraction ≤40%, and have either diabetes or heart failure. I (A)

β-BLOCKERS:

- Start and continue indefinitely in all patients who have had myocardial infarction, acute coronary syndrome, or left ventricular dysfunction with or without heart failure symptoms, unless contraindicated. I (A)

Consider chronic therapy for all other patients with coronary or other vascular disease or diabetes unless contraindicated. IIa (C)

INFLUENZA VACCINATION:

Patients with cardiovascular disease should have an influenza vaccination. I (B)

*Patients covered by these guidelines include those with established coronary and other atherosclerotic vascular disease, including peripheral arterial disease, atherosclerotic aortic disease, and carotid artery disease. Treatment of patients whose only manifestation of cardiovascular risk is diabetes will be the topic of a separate AHA scientific statement. ACE indicates angiotensin-converting enzyme.
†Non-HDL-C = total cholesterol minus HDL-C.
‡Pregnant and lactating women should limit their intake of fish to minimize exposure to methylmercury.
§When LDL-lowering medications are used, obtain at least a 30% to 40% reduction in LDL-C levels. If LDL-C <70 mg/dL is the chosen target, consider drug titration to achieve this level to minimize side effects and cost. When LDL-C <70 mg/dL is not achievable because of high baseline LDL-C levels, it generally is possible to achieve reductions of >50% in LDL-C levels by either statins or LDL-C–lowering drug combinations.
‖Standard dose of statin with ezetimibe, bile acid sequestrant, or niacin.
¶The combination of high-dose statin + fibrate can increase risk for severe myopathy. Statin doses should be kept relatively low with this combination. Dietary supplement niacin must not be used as a substitute for prescription niacin.
#Patients with very high triglycerides should not consume alcohol. The use of bile acid sequestrant is relatively contraindicated when triglycerides are >200 mg/dL.
**Creatinine should be <2.5 mg/dL in men and <2.0 mg/dL in women.
††Potassium should be <5.0 mEq/L
From Smith SC, Allen J, Blair SN, et al. AHA/ACC guidelines for secondary prevention for patients with coronary and other atherosclerotic vascular disease: 2006 update. *Circulation* 2006;113:2364–2365.

References

1. Smith SC, Allen J, Blair SN, et al. AHA/ACC guidelines for secondary prevention for patients with coronary and other atherosclerotic vascular disease: 2006 update. *Circulation* 2006;113:2363–2372.

2. Mosca L, Appel LJ, Benjamin EJ, et al. Evidence-based guidelines for cardiovascular disease prevention in women. *Circulation* 2004;109:672–693.

3. US Department of Health and Human Services. *The health consequences of smoking: a report of the Surgeon General.* Washington: US Department of Health and Human Services, Centers for Disease Control and Prevention, National Center for Chronic Disease Prevention and Health Promotion, Office on Smoking and Health; May 27, 2004. Available at: http://www.surgeongeneral.gov/library/smokingconsequences. Accessed March 15, 2006.

4. Chobanian AV, Bakris GL, Black HR, et al. Seventh report of the Joint National Committee on Prevention, Detection, Evaluation, and Treatment of High Blood Pressure. *Hypertension* 2003;42:1206–1252.

5. Expert Panel on Detection, Evaluation, and Treatment of High Blood Cholesterol in Adults. Executive Summary of the Third Report of The National Cholesterol Education Program (NCEP) Expert Panel on Detection, Evaluation, and Treatment of High Blood Cholesterol in Adults (Adult Treatment Panel III). *JAMA* 2001;285:2486–2497.

6. Grundy SM, Cleeman JI, Merz CN, et al. Implications of recent clinical trials for the National Cholesterol Education Program Adult Treatment Panel III guidelines [published correction appears in *Circulation* 2004;110:763]. *Circulation* 2004;110:227–239.

7. Kris-Etherton PM, Harris WS, Appel LJ, et al. Fish consumption, fish oil, omega-3 fatty acids, and cardiovascular disease [published correction appears in *Circulation* 2003;107:512]. *Circulation* 2002;106:2747–2757.

8. Thompson PD, Buchner D, Pina IL, et al. Exercise and physical activity in the prevention and treatment of atherosclerotic cardiovascular disease: a statement from the Council on Clinical Cardiology (Subcommittee on Exercise, Rehabilitation, and Prevention) and the Council on Nutrition, Physical Activity, and Metabolism (Subcommittee on Physical Activity). *Circulation* 2003;107:3109–3116.

9. UK Department of Health. *At least five a week: evidence on the impact of physical activity and its relationship to health: a report from the chief medical officer.* London, England: Wellington House; April 29, 2004. Available at: http://www.dh.gov.uk/assetRoot/04/08/09/81/04080981.pdf. Accessed March 15, 2006.

10. Pate RR, Pratt M, Blair SN, et al. Physical activity and public health: a recommendation from the Centers for Disease Control and Prevention and the American College of Sports Medicine. *JAMA* 1995;273:402–407.

11. US Department of Health and Human Services. *Physical activity and health: a report of the Surgeon General.* Atlanta, GA: US Department of Health and Human Services, Centers for Disease Control and Prevention, National Center for Chronic Disease Prevention and Health Promotion; 1996. Available at: http://www.cdc.gov/nccdphp/sgr/summary.htm. Accessed March 15, 2006.

12. National Institutes of Health; National Heart, Lung, and Blood Institute. Clinical guidelines on the identification, evaluation, and treatment of overweight and obesity in adults: the evidence report. National Institutes of Health; National Heart, Lung, and Blood Institute; September 1998. Publication No. 98-4083. Available at: http://www.nhlbi.nih.gov/guidelines/obesity/ob_gdlns.pdf. Accessed March 15, 2006.

13. Klein S, Burke LE, Bray GA, et al. Clinical implications of obesity with specific focus on cardiovascular disease: a statement for professionals from the American Heart Association Council on Nutrition, Physical Activity, and Metabolism: endorsed by the American College of Cardiology Foundation. *Circulation* 2004;110:2952–2967.

14. Grundy SM, Cleeman JI, Daniels SR, et al. Diagnosis and management of the metabolic syndrome: an American Heart Association/National Heart, Lung, and Blood Institute Scientific Statement [published correction appears in *Circulation* 2005;112:e297; *Circulation* 2005;112:e298]. *Circulation* 2005;112:2735–2752.

15. American Diabetes Association. Standards of medical care in diabetes. *Diabetes Care* 2004;27(suppl 1):S15–S35.

16. Antman EM, Anbe DT, Armstrong PW, et al. ACC/AHA guidelines for the management of patients with ST-elevation myocardial infarction: a report of the American College of Cardiology/American Heart Association Task Force on Practice Guidelines (Committee to Revise the 1999 Guidelines for the Management of Patients with Acute Myocardial Infarction) [published correction appears in *Circulation* 2005;111:2013–2014]. *Circulation* 2004;110:e82–e292.

17. Gibbons RJ, Abrams J, Chatterjee K, et al. ACC/AHA 2002 guideline update for the management of patients with chronic stable angina—summary article: a report of the American College of Cardiology/American Heart Association Task Force on Practice Guidelines (Committee on the Management of Patients With Chronic Stable Angina). *Circulation* 2003;107:149–158.

18. Smith SC Jr, Feldman TE, Hirshfeld JW Jr, et al. ACC/AHA/SCAI 2005 guideline update for percutaneous coronary intervention: a report of the American College of Cardiology/American Heart Association Task Force on Practice Guidelines (ACC/AHA/SCAI Writing Committee to Update the 2001 Guidelines for Percutaneous Coronary Intervention). *Circulation* 2006;113:e166–e286. Available at: http://circ.ahajournals.org/cgi/reprint/113/7/e166. Accessed March 15, 2006.

19. Eagle KA, Guyton RA, Davidoff R, et al. ACC/AHA 2004 guideline update for coronary artery bypass graft surgery: a report of the American College of Cardiology/American Heart Association Task Force on Practice Guidelines (Committee to Update the 1999 Guidelines for Coronary Artery Bypass Graft Surgery) [published correction appears in *Circulation* 2005;111:2014]. *Circulation* 2004;110:e340–e437.

20. Ferraris VA, Ferraris SP, Moliterno DJ, et al. The Society of Thoracic Surgeons practice guideline series: aspirin and other antiplatelet agents during operative coronary revascularization (executive summary). *Ann Thorac Surg* 2005;79:1454–1461.

21. Braunwald E, Antman EM, Beasley JW, et al. ACC/AHA 2002 guideline update for the management of patients with unstable angina and non–ST-segment elevation myocardial infarction—summary article: a report of the American College of Cardiology/American Heart Association task force on practice guidelines (Committee on the Management of Patients With Unstable Angina). *J Am Coll Cardiol* 2002;40:1366–1374.

22. Hunt SA, Abraham WT, Chin MH, et al. ACC/AHA 2005 guideline update for the diagnosis and management of chronic heart failure in the adult: a report of the American College of Cardiology/American Heart Association Task Force on Practice Guidelines (Writing Committee to Update the 2001 Guidelines for the Evaluation and Management of Heart Failure): developed in collaboration with the American College of Chest Physicians and the International Society for Heart and Lung Transplantation: endorsed by the Heart Rhythm Society. *Circulation* 2005;112:e154–e235.

23. Coull BM, Williams LS, Goldstein LB, et al. Anticoagulants and antiplatelet agents in acute ischemic stroke: report of the Joint Stroke Guideline Development Committee of the American Academy of Neurology and the American Stroke Association (a division of the American Heart Association). *Stroke* 2002;33:1934–1942.

24. Harper SA, Fukuda K, Uyeki TM, et al. Prevention and control of influenza. Recommendations of the Advisory Committee on Immunization Practices (ACIP) [published correction appears in *MMWR Morb Mortal Wkly Rep* 2005;54(30):750]. *MMWR Recomm Rep* 2005;54(RR-8):1–40.

25. LaRosa JC, Grundy SM, Waters DD, et al. Intensive lipid lowering with atorvastatin in patients with stable coronary disease. *N Engl J Med* 2005;352:1425–1435.

26. Pedersen TR, Faergeman O, Kastelein JJ, et al. High-dose atorvastatin vs usual-dose simvastatin for secondary prevention after myocardial infarction: the IDEAL study: a randomized controlled trial [published correction appears in *JAMA* 2005;294:3092]. *JAMA* 2005;294:2437–2445.

27. Baigent C, Keech A, Kearney PM, et al. Efficacy and safety of cholesterol lowering treatment: prospective meta-analysis of data from 90,056 participants in 14 randomised trials of statins [published correction appears in *Lancet* 2005;366:1358]. *Lancet* 2005;366:1267–1278.

28. Ballantyne CM, Abate N, Yuan Z, et al. Dose comparison study of the combination of ezetimibe and simvastatin (Vytorin) versus atorvastatin in patients with hypercholesterolemia: the Vytorin Versus Atorvastatin (VYVA) study [published correction appears in *Am Heart J* 2005;149:882]. *Am Heart J* 2005;149:464–473.

29. de Lemos JA, Blazing MA, Wiviott SD, et al. Early intensive vs a delayed conservative simvastatin strategy in patients with acute coronary syndromes: phase Z of the A to Z trial. *JAMA* 2004;292:1307–1316.

30. Braunwald E, Domanski MJ, Fowler SE, et al. Angiotensin-converting-enzyme inhibition in stable coronary artery disease. *N Engl J Med* 2004;351:2058–2068.

31. Pfeffer MA, McMurray JJ, Velazquez EJ, et al. Valsartan, captopril, or both in myocardial infarction complicated by heart failure, left ventricular dysfunction, or both [published correction appears in *N Engl J Med* 2004;350:203]. *N Engl J Med* 2003;349:1893–1906.

32. McMurray JJ, Ostergren J, Swedberg K, et al. Effects of candesartan in patients with chronic heart failure and reduced left-ventricular systolic function taking angiotensin-converting enzyme inhibitors: the CHARM-Added trial. *Lancet* 2003;362:767–771.

33. Granger CB, McMurray JJ, Yusuf S, et al. Effects of candesartan in patients with chronic heart failure and reduced left-ventricular systolic function intolerant to angiotensin-converting-enzyme inhibitors: the CHARM-Alternative trial. *Lancet* 2003;362:772–776.

34. Cannon CP, Braunwald E, McCabe CH, et al. Intensive versus moderate lipid lowering with statins after acute coronary syndromes [published correction appears in *N Engl J Med* 2006;354:778]. *N Engl J Med* 2004;350:1495–1504.

35. Heart Protection Study Collaborative Group. MRC/BHF Heart Protection Study of cholesterol lowering with simvastatin in 20,536 high-risk individuals: a randomised placebo-controlled trial. *Lancet* 2002;360:7–22. Summary for patients in: *Curr Cardiol Rep* 2002;4:486–487.

36. Shepherd J, Blauw GJ, Murphy MB, et al. PROspective Study of Pravastatin in the Elderly at Risk. Pravastatin in elderly individuals at risk of vascular disease (PROSPER): a randomised controlled trial. *Lancet* 2002;360:1623–1630.

37. ALLHAT Officers and Coordinators for the ALLHAT Collaborative Re-

search Group. The Antihypertensive and Lipid-Lowering Treatment to Prevent Heart Attack Trial. Major outcomes in moderately hypercholesterolemic, hypertensive patients randomized to pravastatin vs usual care: the Antihypertensive and Lipid-Lowering Treatment to Prevent Heart Attack Trial (ALLHAT-LLT). *JAMA* 2002;288:2998–3007.

38. Sever PS, Dahlof B, Poulter NR, et al. Prevention of coronary and stroke events with atorvastatin in hypertensive patients who have average or lower-than-average cholesterol concentrations, in the Anglo-Scandinavian Cardiac Outcomes Trial–Lipid Lowering Arm (ASCOT-LLA): a multicentre randomised controlled trial. *Lancet* 2003;361:1149–1158.

39. Smith, SC. Evidence based medicine: making the grade: miles to go before we sleep. *Circulation* 2006;113:178–179.

CHAPTER 28 ■ OVERVIEW OF THE AHA "GET WITH THE GUIDELINES" PROGRAMS

YULING HONG AND KENNETH A. LABRESH

BARRIERS TO THE USE OF GUIDELINES
PROGRAM ELEMENTS
MEASURE DEFINITIONS
RECOGNITION
GET WITH THE GUIDELINES RESULTS
CHALLENGES AND OPPORTUNITIES

Despite recent advances in scientific knowledge about and improvement of treatment and prevention (primary and secondary) for heart disease and stroke, these conditions remain the number one and three causes of death in the United States (1). Every year there are nearly 500,000 deaths from coronary heart disease (CHD) and over 160,000 from stroke in the country. An estimated 700,000 Americans have new CHD every year, and an additional 500,000 have recurrent CHD events. The corresponding numbers for stroke are 500,000 and 200,000, respectively. The burden of heart failure in the society is also substantial. Deaths attributable to heart failure as the primary or secondary cause total 265,000 per year. In addition, there are one million annual heart failure discharges from hospitals. The combined annual direct and indirect cost for CHD, stroke, and heart failure exceeds $225 billion (1).

This enormous burden of disease is also associated with numerous data collection efforts in hospitals to assess the quality of care delivered in coronary artery disease (CAD), heart failure, and stroke. These include the Joint Commission for the Accreditation of Healthcare Organizations (JCAHO) ORYX data and the Centers for Medicare and Medicaid Services (CMS) measure sets for acute myocardial infarction and heart failure (2–4), the National Registry of Myocardial Infarction (5), the Global Registry of Acute Coronary Events (GRACE) for acute coronary syndromes (6), The Paul Coverdell National Acute Stroke Registry (7), and the ADHERE® Registry for heart failure (8). Table 28-1 presents data from several of these sources that demonstrate, despite wide dissemination of these guidelines, that recommended interventions are frequently not initiated during hospitalization for acute cardiac events, heart failure, and stroke (4,6–8).

BARRIERS TO THE USE OF GUIDELINES

Barriers to the routine use of evidence-based care fall into three general categories: knowledge, attitudes, and behavior (9) (Table 28-2). Knowledge barriers include absence of knowledge of new or updated guidelines or, if known, insufficient familiarity with the guidelines to be willing or able to use them. For example, one hospital seeking to extend CAD prevention measure use to patients with peripheral vascular disease engaged vascular surgeons to initiate lipid and angiotensin-converting enzyme (ACE) inhibitor therapies prior to hospital discharge. Resistance to the plan was substantial until a medical consultant offered to select and initiate these therapies in appropriate patients. On further discussion the initial unwillingness to participate centered on unfamiliarity with specific agents and doses. Guidelines and evidence may be known but not adhered to because of a lack of belief in the concept of evidence-based medicine or lack of belief that the benefits seen in clinical trials really occur in the "real world." These attitudinal barriers may mask knowledge barriers, as illustrated, or may represent concerns about autonomy and control.

The final category, behavioral factors, relates to patients, guidelines, and the organizational environment. Patient preferences may not be consistent with guideline recommendations. Guidelines from multiple organizations may be contradictory, causing confusion. The most common issues relate to the environment, such as organizational constraints in culture, priorities, resources, and systems. Even if physicians know, believe, and intend to use the guidelines every time, this may not result in higher treatment rates. Davis and colleagues have demonstrated that typical didactic presentations may improve knowledge but do not produce increased use of evidence-based therapies (10). In a chart review of primary care practices, selected as practices that were high prescribers of statins, knowledge of the National Cholesterol Education Program (NCEP) guidelines for lipid treatment and the intention of practitioners to use these guidelines were assessed. Although 95% of the physicians could demonstrate complete and accurate knowledge of the guidelines, and 65% stated that they used the guidelines most or all the time, only 18% of their CAD population had low-density lipoprotein (LDL) cholesterol levels of <100 mg/dL, and this was only in their patients who were on treatment (11).

The use of a team approach can help to address patient factors and support patient self-management after discharge. Environmental issues are usually addressed by changes in the underlying culture and systems of care delivery. W. Edwards Demming has said that most problems are 10% about the people and 90% about the systems (12). Systems always produce exactly the result they were designed to produce (Burwick DM, personal communication). It then follows that "trying harder" with the same system will not change practice. This then explains the dichotomy between physicians with knowledge and intention, cited earlier, and yet poor performance of the system to deliver care.

In the hospital setting where the highest-risk patients, those with acute cardiovascular events or stroke, are treated there is a unique opportunity to redesign systems of care. Hospitals

TABLE 28-1

HOSPITAL PERFORMANCE DATA FOR MYOCARDIAL INFARCTION, HEART FAILURE, AND STROKE

Measures	US Medicare (4)	GRACE (6)	ADHERE® (8)	Coverdell (7)
Time Period	2000–2001	1999–2000	2002–2003	2001–2002
Patient Population	AMI	ACS	Heart Failure	Stroke and TIA
Aspirin early	85%	93%	a	b
BB early	69%	81%	a	a
Aspirin discharge	86%	89%	a	94%
BB discharge	79%	71%	b	a
ACE discharge	74%	55%	72%	a
Lipid discharge	40%	47%	a	a
Discharge instruction for HF	a	a	24%	a
LVEF measure for HF	a	a	87%	a
Smoking cessation	b	b	43%	23%
rTPA for stroke	a	a	a	4%
Anticoag for A Fib	a	a	a	79%

[a]Measure not collected for patient population.
[b]Measure not reported.
ACS, acute coronary syndromes; A Fib, atrial fibrillation; AMI, acute myocardial infarction; anticoag, anticoagulation; BB, beta-blocker; GRACE, Global Registry of Acute Coronary Events; HF, heart failure; LVEF, left ventricular ejection fraction; rTPA, recombinant tissue plasmin activator; TIA, transient ischemic attack.

have professionals from a number of disciplines that participate in the care of these patients. System changes, such as the use of preprinted order sets, reduce the reliance on memory that often fails us when there are more urgent, acute treatments to occupy our attention. For this reason preprocedure orders for cardiac catheterization and revascularization procedures are common. Using similar systems for admission orders and a discharge checklist can be helpful in ensuring that key evaluations such as LDL cholesterol measurement, A1C measurement in diabetics, and routine, evidence-based therapies are given for all patients unless there is a specific contraindication. The participation of multidisciplinary teams in the development and implementation of these systems can also lead to the use of all members of the care team to catch the inadvertent omissions that too often characterize secondary prevention.

PROGRAM ELEMENTS

The American Heart Association's (AHA) Get With The Guidelines (GWTG) is a program designed to assist hospitals in redesigning these systems of care. GWTG currently offers quality improvement modules for three disease states. The CAD module (GWTG-CAD) was launched nationally in April 2001 and is currently being implemented in almost every state. The stroke module (GWTG-Stroke) and the heart failure module (GWTG-HF) were launched in May 2004 and March 2005, respectively.

Elements of the program include organizational stakeholder and opinion leader meetings, hospital recruitment, collaborative learning sessions, hospital tool kits, local clinical champions, multidisciplinary teams, and hospital recognition (13). Data collection, decision support, and hospital data feedback via multiple on-demand reports of performance on all key measures are done with an Internet-based Patient Management Tool (PMT).

This program uses a collaborative model to bring together teams from many hospitals in a region to work together to address barriers to care (Fig. 28-1). Learning from each other, hospitals can successfully adapt the successful approaches used by others for their own unique environment. This approach significantly speeds up the improvement process and helps to engage hospital leadership, an important ingredient in producing permanent change, by creating a sense of community. Workshops include didactic presentation of clinical trial evidence and the AHA/American College of Cardiology (ACC), American Stroke Association (ASA) guidelines for acute care and secondary prevention for CHD (14–16), stroke (17–19), or heart failure (20) followed by examples of successful hospital implementation. Observing the successes of other hospitals creates the sense that improvement is achievable. Standardized quality improvement methodology based on the Model for Improvement is presented at each session (21,22).

Hospital teams learn to clearly state their goals for each measure and select a pilot population and location to begin the process. By initially focusing on an area in the hospital where success is most likely, hospital teams can develop positive momentum as they expand to other areas and patient populations. They also learn to use plan-do-study-act (PDSA) cycles to test their ideas for change. These tests are designed to answer two questions. The first is: How will we know that the change is an improvement? This question is designed to provide a framework to quickly evaluate new and creative solutions to defects in their system of care. These change ideas are brought back from GWTG sessions; learned from calls, e-mail lists, and GWTG materials; and developed by the teams themselves (23). Change concepts may be very successful in some environments, but not in others. Even well-developed critical pathways, preprinted orders, and reminders often require adaptation to a specific hospital environment; some may not work at all. Thus after a small test is *planned* (a few patients on 1 or 2 days using a single physician and care team), *done*, and the resulting data *studied*, teams *act* by adopting or adapting the change and doing further tests on a larger scale or abandoning the idea and moving on to another. The small scale of these initial tests gives teams the ability to try new and innovative ideas not previously considered, sorting through many to find the few highly effective concepts that substantially improve performance. There appears to be relationship to the number of tests run and success in improvement (21,22).

TABLE 28-2

BARRIERS TO ADOPTION ADDRESSED BY GET WITH THE GUIDELINES

Barrier	Description	GWTG Solution
Knowledge		
Lack of awareness	Practitioner unaware of guidelines.	AHA/ACC guidelines disseminated at workshops, conferences, and via electronic channels.
Lack of guideline familiarity	Practitioner not knowledgeable enough with interventions to apply.	PMT has decision support, inclusion, exclusion criteria, interventions reviewed in depth in workshops, conference calls.
Attitudes		
Lack of agreement with the guidelines	Practitioner disagrees with expert interpretation of the evidence; lack of cost-effectiveness data.	Rigorous AHA/ACC, ASA guideline development process. In-depth presentation of science in GWTG and embedded in PMT.
Lack of agreement with guidelines in general	Practitioners view as cookbook, challenge to autonomy and authority.	Peer-to-peer interaction with opinion leaders in GWTG workshops and calls. Multidisciplinary teams to build hospital consensus.
Lack of outcome expectancy	Practitioner does not believe guidelines will improve outcomes.	Data linking measure adherence to outcomes presented in GWTG events.
Lack of self-efficacy	Practitioner does not believe he/she can perform the recommendation.	Most measures are prescriptions of basic medication or behavioral intervention that can be referred to experts in the hospital.
Lack of motivation	Habit, routines, belief that performance is already sufficient.	Opinion leaders, AHA/ASA recognition provides motivation. Use prompts, reminders, and critical pathways developed or refined in GWTG process.
Behavior		
Patient factors	Patient preferences differ from guidelines.	Evidence of clear risk/benefit advantage present in most GWTG measures. Patient summary and educational materials in the PMT inform and support patient choices.
Guidelines factors	Presence of contradictory guidelines.	AHA/ACC, ASA guidelines are clear and precise and align with guidelines from other organizations.
Environmental factors	Lack of time, resources, organizational constraints, liability concerns; lack of efficient systems.	Hospital teams develop, test, and implement efficient and effective tools in GWTG program. AHA/ASA recognition helps to engage hospital leadership and align resources with program priorities. Effective and safe systems are created to reduce liability risks. Rigorous science, decision support, and patient eligibility available in the PMT.

Adapted from LaBresh KA, Gliklich R, Liljestrand J, et al. Get With The Guidelines to improve cardiovascular secondary prevention. *Jt Comm J Qual Saf* 2003;29(10):539–550, with permission.
ACC, American College of Cardiology; AHA, American Heart Association; ASA, American Stroke Association; GWTG, Get With The Guidelines; PMT, Patient Management Tool.

The second question is: What change can we make that will result in improvement? This question is the basis of implementing the successful changes previously tested with the emphasis on what *we* can implement. Large-scale implementation requires widespread communication and support. These strategies need to become part of the standard system of care. Here, there is no room for failure. New systems need to be monitored and adjusted by the ongoing collection of key performance measures, and they need to be adapted as needed over time. Implementation requires acceptance of doing things in a

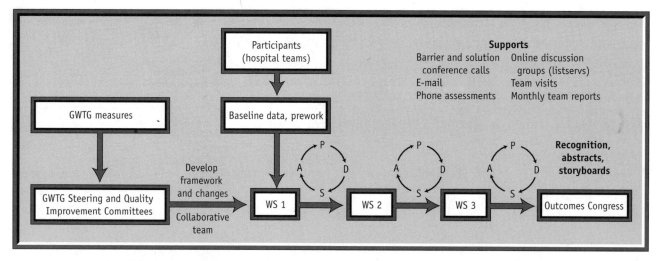

FIGURE 28-1. Get With the Guidelines quality improvement framework. WS, workshop; P, plan; D, do; S, study; A, act. (From LaBresh KA. Using "Get With The Guidelines" to prevent recurrent cardiovascular disease. *Curr Treat Options Cardiovasc Med* 2005;7:287–292, with permission.)

new way. What predicts the successful adoption of change by a diverse group? Everett Rogers (24) described five criteria that predict the successful adoption of change. The demonstration of *relative advantage* implies that the change is better than the system that is being replaced. Because the process of changing routines is difficult, the new system must perform better than the old system to make the effort worthwhile. Successful change should not be overly *complex*, and its advantage should be *observable*. *Trialability* implies that the innovation should have the capacity for testing on a small scale before full-scale implementation. Successfully adopted innovation needs to be *compatible* with individual or institutional values, priorities, and resources. The ability to test a system change and customize it is one way to help address this issue. If stroke is not an important part of a hospital's strategic priorities, it is much less likely that a system change to improve stroke care will be successfully adopted. A system change that uses emergency department physicians to administer recombinant tissue plasmin activator (rTPA) for an acute stroke without the onsite evaluation of a neurologist may be successful in some hospital environments but not feasible in others.

Simultaneous, facilitated breakout sessions, a key part of the GWTG workshops, allow multidisciplinary teams from six to eight hospitals each to discuss barriers and potential solutions, share tools and pathways each has developed, and share results of their small tests of change. The hallmark of these sessions is, "Share openly and steal shamelessly (with attribution)." Each team then develops a plan for testing a new change. Hospital teams present their plans, including the PDSA cycle they will "do by next Tuesday." These brief presentations create a sense of purpose, urgency, and accountability to each other and the program. Between workshops, hospital interactions are continued via conference calls and e-mail exchanges. Results of PDSA cycles are shared by many of the participants. These exchanges provide an opportunity for coaching on cycle design and execution by both faculty and peers. Guest speaker presentations are also included in the calls to communicate new science and guidelines.

One example of a successful systems-based approach is the creation of a practitioner order system that defaults to evidenced-based treatment in all patients with CAD. When this occurs, all patients are treated unless they have a specific contraindication to that therapy. Thus the physician need manage only these exceptions. Such an approach can significantly re-

duce the burden of remembering every appropriate therapy for every patient every time. The role of GWTG program in addressing each of the categories of barriers is illustrated in Table 28-2.

Additional sharing and quality improvement skills are provided in subsequent workshops. These face-to-face meetings provide an important vehicle to exchange specific information on how changes were accomplished and lessons learned (25). Momentum is maintained, and more reluctant participants become motivated by the success of others and the desire not to be left behind (24,26). Teams also learn new skills to maintain the progress they have made and spread success to other areas and with additional patient groups (21,22).

An important tool for the program is the Internet-based PMT that is used to collect data and provide decision support at the point of care (23). This tool provides measure definitions including inclusion and exclusion criteria and decision support with references to the content of the guidelines and references for each measure. Clinical staff at the point of care can do the data collection. Electronic systems with these elements have been shown to significantly reduce medication errors (27). Reminders in the PMT can help to provide a safety net for the discharge measures by providing feedback before the patient leaves the care setting, thus proving the opportunity to correct any unintended omissions (23). Customized patient education materials from the AHA/ASA can be printed for patients along with a treatment summary letter to support patient self-management after discharge, a key element in improving chronic management (28,29). A summary letter can also be prepared within the system and faxed to the patient's physician at the time of discharge to support the transition of care to the office setting.

MEASURE DEFINITIONS

The performance measures assessed in the GWTG-CAD program are indicated in Table 28-3. Indicator-specific inclusion and exclusion criteria were applied so that only eligible patients without contraindications or documented intolerance for that specific indicator remained in the denominators (ideal patients). Measure definitions for early and late aspirin, early and late beta-blockers, and smoking cessation counseling use the

---

TABLE 28-3

PERFORMANCE MEASURES FOR CORONARY ARTERY DISEASE

Measure Definition	Patient Population Applied To[a]	Guidelines Used
Aspirin given in the 24 hours prior to or after admission	ACS	ACC/AHA 2002 Guideline Update for the Management of Patients With Unstable Angina and Non-ST-Segment Elevation Myocardial Infarction (14) and ACC/AHA Guidelines for Management of Patients With ST-Elevation Myocardial Infarction (15)
Beta-blocker given in the first 24 hours	ACS	Same as above
Aspirin prescribed at discharge	All	AHA/ACC Secondary Prevention Guidelines (16)
Beta-blocker prescribed at discharge	All	Same as above
Smoking cessation counseling given at discharge	All patients who have smoked in the 12 months prior to admission	Same as above
ACE inhibitor or ARB prescribed at discharge	All post-MI	Same as above
Lipid-lowering therapy at discharge	All with LDL-c >100mg/dL or on lipid-lowering agents prior to admission	Same as above

[a]Eligible patients are those without contraindications for each of the applicable measures.
ACC, American College of Cardiology; ACE, angiotensin-converting enzyme; ACS, acute coronary syndromes; AHA, American Heart Association; ARB, angiotensin receptor blocker; LDL-c, low-density lipoprotein cholesterol; MI, myocardial infarction.

JCAHO and CMS specifications (2,3); in addition, ACE inhibitor or angiotensin-receptor blocker (ARB) use is collected for all patients with acute myocardial infarction at all levels of left ventricular function. Two lipid indicators are used: the percent of all patients discharged on lipid therapy, LipidRX, and LDL100Rx, defined as the percent of patients who have an LDL cholesterol >100 mg/dL or who enter the hospital on lipid-lowering agents. Measurement of LDL cholesterol for all patients within the first 24 hours of admission is also tracked. The blood pressure measure assesses the percent of patients with the last recorded hospital blood pressure <140/90 mm Hg. The final measure is the percentage of patients referred for cardiac rehabilitation or given formal exercise recommendation by the time of discharge.

Performance measures for the GWTG-Stroke program (Table 28-4) include acute, subacute, and prevention measures and exclude patients with contraindications to the measure. Acute measures are the percent of patients with acute ischemic stroke who present to the hospital within 2 hours of the onset of symptoms and receive rTPA within 60 minutes and the percent of patients with ischemic stroke or transient ischemic attack (TIA) who receive antithrombotic therapy within the first 48 hours of admission. The subacute measure is the use of deep vein thrombophlebitis prophylaxis for nonambulatory patients. The prevention measures, applicable for ischemic stroke or TIA patients, include antithrombotic therapy at discharge, anticoagulation for patients with atrial fibrillation, lipid-lowering therapy for LDL cholesterol >100 mg/dL or on therapy on admission, and smoking cessation counseling for all patients who have smoked within 12 months of admission.

Performance measures for GWTG-HF are the four CMS/JCAHO measures: heart failure discharge instructions, measurement of left ventricular function, ACE inhibitor, or ARB at discharge for patients with LVEF ≤0.40, in absence of documented contraindications or intolerance to both agents (2,3), plus an additional measure, beta-blocker use at discharge for patients with LVEF ≤0.40 in absence of documented contraindications or intolerance (Table 28-5).

RECOGNITION

Each GWTG module offers recognition awards. The first level designates participating hospitals as those that have a multidisciplinary team, a physician champion, orders or protocols that include the GWTG measures, and submission of baseline data from at least 30 consecutive patients. The Performance Achievement Award recognizes the attainment of 85% performance for each of the modules performance measures (Tables 28-3 to 28-5). Sustained achievement at 85% for each of the performance measures is also recognized on an annual basis for consecutive years of achievement.

Recognition awards have been used as a nonfinancial incentive to engage hospital leadership, governance, and the hospital's community in support of the team's efforts. They have played an important role in incorporating the goals of the GWTG modules into the organization's strategic plan and help to mobilize resources to maintain the program over time.

In Hawaii, AHA recognition milestones were incorporated into the pay-for-quality initiative of the state's largest commercial payer, resulting in near universal participation in the CAD program (30).

GET WITH THE GUIDELINES RESULTS

More than 600 hospitals are in the GWTG-CAD program. The GWTG collaborative approach was demonstrated to produce significant improvement in several measures in the initial 24-hospital pilot by the fourth quarter of intervention (31) (Fig.

TABLE 28-4

PERFORMANCE MEASURES FOR ISCHEMIC STROKE AND TIA

Measure Definition	Patient Population Applied To[a]	Guidelines Used
IV rTPA in patients who arrived <2 hr after symptom onset	Ischemic stroke	Guidelines for the Early Management of Patients With Ischemic Stroke (17); ASA/AAN Scientific Statement on Anticoagulants and Antiplatelet Agents in Acute Ischemic Stroke (18)
Antithrombotics <48 hr from admission	All	Same as above
DVT prophylaxis ≤48 hr	All nonambulatory	Same as above
Antithrombotics at discharge	All	Preventing Ischemic Stroke in Patients With Prior Stroke and Transient Ischemic Attack (19)
Anticoagulation for atrial fibrillation at discharge	All with atrial fibrillation	Same as above
Therapy at discharge if LDL-c >100 mg/dL or on therapy at admission	All	Same as above
Smoking cessation counseling given at discharge	All	Same as above

[a]Eligible patients are those without contraindications for each of the applicable measures.
AAN, American Academy of Neurology; ASA, American Stroke Association; DVT, deep vein thrombosis; IV, intravenous; LDL-c, low-density lipoprotein cholesterol; rTPA, recombinant tissue plaminogen activator.

28-2). Significant increases of 10% to 20% compared to baseline in many of the essential acute treatment and secondary prevention measures in less than a year of implementation have been seen in the larger national cohort, with improvement continuing through 2 years in the program (32).

GWTG-Stroke has grown even more rapidly with more than 500 hospitals joining in less than 18 months. The early results from the GWTG-Stroke have indicated nearly a fivefold increase in the use of rTPA, with no increase in rates of complication and even larger increases from lower baseline performance in the prevention measures than seen in the CAD module (33,34). There has been rapid adoption of the heart failure module as well with nearly 200 hospitals participating within the first 6 months of the program.

CHALLENGE AND OPPORTUNITIES

The increased emphasis on data collection by a number of organizations, as discussed earlier, creates great pressure on hospital resources that may detract from the ability to use the data to improve care (35). Although CMS provides process improvement assistance through the Quality Improvement program, most of these efforts provide data feedback only. The design of some of these data collection systems, necessitating retrospective chart review well after care has been delivered, eliminates the possibility of using that feedback to correct "near-misses" in the omission of care. Data collection pro-

TABLE 28-5

PERFORMANCE MEASURES FOR HEART FAILURE

Measure Definition	Patient Population Applied To[a]	Guidelines Used
Complete set of discharge instructions	All	ACC/AHA 2005 Guideline Update for the Diagnosis and Management of Chronic Heart Failure in the Adult (20)
Measure of left ventricular function	All	Same as above
Smoking cessation counseling	Smokers within the last 12 months	Same as above
ACE inhibitor or ARB at discharge	Those with left ventricular ejection fraction ≤0.40	Same as above
Beta-blockers at discharge	Those with left ventricular ejection fraction ≤0.40	Same as above

[a]Eligible patients are those without contraindications for each of the applicable measures.
ACC, American College of Cardiology; AHA, American Heart Association; ACE, angiotensin-converting enzyme; ARB, angiotensin-receptor blocker.

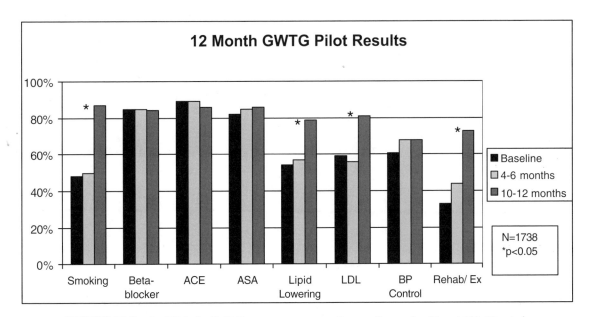

FIGURE 28-2. Get With the Guidelines coronary artery disease pilot results. $N = 1,738$, Hospitals = 24. ACE, angiotensin-converting enzyme inhibitor use at discharge; ASA, aspirin use at discharge; Beta-blocker, beta-blocker at discharge; BP control, blood pressure less than 140/90 mm HG by the time of discharge; LDL, lipid profile measurement in the hospital for determination of low-density lipoprotein; Lipid lowering, use of lipid-lowering agents at discharge; Rehab/Ex, referral to cardiac rehabilitation or exercise recommendations at discharge; Smoking, smoking cessation counseling. Significance (asterisk) based on nonoverlapping confidence intervals compared to the baseline period. (From LaBresh KA, Ellrodt, AG, Gliklich, RG, et al. Get With The Guidelines for Cardiovascular Secondary Prevention: Pilot Results. *Arch Int Med* 2004;164:203–209,with permission.)

grams without robust process change support also tend to document poor care, but may not support rapid improvement in that care. Although data feedback is a necessary part of care improvement, excessive time spent collecting data not related to quality measures may divert resources from improvement activities, particularly in smaller hospitals.

Public reporting of data, emphasis on culture change, and the adoption of health information technology, along with process improvement support, are key strategies to transform the health care system (30). Coupled with potential change in the reimbursement system to reward the investment in quality, these emerging trends will play an important role in enhancing the care of patients with CAD, stroke, and heart failure. GWTG engages medical and administrative leadership, promotes team approaches to care and improvement, and uses electronic technology that can be used during the care process to produce process and cultural change in participating hospitals. Nonfinancial incentives such as AHA/ASA recognition awards also encourage leadership and community support of high-performing systems of care. Expanded participation in such programs, catalyzed by campaigns such as the Institute for Healthcare Improvement's 100,000 lives campaign (36), is encouraging progress toward the goal of providing the right care for every patient, every time.

ACKNOWLEDGMENT

The Centers for Medicare and Medicaid Services provided resources for program development and analysis under contract 500-02-MA03 and have reviewed the manuscript. The conclusions and interpretation of results are the sole responsibility of the author and do not necessarily reflect the position or policy of the government or the American Heart Association.

Get With The Guidelines is partly supported by grants from Merck, GlaxoSmithKline, and Bristol Myers Squibb, who played no role in the preparation of this manuscript.

References

1. American Heart Association. Heart disease and stroke statistics: 2005 update. Dallas, TX: American Heart Association; 2004.
2. Joint Commission on Accreditation of Healthcare Organizations. ORYZ for hospitals. Available at: http://www.jointcommission.org/AccreditationPrograms/Hospitals/ORYX. Accessed September 30, 2005.
3. Centers for Medicare & Medicaid Services. Medicare quality improvement community: priority topics. Available at: http://www.medqic.org/content/nationalpriorities/index.jsp. Accessed September 29, 2005.
4. Jencks SF, Huff ED, Cuerdon T. Changes in the quality of care delivered to Medicare beneficiaries, 1998–1999 to 2000–2001. *JAMA* 2003;289:305–312.
5. Rogers WJ, Canto JG, Lambrew CT, et al. Temporal trends in the treatment of over 1.5 million patients with myocardial infarction in the US from 1990 through 1999. *J Am Coll Cardiol* 2000;36:2056–2063.
6. Fox KAA, Goodman SG, Klein W, et al. Management of acute coronary syndromes. Variations in practice and outcome. Findings from the Global Registry of Acute Coronary Events (GRACE). *European Heart J* 2002;23:1177–1189.
7. Reeves MJ, Arora S, Broderick JP, et al. Acute stroke care in the US: results from 4 pilot prototypes of the Paul Coverdell National Acute Stroke Registry. *Stroke* 2005;36(6):1232–40.
8. Fonarow GC, Yancy CW, Haywood JT, et al. Adherence to heart failure quality-of-care indicators in US hospitals: analysis of the ADHERE Registry. *Arch Intern Med* 2005;165(13):1469–1477.
9. Cabana MD, Rand CS, Powe NR, et al. Why don't physicians follow clinical practice guidelines? A framework for improvement. *JAMA* 1999;282:1458–1465.
10. Davis D, O'Brien MAT, Freemantle N, et al. Impact of formal continuing medical education: do conferences, workshops, rounds, and other traditional continuing education activities change physician behavior or health care outcomes? *JAMA* 1999;82:867–874.
11. Pearson TA, Laurora I, Chu H, et al. The Lipid Treatment Assessment Project (L-TAP): a multicenter study to evaluate the percentages of dyslipidemic patients receiving lipid lowering therapy and achieving low density lipoprotein cholesterol goals. *Arch Int Med* 2000;60:459–467.

12. Deming WE. *Out of the crisis*. Cambridge, MA: MIT Press; 2000, Chapter 2.

13. LaBresh KA, Tyler PA. A collaborative model for hospital-based cardiovascular secondary prevention. *Qual Manag Health Care* 2003;12:20–27.

14. Braunwald E, Antman EM, Beasley JW, et al. ACC/AHA 2002 guideline update for the management of patients with unstable angina and non-ST-segment elevation myocardial infarction—summary article. *J Am Coll Cardiol* 2002;40:1366–1374.

15. Anbe DT, Armstrong PW, Bates ER, et al. ACC/AHA guidelines for the management of patients with ST-elevation myocardial infarction—executive summary. *Circulation* 2004;110:588–636.

16. Smith SC Jr, Blair SN, Bonow RO, et al. AHA/ACC guidelines for preventing heart attack and death in patients with atherosclerotic cardiovascular disease: 2001 update. *Circulation* 2001;104:1577–1579.

17. Adams H, Adams R, Del Zoppo G, et al. Guidelines for the early management of patients with ischemic stroke: 2005 guidelines update. A scientific statement from the Stroke Council of the American Heart Association/American Stroke Association. *Stroke* 2005;36:916–923.

18. Coull BM, Williams LS, Goldstein LB, et al. Anticoagulants and antiplatelet agents in acute ischemic stroke: report of the Joint Stroke Guideline Development Committee of the American Academy of Neurology and the American Stroke Association (a Division of the American Heart Association). *Stroke* 2002;33:1934–1942.

19. Wolf PA, Clagett GP, Easton JD, et al. Preventing ischemic stroke in patients with prior stroke and transient ischemic attack. a statement for healthcare professionals from the Stroke Council of the American Heart Association. *Stroke* 1999;30:1991–1994.

20. Hunt SA, Abraham WT, Chin MH, et al. ACC/AHA 2005 guideline update for the diagnosis and management of chronic heart failure in the adult. *Circulation* 2005;112:1825–1852.

21. Kilo CM. Improving care through collaboration. *Pediatrics* 1999;103(1 suppl E):384–393.

22. Berwick DM. A primer on leading the improvement of systems. *BMJ* 1996, 312:619–622.

23. LaBresh KA, Gliklich R, Liljestrand J, et al. Get With The Guidelines to improve cardiovascular secondary prevention. *Jt Comm J Qual Saf* 2003; 29(10):539–550.

24. Rogers E. *Diffusion of innovations*. New York: The Free Press; 1995.

25. Dixon NM. *Common knowledge*. Boston: Harvard Business School Press; 2000.

26. Berwick DM. Disseminating innovations in health care. *JAMA* 2003;289:1969–1975.

27. Kaushal R, Shojania KG, Bates DW. Effect of computerized order entry and clinical decision support on medication safety: a systematic review. *Arch Int Med* 2003;163:1409–1416.

28. Bodenheimer T, Wagner EH, Grumbach K. Improving primary care for patients with chronic illness. *JAMA* 2002;288:1775–1779.

29. Bodenheimer T, Wagner EH, Grumbach K: Improving primary care for patients with chronic illness: the chronic care model, part 2. *JAMA* 2002; 288:1909–1914.

30. Berthiaume JT, Tyler PA; Ng-Osorio J, et al. Aligning financial incentives with Get With The Guidelines to improve cardiovascular care. *Am J Manag Care* 2004;10:501–504.

31. LaBresh KA, Ellrodt, AG, Gliklich, RG, et al. Get With The Guidelines for cardiovascular secondary prevention: pilot results. *Arch Int Med* 2004;164:203–209.

32. LaBresh KA, Fonarow GC, Tyler PA, et al. Are improvements in cardiovascular care associated with the American Heart Association's Get With The Guidelines program sustained over time? *Circulation* 2004;110:III-784.

33. Schwamm L, LaBresh KA, Albright D, et al. Does Get With The Guidelines-Stroke improve acute intervention in patients hospitalized with ischemic stroke or TIA? *Stroke* 2005;36(2):436.

34. LaBresh KA, Schwamm L, Albright D, et al. Does Get With The Guidelines improve secondary prevention in patients hospitalized with ischemic stroke or TIA? *Stroke* 2005;36(2):454.

35. Centers for Medicare and Medicaid Services. Quality initiatives—general information. Available at: www.cms.hhs.gov/QualityInitiativesGenInfo/. Accessed September 30, 2005.

36. Institute of Healthcare Improvement. 100K lives campaign. Available at: http://www.ihi.org/ihi/programs/campaign/. Accessed September 30, 2005.

CHAPTER 29 ■ CARDIAC REHABILITATION

DANIEL E. FORMAN

HISTORY
ORGANIZATION OF TRADITIONAL CARDIAC
    REHABILITATION
Exercise Training
Risk-Factor Modification
Education
Psychosocial Assessment
DESIGN OF CARDIAC REHABILITATION
SAFETY OF EXERCISE TRAINING
COST EFFICACY
EVIDENCE FOR CARDIAC REHABILITATION
    EFFECTIVENESS
WHAT IS CRITICAL IN CARDIAC REHABILITATION?
SUMMARY

Cardiac rehabilitation is a dynamic and relevant component of the armamentarium for acute coronary syndrome (ACS) management. Because the inflammatory and biological underpinnings of atherosclerotic disease commonly originate from lifestyle and risk factors, the rationale to prioritize exercise and comprehensive secondary prevention has never been more compelling. Nonetheless, cardiac rehabilitation is distressingly underutilized. Adding to such irony, third-party payers are becoming more averse to paying for cardiac rehabilitation. Underutilization may relate to an erroneous perception that cardiac rehabilitation is less important than other ACS interventions, such as revascularization and pharmacological stabilization. Acute interventions provide enhanced myocardial salvage and stability in the short term. Yet, coronary artery disease (CAD) is a chronic process, and unhealthy lifestyle patterns and medical noncompliance in the long term are common and insidious. Functional decline, cognitive impairment, reduced quality of life, recurrent myocardial infarction (MI), angina, heart failure (HF), arrhythmias, and even death are among the many detrimental consequences of CAD, especially when exacerbated by suboptimal lifestyle behaviors. The short-term successes in the management of ACS have led to a growing population of chronic CAD patients who are particularly vulnerable to long-term health consequences. Cardiac rehabilitation is a vital link to a healthier future for ACS patients.

HISTORY

Cardiac rehabilitation was first developed approximately 50 years ago amid shifting views regarding early mobilization and activity for MI patients. Until that time, bed rest and sedentary management were promoted with the logic that they helped to reduce ischemia, arrhythmia, recurrent infarction, ventricular aneurysm, and/or myocardial rupture (1). However, seminal research then began to illuminate the unhealthy effects of extended post-MI bed rest, as well as the beneficial effects of early mobilization and exercise (2). Cardiac rehabilitation was formulated as a means to initiate and then advance exercise safely (3). Programs typically included both in-hospital and outpatient formats. The in-hospital model facilitated transition from bed rest to activity as part of the initial CAD (MI or coronary artery bypass graft [CABG]) hospitalization. After hospital discharge, outpatient programming was developed to advance activity and then to foster regular exercise maintenance (4).

Given this context, for many caregivers cardiac rehabilitation solidified in the medical lexicon as *exercise* supervision (i.e., primarily a means to mobilize safely post-MI or post-CABG patients who were typically feeble and anxious in the midst of prolonged and overwhelming hospitalizations). As such, cardiac rehabilitation was initially endorsed as medically worthwhile because it produced earlier hospital discharge and perhaps even expedited return to work (6).

Justifying cardiac rehabilitation in terms of a vocation probably contributed to a bias that cardiac rehabilitation was suited specifically to employed men. This view overlooked the fact that many others suffered from CAD, and subsequent research showed that return to work after an MI had much more to do with the job itself than to cardiac rehabilitation. Still, patterns quickly became ingrained, and despite multiple studies demonstrating cardiac rehabilitation's substantial benefits for women, older adults, and ethnically diverse populations, underreferral of these groups relative to white, middle-aged men remains disproportionate (6,7).

Over subsequent years, insights and emphasis regarding risk-factor modification evolved, and cardiac rehabilitation programs broadened to include these objectives. In 1994, the American Heart Association (AHA) formally declared that cardiac rehabilitation was reorganizing into comprehensive secondary prevention programs (8). Blood pressure control, smoking cessation, stress reduction, low-density lipoprotein (LDL) lipid reduction, diet modification, medication adherence (typically beta-blockers, aspirin, angiotensin-converting enzyme (ACE) inhibitors, and statins), and weight loss became parts of aggregate cardiac rehabilitation objectives.

Even with formalized integration of exercise training and risk-factor modification, many caregivers and patients continued to see cardiac rehabilitation primarily as exercise training. The persistence of such a perspective has also likely contributed to today's mounting under-referral to cardiac rehabilitation. Contemporary CAD treatment standards have brought about shortened hospitalizations, and in so doing, relatively fewer patients are debilitated and enfeebled as a result of ACS hospitalizations. Referral to cardiac rehabilitation based primarily on functional limitation is no longer as relevant.

Amid these changes, home-based cardiac rehabilitation options have also grown in appeal (9–14). Home-based programs provide some of the beneficial components of traditional cardiac rehabilitation, but in a format that many believe is better suited to today's more rapidly discharged and physically intact ACS patients. Furthermore, home-based training has been touted as better able to extend to patients with logistic constraints (e.g., someone who might not be willing or able to travel to a hospital-based program, such as frail elders who may not drive or who are unable to leave an infirm spouse alone at home). Novel technological advances have added to the appeal of home-based options, as they provide potential to better link home-based patients to one another as well as to hospital personnel (i.e., facilitating community and close supervision without leaving home). Perhaps most significant, many view home-based cardiac rehabilitation as a means to provide key benefits of cardiac rehabilitation with maximal cost efficacy.

Overall, there is a sense of dynamic transition in the field of cardiac rehabilitation. Biological insights about the broad benefits of exercise and risk-factor modification (as both primary and secondary CAD prevention) are escalating just as reimbursements and space allocations within hospitals for cardiac rehabilitation are shrinking. In fact, given many reports of the pleiotropic benefits of exercise (15–17) and risk-factor modification (18–21), the spectrum of patients deemed eligible for cardiac rehabilitation has broadened to include those with HF, peripheral arterial disease (PAD), heart transplant, diabetes, and obesity, as well as those with CAD (ACS patients and/or postrevascularization) (22). Still, most present-day cardiac rehabilitation programs are typically losing money and emphasis, and considerations about the future of cardiac rehabilitation are provoking animated debate. Even among CAD patients, the estimated participation rate is only 10% to 20% of the >2 million eligible patients, and enrollment of patients with other cardiovascular diagnoses is even lower (6). Even among the patients who enroll, 25% to 50% drop out within weeks to months. Home-based cardiac rehabilitation may hold promise for better outreach and application, but these programs have not been standardized, and goals and techniques in home-based cardiac rehabilitation may vary widely from one institution to another.

Given all these complicated currents, we will review standards for traditional outpatient cardiac rehabilitation (i.e., hospital- or clinic-based programs that have been standardized as part of coronary heart disease [CHD] management). Our goal is to consider most worthwhile features that should logically be preserved, even if formats change.

ORGANIZATION OF TRADITIONAL CARDIAC REHABILITATION

In its most recent scientific statement on the issue, the AHA described cardiac rehabilitation as a coordinated, multifaceted intervention designed to optimize a patient's physical, psychological, and social functioning, in addition to stabilizing the underlying atherosclerotic processes (22). The guidelines recognize that although in-patient programs once existed for the most infirm and unstable cardiac patients, these have become rare. In most cases, cardiac rehabilitation now refers to an outpatient model, usually allied with a hospital or medical facility that provides ready access to physicians and medical supervision. Standardized programming includes baseline patient assessments (Table 29-1), nutritional counseling, aggressive risk management (including lipids, hypertension, weight, diabetes, and tobacco), psychosocial and vocational counseling, physical activity and exercise training counseling, and reinforcement of evidence-based cardioprotective medications (18).

Eligibility for cardiac rehabilitation applies to CAD and post-MI patients, including those who are revascularized with CABG or percutaneous coronary intervention (PCI), as well as those who are not revascularized. As indicated, eligibility has expanded to include patients with heart transplant, heart failure, PAD, or other forms of cardiovascular disease, including heart valve repair (22). Third-party reimbursement has typically lagged behind broadened enrollment criteria, often creating an unpleasant dimension of financial tension among patients for whom cardiac rehabilitation is clearly indicated. However, medicare expanded coverage includes heart valve repair/replacement, PTZA or stenting, heart or heart-lung transplant MI, CABG, and stable angina pectoris, even for diagnoses for which cardiac rehabilitation is reimbursed, the duration of subsidization (i.e., number of sessions) has typically been truncated, and copayment costs have usually increased. In the past, programs were usually designed to extend for 36 sessions, usually two to three times a week. Today, reimbursement commonly stops after only 10 to 20 sessions, with no particular scientific rationale used to justify this change.

Exercise Training

Exercise training remains a cornerstone of cardiac rehabilitation. Studies have consistently demonstrated improvement in exercise capacity as the result of participation in cardiac rehabilitation. Clinical impacts include expanded daily living activities, self-confidence, and quality of life. Just as important, symptoms related to CAD typically diminish with exercise training, with exercise contributing, at least in part, to greater work efficiency, such that less cardiac work is required for the same (submaximal) level of activity (e.g., lower heart rate and blood pressure for the same workload) (15,16,23).

American Heart Association guidelines for cardiac rehabilitation emphasize that the key objectives for exercise extend beyond functional gains accrued by exercise and have more to do with improving underlying biological and physiological capacities. Exercise improves central cardiac physiology (favorable remodeling along with increased stroke work and cardiac output) as well as peripheral physiology (vascular, skeletal muscle, and endothelial enhancements). Exercise training also modifies atherosclerosis, including inflammation (24–30). Exercise induces ischemic preconditioning, building resistance to subsequent episodes of ischemic stress (31–32), and reducing thrombotic risk by enhancing intrinsic fibrinolysis (33). Exercise brings about indirect benefits via improvements in blood pressure, lipids, glucose metabolism, weight reduction, and autonomic function (34–39).

Exercise training regimens are explicit, with specific modifications for different patient scenarios (e.g., high versus low risk, obesity, deconditioning, advanced age and/or frailty, heart failure/transplant, stroke, and PAD) (40). Both aerobic and resistance training modalities are utilized. Training goals include increasing exercise capacity as well as improved work efficiency, such that myocardial work demands are reduced for a given workload. Furthermore, training objectives now include goals for behavior modification such that long-term exercise adherence is prioritized and more likely achieved.

Exercise is typically prescribed two to four times a week, 30 to 45 minutes a session, at a training intensity based on 60% to 85% of the peak heart rate (HR) or heart rate reserve (an HR training target based on the peak HR assessed relative to the resting HR). Based on traditional 3-month aerobic exercise programs, exercise tolerance on the treadmill increases by 30% to 50% and peak VO_2 by 15% to 20% (41). Variations of duration, intensity, and training modalities are anticipated, especially as cardiac rehabilitation has been modified to be

TABLE 29-1

REQUISITE COMPONENTS OF CARDIAC REHABILITATION

	Evaluation	Interventions
Assessment: evaluating patient and developing Prevention plan	Medical history: cardiovascular, comobordities, Symptoms, risk factors, medications, compliance Physical exam Testing: ECG, exercise testing, quality of life assessment questionnaire (e.g., SF36), affective questionnaire (e.g., Beck's depression scale), fasting glucose, fasting lipids, HgAIC	Patient care plan, clarifying priorities for exercise, physical activity, risk reduction, education, improved quality of life, stress, reduction; communicate plan with patient and primary care provider Assess readiness to change in regards to cardiac rehabilitation itself as well as specific therapeutic goals (medication compliance, diet, exercise, risk reduction, stress reduction); reinforce with encouragement, education, cohesive programming
Nutritional Counseling: evaluating dietary patterns and goals for change	Obtain estimates of total daily caloric intake Assess eating habits: meals, snacks, dining out, alcohol Assess targets for nutrition intervention in context of comorbid issues (HTN, weight, diabetes, HR, renal disease)	Prescribe specific dietary modifications that are individualized according to specific target areas (calori goals, fats, cholesterol, other nutrients) Education and counsel of patient/family regarding diet and strategies to achieve it Incorporate behavior-change models and compliance strategies Generate plan to address eating-behavior problems
Management of Lipid Levels: assess and modify diet, medications, and physical activity	Obtain fasting measures LDL, HDL, tryglyceride Assess current treatment and compliance	Nutrition counseling and weight management for AHA Step II diet in those patients with LDL ≥70 mg/dL. Likely pharmacological Rx for patients with LDL ≥100 mg /dL in concert with the primary care provider Incorporate behavior-change models and compliance strategies Overall lipid goals: LDL <70 mg/dL; HDL >45; TG <200 Plan for routine reassessment and surveillance
Management of HTN: assess and modify medications, diet, and physical activity	Measurement of BP on at least two visits Assess current treatment and compliance	If systolic 130-139 or diastolic 85-89, initiate lystyle changes If systolic ≥140 or diastolic ≥90, initiate pharmacological therapy in convert with the primary care provider Overall goals: BP systolic <130 mmHg; BP diastolic <85 mmHg Incorporate behavior-change modes and compliance strategies Plan for routine reassessment and surveillance
Smoking Cessation: plan to quit, behavioral supports, medications, exercise	Document smoking status and any pertinent history of efforts to curb smoking (i.e.,relapse, etc); assess use of tobacco equivalents (chewing tobacco, pipe, secondhand smoke) Assess confounding psychosocial issues	When readiness to change is confirmed, set a quit date and select appropriate treatment strategy (preparation) Education and encouragement; consider formal smoking cessation program, with group or individual counseling; consider supplemental strategies (accupuncture, hypnosis) Provide pharmacological support as needed in concert with primary care provider Incorporate behavior-change models and compliance strategies Plan for routine reassessment and suveillance
Weight Management: plan to change weight, behavioral supports, exercise, consider medications, and other interventions	Measure weight, height, and waist circumference; calculate BMI	In patients with BMI >25kg/m² and wait >40 inches in men and >35 inches in women Short-term and long-term goals individualized to patient and risk factors; goals to reduce weight by at least 10%, at 1-2 lb/wk over a period of time Develop integrated exercise, behavioral, diet program that maintains appropriate intake of nutrients, fiber, and which emphasize increased energy expenditure

TABLE 29-1

CONTINUED

	Evaluation	Interventions
Diabetes Management: identify candidates and refine therapy	Identify patients with diabetes; note medications (type, dose, frequency) and monitoring schedule (type and frequency); note history of hypoglycemia Obtain fasting plasma glucose and HbA1C	Aim for energy deficit 500-1,000 kcal/day Incorporate behavior-change models and compliance strategies Plan for routine reassessment and surveillance Develop regimen of dietary adherence and weight control that includes exercise and medications, and optimal control of risk factors; close coordination with primary care provider Monitor glucose before and after exercise sessions; instruct patients regarding identification and treatment of postexercise hypoglycemia; limit or prohibit exercise if blood glucose ≥ 300 mg/dL
Psychosocial Management: assessment of affective state	Using interview or standardized assessment tools, identify psychosocial distress (depression, anxiety, anger, hostility, social isolation, sexual dysfunction/ maladjustment) and/or substance abuse (ETOH psychotropics)	Offer individual or small group education and counseling regarding adjustment to CHD, stress reduction, and health-related lifestyle change; when possible, include family members and significant others in these sessions Develop supportive rehabilitation environment and community resources to enhance patient's and family's level of social support Teach and support self-help strategies Work with primary car provider to refer patients at risk to appropriate mental health specialists for further diagnosis and treatment
Physical Activity Counseling: assess current activity, barriers to activity, and goals	Assess current physical activity; assess domestic, occupational, and recreational goals	Education, advice, support, counseling Set goals to increase physical activity (e.g., 30 minutes a day of moderate appealing physical activity 5 d/wk; may be less intensive or in shorter to suggest how to incorporate increased activity into a daily routine
Exercise Training: exercise prescription based on a stress test	Obtain exercise test (or other standard assessment of exercise capacity) before participation. Test should include assessment of HR, rhythm, signs, symptoms, ST changes, and exercise capacity	Proper warm-ups and cool downs; proper stretching; teaching regarding optimal breathing, safe exercise ECG monitoring when deemed appropriate by intake evaluation Develop documented individualized exercise prescription for aerobic and resistance training that is base on initial evaluation, risk stratification, patient goals, resources; exercise prescription should specify frequency, intensity, duration, and modality Aerobic goals: 3–5 d/wk, 1 50–80% of exercise capacity; 30–60 min; using walking, treadmill, cycling, rowing, stair climber, arm ergometry Resistance training: 2–3 d/wk; 8–15 repetitions max for each muscle group (where repetitive max is the maz number of times a load can be lifted before fatigue); 1–3 sets of 8–10 different upper and lower body exercises (20–30 min); using elastic bands, cuff/hand weights, dumbbells, free weights, wall pulleys, weight machines

From Balady GJ, et al. Core components of cardiac rehabilitation in secondary prevention: a statement for healthcare professional from the American Heart Association and the American Association of Cardiovascular and Pulmonary Rehabilitation. *Circulation* 2000;102:1069–1073.

more accessible and effective for a wider range of patients and with more diverse underlying cardiovascular pathologies. Shorter, lower-intensity regimens have been demonstrated to yield significant physiological benefits at the level of the endothelium and skeletal muscle and greater patient adherence. Such considerations may be particularly useful to older patients and or those with HF. Likewise, resistance training provides a key means to modify the weakness and frailty that may otherwise hinder many older rehabilitation patients at the onset of their exercise training (40).

Risk-Factor Modification

The AHA guidelines also emphasize the importance of risk-factor modification. Although exercise alone has some impact on risk factors (i.e., favorable impact on high-density lipoprotein [HDL] cholesterol and insulin resistance) (42–44), the addition of specific risk-factor modifying strategies adds to efficacy. Among the risk-factor modifying goals are smoking cessation, lipid modification, weight reduction, blood pressure reduction, diabetes control, and stress management. Focus on risk modification is typically integrated into the exercise-training program. In fact, these two concerns can be blended synergistically when exercise becomes part of the strategy to achieve a healthful lifestyle (i.e., exercise training as a means to reinforce weight loss, smoking cessation, blood pressure reduction, and glucose control).

Patient evaluations are utilized as a means to initially assess risk factors and to identify therapeutic goals and strategies. Although sometimes these priorities overlap with those of the primary caregivers, cardiac rehabilitation provides a mechanism of extensive monitoring (both qualitative and quantitative) over the weeks of the program that is usually viewed as an augmentation of caregiving efficacy.

Education

Strong orientation to education is blended with exercise and risk-factor modification. Several layers of learning overlap as part of a cardiac rehabilitation experience. On the most basic level, cardiac rehabilitation provides an opportunity to modify common misconceptions and anxieties among cardiovascular patients, particularly at the outset of the program. Often reeling from fears and anxiety after an MI, many patients present to cardiac rehabilitation with distorted impressions and beliefs. A few of the many examples of such misunderstanding include patients who express fear that "any activity is dangerous," that their "heart function is only 50% of normal" (when in fact they were told that ejection fraction is 50%), that their "family has heart disease so there is nothing I can do to help myself," and/or that "heart failure means I have failed." Although such examples may seem excessive, in reality many patients are overwhelmed with notions of mortality and loss of control, feelings that are then made worse in the haze of foreshortened hospitalizations in which life and death dynamics are squeezed together with rapid revascularization and discharge. Many patients often report to rehabilitation with little recall of their incident hospitalization and/or medical instructions, as both emotions and anesthesia (for those who were revascularized) commonly blur their memories.

These examples demonstrate situations in which even basic explanations help to catalyze improved wellness behaviors and compliance, as well as to reduce stress. Furthermore, education plays a key role in modifying cardiovascular risk, particularly diabetes, hypertension, weight reduction, and smoking cessation. Nutrition education is similarly key, modifying intake of high-lipid foods, high caloric intake, as well as excessive salt.

Many programs incorporate shopping or restaurant expeditions and cooking classes into the cardiac rehabilitation curriculum, providing key learning opportunities for patients and their families.

Beyond these overt issues, education relates to a more fundamental set of behavioral modifications. Adults participating in cardiac rehabilitation are typically at a point in their health and recovery in which they are often exceptionally receptive to new lifestyle patterns. Stages of patients' readiness for healthful behavior change have been described in terms of (a) precontemplation, (b) contemplation, (c) preparation and action, and (d) maintenance. Cardiac rehabilitation staff members are trained to identify the readiness for changes of each patient and then formulate strategies to best help each patient advance toward durable behavior modifications. Personalized education interventions are then aimed at improving cardiac risk, managing emergencies, understanding the disease process, maintaining psychosocial health, and adapting to limitations imposed by the disease process (45). These sophisticated objectives are consistent with advanced theories of adult learning (i.e., creating a learning environment in which adults feel self-directed and actively involved in their own learning experience) (46).

Physician involvement in the education process is highly effective. Although cardiac rehabilitation depends on a team with wide-ranging skills and expertise, the physician's presence and recommendations are powerful contributors to healthful behaviors (47).

In addition to individual feedback and clarifications, educational talks are usually presented to patients as a group. Pertinent topics include guidelines about exercise at home, better understanding of cardiovascular physiology and disease, lipid management, stress reduction, explanations of common medicines and adherence recommendations, and more. Even for patients who feel that they are already well informed, cardiac rehabilitation provides a forum to resolve uncertainties created by discrepant information from different sources and to become aware of research developments.

Psychosocial Assessment

In addition to exercise training and risk-factor modification, psychosocial interventions are a fundamental feature of cardiac rehabilitation. Depression, anger, and social isolation are among the affective issues that exacerbate cardiovascular disease and diminish medical compliance. Therefore, cardiac rehabilitation includes psychosocial screening, as well as mechanisms to modify these problems by a physician or ancillary clinical specialists, such as psychologists and social workers. The value of these interventions is reinforced by concomitant exercise, nutrition counseling, and medication surveillance.

DESIGN OF CARDIAC REHABILITATION

A case manager is a critical part of the cardiac rehabilitation organization. This person usually works with the supervising physician to identify, stratify, and implement a risk-reduction strategy for each cardiac rehabilitation patient. The case manager also plays a key role coordinating care among the comprehensive cardiac rehabilitation staff (i.e., physician, nurses, exercise physiologists, nutritionists, and psychosocial specialists). Close links are also maintained with the referring physician, especially as medication adjustments are often indicated as patients advance toward more active routines or dietary changes. Whereas the exact responsibilities and visibility of the supervising physician may vary from one program to another, the physician usually performs an initial medical evaluation and stress test and formulates an exercise prescription based on baseline capacity and cardiovascular risks. The physician's role also includes regular medical surveillance, teaching, and reinforcement of the instructions provided by others in the cardiac rehabilitation program.

Beyond such organizational details, key features of cardiac rehabilitation often extend to interpersonal dynamics among the patients. Much of the success of cardiac rehabilitation seems to relate to the social connections that form in the course of patients' participation. Research is validating that interpersonal bonds and community play a key role in attaining and then maintaining healthful lifestyle choices (48). Therefore, the process itself affords cathartic value, in catalyzing healthful behaviors, exercise and medication adherence, and in overcoming some of the notorious affective contributors (e.g., anger and depression) that may have triggered coronary instability in the first place. Many programs even organize special disease-, age-, or gender-specific cardiac rehabilitation experiences that bolster opportunities for such connections and support to accrue. For example, cardiac rehabilitation sessions that are particularly oriented to diabetes, older patients, PAD, and/or HF have been demonstrated to be particularly effective in promoting ties among the participating patients.

SAFETY OF EXERCISE TRAINING

At entry, many cardiac rehabilitation programs entail a comprehensive exam as well as a stress test as a key means to ensure exercise safety. Exercise prescription is based on the strategy of incremental changes that are of moderate intensity at the outset, but then advance in intensity and duration as safely tolerated. Even risk-factor modifications are modulated to ensure that lifestyle changes are not cumulatively overwhelming, especially in the context of stresses from illness and anxieties about work and other responsibilities.

Given these routines and precautions, cardiac rehabilitation has proven to be remarkably safe. In a survey of 167 supervised programs, the rate of cardiac arrest was 1 per 112,000 patient-hours, and the rate of nonfatal MI was 1 per 294,000 patient-hours; the mortality rate was 1 per 784,000 patient-hours (49). These numbers are considerably smaller than events typically reported for unsupervised exercise.

Even as indications for cardiac rehabilitation have broadened to include patients who raise additional medical concerns (e.g., low ejection fraction and/or very elderly), safety has been preserved (50). Telemetry is often utilized during exercise for patients who are assessed to be at highest risk for arrhythmia or ischemia, but this varies to some extent among institutions.

The safety of strength training in cardiac rehabilitation has been well demonstrated, even for very old CAD and HF patients, and has helped allay concerns that this training modality would be associated with disproportionate risk. In fact, successful strength training leads to improved muscle strength and endurance without increases in ischemia, arrhythmias, or hemodynamic instability.

COST EFFICACY

Cost-effectiveness has been a major concern of caregivers and researchers even since the earliest days of cardiac rehabilitation. Early studies rationalized costs in terms of earlier discharge after MI or CABG (23), but were based on predominantly weak and debilitated patients. A related body of literature asserted that cardiac rehabilitation's cost benefits

should be assessed as a means to facilitate earlier return to work and re-employment (51).

More recently, Ades et al (52) evaluated cost efficacy relative to other ACS treatment modalities. This analysis demonstrated that cardiac rehabilitation improved life expectancy by 0.202 years during a 15-year period and was associated with a cost-effectiveness value of $2,130 to $4,950 (depending on the year) per life-year saved. The results compared favorably with other aspects of ACS management, including thrombolysis, CABG, and cholesterol-lowering medications.

Many see home-based cardiac rehabilitation options as among the most cost-effective strategies. Carlson et al (13) compared traditional cardiac rehabilitation to off-site exercise, educational support, and telephone follow-up. The off-site program yielded relatively higher indices of exercise performance at 3 and 6 months, with $830/patient cost savings compared to traditional hospital-based programs.

EVIDENCE FOR CARDIAC REHABILITATION EFFECTIVENESS

Although the conceptual benefits of exercise training, risk-factor modification, and even psychosocial intervention from cardiac rehabilitation may seem obvious, a lack of unambiguous data demonstrating mortality and morbidity benefits of comprehensive cardiac rehabilitation programs has fueled debate and controversy. Although numerous randomized trials of predominantly *exercise-based* cardiac rehabilitation have been completed over the past 30 years, none has had sufficient statistical power to prove survival benefit. Therefore, several meta-analyses have tried to integrate smaller trials to formulate more definitive conclusions. Two meta-analyses integrated data from more than 21 randomized, controlled trials performed in the 1970s and 1980s involving more than 4,000 patients (53–54). Both showed significantly reduced mortality for patients in cardiac rehabilitation programs compared with usual care (25% reduced total mortality and cardiovascular mortality at 3 years). However, neither demonstrated reduction in rates of reinfarction.

Not only do these meta-analyses depend on smaller trials that were completed years before revascularization or other contemporary therapies had been standardized, but they also focused predominantly on subjects who were generally low-risk, middle-aged white men, thus blunting their generalizability to women, older adults, ethnic minorities, and revascularized patients. A more recent meta-analysis by Taylor et al (56) analyzed benefits of *exercise-based* cardiac rehabilitation, and also showed lower total and cardiac mortality rates with cardiac rehabilitation compared with usual care. Favorable trends were also evident for nonfatal MI and revascularization among the cardiac rehabilitation patients. Moreover, breakdown of Taylor's study showed no differences between trials completed after 1995 to those that were completed earlier, suggesting that the favorable impact of cardiac rehabilitation persisted even in the context of more contemporary management. Efficacy of cardiac rehabilitation was further substantiated by the fact that Taylor's analysis included significant proportions of women, elderly, and revascularized CAD patients. Surprisingly, subgroup analysis showed no significant differences in mortality benefits between programs limited to exercise and those providing more comprehensive secondary interventions.

An even more recent meta-analysis by Joliffe et al (57) studied 8,500 patients from 36 trials to compare exercise-only and comprehensive cardiac rehabilitation programs. The analysis showed 27% reduction in total mortality for the exercise-only programs (OR 0.73; 95% CI, 0.54 to 0.98) and 13% reduction in the comprehensive programs (OR, 0.87; 95% CI, 0.71 to 1.05). The exercise-only intervention also reduced cardiac mortality slightly more than the comprehensive interventions (OR, 0.69; 95% CI, 0.51 to 0.94 for exercise only, versus OR, 0.74; 95% CI, 0.57 to 0.96 for comprehensive programs). Neither had an effect on nonfatal MI.

These meta-analyses demonstrated the value of exercise-based cardiac rehabilitation programs to modify mortality and morbidity. Although both Taylor's and Joliffe's meta-analyses failed to show the expected superiority of comprehensive cardiac rehabilitation, the studies were based primarily on trials that antedated widespread revascularization and most essentials of contemporary medical management. It seems probable that if comprehensive management included beta-blockers, ACE inhibitors, statins, and other features of today's standards for care, this strategy would more significantly reduce total and cardiovascular mortality, as well as recurrent MI (58).

The rationale for comprehensive risk-factor reduction using the case-management model is substantiated by data from the MULTIFIT (59) and SCRIP (19) studies. In the former, a case-management program was utilized for men and women after MI. An intervention of risk reduction including a nurse case-manager, education, and risk reduction counseling brought about improved function as well as reduced risk indices. In the SCRIP study, a similar intervention for CAD patients demonstrated not only significant risk reduction, but also improvements in rates of coronary angiography and rehospitalization and reduced recurrent cardiac events.

Although some authorities have asserted that effective risk reduction can be achieved without a formalized program, a strongly worded manuscript by Ades, Balady, and Berra argues to the contrary (60). These authors emphasize that physicians in clinical practice have not been particularly effective in assisting CAD patients to attain well-defined risk-factor goals and refer to the fact that only 9% to 25% of CAD patients in practice settings have met the NCEP guidelines for lipid management. Likewise, a significant percentage of patients treated only by their primary physicians were not taking preventive medications that have been shown to improve long-term outcomes. They conclude that focused and well-organized risk-factor reduction as provided in a formal program of cardiac rehabilitation is a critical part of clinical effectiveness.

WHAT IS CRITICAL IN CARDIAC REHABILITATION?

Given this orientation to comprehensive cardiac rehabilitation, multiple challenges will inevitably arise over the next several years. A key question to be addressed is, What are the critical elements in cardiac rehabilitation, and, in particular, What are the elements that should be preserved even if formats change?

Exercise training is a vital component. Although patients with CAD are no longer as debilitated and frail as in the past, it still remains difficult for most people to initiate an exercise routine. Even for patients who claim they already exercise, guidance remains crucial in knowing how to exercise safely and effectively, especially in the period following an ACS event. Cardiac rehabilitation provides critical assessment, supervision, education, and monitoring to ensure safety, confidence, and maximal comfort as patients adapt to new medical complexities or exercise behaviors. These challenges are most conspicuous in the caregiving provided to frail populations (i.e., people for whom unsupervised exercise would likely be the most upsetting and dangerous). Among the many benefits of cardiac rehabilitation is direct supervision of exercise, providing ample opportunity to learn and practice techniques that

avoid musculoskeletal injury, Valsalva, and hemodynamic instability, as well as opportunity to intervene if any medical instability develops. These benefits are particularly useful in the application of strength training and the growing array of exercise modalities that are now used synergistically with traditional aerobic exercise. Furthermore, cardiac rehabilitation offers opportunities to link exercise with other risk-reduction goals, potentially reinforcing smoking cessation, weight loss, glycemic control, and blood pressure reduction.

Comprehensive risk modification is also a critical component of cardiac rehabilitation. Risk reduction under the supervision of a case manager significantly affects morbidity and mortality for CAD as well as other cardiovascular diseases. Surprisingly, there are no unambiguous data to prove the superiority of cardiac rehabilitation as an exercise and comprehensive risk reduction program, but most assume it to be true, based on the proven benefits of exercise alone, risk reduction alone, and the intuitive rationale for their combination.

Even less tangible but just as significant are those benefits of cardiac rehabilitation derived from education, from the relationships and community that develop among patients to the interventions taken to mitigate underlying psychosocial pressures. The value of such gains is extensive, especially because cardiac rehabilitation patients often begin the program overwhelmed by emotion, confusion, and financial turmoil as they struggle with the circumstances of recent coronary events, revascularization, and/or new medications. Furthermore, cardiac rehabilitation often helps catalyze a narrow window of opportunity toward fundamental behavior shifts and healthful choices. Expertise at behavior modification is an essential component in a successful program.

As an outpatient model, cardiac rehabilitation has evolved over 20 years into a refined curriculum with a multifaceted staff that integrates exercise-inducing strategies to overall health and risk-factor modification. Furthermore, cardiac rehabilitation is remarkably safe. Technologies applied to home-based programs may recreate some of these attributes in a model that it is more cost effective and may even afford unique capacities to circumvent logistical constraints and thereby reach more patients. Still, it remains unclear if home-based programs can still offer the same utility and safety as today's outpatient program models.

SUMMARY

Cardiac rehabilitation is a comprehensive secondary prevention program that links exercise training goals to other aspects of risk-factor modification. It has proven therapeutic for both quality and duration of life in the ACS patient, including men, women, elderly, and ethnic minorities. The rationale for exercise and risk-factor modification is consistent with our newest paradigms of cardiovascular pathophysiology. Future research is essential to explore the efficacy of home-based and other novel alternatives.

References

1. White PD, Rusk HA, Lee PR, et al. *Rehabilitation of the cardiovascular patient.* New York: McGraw-Hill; 1958.
2. Levine SA, Lown B. Armchair treatment of acute coronary thrombosis. *JAMA* 1952;148:1365.
3. Wenger NK, Hellerstein HK, Blackburn H, Castranova SJ: Uncomplicated myocardial infarction. Current physician practice in patient management. *JAMA* 1973;224:511.
4. American Association of Cardiovascular & Pulmonary Rehabilitation, ed. *Guidelines for cardiac rehabilitation and secondary prevention programs,* 3rd ed. Champaign, IL: Human Kinetics; 2004.
5. 20th Bethesda Conference: insurability and employability of the patient with

ischemic heart disease. October 3–4, 1988, Bethesda, MD. *J Am Coll Cardiol* 1989;14:1003–1044.

6. Ades PA. Cardiac rehabilitation and secondary prevention of coronary heart disease. *N Engl J Med* 2001;345:892–901.
7. Allen JK, Scott LB, Stewart KJ, et al. Disparities in women's referral to and enrollment in outpatient cardiac rehabilitation. *J Gen Intern Med* 2004;19:747–753.
8. Cardiac rehabilitation programs: a statement for healthcare professionals from the American Heart Association. *Circulation* 1994;90:1602–1610.
9. Miller NH, Haskell WL, Berra K, et al. Home versus group exercise training for increased functional capacity after myocardial infarction. *Circulation* 1984;70:645–649.
10. Southard BH, Southard DR, Nuckolls J. Clinical trials of an internet-based case management system for secondary prevention of heart disease. *J Cardiopulm Rehabil* 2003;23:341–348.
11. Arthur HM, Smith KM, KIodis J, et al. A controlled trial of hospital versus home-based exercise in cardiac patients. *Med Sci Sports Exerc* 2002;34:1544.
12. Gordon NF, English CD, Contractor AS, et al. Effectiveness of three models for comprehensive cardiovascular disease risk reduction. *Am J Cardiol* 2002;89:1263.
13. Carlson JJ, Johnson JA, Franklin BA, VanderLaan RL. Program participation, exercise adherence, cardiovascular outcomes, and program cost of traditional versus modified cardiac rehabilitation. *Am J Cardiol* 2000;86:17.
14. King AC, Pruitt LA, Phillips W, et al. Comparative effects of two physical activity programs on measured and perceived physical functioning and other health-related quality of life outcomes in older adults. *J Gerontol A Biol Sci Med Sci* 2000;55(2):M74–M83.
15. Thompson PD, Buchner D, Piña IL, et al. Exercise and physical activity in the prevention and treatment of atherosclerotic cardiovascular disease: a statement from the Council on Clinical Cardiology (Subcommittee on Exercise, Rehabilitation, and Prevention) and the Council on Nutrition, Physical Activity, and Metabolism (Subcommittee on Physical Activity). *Circulation* 2003;107:3109–3116.
16. Shephard RJ, Balady GJ. Exercise as cardiovascular therapy. *Circulation* 1999;99:963–972.
17. Lakka TA, Venäläinen JM, Rauramaa R, et al. Relation of leisure-time physical activity and cardiorespiratory fitness to the risk of acute myocardial infarction. *N Engl J Med* 1994;330:1549–1554.
18. Balady GJ, Ades PA, Comoss P, et al. Core components of cardiac rehabilitation/secondary prevention programs: a statement for healthcare professionals from the American Heart Association and the American Association of Cardiovascular and Pulmonary Rehabilitation Writing Group. *Circulation* 2000;102(9):1069–1073.
19. Haskell WL, Alderman EL, Fair JM, et al. Effects of intensive multiple risk factor reduction on coronary atherosclerosis and clinical cardiac events in men and women with coronary artery disease. The Stanford Coronary Risk Intervention Project (SCRIP). *Circulation* 1994;89:975–990.
20. Smith SC, Blair SN, Criqui MH, et al. Preventing heart attack and death in patients with coronary disease. *Circulation* 1995;92:2–4.
21. Expert Panel on Detection, Evaluation, and Treatment of High Blood Cholesterol in Adults. Executive Summary of The Third Report of The National Cholesterol Education Program (NCEP) Expert Panel on Detection, Evaluation, And Treatment of High Blood Cholesterol In Adults (Adult Treatment Panel III). *JAMA* 2001;285(19):2486–2497.
22. Leon AS, Franklin BA, Costa F, et al. Cardiac rehabilitation and secondary prevention of coronary heart disease: an American Heart Association scientific statement from the Council on Clinical Cardiology (Subcommittee on Exercise, Cardiac Rehabilitation, and Prevention) and the Council on Nutrition, Physical Activity, and Metabolism (Subcommittee on Physical Activity), in collaboration with the American association of Cardiovascular and Pulmonary Rehabilitation. *Circulation* 2005;111(3):369–76. Erratum in: *Circulation* 2005;111(13):1717.
23. Ades PA, Maloney A, Savage P, et al. Determinants of physical functioning in coronary patients: response to cardiac rehabilitation. *Arch Intern Med* 1999;159:2357–2360.
24. Niebauer J, Hambrecht R, Velich T, et al. Attenuated progression of coronary artery disease after 6 years of multifactorial risk intervention: role of physical exercise. *Circulation* 1997;96:2534–2541.
25. Tanaka H, Dinenno FA, Monahan KD, et al. Aging, habitual exercise, and dynamic arterial compliance. *Circulation* 2000;102:1270–1275.
26. Dimmeler S, Zeiher AM. Exercise and cardiovascular health: get active to "AKTivate" your endothelial nitric oxide synthase. *Circulation* 2003;107:3118–3120.
27. Hambrecht R, Adams V, Erbs S, et al. Regular physical activity improves endothelial function in patients with coronary artery disease by increasing phosphorylation of endothelial nitric oxide synthase. *Circulation* 2003;107:3152–3158.
28. Fukai T, Siegfred MR, Ushio-Fukai M, et al. Regulation of the vascular extracellular superoxide dismutase by nitric oxide and exercise training. *J Clin Invest* 2000;105:1631–1639.
29. Milani RV, Lavie CJ, Mehra MR. Reduction in C-reactive protein through cardiac rehabilitation and exercise training. *J Am Coll Cardiol* 2004;43(6):1056–1061.
30. Kaspis C, Thompson PD. The effects of physical activity on serum C-reactive protein and inflammatory markers: a systematic review. *J Am Coll Cardiol* 2005;45(10):1563–1569.
31. Murry CE, Jennings RB, Reimer KA. Preconditioning with ischemia: a delay of lethal cell injury in ischemic myocardium. *Circulation* 1986;74:1124–1136.
32. Bolli R. The late phase of preconditioning. *Circ Res* 2000;87:972–983.
33. Rauramaa R, Li G, Vaisanen SB. Dose-response and coagulation and hemostatic factors. *Med Sci Sports Exerc* 2001;33:S516–S520, S528–S529.
34. Fagard RH. Exercise characteristics and the blood pressure response to dynamic physical training. *Med Sci Sport Exerc* 2001;33:S484–S492.
35. Pescatello LS, Franklin BA, Fagard R, et al. American College of Sports Medicine position stand: exercise and hypertension. *Med Sci Sports Exerc* 2004;36(3):533–553.
36. Kraus WE, Houmard JA, Duscha BD, et al. Effects of the amount and intensity of exercise on plasma lipoproteins. *N Engl J Med* 2002;347:1483–1492.
37. Stewart KJ. Exercise training and the cardiovascular consequences of type 2 diabetes and hypertension: plausible mechanisms for improving cardiovascular health. *JAMA* 2002;288:1622–1631.
38. Ross R, Janssen I. Physical activity, total and regional obesity: dose-response considerations. *Med Sci Sports Exerc* 2001;33:S521–S527.
39. Kingwell BA, Dart AM, Jennings GL, et al. Exercise training reduces the sympathetic component of the blood pressure-heart rate baroreflex in man. *Clin Sci* 1992;82:357–362.
40. Modifiable cardiovascular risk factors. In: American Association of Cardiovascular & Pulmonary Rehabilitation, ed. *Guidelines for cardiac rehabilitation and secondary prevention programs*. 3rd ed. Champaign, IL: Human Kinetics; 2004.
41. Wenger NK, Froehlicher ES, Smith LK, et al. Cardiac rehabilitation: clinical practice guidelines. Rockville, MD: Agency for Health Care Policy and Research and the National Heart, Lung, and Blood Institute; 1995, AHCPR publication no. 96-0672.
42. Leon AS, Rice T, Mandel S, et al. Blood lipid response to 20 weeks of supervised exercise in a large biracial population: the HERITAGE Family Study. *Metabolism* 2000;49:513–520.
43. Leon AS, Sanchez OA. Response of blood lipids to exercise training alone or combined with dietary intervention. *Med Sci Sports Exerc* 2001;33:S502–S515.
44. Durstine JL, Grandjean PW, Davis PG, et al. Blood lipid and lipoprotein adaptations to exercise: a quantitative analysis. *Sports Med* 2001;31:1033–1062.
45. Marcus BH, Simkin LR. The transtheoretical model: applications to exercise behavior. *Med Sci Sports Exerc* 1994;26(11):1400–1404.
46. Education and behavior modification for risk-factor modification. In: American Association of Cardiovascular & Pulmonary Rehabilitation, ed. *Guidelines for cardiac rehabilitation and secondary prevention programs*, 3rd ed. Champaign, IL: Human Kinetics; 2004.
47. Manley MW, Epps RP, Glynn TJ. The clinician's role in promoting smoking cessation among clinic patients. *Med Clin North Am* 1992;76:2,477–494.
48. Schulz AJ, Zenk S, Odoms-Young A, et al. Healthy eating and exercising to reduce diabetes: exploring the potential of social determinants of health frameworks within the context of community-based participatory diabetes prevention. *Am J Public Health* 2005;95(4):645–651.
49. Van Camp SP, Peterson RA. Cardiovascular complications of outpatient cardiac rehabilitation programs. *JAMA* 1986;256:1160–1163.
50. Franklin BA, Bonzheim K, Gordon S, et al. Safety of medically supervised outpatient cardiac rehabilitation therapy: a 16-year follow-up. *Chest* 1998;114:902–906.
51. Dugmore LD, Tipson RJ, Phillips MH, et al. Changes in cardiorespiratory fitness, psychological well-being, quality of life, and vocational status following a 12 month cardiac exercise rehabilitation programme. *Heart* 1999;81:359–366.
52. Ades PA, Pashkow FJ, Neston JR. Cost-effectiveness of cardiac rehabilitation after myocardial infarction. *J Cardiopulmonary Rehab* 1997;17:222–231.
53. O'Connor GT, Buring JE, Yusuf S, et al. An overview of randomized trials of rehabilitation with exercise after myocardial infarction. *Circulation* 1989;80:234–244.
54. Oldridge NB, Guyatt GH, Fischer ME, et al. Cardiac rehabilitation after myocardial infarction: combined experience of randomized clinical trials. *JAMA* 1988;260:945–950.
55. Kaillio V, Hamalainen H, Hakkila J, et al. Reduction in sudden deaths by a multifactorial intervention programme after acute myocardial infarction. *Lancet* 1979;2:1081–1094.
56. Taylor RS, Brown A, Ebrahim S, et al. Exercise-based rehabilitation for patients with coronary heart disease: systemic review and meta-analysis of randomized controlled trials. *Am J Med* 2004;116:682–692.
57. Jolliffe JA, Fees K, Taylor RS, et al. Exercise-based rehabilitation for coronary heart disease. *The Cochrane Library* 2005;3:1–85.
58. Pasternack R. Comprehensive rehabilitation of patients with cardiovascular disease. In: Zipes DP, Libby P, Bonow RO, et al, ed. *Braunwald's heart disease.* Philadelphia: Elsevier Saunders; 2005:1085–1102.
59. DeBurske RF, Houston-Miller N, Superko HR, et al. A case-management system for coronary risk factor modification after acute myocardial infarction. *Ann Intern Med* 1994;120:721–729.
60. Ades PA, Balady GJ, Berra K. Transforming exercise-based cardiac rehabilitation programs into secondary prevention centers: a national imperative. *J Cardiopulm Rehabil* 2001;21:263–272.

Page numbers followed by a t indicate a table, those followed by f indicate a figure.

A

Abciximab
  for cardiogenic shock, 95
    before PCI, 95, 96f
    with reteplase, 95
    before primary PCI, 102
  for STEMI in ED, 41–42
Acarbose, for type 2 diabetes, 255t, 256, 256t
Accelerated diagnostic protocols (ADPs)
  for chest pain, 82
  exercise testing as
    evolution of, 82–83, 83t
    use of, 83, 84f
Activated factor VII, recombinant, for hemorrhage in acute MI, 154
Acute aortic syndromes (AAS), 166–172
  clinical presentation of, 167–169, 168f, 168t
  conditions associated with increased risk of, 166, 166t
  diagnosis of, 169–170, 169f, 170t, 171f
  epidemiology and pathophysiology of, 166–167, 166t
  management of, 170–171
    clinical pathway for, 171–172, 172f
  natural history of, 167
Acute coronary syndrome (ACS)
  definition of, 129
  glucose insulin potassium infusions in, 178
  ST-elevation (See ST-elevation coronary syndromes; ST-elevation myocardial infarction (STEMI))
Acute coronary syndrome (ACS), hyperglycemia in
  intensive management of, 174–179
    background on, 174
    epidemiology of, 174–175
    glucose control in, clinical evidence of, 176–178, 177t
    insulin infusion protocols in, 178–179, 179t
    mechanism of, 175–176
    recommendations for, 178–179
  newly noted, metabolic implications of, 175
Acute coronary syndrome (ACS) in ED, non–ST elevation, 27–37, 133, 133t
  ACC/AHA 2003 guidelines for diagnosis and treatment in, 30, 31f
    benefits of, 37
  ACC/AHA classification of recommendations and levels of evidence in, 27, 28t
  cardiac markers in, 28, 33t
  critical pathways in, 33–37, 34f–36f
  diagnosis and risk stratification of, 27, 28t
  ECG in, 28, 33t
  epidemiology of, 27

history and physical examination in, 27–28, 29t
in-hospital death from, predictors of, 133, 133t
management of
  early conservative, 31f, 32
  early invasive, 31f, 32–33
  medications in, 30–32
  need for, 27
  other tests in, 30
  point-of-care testing of cardiac markers in, 28–30
  quality improvement in, 37
  risk of death or nonfatal MI in, 32, 33t
Acute decompensated heart failure (ADHF), in ED, 46–52. See also Heart failure, in ED
Acute ischemic stroke. See Stroke, acute ischemic (AIS)
Acute myocardial infarction (AMI). See also Myocardial infarction (MI)
  AHA guidelines for, 291–297 (See also AHA Get With the Guidelines Program (GWTG))
  ambulance management of, 9, 10f
  diabetes and
    epidemiology of, 174
    risk of developing, 175
  ED protocol for, in community hospitals, 116, 117t
  hemodynamic parameters in, 141f
  hospital performance data for, 291, 292t
  hyperglycemia first noted with, on morbidity, 174–175
  Killip classification of, 138, 140t
  level 1 protocol for, 15, 16f
  portable box for, 115
  prehospital protocol for, in community hospitals, 114, 114t
  primary percutaneous intervention for, 100–106 (See also Percutaneous coronary intervention (PCI), primary)
Acute myocardial infarction (AMI), complicated, 129–154, 130t
  coronary angiography for, 135, 135f, 136t
  early risk characterization in, 131–133
    identifying high risk patients in, 131–132, 131f, 132f, 133t
    with non–ST-segment elevation MI, 133, 133t
  fundamental concepts of, 129
  mechanical complications of, 143–146
    echocardiogram of, 143, 144f
    left ventricular dilation and aneurysm formation, 145–146
    left ventricular free-wall rupture, 144–145
    mitral regurgitation, 145, 145f

pseudoaneurysm, 145–146
ventricular septal rupture, 143–144
myocardial complications of, 135–143
  cardiogenic shock, 138–139, 140t, 141t
  diastolic dysfunction, 139–142, 142t, 143f
  left ventricular dysfunction, 138–139, 140f, 140t, 141t
  right ventricular infarction, 135, 137t
  management of, 136–138, 138t, 139f
necrotic process in, 129
pathobiologic and clinical sequence of events in, 130f
percutaneous coronary interventions for, 135, 135f, 136t
pericardial complications of, 146–148
  pericarditis, 146, 146t
  postmyocardial infarction (Dressler's) syndrome, 146t, 147
  pulmonary embolism, 147
  systemic embolism, 147, 147f
  thromboembolic, 147
recurrent ischemia in, 133–134, 134f
reinfarction in, 134, 135f
rhythm and conduction disturbances in, 149, 150t, 151t
surgical revascularization for, 135, 135f, 137t
treatment complications of, hemorrhage, 149–154
  from antiplatelet therapy, 149–152, 152t
  from fibrinolytic therapy, 153–154, 153f
  from heparin compounds, 152, 152t, 153f
  from hirudin and other direct thrombin antagonists, 152–153
  recombinant activated factor VII for, 154
  from warfarin, 153, 153f
  wound healing in, cellular characteristics of, 129–131
ADHERE registry/program, 190, 193, 194f, 207
ADHERE-EM, 47–48, 47t, 48t
  disease management on outcome in, 51–52, 52t
Advanced cardiac life support (ACLS), early, 19
AFFIRM trial, 187
AHA Get With the Guidelines Program (GWTG), 291–297
  challenge and opportunities in, 296–297
  measure definitions in, 294–295, 295t
  program elements in, 292–294, 294f
  recognition awards in, 295
  results of, 295–296, 297f

AHA guidelines, barriers to use of, 291–292, 293t
Airline flight attendants, defibrillation by, 21
Airport personnel, defibrillation by, 21
Aldosterone antagonists. See also specific agents
  for atherosclerotic disease prevention, 285, 288t
  for heart failure, 204, 206t
  for left ventricular dilation and aneurysm formation after acute MI, 146
α-glucosidase inhibitors (AGIs), for type 2 diabetes, 255t, 256, 256t
Alteplase. See also Tissue plasminogen activator (tPA)
  for acute ischemic stroke, 69f–71f
    dosing of, 70f–71f
    prehospital, 10
  for STEMI in ED, 41, 42t
American Heart Association. See AHA
Amiodarone
  for atrial fibrillation, 56, 58t
    and atrial flutter, 186–187, 187f, 188f
    with CABG, 165
    with congestive heart failure, 56
    with pre-excitation conditions, 56
  for atrial flutter, 186–187, 187f, 188f
  for ventricular tachyarrhythmias, 148t, 149t
Amrinone, for left ventricular dysfunction, 141
Amylin mimetics. See also specific agents
  for type 1 diabetes, 253
  for type 2 diabetes, 255t, 256, 256t
Aneurysm, false, after acute MI, 146
Angiography, coronary. See Catheterization, cardiac
Angioplasty
  for acute MI, 103
  for cardiogenic shock, 96
  for right ventricular infarction, 136, 138f
Angiotensin receptor blockers (ARBs). See also specific agents
  for atherosclerotic disease preventionfor atherosclerotic disease prevention, 285, 288t
  for heart failure, 200–202, 203t
  for hypertension, 268, 269f
Angiotensin renin blockers. See also specific agents
  for acute coronary syndrome, non–ST elevation, 30
Angiotensin-converting enzyme (ACE) inhibitors. See also specific agents
  for acute coronary syndrome, non–ST elevation, 30

Angiotensin-converting enzyme (ACE) inhibitors (continued)
for atherosclerotic disease prevention, 285, 288t
for heart failure, 200, 202t, 203t
for hypertension, 268, 268f
for left ventricular dilation and aneurysm formation after acute MI, 146

Antiarrhythmic agents. See also specific agents
for atrial fibrillation and atrial flutter, 186–187, 187f, 188f
for atrial fibrillation with CABG, 165
for ventricular tachyarrhythmias, 148t

Anticoagulation. See also specific agents
for atrial fibrillation in ED, oral, 60–61, 60t
for atrial fibrillation with CABG, 165
for embolic stroke prevention with atrial flutter/fibrillation, 185–186, 186f

Antiplatelet agents. See also specific agents
for acute coronary syndrome, non–ST elevation, 30
for acute MI, 103
for atherosclerotic disease prevention, 285, 288t
hemorrhage from, in acute MI, 149–152, 152t
for recurrent ischemia, 133, 134f

Antithrombin agents. See also specific agents
for acute coronary syndrome, non–ST elevation, 32

Antithrombotic therapy. See also specific therapies
for atrial fibrillation, in ED, 60–61, 60t, 61f

Anxiolytics. See also specific agents
for recurrent ischemia, 133, 134f

Aortic dissection, 166–172
clinical presentation of, 167–169, 168f, 168t
conditions associated with increased risk of, 166, 166t
diagnosis of, 169–170, 169f, 170t
epidemiology and pathophysiology of, 166, 166t
management of, 170–171
clinical pathway for, 171–172, 172f
natural history of, 167

Aortic intramural hematoma. See Intramural hematoma (IMH)
Aortic syndromes, acute, 166–172. See also Acute aortic syndromes (AAS)
Aortic ulcer, penetrating (PAU), 166–172
clinical presentation of, 167–169, 168f, 168t
conditions associated with increased risk of, 166, 166t
diagnosis of, 169–170, 170t
epidemiology and pathophysiology of, 166–167, 166t
management of, 170–171
clinical pathway for, 171–172, 172f
natural history of, 167

Aortocoronary bypass surgery. See also Coronary artery bypass graft (CABG) surgery
angiography selection criteria for, at community hospitals with off-site backup, 109, 110t

ApoE, in hypertriglyceridemia, 245

Apolipoproteins, 241

Argatroban. See also Direct thrombin antagonists/inhibitors
for coagulopathy in intracerebral hemorrhage, 73
for deep vein thrombosis, 228

Arrhythmia
atrial (See Atrial fibrillation; Atrial flutter)
brady-, 149, 151t
in cardiac catheterization laboratory, management of, 105, 105t
supraventricular, 149, 150t
ventricular
automatic, 131
reentrant, 131
tachyarrhythmia management in, 148t–149t

Arrhythmogenic right ventricular dysplasia/cardiomyopathy, ICD therapy for primary prevention of sudden cardiac death with, 215

Aspiration pneumonia, with stroke, prevention of, 78–79

Aspirin
for acute coronary syndrome, non–ST elevation, 30
for atherosclerotic disease prevention, 285, 288t
for atrial fibrillation, in ED, 60–61, 60t
for embolic stroke prevention in atrial flutter/fibrillation, 185–186, 186f
for fibrinolysis, prehospital, 11
hemorrhage from, in acute MI, 153–154, 153f
for left ventricular dilation and aneurysm formation after acute MI, 146
before primary percutaneous coronary intervention, 101
for recurrent ischemia, 133, 134f
for thrombolysis, as adjunctive therapy, 42–43, 43t

Atheroembolism, after acute MI, 147–149, 148t–149t

Atherogenic dyslipidemia, agents for, 244, 244t

Atherosclerotic vascular disease, secondary prevention of, 285, 286t–288t

Atorvastatin, for hyperlipidemia, 244

Atrial fibrillation, 181–188
48 + hours after, 183, 185f
anticoagulation for embolic stroke prevention in, 185–186
cardiac imaging in, 184–185, 186f
cardioversion to restore sinus rhythm in, 183
duration of, assessing, 183
epidemiology of, 181
etiology and pathophysiology in, 182, 183f
hemodynamic stability in, assessing, 182, 183f
initial assessment in, 181, 182f
lone, 53
management of, 164–165
with permanent fibrillation, 183–184, 185f
rate control medication in, 186, 187f
rhythm control and antiarrhythmic drugs in, 186–187, 187f, 188f
paroxysmal (recurrent), 53
persistent, 53
RACE pathway for, 181, 182f

goals and strategies based on, 181–182, 182f, 183f
up to 48 hours after, 183, 184f
Atrial fibrillation, in ED, 53–61
classification of, 53
epidemiology of, 53
initial evaluation of, 54–55
management of, 56–61
with acute onset AF, 56–58
with acute onset AF, drug and electrical (observation unit) protocols in, 58–60, 59t
antithrombotic therapy in, 60–61, 60t, 61f
emergent electrical cardioversion in, 56
heart rate–controlling medications in, 56, 57t
heart rhythm–controlling medications in, 56, 58t
overview of, 54, 55f
with unstable AF, 56
pathophysiology of, 53–54, 54t

Atrial flutter, 181–188
48 + hours after, 183, 185f
anticoagulation for embolic stroke prevention in, 185–186
cardiac imaging in, 184–185, 186f
cardioversion to restore sinus rhythm in, 183
duration of, assessing, 183
epidemiology of, 181
etiology and pathophysiology in, 182, 183f
hemodynamic stability in, assessing, 182, 183f
initial assessment in, 181, 182f
management of, 184
rate control medication in, 186, 187f
rhythm control and antiarrhythmic drugs in, 186–187, 187f, 188f
RACE pathway for, 181, 182f, 184
goals and strategies based on, 181–182, 182f, 183f
up to 48 hours after, 183, 184f

Attitude barriers, to AHA guideline implementation, 291, 293t
Automated external defibrillators (AEDs), public access, 19–23. See also Defibrillation, public access
Automatic ventricular arrhythmias, 131

B
Baseline patient assessments, in cardiac rehabilitation, 300, 300t
Behavior barriers, to AHA guideline implementation, 291, 293t
Benzodiazepines, for recurrent ischemia, 133, 134f
Beta blockers. See also specific agents
for acute coronary syndrome, non–ST elevation, 30
for aortic dissection, 170
for atherosclerotic disease prevention, 285, 288t
for atrial fibrillation, 56, 57t
prophylaxis against, in CABG, 164
for atrial fibrillation/flutter, rate control in, 186, 187f
contraindications to, 203, 203t
dosing of, 203, 203t
for heart failure, 202–204, 203t, 204t, 205f
important issues with, 204, 204t
for left ventricular diastolic dysfunction in acute MI, 139

for left ventricular dilation and aneurysm formation after acute MI, 146
for myocardial reinfarction, 134, 135f
on myocardial reinfarction risk, 134
OPTIMIZE-HF algorithm for, 204, 205f
before primary percutaneous coronary intervention, 103, 103t
for recurrent ischemia, 133, 134f
side effects of, management of, 204, 204t
for thrombolysis, as adjunctive therapy, 43, 43t
for ventricular tachyarrhythmias, 149t

Biguanides, for type 2 diabetes, 254, 255t, 256t
Bile acid sequestrants, for hyperlipidemia, 244
Biochemical markers, for complicated acute MI, 131–132
Bisoprolol, for heart failure, 202–204, 203t, 204t, 205f
Bivalirudin, for coagulopathy in intracerebral hemorrhage, 73
Biventricular device, echocardiography for optimization of, 219–221
Biventricular failure, hemodynamic parameters in, 141t
Biventricular pacemaker, for heart failure, 216
Blood pressure
cardiovascular events and, 260–261, 261f, 262f, 262t
high (See Hypertension)
systolic, in acute MI, mortality and, 131, 132f
Blood pressure control. See also specific agents
for acute ischemic stroke, 74
for atherosclerotic disease prevention, 285, 286t
in cardiac rehabilitation, 301
Bradyarrhythmias, 149, 151t
Brain natriuretic peptide (BNP), in pulmonary embolism, 229
Bridging therapy, 71
B-type natriuretic peptide (BNP), for heart failure
decision making in, 49–50
diagnosis of, 48–49, 49t
Bupropion, for smoking cessation, 280t

C
Calcium channel blockers. See also specific agents
for atrial fibrillation, 56, 57t
with CABG, 165
for atrial fibrillation/flutter, rate control in, 186, 187f
for hypertension, 267
on myocardial reinfarction risk, 134
for recurrent ischemia, 133, 134f
Candesartan, for heart failure, 200–202, 203t
Captopril, for heart failure, 200, 202t, 203t
Cardiac biomarkers, for pulmonary embolism, 228–229
Cardiac catheterization. See Catheterization, cardiac
Cardiac catheterization laboratory arrhythmia management in, 105, 105t
direct admission to, 15, 17f
Cardiac checklist, 3, 3t
Cardiac death, sudden, ICD therapy for

primary prevention of, 212–215, 214t, 215t
  with arrhythmogenic RV dysplasia/cardiomyopathy, 215
  with hypertrophic cardiomyopathy, 215
secondary prevention of, 211–212, 213t
Cardiac dyssynchrony, 216, 216t
Cardiac enzymes, for complicated acute MI, 131–132
Cardiac markers
  in acute coronary syndrome, non-ST elevation, 28, 33t
  point-of-care testing of, 28–30
Cardiac rehabilitation, 299–304. See also Rehabilitation, cardiac
Cardiac resynchronization therapy (CRT), for heart failure, 216–222
  beneficial effects of, 216, 216t
  biventricular pacemaker design and implantation in, 216
  for cardiac dyssynchrony, 216, 216t
  decision tree for, vs. ICD, 219, 220f
  noninvasive imaging during, 219–222
    cardiovascular magnetic resonance in, 221f, 222
    echocardiography for assessment of dyssynchrony in, 219, 220t, 221f
    echocardiography for biventricular device optimization in, 219–221
    multislice CT in, 221–222
  recommendations for use of, 219, 219t
  trials of, 216–219, 217t–219t
Cardiac tamponade, hemodynamic parameters in, 141t
Cardiogenic shock. See Shock, cardiogenic
Cardiovascular magnetic resonance (CMR), for assessment of resynchronization therapy for heart failure, 221f, 222
Cardioversion
  of atrial fibrillation
    with CABG, direct current, 165
    emergent electrical, 56
    pharmacological, 56, 57t, 58t
  of atrial fibrillation, acute onset drug and electrical (observation unit), 58–60, 59t
    electrical, 57–58
    pharmacological, 57–58
  of atrial flutter/fibrillation, to restore sinus rhythm, 183
  of ventricular tachyarrhythmias, 148t–149t
Cardioverter-defibrillator, implantable
  for heart failure, 204
  for ventricular tachyarrhythmias, 148t, 149t
Carotid endarterectomy (CEA), for stroke and transient ischemic attack, 73
Carvedilol, for heart failure, 202–204, 203t, 204t, 205f
Catheter-based embolectomy, for venous thromboembolism, 230
Catheter-directed thrombolysis, for deep vein thrombosis, 228
Catheterization, cardiac, 155–158
  for acute MI, complicated, 135, 136f
  for cardiogenic shock, 96

indications for, 155–156
informed consent for, 156–157, 157t
patient management in
  after procedure, 158
  during procedure, 158
patient preparation in, 157–158
preoperative evaluation for, 156
risks in, 156–157, 157t
Catheterization laboratory, cardiac
  arrhythmia management in, 105, 105t
  direct admission to, 15, 17f
  protocol for primary PCI at community hospitals in, 116, 120t
Chain of stroke survival, pathways organization into, 77–79, 79f
Chain of survival, 19
Chest pain
  epidemiology and cost of, 81
  identifying low clinical risk with, 81
  spectrum of patients with, 81, 82f
Chest pain units, 81
  accelerated diagnostic protocols in, 82
  concept of, 82
Chest pain units, exercise testing in, 84–88. See also Exercise testing
  immediate (UC Davis method), 86–87, 86t, 87t
    further issues with, 86t, 88
    in special populations, 87–88
  vs. myocardial stress scintigraphy, 87
  safety and efficacy of, 83t, 84
  studies of, 83t, 84–86, 85f, 86f
Cholesterol
  HDL, low, 246–247
  high (See Hyperlipidemia)
  lowering of, rationale for strategies for, 241–243
  target LDL-C level ascertainment in, 244, 244f
Cholesteryl ester transfer protein (CETP), 241
Cholesteryl transferase protein (CETP) inhibitors, for low HDL cholesterol, 247
Cholestyramine, for hyperlipidemia, 244
Chronic venous insufficiency, 228
Circulatory phase, 19
CK-MB, point-of-care testing of, 28–30
Clofibrate, for hypertriglyceridemia, 245
Clopidogrel
  for acute coronary syndrome, non–ST elevation, 30, 33
  for acute MI, 103
  for atherosclerotic disease prevention, 285, 288t
  for fibrinolysis, prehospital, 11
  before primary percutaneous coronary intervention, 102
  for recurrent ischemia, 133, 134f
  for thrombolysis, as adjunctive therapy, 43, 43t
Coagulopathy treatment, in intracerebral hemorrhage, 73
Colesevelam, for hyperlipidemia, 244
Colestipol, for hyperlipidemia, 244
Community hospitals without on-site surgery, primary PCI at, 108–127. See also under Percutaneous coronary intervention (PCI), primary
Computed tomography (CT), for stroke, 74

Conduction disturbances, in acute MI, 149, 151t
COPERNICUS, 202–203
Cor pulmonale, hemodynamic parameters in, 141t
Coronary angiography. See Catheterization, cardiac
Coronary arteriography, 155. See also Catheterization, cardiac; Percutaneous coronary intervention (PCI)
Coronary artery bypass graft (CABG) surgery
  for cardiogenic shock, 96
  for recurrent MI, 135, 137t
Coronary artery bypass graft (CABG) surgery pathways, 160–165
  atrial fibrillation management in, 164–165
  background on, 160–161
  extubation guidelines in, 163–164, 163t
  goals for, 160, 160t
  key outcomes in, 160, 161t
  postoperative, 162–163, 162t
  preoperative, 161–162, 161t
  transfer to step-down order set in, 163, 164t
Coronary artery disease (CAD)
  AHA guidelines for, 291–297 (See also AHA Get With the Guidelines Program (GWTG))
  diabetes and, 174
  performance measures for GWTG for, 294–295, 295t
Coronary bypass surgery (CABG)
  emergency, 105, 105t
  emergency transfer for, from community hospitals without on-site surgery, 112
Coronary care unit
  overutilization of, 2
  reducing length of stay in, after thrombolysis, 97–98, 97f
Coronary catheterization. See Catheterization, cardiac
Coronary heart disease (CHD). See also specific types
  AHA guidelines for, 291–297 (See also AHA Get With the Guidelines Program (GWTG))
  epidemiology of, 291
Coronary vascular disease, secondary prevention for patients with, 285, 286t–288t
Creatine kinase (CK), in acute MI, complicated, 131–132
Critical illness, hyperglycemia on, 176–178, 177t
Critical pathways. See also specific disorders and pathways
  cardiac checklist in, 3, 3t
  vs. clinical protocols, 1
  development of, methods for, 2, 2t
  evidence for benefit of, 3–5, 4f
  goals of, 1, 1t
  implementation of, methods for, 2–3, 2t
  need and rationale for, 2
  reducing hospital stay with, 2
  reducing overutilization of intensive care with, 2

D
Dalteparin, for venous thromboembolism prophylaxis, 233
Danaparoid, for coagulopathy in intracerebral hemorrhage, 73

DDAVP, for intracerebral hemorrhage from platelet disorders, 73
Deep vein thrombosis (DVT). See also Venous thromboembolism (VTE)
  diagnosis of, 225–226, 225f, 225t
  oral anticoagulant therapy for, 231–233
    epidemiologic approach to, 232, 232t
    newer drugs in, 231
    optimal duration of, 231–232, 232t
    warfarin in, 231
  prevention of, 233–235, 233t, 234f, 234t
    with stroke, 79
  treatment of, initial, 227–228, 228f
Defibrillation
  home, 22
  time to, importance of, 19
Defibrillation, public access, 19–23
  by airline flight attendants, 21
  by airport personnel, 21
  cost benefit of, 22
  early, by public safety personnel, 19–20, 21
  fundamentals of, 19
  history and concept of, 20–21
  at home, 22
  by lay persons, 21–22
  by security officers in Las Vegas gaming casinos, 21
  time to defibrillation in, 19
Diabetes mellitus, 249–257
  acute coronary syndrome with, 174 (See also Acute coronary syndrome (ACS), hyperglycemia in)
  after myocardial infarction, risk of, 175
  categories of, 249, 249t
  control of, education on, 301
  coronary artery disease and, 174
  epidemiology of, 249
  myocardial infarction and, epidemiology of, 174
  prediabetes, 250, 250f
  prevention of
    complications of, 252
    type 1, 250
    type 2, 250–252, 251t
  treatment of hyperglycemia in, 252–257
    for atherosclerotic disease prevention, 285, 287t
    combination therapy for, 257
    DPP-IV inhibitors, 257
    glitazars, 257
    glycemic goals in, 252, 252t
    with type 1 diabetes, amylin mimetics, 253
    with type 1 diabetes, insulin, 252–253, 253t
    with type 2 diabetes, 254–257
    with type 2 diabetes, insulin and insulin analogues, 254
    with type 2 diabetes, noninsulin therapies, 254–257, 255t, 256t
  type 1, 252–253
  type 2, 254
Diabetes Mellitus and Acute Myocardial Infarction (DIGAMI) studies, 178
Diabetic retinopathy, prevention of, 252
Diagnosis. See also specific disorders
  accelerated protocols for (See Accelerated diagnostic protocols (ADPs))
  optimal prehospital, 9–10, 10f

Diastolic dysfunction, with acute MI, 139–142, 142t, 143f
Dietary modification
    for hyperlipidemia, 243
    for hypertriglyceridemia, 245
Digoxin
    for atrial fibrillation, 56, 57t
        with congestive heart failure, 56
    for atrial fibrillation/flutter, rate control in, 186, 187f
    for congestive heart failure, 56
    for heart failure, 206, 207t
Diltiazem
    for atrial fibrillation, 56, 57t
        with CABG, 165
        with congestive heart failure, 56
        rate control in, 186, 187f
    for atrial flutter, rate control in, 186, 187f
Dipeptidyl peptidase IV (DPP-IV) inhibitors. See also specific agents
    for diabetes mellitus, 257
Direct current cardioversion (DCCV), for atrial fibrillation with CABG, 165
Direct thrombin antagonists/ inhibitors. See also specific agents
    for acute MI, 104
        hemorrhage from, 152–153
    for coagulopathy in intracerebral hemorrhage, 73
    for deep vein thrombosis, 228
Disease management, 1
Diuretics
    for congestive heart failure, 140–141
    for heart failure, 206, 207t, 208t
Dobutamine
    for congestive heart failure, 140
    for heart failure, early use of, 50–51, 51f
    for hypotension with right ventricular infarction, 137
    for ventricular septal rupture, 144
Dofetilide
    for atrial fibrillation, 56, 58t, 186–187, 187f, 188f
    for atrial flutter, 186–187, 187f, 188f
Door-to-balloon times, 109, 114
    community hospital programs to improve, 116–117, 120–121, 121t
Dopamine
    for congestive heart failure, 140
    for heart failure, early use of, 50–51, 51f
    for hypotension with right ventricular infarction, 137
    for ventricular septal rupture, 144
Dressler's syndrome, 146t, 147
Dyslipidemia
    atherogenic, agents for, 244, 244f
    secondary prevention of atherosclerotic disease and, 285, 286t–287t
Dysmetabolic syndrome. See Metabolic syndrome

E
Echocardiography
    for assessment of dyssynchrony, 219, 220t, 221f
    for biventricular device optimization, 219–221
    for cardiogenic shock, reducing, 97
    of mechanical complications of acute MI, 143, 144f
    of pulmonary embolism, 229

Education
    community, on stroke, 77
    patient, in cardiac rehabilitation, 301–302, 304
Electrical phase, 19
Electrocardiogram (ECG)
    of acute coronary syndrome, non–ST elevation, 28, 33t
    of acute MI, complicated, 131, 132f
    of atrial fibrillation, 181
    of atrial flutter, 181
    of patients with chest pain, to identify low clinical risk, 81
    prehospital, 13
    of ST-elevation myocardial infarction, 39, 40f, 41t
Embolectomy, for venous thromboembolism, 230–231
Embolic stroke, anticoagulation to prevent atrial flutter/ fibrillation in, 185–186, 186f
Embolism, after acute MI
    pulmonary, 147, 147f
    systemic, 147, 147f, 149
Emergency department (ED), non–ST elevation acute coronary syndrome in, 27–37. See also Acute coronary syndrome (ACS) in ED, non–ST elevation
Emergency medical services (EMS)
    early defibrillation by, 19–20
    effective communication with, for stroke, 77–78
Emergent carotid endarterectomy, for stroke and transient ischemic attack, 73
Emergent electrical cardioversion, for atrial fibrillation, 56
Enalapril, for heart failure, 200, 202t, 203t
Endarterectomy, emergent carotid, for stroke and transient ischemic attack, 73
Endovascular therapy. See also specific therapies
    for aneurysmal spontaneous intracerebral hemorrhage, 73
Enoxaparin
    for acute coronary syndrome, non–ST elevation, 32
    for deep vein thrombosis, 227
    for fibrinolysis, prehospital, 11
    prehospital, 11
    protamine for anticoagulant effects of, 152, 152t
    for thrombolysis, as adjunctive therapy, 43–44, 43t
Eplerenone, for heart failure, 204, 206t
Eptifibatide, for acute coronary syndrome, non–ST elevation, 30–32
Esmolol
    for atrial fibrillation, 56, 57t
    for atrial fibrillation/flutter, rate control in, 186, 187f
Estrogen replacement therapy, for hyperlipidemia, 243–244
Exenatide, for type 2 diabetes, 255t, 256–257, 256t
Exercise testing
    in accelerated diagnostic protocols, 82
    early
        evolution of, 82–83, 83t
        use of, 83, 84f
Exercise testing, in chest pain units, 84–88
    immediate (UC Davis method), 86–87, 86t, 87f
        further issues with, 86t, 88
        in special populations, 87–88

vs. myocardial stress scintigraphy, 87
    safety and efficacy of, 83t, 84
    studies of, 83t, 84–86, 85f, 86f
Exercise training, in cardiac rehabilitation, 301, 303
    safety of, 302
Extubation, after coronary artery bypass surgery, 163–164, 163t
Ezetimibe, for hyperlipidemia, 244

F
Facilitated percutaneous coronary intervention (PCI), 40–41, 94–95. See also Percutaneous coronary intervention (PCI)
Factor Xa inhibitors. See also specific agents
    for acute coronary syndrome, non–ST elevation, 32
Fagerstrom test for nicotine dependence, 274, 277t
False aneurysm, after acute MI, 146
Fenofibrate, micronized, for hypertriglyceridemia, 245
Fibrates. See also specific agents
    for hypertriglyceridemia, 245
Fibrillation
    atrial (See Atrial fibrillation)
    ventricular, management of, 148t–149t
Fibrinolysis
    on myocardial reinfarction risk, 134
    for right ventricular infarction, 136, 138f
    stroke from, risk factors and predictors of, 132, 133t
Fibrinolysis, prehospital, 9–12. See also Thrombolysis; specific agents
    adjunctive therapy in, 11
    alternative reperfusion strategies in ambulance in, 11–12, 11f
    diagnosis for, optimal, 9, 10f, 11f
    drug administration in, 10–11
    reperfusion therapy in, 9
Fibrinolytic therapy. See also specific therapies
    full-dose, for cardiogenic shock, 95, 95f
    with GP IIb/IIIa inhibition, for cardiogenic shock, 95
    hemorrhage from, in acute MI, 153–154, 153f
Fish oils, for hypertriglyceridemia, 246
Flecainide
    for atrial fibrillation, 56, 58t
        with pre-excitation conditions, 56
    for atrial fibrillation and atrial flutter, 186–187, 187f, 188f
Flight attendants, airline, defibrillation by, 21
Fluvastatin, for hyperlipidemia, 244
Fondaparinux
    for acute coronary syndrome, non–ST elevation, 32
    for coagulopathy in intracerebral hemorrhage, 73
    for deep vein thrombosis, 227
    for pulmonary embolism, 230
    for venous thromboembolism prophylaxis, 233–234
Fosinopril, for heart failure, 200, 202t, 203t
Fresh frozen plasma (FFP), for coagulopathy in intracerebral hemorrhage, 73

G
Gemfibrozil, for hypertriglyceridemia, 245

Get with the Guidelines Program, AHA, 291–297. See also AHA Get With the Guidelines Program (GWTG)
Glimepiride, for type 2 diabetes, 254, 255t, 256t
Glipizide, for type 2 diabetes, 254, 255t, 256t
Glitazars, for diabetes mellitus, 257
Glucose, impaired fasting, 250, 250f
Glucose control, in critical illness and acute coronary syndrome, 176–178, 177t
Glucose insulin potassium (GIK), in acute coronary syndrome, 178
Glucose tolerance
    categories of, 249–250, 249t, 250f
    impaired, 250, 250f
Glyburide, for type 2 diabetes, 254, 255t, 256t
Glycemic goals, in hyperglycemia treatment, 252, 252t
Goals, of critical pathways, 1, 1t. See also specific diorders and pathways
GP IIb/IIa inhibitors, for cardiogenic shock, before PCI, 95–97, 96f
GP IIb/IIIa receptor inhibitors. See also specific agents
    for acute coronary syndrome, non–ST elevation, 30–32
    for acute MI, 104
    for cardiogenic shock, 95
    on myocardial reinfarction risk, 134
    before primary percutaneous coronary intervention, 102
    for recurrent ischemia, 133, 134f
Guidelines, AHA. See also AHA Get With the Guidelines Program (GWTG); specific disorders
    barriers to use of, 291–292, 293t
    encouraging use of, 291–297 (See also AHA Get With the Guidelines Program (GWTG))

H
Heart failure, 183, 190–209
    ADHERE program on, 193, 194f
    AHA guidelines for, 291–297 (See also AHA Get With the Guidelines Program (GWTG))
    critical pathway tools for, 193–200
        admission checklist in, 193, 195f–196f
        critical pathways grid in, 197, 198f
        discharge summary checklist in, 197, 199f
        rationale for, 193
        standard orders in, 193, 197, 197f
        success of, 197, 200, 201f, 202f
    epidemiology of, 190, 291
    hospital performance data for, 291, 292t
    JCAHO core performance measures for, 190, 191t
    next steps in, 207
    patient education in, 206–207
    performance measures for GWTG for, 294–295, 296t
    risks with, 210
    risk-treatment mismatch in, 192–193, 193f, 194f
    treatment for, in-hospital initiation of, 192–193, 193f

treatment for, optimal, 200–206
  ACE inhibitors in, 200, 202t,
    203t
  aldosterone antagonists in,
    204, 206t
  angiotensin II receptor blockers
    in, 200–202, 203t
  beta blockers in, 202–204,
    203t, 204t, 205f
  digoxin in, 206, 207t
  diuretics in, 206, 207t, 208t
  nonpharmacologic, 204
  with preserved systolic
    function, 204
  symptomatic, 206, 207t
  underutilization of standard-of-
    care therapies for, 190–191,
    191t, 192f
  reasons for, 193
Heart failure, cardiac
  resynchronization therapy
  for, 216–222
  beneficial effects of, 216, 216t
  biventricular pacemaker design
    and implantation in, 216
  for cardiac dyssynchrony, 216,
    216t
  vs. ICD, decision tree for, 219,
    220f
  noninvasive imaging during,
    219–222
  cardiovascular magnetic
    resonance in, 221f, 222
  echocardiography for
    assessment of dyssynchrony
    in, 219, 220t, 221f
  echocardiography for
    biventricular device
    optimization in, 219–221
  multislice CT in, 221–222
  recommendations for use of, 219,
    219t
  trials of, 216–219, 217t–218t
Heart failure, implantable
  cardioverter-defibrillator
  (ICD) for, 210–215
  background on, 210
  components and function of,
    210–211, 212rf
  vs. CRT, decision tree for, 219,
    220f
  goals and rationale of, 210, 211t
  implantation of, 211
  for sudden cardiac death
    prevention
    primary, 212–215, 214t, 215t
    primary, with arrhythmogenic
      RV dysplasia, 215
    primary, with hypertrophic
      cardiomyopathy, 215
    secondary, 211–212, 213t
  use of, 210, 211f
Heart failure, in ED, 46–52
  ADHERE-EM observations on,
    47–48, 47t, 48t
  demographics of, 46–47, 46t
  diagnosis of
    chest radiography in, 48
    history and physical findings
      in, sensitivity of, 48, 48t
    troponin in, 47, 47t
  disease management for, 47, 47t
    ADHERE-EM, on outcome,
      51–52, 52t
  hemodynamic mismatch vs.
    volume overload in, 50
  natriuretic peptides in
    for decision making, 49–50
    for diagnosis, 48–49, 49t
  risk stratification for, 50, 51f
    early vasoactive use in, 50–51,
      51f
Hematoma, intramural (IMH). See
  Intramural hematoma (IMH)

Hemodynamic parameters, in
  commonly encountered
  clinical situations, 141t
Hemorrhage
  from acute MI treatment,
    149–152, 152t
  intracerebral, treatment of
    for coagulopathy, 73
    with spontaneous hemorrhae,
      73
    surgery or endovascular
      therapy in, 73
  intracranial, from thrombolysis
    for STEMI in ED, 43f, 44
  subarachnoid, treatment of, 73
Heparin
  for acute coronary syndrome,
    non–ST elevation, 32
  for atrial fibrillation with CABG,
    165
  for fibrinolysis, prehospital, 11
  hemorrhage from, in acute MI,
    152, 152t, 153f
  low molecular weight
    for acute MI, 104
    for coagulopathy in
      intracerebral hemorrhage, 73
    for deep vein thrombosis, 227
    on myocardial reinfarction
      risk, 134
    protamine sulfate on, 73
    for pulmonary embolism, 230
    for recurrent ischemia, 133,
      134f
    for thrombolysis, as adjunctive
      therapy, 43–44, 43t
    for venous thromboembolism
      prophylaxis, 233–234
  with percutaneous coronary
    intervention
    preprocedural, 101
    procedural, 104
  for STEMI in ED, 41
  unfractionated
    for coagulopathy in
      intracerebral hemorrhage, 73
    for pulmonary embolism,
      229–230
    for recurrent ischemia, 133,
      134f
    for thrombolysis, as adjunctive
      therapy, 43–44, 43t
    for venous thromboembolism
      prophylaxis, 233
Hepatic lipase, 241
Hirudin, hemorrhage from, in acute
  MI, 152–153
Home defibrillation, 22
Hormone replacement therapy
  (HRT), for hyperlipidemia,
  243–244
Hospital length of stay, reducing, 2
  after thrombolysis, 97–98, 97f
Hospital performance data, for MI,
  heart failure, and stroke,
  291, 292t
Hypercholesterolemia. See
  Hyperlipidemia
Hyperglycemia
  in acute coronary syndrome,
    intensive management of,
    174–179
    background on, 174
    epidemiology of, 174–175
    glucose control in, clinical
      evidence of, 176–178, 177t
    insulin infusion protocols in,
      178–179, 179t
    mechanism of, 175–176
    recommendations for, 178–179
  on critical illness, 176–178, 177t
  electrophysiological abnormalities
    with, 176

first noted
  with acute coronary syndrome,
    metabolic implications of,
    175
  with myocardial infarction, on
    morbidity, 174–175
  on myocardial energy, 175–176
  on myocardial function, 176,
    177t
  stress, 175
  vascular function and
    inflammation in, 176
Hyperlipidemia, 241–247
  epidemiology of, 241
  genetic disorders in, 245
  hypertriglyceridemia with,
    245–246, 246f
  lipid modifying enzymes and
    transport proteins in, 241
  lipoprotein metabolism and, 241
  with low HDL, 246–247
  nonpharmacologic therapy for,
    243–244
  pharmacologic therapy for, 244,
    244f, 245f
  rationale for cholesterol lowering
    strategies in, 241–243
  risk factor evaluation with, 244,
    244f
  target LDL-C level ascertainment
    in, 244, 244f
Hyperlipoproteinemia, 245. See
  also Hyperlipidemia
Hypertension, 260–271
  blood pressure approach to,
    260–261, 261f, 262f, 262t
  definitions of, 260–261
    more fundamental, 263–264,
      263f
  evaluation of patient with, 264
  history of, 260
  idiopathic pulmonary,
    hemodynamic parameters in,
    141t
  staging of, 261–263
  treatment of, 264–271
    ACE inhibitors in, 268, 268f
    angiotensin receptor blockers
      in, 268, 269f
    calcium channel blockers in,
      267
    in children, 268–269
    compelling indications for,
      266–267, 266t
    conflicting nonantihypertensive
      drugs in, 269–270
    drug, favoring particular agents
      in, 267–268, 268f
    drug, starting, 265–267, 265f,
      266t
    drug combinations in, 267
    drug combinations in,
      inappropriate, 269
    effectiveness of, 270–271
    for hypertensive emergencies
      and urgencies, 270
    inadequate responses to,
      269–270
    JNC 7 algorithm for, 265–266
    lifestyle modifications in,
      264–265, 265f, 265t
    in pregnancy, 268–269
    with secondary hypertension,
      270, 270t
Hypertensive emergencies,
  treatment of, 270
Hypertensive urgencies, treatment
  of, 270
Hypertriglyceridemia, 245–246,
  246f
Hypertrophic cardiomyopathy, ICD
  therapy for prevention of
  sudden cardiac death with,
  215
Hypoalphalipoproteinemia,
  246–247

Hypovolemic shock, hemodynamic
  parameters in, 141t
Hypoxia, on myocardial energy,
  175–176

I
Ibutilide, for atrial fibrillation, 56,
  58t
Idiopathic pulmonary hypertension,
  hemodynamic parameters in,
  141t
IMPACT-HF, 200, 203
Impaired fasting glucose (IFG), 250,
  250f
Impaired glucose tolerance (IGT),
  250, 250f
Implantable cardioverter-
  defibrillator (ICD)
  implantation of, 211
  for ventricular tachyarrhythmias,
    148t, 149t
Implantable cardioverter-
  defibrillator (ICD), for heart
  failure, 204, 210–222
  background on, 210
  components and function of,
    210–211, 212f
  decision tree for, vs. CRT, 219,
    220f
  goals and rationale of, 210, 211t
  implantation of, 211
  sudden cardiac death prevention
    in
    primary, 212–215, 214t, 215t
    primary, with arrhythmogenic
      RV dysplasia/
      cardiomyopathy, 215
    primary, with hypertrophic
      cardiomyopathy, 215
    secondary, 211–212, 213t
  use of, 210, 211f
Incretin mimetics, for type 2
  diabetes, 255t, 256–257,
  256t
Infarct wave front, 9
Infarction, recurrent, 134, 135f
Inferior vena caval filters, for
  venous thromboembolism,
  230
Inflammation, in hyperglycemia,
  176
Inflammatory markers, for
  complicated acute MI, 132
Influenza vaccination, for
  atherosclerotic disease
  prevention, 285, 288t
Insulin
  infusion protocols for, 178–179,
    179t
  for type 1 diabetes, 252–253,
    253t
  for type 2 diabetes, 254
Insulin analogues, for type 2
  diabetes, 254
Insulin resistance syndrome. See
  Metabolic syndrome
Insulin sensitizers. See also specific
  agents
  for type 2 diabetes, 254–256,
    255t, 256t
Intensive care. See also specific
  types and disorders
  overutilization of, 2
International Normalized Ratio
  (INR)
  for atrial fibrillation patients, 61,
    61f
  bleeding rate and intensity of,
    232, 232t
Intra-aortic balloon
  counterpulsation, for
  ventricular septal rupture,
  144

Intra-aortic balloon pump (IABP)
    for acute MI, 104
    for recurrent ischemia, 133–134,
        134f
Intracerebral hemorrhage
    spontaneous
        treatment of, 73
    surgery or endovascular therapy
        for, 73
    treating coagulopathy in, 73
Intracranial hemorrhage, from
    thrombolysis for STEMI in
    ED, 43f, 44
Intramural hematoma (IMH),
    166–172
    clinical presentation of, 167–169,
        168f, 168t
    conditions associated with
        increased risk of, 166, 166t
    diagnosis of, 169–170, 170t,
        171f
    epidemiology and
        pathophysiology of,
        166–167, 166t
    management of, 170–171
        clinical pathway for, 171–172,
            172f
    natural history of, 167
Irbesartan, for heart failure,
    200–202, 203t
Ischemia, recurrent, 133–134, 134f
Ischemic stroke. See Stroke, acute
    ischemic (AIS)

J
JNC 7 algorithm, for hypertension,
    265–266

K
Killip classification, 138, 140t
Knowledge barriers, to AHA
    guideline implementation,
    291, 293t
Kussmaul's sign, 136

L
Las Vegas gaming casinos,
    defibrillation by security
    officers in, 21
Lecithin-cholesterol acyltransferase
    (LCAT), 241
Left ventricular aneurysm
    formation, after acute MI,
    145–146
Left ventricular assist device,
    percutaneous, for acute MI,
    104
Left ventricular dilation, after acute
    MI, 145–146
Left ventricular dysfunction
    with acute MI, 138–139, 140f,
        140t, 141t
    diastolic, with acute MI,
        139–142, 142t, 143f
Left ventricular failure,
    hemodynamic parameters in,
    141t
Left ventricular free-wall rupture,
    after acute MI, 144–145
Left ventricular thrombus, after
    acute MI, 147–149, 147f,
    148t–149t
Lepirudin. See also Direct thrombin
    antagonists/inhibitors
    for coagulopathy in intracerebral
        hemorrhage, 73
    for deep vein thrombosis, 228
Lidocaine, for ventricular
    tachyarrhythmias, 148t
Lipid disorders. See Hyperlipidemia
Lipid modification, in cardiac
    rehabilitation, 301
Lipoprotein lipase, 241
Lipoproteinemia, hypoalpha-,
    246–247

Lipoproteins
    families of, 241
    metabolism of, 241
Lisinopril, for heart failure, 200,
    202t, 203t
Lone atrial fibrillation, 53
Lopressor, before primary
    percutaneous coronary
    intervention, 84t, 103
Losartan, for heart failure,
    200–202, 203t
Lovastatin, for hyperlipidemia, 244
Low molecular weight heparin
    (LMWH)
    for acute MI, 104
    for coagulopathy in intracerebral
        hemorrhage, 73
    for deep vein thrombosis, 227
    on myocardial reinfarction risk,
        134
    protamine sulfate on, 73
    for pulmonary embolism, 230
    for recurrent ischemia, 133, 134f
    for thrombolysis, as adjunctive
        therapy, 43–44, 43t
    for venous thromboembolism
        prophylaxis, 233–234

M
Magnesium, for atrial fibrillation,
    56, 57t
Magnetic resonance, cardiovascular,
    for resynchronization
    therapy assessment for heart
    failure, 221f, 222
Magnetic resonance imaging (MRI),
    for stroke, 74
Mechanical embolectomy device,
    for ischemic stroke, 71
Mechanical embolectomy removal
    in cerebral ischemia
    (MERCI), for ischemic
    stroke, 71
Meglitinides, for type 2 diabetes,
    254, 255t, 256t
MERIT-HF, 203
Metabolic phase, 19
Metabolic syndrome, 249–257
    definition and synonyms for, 250
    epidemiology of, 249
    risk factor approach and, 263
    risks associated with, 250
Metformin, for type 2 diabetes,
    254, 255t, 256t
Metoprolol
    for atrial fibrillation, 56, 57t
        with CABG, 165
        with CABG, prophylaxis
            against, 164
        rate control in, 186, 187f
    for atrial flutter, rate control in,
        186, 187f
    for heart failure, 202–204, 203t,
        204t, 205f
    for thrombolysis, as adjunctive
        therapy, 43, 43t
Micronized fenofibrate, for
    hypertriglyceridemia, 245
Miglitol, for type 2 diabetes, 255t,
    256, 256t
Milrinone, for left ventricular
    dysfunction, 141
Ministroke. See Transient ischemic
    attack (TIA)
Mitral regurgitation, after acute
    MI, 145, 145f
Morphine
    for acute coronary syndrome,
        non–ST elevation, 30
    for thrombolysis, as adjunctive
        therapy, 42, 43t
Morphine sulfate, for recurrent
    ischemia, 133, 134f
Multislice computed tomography
    (MSCT), of cardiac

resynchronization therapy
    for heart failure, 221–222
Myocardial energy balance,
    175–176
Myocardial infarction (MI). See
    Acute myocardial infarction
    (AMI); ST-elevation
    myocardial infarction
    (STEMI)
Myocardial ischemia, early
    recurrent, coronary
    angiography and PCI for,
    135, 136t
Myocardial stress scintigraphy,
    exercise testing vs., 87

N
Nateglinide, for type 2 diabetes,
    254, 255t, 256t
Natriuretic peptides. See also
    specific agents
    for heart failure
        decision making in, 49–50
        diagnosis of, 48–49, 49t
        with pulmonary embolism, 229
Nesiritide, for heart failure, early
    use of, 50–51, 51f
Niacin
    for hypertriglyceridemia,
        245–246
    for low HDL cholesterol, 247
Niaspan, for hypertriglyceridemia,
    246
Nicotine dependence, 274, 277t.
    See also Smoking cessation
Nicotine replacement therapy
    (NRT), 278, 280t–281t
    in cardiac patients, 279
    for smoking cessation, 280t–281t
Nicotinic acid, for
    hypertriglyceridemia,
    245–246
Nitrates. See also specific agents
    for acute coronary syndrome,
        non–ST elevation, 30
    for congestive heart failure,
        140–141
Nitroglycerin
    for heart failure, early use of,
        50–51, 51f
    for left ventricular dysfunction,
        141
    diastolic, in acute MI, 140
    for thrombolysis, as adjunctive
        therapy, 42, 43t
Nitroprusside
    for aortic dissection, 170
    for heart failure, early use of,
        50–51, 51f
    for left ventricular dysfunction,
        141
    diastolic, in acute MI,
        139–140
    for ventricular septal rupture,
        144
No reflow, management of, 104,
    104t
Non–ST elevation myocardial
    infarction (NSTEMI), in ED,
    27–37, 133, 133t. See also
    Acute coronary syndrome
    (ACS) in ED, non–ST
    elevation
Non-sulfonylurea secretagogues. See
    also specific agents
    for type 2 diabetes, 254, 255t,
        256t

O
OPTIME-CHF, 192–193
OPTIMIZE-HF, 200, 201f, 202f,
    205f, 207
Out-of-hospital cardiac arrest
    (OOH-CA), epidemiology of,
    19

Oxygen, with thrombolysis, as
    adjunctive therapy, 42, 43t

P
Paroxysmal atrial fibrillation, 53
Patient assessments, baseline, in
    cardiac rehabilitation, 300,
    300t
Patient factors, in following AHA
    guidelines, 291, 293t
Patient Management Tool (PMT),
    292–294, 293t
Penetrating aortic ulcer (PAU). See
    Aortic ulcer, penetrating
    (PAU)
Percutaneous coronary intervention
    (PCI), 13, 100–106, 108,
    155–159
    adjunctive pharmacology for
        postprocedural, 105
        preprocedural, 101–103, 101f,
            103t
        procedural, 104
    AHA/ACC guidelines on, 100
    angiographic exclusions
        precluding, 105, 105t
    angioplasty vs. stenting in, 103
    for cardiogenic shock, 96
    coronary bypass surgery with,
        emergency, 105, 105t
    door-to-balloon times in, 109,
        114
    facilitated, 40–41, 94–95
    GP IIb/IIIa inhibitors for
        cardiogenic shock before,
        95–96, 96f
    history of, recent, 100
    indications for, 156
    informed consent for, 156–157,
        157t
    no reflow management in, 104,
        104t
    patient management in
        after procedure, 158–159
        during procedure, 158
    patient preparation in, 157–158
    postprocedural pathways in,
        101f, 105–106
    preoperative evaluation for, 156
    preprocedural pathways in, 82f,
        100–101
    procedural pathways in, 101t,
        103–104
    for recurrent MI, 135, 136t
    reperfusion injury management
        in, 104–105, 105t
    rescue, 94, 94f
        after failed thrombolysis, 44
    risks in, 156–157, 157t
    vs. thrombolysis, 100
        for STEMI, 39–41, 42t
    time to reperfusion on, 100–101
    transfer for, 83f, 101
        barriers to, 108–109
        regional programs of, 13–18
            (See also Transfer programs,
            for primary percutaneous
            coronary intervention)
Percutaneous coronary intervention
    (PCI), at community
    hospitals without on-site
    surgery, 108–127
    acuity-based procedure-bumping
        protocol in, 121–122, 122t
    acute MI protocol for
        ED, 116, 117t
        prehospital, 114, 114t
        team for, 110–111
    cardiac transfer agreement and
        hospital collaboration for,
        115, 116t
    case review processes and
        tracking tools in, 127
    catheterization laboratory
        protocol for, 116, 120t

data gathering and analysis processes and tracking tools in, 127

door-to-balloon time improvement program in, 116–117, 120–121, 121t

ED emergency triage system for, 111f, 114–116, 114t–116t, 118f–119f

emergency transfer in
for CABG, 112
cardiac surgery center protocol for, 115, 115t
formal agreements on, 115t, 122–124
protocol for, 115t, 122–124, 123f

emergent coronary angiography criteria in, 109, 109t

equipment requirements for, 112, 112t

essential elements of, 110

in-hospital management pathways in, 124–127, 124t, 125f, 126f

intensive staffing on shoestring budget in, 113–114

operator and institutional criteria for, 109, 109t, 112, 112t, 113t

position profiles, expectations, and training programs for, 112–113, 112t, 113t

primary PCI critical pathway for, 111–112, 111f

quality assurance processes and tracking tools in, 127

rationale for, 108–110, 109t

selection criteria for
angiography, 109, 110t
clinical and angiographic, 109t, 110t, 112
studies on, 109–110

training/performance requirements for staffing for, 112, 113t

Percutaneous left ventricular assist device (p-VAD), for acute MI, 104

Performance data, hospital, for MI, heart failure, and stroke, 291, 292t

Performance measures, for AHA Get With the Guidelines Program, 294–295, 295t, 296t

Pericarditis, early postinfarction, 146, 146t

Persistent atrial fibrillation, 53

D-Phenylalanine derivatives. See also specific agents
for type 2 diabetes, 254, 255t, 256t

Physical activity, for atherosclerotic disease prevention, 285, 287t

Pioglitazone, for type 2 diabetes, 254–256, 255t, 256t

Platelet disorders, treating intracerebral hemorrhage in, 73

Platelet glycoprotein IIb/IIIa, for prehospital fibrinolysis, 11–12

Point-of-care (POC) testing, of cardiac markers, 28–30

Polacrilex, for smoking cessation, 280t

Postmyocardial infarction syndrome, 146t, 147

Postphlebitis syndrome, prevention of, 233

Pramlinitide
for type 1 diabetes, 253
for type 2 diabetes, 255t, 256, 256t

Pravastatin, for hyperlipidemia, 244

Prediabetes, 250, 250f

Pre-excitation syndromes, cardioversion for, emergent electrical, 56

Prehospital electrocardiogram, 13

Prehospital fibrinolysis, 9–12
adjunctive therapy in, 11
alternative reperfusion strategies in ambulance in, 11–12, 11f
diagnosis for, optimal, 9, 10f, 11f
drug administration in, 10–11
reperfusion therapy in, 9

Prevention, secondary, 285, 286t–288t
of heart failure, implantable cardioverter-defibrillator for, 211–212, 213t

Procainamide
for atrial fibrillation with pre-excitation conditions, 56
for ventricular tachyarrhythmias, 148t

Propafenone
for atrial fibrillation, 56, 58t, 186–187, 187f, 188f
with pre-excitation conditions, 56
for atrial flutter, 186–187, 187f, 188f

Propanolol, for atrial fibrillation, 56, 57t

Protamine (sulfate)
for anticoagulant effects of enoxaparin, 152, 152t
on low molecular weight heparin, 73

Pseudoaneurysm, after acute MI, 145–146

Psychosocial assessment, in cardiac rehabilitation, 302

Public access defibrillation (PAD), 19–23. See also Defibrillation, public access

Public safety personnel, early defibrillation by, 19–20, 21

Pulmonary embolism (PE). See also Venous thromboembolism (VTE)
after acute MI, 147
cardiac biomarkers for, 228–229
chest CT of, 229
diagnosis of, 226–227, 226f, 226t
echocardiography of, 229
hemodynamic parameters in, 141t
initial treatment of, 228–230, 228f
oral anticoagulant therapy for, 231–233
epidemiologic approach to, 232, 232t
individual approach to, 232–233
newer drugs in, 231
optimal duration of, 231–232, 232t
warfarin in, 231
prevention of, 233–235, 233t, 234f, 234t
risk stratification in, 228
with stroke, prevention of, 79
thrombolysis for, 229–231

Pulmonary hypertension, idiopathic, hemodynamic parameters in, 141t

Pulmonary thromboendarterectomy, 230

Q
Quinapril, for heart failure, 200, 202t, 203t

Quinidine, for atrial fibrillation, 56, 58t

R
RACE pathway, for atrial fibrillation/flutter, 181, 182f, 184
goals and strategies based on, 181–182, 182f, 183f
rhythm control and antiarrhythmic drugs in, 187

Ramipril, for heart failure, 200, 202t, 203t

Recognition, in AHA Get With the Guidelines Program, 295

Recombinant activated factor VII, for hemorrhage in acute MI, 154

Recombinant tissue-type plasminogen activator (rtPA)
for acute ischemic stroke, IV, 63–71
algorithm for, 64, 71, 72f
critical pathway for, 64, 65f–71f
dosing of, 70f–71f
research on, 63–64
for pulmonary embolism, 229–230

Recurrent atrial fibrillation, 53

Recurrent ischemia, 133–134, 134f
coronary angiography and PCI for, 135, 136t

Reentrant ventricular arrhythmias, 131

Regional transfer programs, for primary percutaneous coronary intervention, 13–18. See also Transfer programs, for primary percutaneous coronary intervention

Rehabilitation, cardiac, 299–304
cost efficacy of, 302–303
critical factors in, 303–304
definition of, 299
design of, 302
education in, 301–302, 304
effectiveness of, 303
eligibility for, 300–301
exercise training in, 301, 303
safety of, 302
history of, 299–300
organization of, traditional, 300–302, 300t
risk-factor modification in, 301, 303–304

Reinfarction, 134, 135f

Repaglinide, for type 2 diabetes, 254, 255t, 256t

Reperfusion
alternative in-ambulance therapies for, 11–12, 11f
early, assessment of, 93–94, 93t
management of injury from, 104–105, 105t
time to
improving, 101, 102f
on percutaneous coronary intervention, primary, 100–101

Reperfusion therapy. See also Thrombolysis; specific agents; specific therapies
prehospital, 9
for ST-elevation coronary syndromes, 9

Rescue PCI, 94, 94f
for thrombolytic agent–treated STEMI, 44

Reteplase
with abciximab, for cardiogenic shock, 95
for STEMI in ED, 41–42, 42t

Retinopathy, diabetic, prevention of, 252

Return of spontaneous circulation (ROSC), 19, 20

Revascularization, for recurrent MI, 135, 137t

rFVIIa, for hemorrhage from treatment of acute MI, 149–152, 152t

Rhythm control, for atrial fibrillation and atrial flutter, 186–187, 187f, 188f

Rhythm disturbances, in acute MI, 149, 150t

Right ventricular (RV) infarction, 135, 137t
hemodynamic parameters in, 141t
management of, 136–138, 138t, 139f

Risk-factor modification, in cardiac rehabilitation, 301, 303–304

Rosiglitazone, for type 2 diabetes, 254–256, 255t, 256t

Rosuvastatin, for hyperlipidemia, 244

S
Scintigraphy, myocardial stress, exercise testing vs., 87

Secondary prevention, 285, 286t–288t
of heart failure, implantable cardioverter-defibrillator for, 211–212, 213t

Septic shock, hemodynamic parameters in, 141t

Shock, cardiogenic, 141–142, 282f
with acute MI, 138–139, 140t, 141t
angioplasty for, 96
hemodynamic parameters in, 141t
thrombolysis for, 94–97
combination fibrinolytic therapy and GP IIb/IIa inhibition in, 95
conservative strategy for, 96–97
facilitated PCI in, 94–95
full-dose fibrinolytic therapy alone in, 95, 95f
GP IIb/IIa inhibition alone in, 95–97, 96f
reducing other cardiac testing in, 97
routine invasive vs. conservative strategy for, 96

Simvastatin, for hyperlipidemia, 244

Simvastatin-niacin, for low HDL cholesterol, 247

Smoking, on health, 273

Smoking cessation, 273–283
for atherosclerotic disease prevention, 285, 286t
books and other self-help resources in, 279–281, 281t
for cardiac patients, 273
in cardiac rehabilitation, 301
nicotine replacement therapy in, 278, 280t–281t
in cardiac patients, 279
pharmacologic therapies for, 278, 280t–281t
physician interventions for, 273
program referral in, 279, 282t
relapse prevention in, 281
summary and conclusions on, 282–283
treatment approaches to, 273–278
assessing readiness to quit in, 274, 276f
benefits of quitting smoking in, 276–277, 279f

Smoking cessation (continued)
    Fagerstrom test for nicotine
        dependence in, 274, 277t
    five As of, 274–279
    key principles in, 273–274
    reasons to stop now in,
        276–277, 278t
    web sites on, 281–282
Sodium nitroprusside. See
    Nitroprusside
Sotalol
    for atrial fibrillation, 186–187,
        187f, 188f
    with pre-excitation conditions,
        56
    for atrial flutter, 186–187, 187f,
        188f
Spironolactone, for heart failure,
    204, 206t
Statin-niacin, for low HDL
    cholesterol, 247
Statins. See also specific agents
    for hyperlipidemia, 244
    before primary percutaneous
        coronary intervention, 103
ST-elevation coronary syndromes,
    reperfusion therapy for, 9,
    10f, 11f
ST-elevation myocardial infarction
    (STEMI)
    initial evaluation of, 39, 40f, 41t
    percutaneous coronary
        intervention for, 13 (See also
        Percutaneous coronary
        intervention (PCI), primary)
    reperfusion therapy for, 9, 10f,
        11f
    standardized protocol for, 15,
        16f
ST-elevation myocardial infarction
    (STEMI), ED thrombolysis
    for, 39–44
    adjunctive therapy in, 42–44,
        43f, 43t
    initial evaluation of, 39, 40f, 41t
    intracranial hemorrhage from,
        43f, 44
    overview of, 39
    vs. percutaneous coronary
        intervention, 39–41, 42t
    rescue PCI with, 44
    thrombolytic agent choice in,
        41–42, 42t
Stenting, for acute MI, 103
Streptokinase
    prehospital, 10
    for STEMI in ED, 41, 42t
Stress management, in cardiac
    rehabilitation, 301
Stroke, 63–79. See also Stroke,
    acute ischemic (AIS);
    Transient ischemic attack
    (TIA)
    AHA guidelines for, 291–297
        (See also AHA Get With the
        Guidelines Program
        (GWTG))
    clinical diagnosis of, 63, 64f
    complications from, prevention
        of, 78–79
    critical pathways committee for,
        75, 77f
    critical pathways for
        IV tPA thrombolysis for, 64,
            65f–71f
        rationale for, 74–75
    epidemiology of, 63, 291
    with fibrinolytic therapy for
        copmlicated acute MI, risk
        factors and predictors of,
        132, 133t
    hospital performance data for,
        291, 292t
    neuroimaging pathways for, ED,
        74

neurology admit order templates
    for, 75, 76f–77f
pathways organization into chain
    of stroke survival for,
    77–79, 79f
performance measures for
    GWTG for, 294–295, 296t
quality improvement
    infrastructure for, 75–76,
    76f–78f
variability in care for, 74
Stroke, acute ischemic (AIS), 61,
    61f
    antithrombotics for, 71
    with atrial fibrillation, risk for,
        60–61, 60t, 61f
    blood pressure control for, 74
    emergent carotid endarterectomy
        for, 73
    IA tPA thrombolysis for, 71
    IV tPA thrombolysis for, 63–71
        algorithm for, 64, 71, 72f
        critical pathway for, 64,
            65f–71f
        dosing of, 70f–71f
        research on, 63–64
    mechanical embolectomy device
        for, 71
    thrombolysis for, 63–66, 65f–71f
Stroke, hemorrhagic
    evidence-based interventions for,
        73
    from fibrinolysis for acute MI,
        risk for, 132, 133t
Subarachnoid hemorrhage,
    treatment of, 73
Sudden cardiac death, ICD therapy
    for
    primary prevention of, 212–215,
        214t, 215t
        with arrhythmogenic RV
            dysplasia/cardiomyopathy,
            215
        with hypertrophic
            cardiomyopathy, 215
    secondary prevention of,
        211–212, 213t
Sulfonylureas (SUs), for type 2
    diabetes, 254, 255t, 256t
Supraventricular arrhythmias, 149,
    150t
Survival, chain of, 19
Syndrome X. See Metabolic
    syndrome
Systems-based approach, to AHA
    guidelines implementation,
    294

T
Tachyarrhythmias, ventricular,
    management of, 148t–149t
Tangier disease, 247
Telemedicine, for stroke, 77, 79f
Telmisartan, for heart failure,
    200–202, 203t
Tenecteplase
    full-dose, for cardiogenic shock,
        95, 95f
    for STEMI in ED, 41–42, 42t
Thiazolidinediones, for type 2
    diabetes, 254–256, 255t,
    256t
30-30-30 goal, 14–15, 15t
Thrombectomy, for acute MI,
    103–104
Thrombin inhibitors, direct. See
    also specific agents
    for acute MI, 104
Thrombocytopenia, with
    intracerebral hemorrhage,
    treatment of, 73
Thromboembolism. See Thrombus
    and thomboembolism
Thromboendarterectomy,
    pulmonary, 230

Thrombolysis. See also Reperfusion
    therapy; specific therapies
    adjunctive therapy for, 42–44,
        43f, 43t
    catheter-directed, for deep vein
        thrombosis, 228
    early discharge after, strategy for,
        97–98
    failed, rescue PCI for, 44
    identifying low-risk patients with,
        97
    vs. PCI, 100
        for STEMI, 39–41, 42t
    prevention and follow-up for, 98
    for pulmonary embolism,
        229–231
Thrombolysis, critical pathway
    after, 93–99
    for cardiogenic shock, 94, 96
        combination fibrinolytic
            therapy and GP IIb/IIIa
            inhibition in, 95
        conservative strategy in, 96–97
        facilitated PCI in, 94–95
        full-dose fibrinolytic therapy
            alone in, 95, 95f
        GP IIb/IIIa inhibition alone in,
            95–97, 96f
        reducing other cardiac testing
            in, 97
        routine invasive vs.
            conservative strategy in, 96
    early reperfusion in, assessment
        of, 93–94, 93t
    reducing hospital and ICU length
        of stay in, 97
    rescue PCI in, 94, 94f
Thrombolysis, for ST-elevation
    myocardial infarction
    (STEMI) in ED, 39–44
    adjunctive therapy in, 42–44,
        43f, 43t
    choice of agent for, 41–42, 42t
    intracranial hemorrhage from,
        43f, 44
    overview of, 39
    vs. percutaneous coronary
        intervention, 39–41, 42t
    rescue PCI with, 44
Thrombolytic agents. See also
    specific agents
    before primary percutaneous
        coronary intervention, 102
    for STEMI in ED, 41–42, 42t
Thrombus and thromboembolism
    in acute MI, management of,
        103–104, 104t
    after acute MI, 147
    with atrial fibrillation, 60–61,
        60t, 61f
    venous (See Venous
        thromboembolism (VTE))
TIA. See Transient ischemic attack
    (TIA)
TIMI flow grade classification, for
    assessing early reperfusion,
    93, 93t
Tirofiban
    for acute coronary syndrome,
        non–ST elevation, 30–32
    for cardiogenic shock, before
        PCI, 95, 95f
Tissue plasminogen activator (tPA)
    IA, for acute ischemic stroke, 71
    IV, for acute ischemic stroke,
        63–71
        algorithm for, 64, 71, 72f
        critical pathway in, 64,
            65f–71f
        dosing of, 70f–71f
        research on, 63–64
tPA. See Tenecteplase; Tissue
    plasminogen activator (tPA)

Transfer
    to cardiac surgery center for
        acute MI, emergency
        protocol for, 115, 115t
    cardiac transfer agreement and
        inter-hospital collaboration
        for, 115, 116t
    improving delays in, 101, 102f
Transfer programs, for primary
    percutaneous coronary
    intervention, 13–18
    challenges to implementation of,
        16
    direct admission to cardiac
        catheterization lab in, 15,
        17f
    education and training in, 15
    empowering ED physician in, 15,
        16f
    feasibility of, in U.S., 14
    feedback and quality
        improvement in, 15–16
    individualized transfer
        agreements in, 15
    organizing system for, 14–15,
        15t
    results of, 16
    standardized protocol in, 15, 16f
    trials on, 13–14, 14f
Transient ischemic attack (TIA), 63.
    See also Stroke
    AHA guidelines for, 291–297
    clinical diagnosis of, 63
    emergent carotid endarterectomy
        for, 73
    initial management of, 64f
    performance measures for
        GWTG for, 294–295, 296t
    rationale for critical pathways
        for, 74–75
TRAPS, 53, 54t, 182
Trialability, 294
Troponin
    in acute coronary syndrome, non-
        ST elevation, 28, 33t
    in acute decompensated heart
        failure, 47, 47t
    point-of-care testing of, 28–30
    in pulmonary embolism, 229
Troponin I, in complicated acute
    MI, 131–132
Troponin T, in complicated acute
    MI, 131–132

U
Unfractionated heparin (UFH)
    for coagulopathy in intracerebral
        hemorrhage, 73
    for pulmonary embolism,
        229–230
    for recurrent ischemia, 133, 134f
    for thrombolysis, as adjunctive
        therapy, 43–44, 43t
    for venous thromboembolism
        prophylaxis, 233

V
Valsartan, for heart failure,
    200–202, 203t
Vascular disease. See also specific
    diseases
    secondary prevention for patients
        with, 285, 286t–288t
Vascular function
    hyperglycemia on, 176, 177t
    inflammation in hyperglycemia
        and, 176
Vasoactive therapy. See also specific
    agents
    for heart failure, early use of,
        50–51, 51f
Vasodilators. See also specific
    agents
    for heart failure, 206, 207t
Vena caval filters, for venous
    thromboembolism, 230

Venous insufficiency, chronic, 228
Venous thromboembolism (VTE), 224–235
    after acute MI, 147
    diagnosis of, 225–227
        for deep vein thrombosis, 225–226, 225f, 225t
        for pulmonary embolism, 226–227, 226f, 226t
    epidemiology of, 224–225, 225t
    oral anticoagulant therapy for, 231–233
        epidemiologic approach to, 232, 232t
        individual approach to, 232–233
        newer drugs in, 231
        optimal duration of, 231–232, 232t
        warfarin in, 231

prevention of, 233–235, 233t, 234f, 234t
risk factors for, 224–225, 225t
treatment of, initial, 227–231
    for deep vein thrombosis, 227–228, 228f
    embolectomy in, 230–231
    for pulmonary embolism, 228–230, 228f
Ventricular arrhythmias
    automatic, 131
    reentrant, 131
    tachyarrhythmia management in, 148t–149t
Ventricular fibrillation (VF), management of, 148t–149t
Ventricular rate control, in atrial fibrillation/flutter, 186, 187f
Ventricular septal rupture (VSR) after acute MI, 143–144

hemodynamic parameters in, 141t
Ventricular tachyarrhythmias, management of, 148t–149t
Verapamil, for atrial fibrillation/atrial flutter, 56, 57t
    rate control in, 186, 187f
Vitamin K, for coagulopathy in intracerebral hemorrhage, 73
von Willebrand syndromes, for intracerebral hemorrhage treatment, 73

W
Warfarin
    for atherosclerotic disease prevention, 285, 288t
    for atrial fibrillation with CABG, 165
    for coagulopathy in intracerebral hemorrhage, 73

for embolic stroke prevention, 185–186, 186f
hemorrhage from, in acute MI, 153, 153t
for venous thromboembolism, 231
Weight management, for atherosclerotic disease prevention, 285, 287t
Weight reduction, in cardiac rehabilitation, 301
Wolff-Parkinson-White syndrome, emergent electrical cardioversion for, 56
Wound healing, in acute MI, cellular characteristics of, 129–131

X
Ximelagatran, for coagulopathy in intracerebral hemorrhage, 73